AF687507

Diagnosis and Management of Rheumatic Diseases

Diagnosis and Management of Rheumatic Diseases

Editor: Nicholas Greyson

AMERICAN
MEDICAL PUBLISHERS
www.americanmedicalpublishers.com

AMERICAN
MEDICAL PUBLISHERS
www.americanmedicalpublishers.com

Cataloging-in-Publication Data

Diagnosis and management of rheumatic diseases / edited by Nicholas Greyson.
p. cm.
Includes bibliographical references and index.
ISBN 979-8-88740-056-3
1. Rheumatology. 2. Joints--Diseases--Diagnosis. 3. Joints--Diseases--Treatment.
4. Connective tissues--Diseases--Diagnosis. 5. Connective tissues--Diseases--Treatment.
I. Greyson, Nicholas.
RC927 .D53 2023
616.723--dc23

© American Medical Publishers, 2023

American Medical Publishers,
41 Flatbush Avenue,
1st Floor, New York,
NY 11217, USA

ISBN 979-8-88740-056-3 (Hardback)

This book contains information obtained from authentic and highly regarded sources. Copyright for all individual chapters remain with the respective authors as indicated. All chapters are published with permission under the Creative Commons Attribution License or equivalent. A wide variety of references are listed. Permission and sources are indicated; for detailed attributions, please refer to the permissions page and list of contributors. Reasonable efforts have been made to publish reliable data and information, but the authors, editors and publisher cannot assume any responsibility for the validity of all materials or the consequences of their use.

Trademark Notice: Registered trademark of products or corporate names are used only for explanation and identification without intent to infringe.

Contents

Preface

Every book is initially just a concept; it takes months of research and hard work to give it the final shape in which the readers receive it. In its early stages, this book also went through rigorous reviewing. The notable contributions made by experts from across the globe were first molded into patterned chapters and then arranged in a sensibly sequential manner to bring out the best results.

Rheumatic diseases are the conditions that cause chronic and intermittent pain, and affect the joints and the connective tissue. Some rheumatic diseases are autoimmune in origin such as rheumatoid arthritis, scleroderma, systemic lupus erythematosus, ankylosing spondylitis, etc. Different rheumatic disorders are caused due to different reasons and all require different kinds of treatment. The most common symptoms include intermittent pain, swelling, warmth, and stiffness. Rheumatism severely affects vital organs such as heart, kidney, nervous system, lungs, etc. Rheumatic disorders are diagnosed using physical examination followed by specialized laboratory and imaging tests. The initial therapy of rheumatological diseases is usually through analgesics, such as non-steroidal anti-inflammatory drugs (NSAIDs), disease-modifying anti-rheumatic drugs (DMARDs), etc. Physiotherapy and occupational therapy are other recommended treatment techniques for these diseases. The topics included in this book on the diagnosis and treatments of rheumatic diseases are of utmost significance and bound to provide incredible insights to readers. Through it, an attempt has been made to further enlighten the readers about the new concepts on these diseases.

It has been my immense pleasure to be a part of this project and to contribute my years of learning in such a meaningful form. I would like to take this opportunity to thank all the people who have been associated with the completion of this book at any step.

Editor

1

Differential Diagnosis of Inflammatory Arthropathies by Musculoskeletal Ultrasonography

Garifallia Sakellariou[1], Carlo Alberto Scirè[2,3], Antonella Adinolfi[4], Alberto Batticciotto[5], Alessandra Bortoluzzi[2], Andrea Delle Sedie[6], Orazio De Lucia[7], Christian Dejaco[8,9], Oscar Massimiliano Epis[4], Emilio Filippucci[10], Luca Idolazzi[11], Andrea Picchianti Diamanti[12], Alen Zabotti[13], Annamaria Iagnocco[14] and Georgios Filippou[2]*

[1] Division of Rheumatology, IRCCS Policlinico San Matteo Foundation, University of Pavia, Pavia, Italy, [2] UOC e Sezione di Reumatologia - Dipartimento di Scienze Mediche, Università degli Studi di Ferrara, Ferrara, Italy, [3] Società Italiana di Reumatologia, Unità Epidemiologica, Milan, Italy, [4] Rheumatology Unit, Grande Ospedale Metropolitano Niguarda, Milan, Italy, [5] Rheumatology Unit, Department of Internal Medicine, ASST-Settelaghi, "Ospedale di Circolo - Fondazione Macchi", Varese, Italy, [6] Rheumatology Unit, University of Pisa, Pisa, Italy, [7] Unit of Clinical Rheumatology, Department of Rheumatology and Clinical Sciences, ASST Centro Traumatologico Ortopedico G. Pini - CTO, Milan, Italy, [8] Department of Rheumatology, Medical University of Graz, Graz, Austria, [9] Department of Rheumatology, Hospital of Bruneck, Bruneck, Italy, [10] Rheumatology Unit, Department of Clinical and Molecular Sciences, Carlo Urbani Hospital, Polytechnic University of Marche, Ancona, Italy, [11] Rheumatology Unit, Ospedale Civile Maggiore, University of Verona, Verona, Italy, [12] Department of Clinical and Molecular Medicine, S. Andrea University Hospital, "Sapienza" University, Rome, Italy, [13] Department of Medical and Biological Science, Rheumatology Clinic, Azienda Sanitaria Universitaria Integrata, Udine, Italy, [14] Academic Rheumatology Centre, Università degli Studi di Torino, Turin, Italy

***Correspondence:**
Carlo Alberto Sciré
c.scire@reumatologia.it

Background: Differential diagnosis in early arthritis is challenging, especially early after symptom onset. Several studies applied musculoskeletal ultrasound in this setting, however, its role in helping diagnosis has yet to be clearly defined. The purpose of this work is to systematically assess the diagnostic applications of ultrasonography in early arthritis in order to summarize the available evidence and highlight possible gaps in knowledge.

Methods: In December 2017, existing systematic literature reviews (SLR) on rheumatoid arthritis (RA), osteoarthritis (OA), psoriatic arthritis (PsA), polymyalgia rheumatica (PMR), calcium pyrophosphate deposition disease (CPPD), and gout were retrieved. Studies on ultrasound to diagnose the target conditions and detecting elementary lesions (such as synovitis, tenosynovitis, enthesitis, bone erosions, osteophytes) were extracted from the SLRs. The searches of the previous reviews were updated and data from new studies fulfilling the inclusion criteria extracted. Groups of reviewers worked separately for each disease, when possible diagnostic accuracy (sensitivities, specificities) was calculated from primary studies. When available, the reliability of ultrasound to detect elementary lesions was extracted.

Results: For all the examined disease, recent SLRs were available. The new searches identified 27 eligible articles, with 87 articles included from the previous SLRs. The diagnostic performance of ultrasound in identifying diseases was addressed by 75 studies; in most of them, a single elementary lesion was used to define diagnosis, except for PMR. Only studies on RA included consecutive patients with new onset of arthritis, while studies on gout and CPPD often focused on subjects with mono-arthritis. Most of the remaining studies enrolled patients with a defined diagnosis. Synovitis was the most frequently detected lesion; clinical diagnosis was the most common reference standard. The diagnostic performance of ultrasound across different conditions was extremely variable. Ultrasound to identify elementary lesions was assessed in 38 studies in OA, gout and CPPD. Its performance in OA was very variable, with better results in CPPD and gout. The reliability of ultrasound was moderate to good for most lesions.

Conclusions: Although a consistent amount of literature investigated the diagnostic application of ultrasound, in only a minority of cases its additional value over clinical diagnosis was tested. This SLR underlines the need for studies with a pragmatic design to identify the placement of ultrasound in the diagnostic pathway of new-onset arthritis.

Keywords: early arthritis, ultrasonography, diagnosis, systematic review, imaging

INTRODUCTION

With effective treatment strategies for inflammatory arthropathies becoming extensively available, in the last decade a prompt diagnosis, allowing intervention within the window of opportunity, has become a critical point in the management of early arthritis (1). However, in rheumatology diagnosis can be achieved with certainty in a minority of cases, and this is particularly true when patients are assessed at very early stages of diseases. While in some cases the presence of valuable biomarkers, such as anticyclic citrullinated peptides antibodies (ACPA), drives the diagnostic process, in seronegative early arthritis the degree of uncertainty remains high. Moreover, the current classification criteria for the main rheumatic diseases, which are often inappropriately used to help diagnosis, require differential diagnosis to be performed before they are applied (2). This difficulty in the correct definition of diagnoses at early stages might lead to inappropriate management, delaying the start of effective treatment but also exposing patients to useless and potentially toxic drugs. In addition, also in a research setting, an imprecise diagnosis implies the impossibility to measure reliably the effect of innovative treatments in early phases. In this context, there is a great interest in the research of new biomarkers and new tools to help the diagnostic process.

Musculoskeletal ultrasonography has been widely applied in rheumatic diseases, demonstrating to be a valid and reproducible tool in both inflammatory and non-inflammatory pathologies. The relevance of this instrument has also been recognized by the European League Against Rheumatism (EULAR), that recommends ultrasound among the imaging which can be considered to help the clinical management of several conditions (3–5). The applications of ultrasound cover the areas of diagnosis, assessment of prognosis, follow-up of diseases and guide for intra-articular and peri-tendinous procedures. In the field of diagnosis, most of the studies on ultrasound investigated the frequency of elementary lesions characteristics of diseases, thus providing information on the diagnostic performance of this tool to detect single abnormalities or on the performance of single lesions to diagnose a disease. On the other hand, only a minority of studies tests the diagnostic value of combinations of lesions, assessed at the same time. Moreover, in this context elementary lesions are not selected based on their diagnostic properties and specificity for a certain condition. Only a minority of studies, in which the added value of ultrasound is tested jointly with clinical evaluation (6, 7), apply a pragmatic design that reproduces the clinical context. The lack of information on the application of ultrasound in a realistic clinical process of diagnosis translates into the limited weight given to this imaging in classification criteria. For instance, the only role for ultrasound in Rheumatoid Arthritis (RA) classification is the possible confirmation of the presence of synovitis (2), while to date the only classification criteria including ultrasound are those for polymyalgia rheumatica (PMR) (8).

Given the limited availability of methodologically sound studies to address the diagnostic performance of ultrasound in a realistic clinical context of differential diagnosis of inflammatory arthropathies, the Ultrasound Study Group of the Italian Society for Rheumatology (SIR) prioritized its research on this subject. The present study represents the first step of such project. The aim of the present work was the evaluation of the available literature on the diagnostic application of ultrasound in inflammatory arthropathies.

MATERIALS AND METHODS

As a first step, the most relevant differential diagnoses in patients with suspected inflammatory arthropathies were identified, including also osteoarthritis (OA) as a relevant differential diagnosis. We afterwards individuated two research questions, rephrased following the PICOs (Patient, Intervention, Comparator, Outcome, Study type) methodology to provide inclusion and exclusion criteria (**Table 1**). On this basis, we planned separate systematic literature reviews (SLR) to assess the diagnostic performance of ultrasound to diagnose OA, RA, psoriatic arthritis (PsA), PMR, gout, calcium pyrophosphate deposition disease (CPPD). The SLRs were not registered, but a common protocol was available for all researchers before

TABLE 1 | Inclusion criteria for research questions.

	Population	Intervention	Comparators (reference standard)	Outcomes	Study type
What is the added value of ultrasound to diagnose the target diseases?	People presenting with joint symptoms	Ultrasound	Clinical diagnosis (without imaging) Other imaging	Confirmation of the diagnosis	Systematic literature reviews, meta-analyses, RCTs, controlled trials, non-controlled trials, diagnostic accuracy studies, cohort studies, cross-sectional studies, case-control studies
What is the accuracy of ultrasound for detecting elementary lesions of the target diseases?	Patients with confirmed diagnosis of the target disease	Ultrasound	Physical examination Surgery Other imaging	Sensitivity, specificity, Likelihood ratios, Diagnostic Odds Ratio, AUC, negative predictive value, positive predictive value Inter-reader and intra-reader reliability	Systematic literature reviews, meta-analyses, RCTs, controlled trials, non-controlled trials, diagnostic accuracy studies, cohort studies, cross-sectional studies, case-control studies

the beginning of the process. The diagnostic performance of ultrasound in detecting elementary lesions was also addressed. If studies on diagnostic performance reported also data on intra and inter-reader reliability on elementary lesions, that information was also extracted. Working groups composed by supervisors and fellows were created to work separately on each topic, participants were selected based on the expertise on the specific disease and on SLR methodology to create uniform groups. The most recent SLRs on ultrasound in the same diseases were first sought in electronic databases (5, 9–13). Some of the authors involved in the present project were also co-authors of these SLR and could provide background material (AA, ABa, AI, AZ, CS, EF, GF, GS). Since many of the existing SLR had a broader focus, only primary studies focusing on the diagnostic use of ultrasound were taken into account for the present work.

The search strategies of the previous SLR were applied in PubMed and Embase, starting from the date of the last search of the previous reviews (5, 9–13). Searches were last run on November 30th 2017. The search on PubMed and Embase was selected because we expected that all the relevant literature would be retrieved, and we did not expect to find further evidence including other databases. The records retrieved from the new searches were transferred into a bibliographic manager software (Zotero, RRID:SCR_013784) and libraries shared with each working group. The titles and abstracts of the retrieved records were evaluated by pairs of reviewers to assess the eligibility for full-text review according to the pre-specified criteria. Full-texts were afterwards evaluated by the same criteria and data from the included studies extracted into a standardized form, including 2 × 2 tables of diagnostic performance. A flow-chart describing the selection process was separately generated for each SLR. Results were summarized through summary of findings tables, describing both studies included in the previous reviews and those identified by the present ones.

RESULTS

In total, all search strategies retrieved 943 references since the date of the last search of the previous SLRs. The higher number of references belonged to the fields of PsA and gout (Additional Online File). After reviewing the abstracts, 27 papers were finally included, together with 87 articles from previous SLRs meeting the inclusion criteria, for a total of 114 papers included in the present SLR (**Table 2**). The PRISMA flow-chart of the SLR for each disease is available in the Additional Online File, as well as the full results, presented through summary of findings tables.

Ultrasound for the Clinical Diagnosis of Inflammatory Arthropathy

Information regarding the value of ultrasound to diagnose diseases could be extracted from 75 studies. The greatest amount of evidence was available for PsA, with 29 studies assessing the diagnostic performance of ultrasound.

There were meaningful differences in terms of enrolled populations across different diseases. In fact, in studies addressing PsA and OA, the primary aim was mostly to report the prevalence of different lesions. The frequency of each lesion was compared in patients with already known PsA or OA and healthy controls or patients with other definite diseases. A realistic clinical scenario of consecutive patients referred for suspicion of inflammatory arthropathy was rarely available (6).

Conversely, studies on RA evaluated the added value of ultrasound over classification criteria (14–17), the added value for diagnosis on top of clinical findings (18–20) or its prognostic value over the future development of RA (21–25) by cross-sectional or longitudinal study design.

Studies dealing with PMR mostly included populations of consecutive patients with shoulder pain (8, 13, 26) and some of them evaluated the additional value of ultrasound on the diagnostic performance of the 2012 classification criteria (8, 26, 27).

In the fields of both gout and CPPD, most of the studies included patients presenting with mono-arthritis and with suspect crystal-related arthritis.

Despite these discrepancies across different conditions, there were only a few studies, mainly focused on RA, that enrolled a population of consecutive patients with joint pain (6, 16–20, 22, 24, 28).

TABLE 2 | Features of the SLRs used as a basis for the present work.

Target disease	References	Aim of the SLR	Last searches	Number of studies included in the present SLR
RA	(12)	To evaluate the added value of ultrasound over clinical findings to the diagnosis of RA in patients with suspected arthritis	November 2015	11
OA	(5)	To provide evidence for the development of the EULAR recommendations for the use of imaging for the clinical management of OA. The SLR does not focus only on ultrasound	December 2015	18
PsA	(9)	To provide evidence for the selection and design of an observational study of the Ultrasound Study Group of the SIR. The SLR focuses on ultrasound	September 25th 2015	24
CPPD	(10)	To provide evidence on the diagnostic performance of ultrasound to diagnose CPPD and to retrieve all the ultrasound definitions of CPPD. The SLR focuses on ultrasound.	31 December 2014	18
PMR	(13)	To review the accuracy of imaging to diagnose PMR	October 2nd 2013	10
Gout	(11)	To provide evidence on the diagnostic performance of ultrasound to help clinicians in the choice of imaging. The SLR does not focus only on ultrasound	February 2016	6

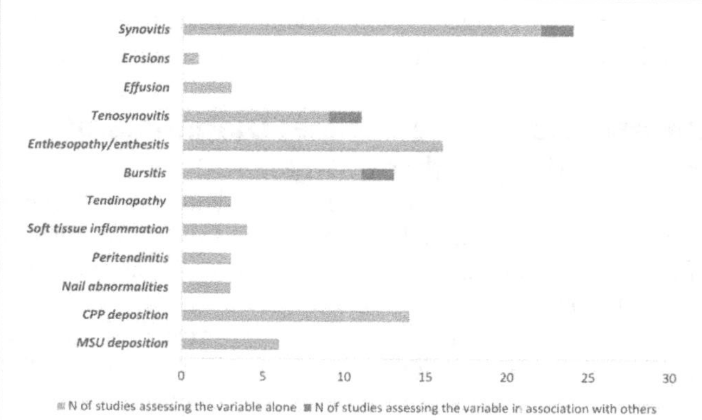

GRAPH 1 | Number of studies using each single elementary lesion to establish diagnoses, alone or in combination. CPP, calcium pyrophosphate; MSU, monosodium urate.

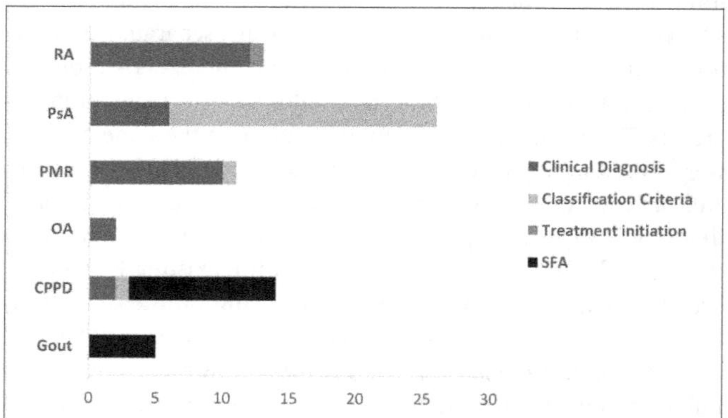

GRAPH 2 | Reference standards adopted to confirm diagnoses. PMR, polymyalgia rheumatica; CPPD, calcium pyrophosphate deposition disease; OA, osteoarthritis; PsA, psoriatic arthritis; RA, rheumatoid arthritis; SFA, synovial fluid analysis.

The interventions used to help diagnosis were also variable. Since most of the studies did not have diagnostic accuracy as primary objective, data on the diagnosis of disease were based on single elementary lesions. A relevant exception was represented by PMR, for which some studies addressed different lesions (tenosynovitis, bursitis and synovitis) in combination (8, 26, 27). **Graph 1** summarizes all the different lesions used to define diagnosis.

The confirmation of the diagnosis was based on a variety of reference standards, which depended on the diagnostic suspicion, as expected. While clinical diagnosis was frequently considered in RA and PMR, for PsA the confirmation of diagnosis mostly relied on clinical diagnosis and classification criteria, while synovial fluid analysis was frequently considered in crystal-related arthropathies (**Graph 2**).

The study design adopted to define diagnostic accuracy was also widely variable. While studies aiming to diagnose RA were mainly cohort studies (15–24, 28), in the field of PsA emerged a significant prevalence of studies with a case-control design; controls were represented mostly by patients with RA (29–37), while in some studies also healthy controls were included (29, 31, 33, 38–43). For the remaining diseases, the type of study was more variable (**Graph 3**).

In OA, adding ultrasound information to the clinical evaluation increased the certainty of the diagnosis made by the clinician (6), while the likelihood of OA, compared to being healthy, increased with the finding of bone erosions (44).

In the field of RA, some studies supported the possibility to integrate clinical and ultrasound findings to reclassify undifferentiated arthritis (14–17, 21), while in other studies ultrasound information was applied to confirm a diagnosis of RA or tested against a clinical diagnosis (18–20), leading in general to an increase in diagnostic performance. The prognostic value of ultrasound in predicting the future development of the disease or the need for specific treatment has also been tested, once again with positive results supporting this application (22–24, 28) (**Tables 3, 4**). The most specific lesion to diagnose RA were bone erosions, with the specificity of 1 reported by a single study (19), although also the specificity of PD positive synovitis was high (ranging from 0.88 to 0.93).

Despite a higher number of studies with a focus on PsA, in this area there was a greater variability, due to many different lesions, tissues and sites assessed. Many studies (14 studies) focused on the assessment of entheseal abnormalities (30, 34, 35, 39, 40, 42, 45–52) and the joints (6 studies) (29, 32, 33, 38, 41, 53), while only a few studies assessed the fingers (considering joints, tendons, soft tissues and entheses) (31, 36, 37) or the nails (43, 54, 55). The primary aim of the included studies rarely addressed the diagnostic accuracy. In fact, most of the studies compared the prevalence of lesions in PsA and other diseases. Also, for this, the diagnostic performance of ultrasound findings, which were usually considered alone and not in combination or in addition to clinical findings, was extremely variable across lesions and sites (**Table 5**). Among the tested lesions, those proving to be more specific to detect PsA were those at the level of the entheses. In fact, the specificity of entheseal PD ranged from 0.33 to 0.99, of enthesophytes from 0.52 to 1 and of calcifications from 0.86 to 0.97. Peritenonitis was also very specific (from 0.95 to 1 when PD signal was present).

Studies focusing on ultrasound of the hips and the shoulders in PMR had a more variable design. In fact, along with some older studies with a case-control design (8, 56–59) several cohort studies, including that on which the current classification criteria are based (8), included consecutive patients with shoulder pain (34, 60). Moreover, several recent studies provided external validation for the classification criteria (26). Again, in terms of accuracy, studies yielded very heterogeneous results (**Table 6**). In general, bilateral findings seemed to be more specific for PMR. The specificity of bilateral subacromiodeltoid bursitis ranged from 0.68 to 0.99, while for bilateral long head of the biceps tenosynovitis ranged from 0.62 to 0.98.

Studies in CPPD evaluated several different sites, including the knees (61–68), the wrist (69, 70), the affected joint or all joints (71). Study design was variable, including both case-control and cohort studies. The diagnosis of CPPD was confirmed more frequently by synovial fluid analysis, while in some cases a clinical diagnosis (70, 71) or histology (68) were used as references. In general, ultrasound seemed to perform well in identifying this condition, especially at the knee and the wrist. The specificity to confirm CPPD at the knee (considering all the assessed sites) ranged from 0.66 to 1, while at the wrist from 0.81 to 0.91.

In the field of gout, the type of joint under investigation was widely variable, all studies (72–74) but two (75, 76) adopted synovial fluid analysis as reference standard to diagnose the

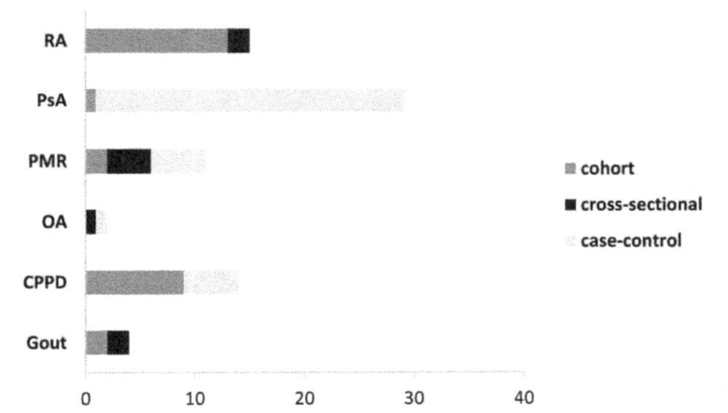

GRAPH 3 | Study design of the included studies, depending on the assessed disease. PMR, polymyalgia rheumatica; CPPD, calcium pyrophosphate deposition disease; OA, osteoarthritis; PsA, psoriatic arthritis; RA, rheumatoid arthritis; SFA: synovial fluid analysis.

TABLE 4 | Performance of ultrasound to predict RA by elementary lesions by site.

	Sensitivity	
GS SYNOVITIS	**Sensitivity**	**Specificity**
Wrist	0.79	0.69
MCP	0.9	0.48
PIP	0.79	0.66
PD SYNOVITIS		
Wrist	0.9	0.48
MCP	0.9	0.66
PIP	0.66	0.76

Summary of sensitivities, specificities across studies assessing the performance of ultrasound to predict RA by elementary lesions by site. Only Filer reports sensitivity and sensitivity for every joint. Gray Scale and power Doppler ≥ 2. MCP, Metacarpophalangeal; PIP, Proximal interphalangeal.

TABLE 3 | Performance of ultrasound to detect RA by elementary lesions and reliability.

Lesion*	**Sensitivity**		**Specificity**		**Intra-reader kappa**		**Inter-reader kappa**	
	Min	**Max**	**Min**	**Max**	**Min**	**Max**	**Min**	**Max**
Erosions	–	0.38	–	1	–	0.93	–	–
GS synovitis	0.69	0.94	0.5	0.86	0.83	0.94	0.56	0.86
PD synovitis	0.72	0.89	0.88	0.93	0.87	0.99	0.64	0.89

*Summary of sensitivities, specificities and reliability across studies assessing the performance of ultrasound to diagnose RA elementary lesions. Of the 13 papers included,only four reported sensibility-sensitivity by using gray scale (GS) and/or power Doppler (PD) ≥ 2. *Hands (including proximal interphalangeal joints) and wrists.*

TABLE 5 | Performance of ultrasound lesions to detect PsA and reproducibility.

Lesion	Sensitivity		Specificity		Intra-reader kappa		Inter-reader kappa	
	Min	Max	Min	Max	Min	Max	Min	Max
Synovial hypertrophy	0.16	0.76	0	1	–	–	0.78–1	–
Joint effusion	0.07	0.61	0.33	0.82	–	–	–	–
Erosions	0.04	0.58	0.40	1	–	–	–	–
Enthesopathy	0.22	1	0.20	1	–	–	–	–
Entheseal PD	0.05	0.3	0.30	0.99	0.91	0.97	–	–
Entheseal erosions	0.05	0.20	0.96	1	–	–	–	–
Enthesophytes	0.15	0.55	0.52	1	–	–	–	–
Entheseal calcifications	0.02	0.19	0.86	0.97	–	–	–	–
Peritenonitis PD	0.36	0.65	0.95	1.00	–	–	–	–
Peritenonitis GS	0.54	0.60	0.95	0.97	–	–	–	–
Soft tissue oedema	0.29	0.42	0.90	1	–	–	–	–
Bursitis	0.02	0.10	0.90	0.99	0.96	–	0.87	–

Summary of sensitivities, specificities and reliability across studies assessing the performance of ultrasound to diagnose PsA. Min, minimal; Max, maximal; PD, power Doppler; GS, gray scale.

TABLE 6 | Performance of ultrasound lesions to detect PMR.

Lesion	Sensitivity		Specificity	
	Min	Max	Min	Max
SAD bursitis at least monolateral	0.09	0.96	0.59	0.90
SAD bursitis bilateral	0.32	0.93	0.68	0.99
LHB tenosynovitis at least monolateral	0.14	0.81	0.47	0.59
LHB tenosynovitis bilateral	0.30	0.37	0.62	0.98
GH synovitis at least monolateral	0.20	0.77	0.34	0.78
GH synovitis bilateral	0.03	0.52	0.66	0.90
Hip synovitis at least monolateral	0.24	0.45	0.55	0.88
Hip synovitis bilateral	0.18	0.38	0.83	0.92
Trochanteric bursitis at least monolateral	0.21	0.98	0.70	0.91

Summary of sensitivities, specificities across studies assessing the performance of ultrasound to diagnose PMR. Min, minimal; Max, maximal; SAD, subacromiodeltoid; LHB, long head of the biceps; GH, gleno-humeral.

disease. 4/6 studies had a cross-sectional design, while the two remaining were a prospective (73) and a retrospective (72) study. While 4 studies reported a satisfactory performance of ultrasound (73–75, 77), for 2 studies sensitivity was low (72, 76). Considering the combination of all possible elementary lesions (e.g., double contour, aggregates, tophi), the specificity of ultrasound to diagnose gout ranged from 0.42 to 0.87.

Ultrasound to Diagnose Elementary Lesions

Data on the accuracy of ultrasound to detect elementary lesions were extracted only for OA, CPPD and gout, with 20 (78–96), 12 (68–70, 97–104), and 6 (105–110) studies addressing this aspect, respectively (**Tables 7–10**).

The typical population enrolled was represented by subjects with confirmed disease, in which ultrasound was compared to a reference standard to confirm the presence of a lesion.

As expected, also the reference standard was variable, in particular for OA. For CPPD, the only assessed target lesion was CPP deposition, which was evaluated by conventional radiography (2 studies), synovial fluid analysis (6 studies), microscopic analysis (2 studies). All studies on gout but one (107), in which conventional radiography was used, adopted synovial fluid analysis as reference standard.

Most of the studies assessing ultrasound to detect elementary lesions had a cross-sectional design, in particular, all the studies on OA, 4 (74–77) and 9 (62, 69, 70, 99–101, 103) studies for gout and CPPD, respectively, while the remaining studies for these two conditions had a cohort design.

In OA, results on the performance of ultrasound were once again widely variable across studies. This was also due to the variability of the reference standards adopted to define each separate lesion and the assessment of different anatomical areas.

Most of the studies on CPPD reported good performance of ultrasound to detect deposits, and this was true especially for specificity. The same conclusions can be drawn from the included articles on gout.

Reliability

Most of the studies on OA in which reliability data were presented reported good reliability for the assessment of osteophytes, erosions, effusion, cartilage damage, synovitis and cysts (**Table 7**).

In RA, the available evidence supported a good intra-reader and inter-reader reliability for erosions, GS and PD synovitis across all the assessed sites (**Tables 3, 4**).

There was less information about reliability in the ultrasound assessment of PsA; entheseal PD, synovial hypertrophy and bursitis were the only lesions for which reliability was available. Inter-reader reliability was good for synovial hypertrophy and bursitis, as well as intra-reader for entheseal PD and bursitis (**Table 5**).

TABLE 7 | Performance of ultrasound to detect osteoarthritis elementary lesions and reliability.

Site/lesion	Sensitivity		Specificity		Intra-reader kappa		Inter-reader kappa	
	Min	**Max**	**Min**	**Max**	**Min**	**Max**	**Min**	**Max**
Knee osteophytes								
Vs CR	0.95	0.99	0.57	0.94	0.82	0.87	–	–
Vs hist.	0.7	0.9	–	–				
Hand osteophytes								
Vs CR	0.83	0.96	0.65	0.76	0.087	1	0.53	0.69
Vs MRI	0.82	0.9	0.75	0.95				
Vs PE	0.89	–	0.68	–				
Foot osteophytes								
Vs CR	0.62	–	0.86	–	–	–	–	–
Hand JSN								
Vs CR	0.82	–	0.72	–	–	–	–	–
Knee cartilage damage								
Vs CR	1	–	1	–	–	–		–
Vs hist.	0.78	0.89	–	–			0.67	
Hand erosions								
Vs CR	0.73	0.94	0.90	1	0.81	–	0.69	0.90
Vs MRI	0.65	0.88	0.90	0.96				
Knee erosions								
Vs CR	0.33	–	0.99	–	–	–	–	–
Foot erosions								
Vs CR	0.33	–	0.98	–	–	–	–	–
Knee effusion								
Vs PE	0.74	1	0	0.52	–	–	–	–
Vs JA	1	–	0	–				
Vs MRI	0.81	–	–	–				
Hand effusion								
Vs PE	1	–	–	–	0.81	–	0.69	–
Vs MRI	0.92	–	0.98	–				
Popliteal cyst								
Vs PE	0.36	0.67	0.89	0.98	–	–	–	–
Vs scint.	0.29	–	0.90	–				
Hand cysts								
Vs MRI	0.87	–	0.97	–	0.81	–	0.69	–
Hand synovitis								
Vs PE	0.15	–	0.96	–	0.81	–	0.69	–
Vs MRI	0.84	–	0.96	–				
Knee synovitis								
Vs PE	0.67	–	0.50	–	–	–	–	–
Pes anserinus bursitis								
Vs PE	0.50	–	0.96	–	–	–	–	–

Summary of sensitivities, specificities and reliability across studies assessing the performance of ultrasound to diagnose OA elementary lesions. Min, minimal; Max, maximal; CR, conventional radiography; hist, histology; MRI, magnetic resonance imaging; PE, physical examination; JA, joint aspiration; scint, scintigraphy.

Among the included studies on PMR, none reported information on the reliability for the assessed lesions.

For CPPD, some studies reported a good inter-reader reliability to assess both the meniscal fibrocartilage and the hyaline cartilage at the level of the knee (**Table 8**). In gout during acute attacks, very good intra-reader reliability was reported for double contour, aggregates, erosions and hypervascularisation. Inter-reader reliability was assessed for tophi, erosions, double contour, hypervascularisation and aggregates, still with good values (**Table 9**). The reliability on the same lesions was also assessed in the intercritical phases, with still good, although in general lower, results (**Table 10**).

TABLE 8 | Performance of ultrasound to detect CPPD elementary lesions and reproducibility.

Site/lesion	Sensitivity		Specificity		Intra-reader kappa		Inter-reader kappa	
	Min	Max	Min	Max	Min	Max	Min	Max
Knee FC	0.007	0.96	0.50	1.00	–	–	0.68	0.81
Knee HC	0.59	1.00	0.00	1.00	–	–	0.55	0.81
Wrist TFCC	0.78	0.81	0.85	0.91	–	–	–	–

Summary of sensitivities, specificities and reliability across studies assessing the performance of ultrasound to diagnose CPPD elementary lesions. FC, fibrocartilage; HC, Hyaline Cartilage; TFCC, Triangular Fibrocartilage Complex.

TABLE 9 | Performance of ultrasound to detect gout elementary lesions and reproducibility (acute attack).

Site/lesion	Sensitivity		Specificity		Intra-reader kappa		Inter-reader kappa	
	Min	Max	Min	Max	Min	Max	Min	Max
Knee/DC	–	0.75	–	–	–	–	–	–
Knee/tophi	–	0.62	–	–	–	–	–	–
1st MTP/DC	0.62	0.87	–	–	–	–	–	–
1st MTP/tophi	0.71	0.87	–	–	–	–	–	0.82
1st MTP/erosion	0.52	–	–	–	–	–	–	0.83
1st MTP/effusion	0.29	–	–	–	–	–	–	–
Knee/1st MTP erosion	0.31	0.48	0.53	0.79	–	–	–	–
Knee/1st MTP DC	0.34	0.51	0.91	0.99	–	–	–	0.87
Knee/1st MTP tophi	0.21	0.65	0.96	1.0	–	–	0.47	0.83
Knee/1st MTP echogenic foci	0.71	0.85	0.56	0.73	–	–	–	–
Symptomatic joint or tendon/erosion	0.11	0.33	0.03	0.81	1.0	–	0.86	–
Symptomatic joint or tendon/hypervascularization	0.88	0.98	0.39	0.66	0.83	-	0.67	–
Symptomatic joint or tendon/HCA	0.25	0.87	0.18	0.99	0.81	–	0.58	0.71
Symptomatic joint or tendon/DC	0.36	0.52	0.83	0.96	1.0	–	0.63	0.71
Symptomatic joint or tendon/tophi	0.29	0.52	0.95	1.0	–	–	0.74	–

Summary of sensitivities, specificities and reliability across studies assessing the performance of ultrasound to diagnose gouty elementary lesions (acute attack). Min, minimal; Max, maximal; MTP, metatarsophalangeal; DC, double contour; HCA, hyperechoic cloudy area.

DISCUSSION

The aim of our SLR was that of retrieving all the available evidence to support future studies on the integration of the information provided by ultrasound in the diagnostic process. Several groups had already focused on this aspect, since recent SLRs were available for all of the conditions of our interest (5, 9, 11, 13, 104). The existing reviews presented a summary of the diagnostic use of ultrasound deriving from a relevant number of studies for each considered disease. Despite all the reviews being relatively recent, we found additional studies in the subsequent literature from which we could retrieve further evidence. The number of SLRs and eligible studies represents a clue of the interest that ultrasound as diagnostic tool has raised. The easier availability of high-end ultrasound equipment, the accessibility to training and the possibility to apply directly the information provided by ultrasound during a routine visit are likely the features that have driven the enthusiasm about the technique. However, when analyzing in depth the available literature, there is an evident gap between the interest in the diagnostic applications of ultrasound and the quality of the studies produced so far in this field. In fact, with some important exceptions, the main objective of the studies was that of describing the prevalence of different lesions and comparing groups of patients in terms of ultrasound findings. Although information on diagnostic accuracy can be retrieved also from such study design, these results cannot be generalized to external populations, since a realistic clinical setting is not reproduced.

Many studies, in fact, included patients with definite and longstanding diagnosis and adopted a case-control design, with controls that were unlikely to be very similar to the true differential diagnoses of disease. This is particularly true for PsA, for which most of the studies had a case-control design.

There was limited evidence regarding the diagnosis of OA (6), while for RA and PMR the studies reproduced a more pragmatic context. In fact, in RA, some studies evaluated patients with new-onset arthralgia and tested the ability of ultrasound to help confirm diagnosis (19), while some others integrated ultrasound on top of classification criteria (16, 17). There were also some studies testing the prognostic value of ultrasound on the future development of RA (22).

In the context of PMR, some older studies still adopted a case-control design (56), however, since the development of the new classification criteria (8), the interest has shifted to the

TABLE 10 | Performance of ultrasound to detect gout elementary lesions and reproducibility (intercritic phase).

Site/lesion	Sensitivity		Specificity		Intra-reader kappa		Inter-reader kappa	
	Min	Max	Min	Max	Min	Max	Min	Max
Knee effusion	0.92	1.0	0.77	0.95	–	–	–	–
Knee synovial hypertrophy	0.49	0.74	0.92	1.0	–	–	–	–
Knee intra-articular PD	0.20	0.45	0.92	1.0	–	–	–	–
Midtarsal joints /effusion, synovial hypertrophy, erosion, tophi	0.91	0.94	0.93	0.96	–	–	–	–
MTP joints/effusion, synovial hypertrophy, erosion, tophi	0.90	0.95	0.78	0.85	–	–	–	–
Multiple sites/intra-articular or intrabursal HAG	0.78	0.91	0.65	0.91	–	0.67	0.50	0.54
Tendon/ligament HAG	0.55	0.72	0.84	0.95	–	0.67	0.50	0.54
Tendon/hyperechoic linear band	0.47	0.64	0.65	0.91	–	0.70	0.35	0.36
Cartilage/DC	0.66	0.82	0.76	0.89	–	0.88	0.69	0.74
1st MTP erosion	0.51	0.77	0.84	0.98	–	–	0.29	0.74
1st MTP DC	0.53	0.84	0.59	1.0	–	–	0.37	0.61
1st MTP tophi	0.26	0.77	0.88	1.0	–	–	0.26	0.78
1st MTP effusion	0.09	0.30	0.51	0.77	–	–	0.23	0.60
1st MTP synovial hypertrophy	0.03	0.19	0.92	1.0	–	–	0.36	0.81
1st MTP synovitis	0.01	0.14	0.73	0.93	–	–	0.48	0.83

Summary of sensitivities, specificities and reliability across studies assessing the performance of ultrasound to diagnose gouty elementary lesions (intercritic phase). Min, minimal; Max, maximal; PD, power Doppler; MTP, metatarsophalangeal; DC, double contour; HAG, hyperechoic aggregate.

evaluation of the additional impact of ultrasound on classification (26). The performance of US in this context was highly variable. Such heterogeneous results might be due to the disease, which may present with variable abnormalities, thus affecting the US sensitivity. Bilateral pathologic conditions appear to be the most specific US findings.

In the field of crystal-related arthropathies, several studies evaluated both patients during the acute presentation and the inter-critical periods. The population of interest was that of patients presenting with monoarthritis, representing a realistic clinical scenario for this diagnostic suspicion, although quite specific.

The ability of ultrasound to correctly identify elementary lesions typical of each disease seemed to be good, and this was especially true for inflammatory lesions. When a suboptimal performance was achieved, it must be kept in mind that in several studies the reference standard adopted to define a lesion (e.g., physical examination) could not be considered the optimal one for the specific lesion.

Although this was not the primary objective of this SLR, we extracted information on intra and inter-reader reliability, if available. The information from the primary studies supported good reliability of ultrasound to identify inflammatory lesions, as well as signs of damage, at the level of joints and entheses, as well as deposition of crystals. It must however be considered that rheumatologists taking part in ultrasound studies might have greater expertise on a specific lesion or disease than average, so that such reliabilities could not be reproduced in a clinical setting.

The present SLR has some limitations. First, only two databases were searched, and, although probably the greatest part of the literature has been covered, we cannot exclude the presence of further studies, even among gray literature. Due to the clinical heterogeneity of the results, we did not perform a pooled estimate of the diagnostic performance. Moreover, a formal assessment of quality and risk of bias was not performed. However, the present work is, to our knowledge, the first one to provide a comprehensive overview on the diagnostic use of ultrasound in arthritis, with a focus on the general question and without concentrating on a single disease.

What emerges from the overview of the results of our SLR is that a very few studies (6, 16, 19, 22, 24) investigated the additional impact of ultrasound findings in making a diagnosis in consecutive patients presenting with joint symptoms, which is indeed the typical scenario of every day's rheumatologist work.

In most studies, clinical and ultrasound assessments were performed separately, and ultrasound findings were not evaluated on top of clinical findings but validated against clinical diagnosis. With this being almost the only evidence available today, it is of no surprise that so far, the relevance of ultrasound in recommendations on the diagnosis and management of rheumatic diseases and in classification criteria is so limited. This happens despite ultrasound being an ideal tool in this context: adequate ultrasound equipment can now be easily accessible, they can be used during scheduled visits and provide immediately helpful information. Multiple sites can be assessed at the same time with good acceptability by the patients. Several other modern imaging have been applied in the setting of early arthritis, such as magnetic resonance imaging (MRI), positron emission tomography (PET) od dual energy CT (DECT), however they present a limited feasibility compared to ultrasound, limited availability, higher costs and, in some cases, limited data in the clinical setting. Since the accuracy of ultrasound in detecting elementary lesions has been established and the increasing ultrasound expertise across rheumatologists allows at least some findings to be detected reliably, the time has come to test the real potentialities of ultrasound during the first evaluation for the suspicion of inflammatory arthropathy. The Musculoskeletal ultrasound Study Group of the Italian Society for Rheumatology has recently focused on the design of such study, which implies the definition of the ideal combination of joints to be assessed based on the clinical suspicion and confirming diagnoses after a follow-up. Before the application of ultrasound, an initial set of differential diagnoses should be defined for each patient, based on clinical features. The additional value of an ultrasound examination, targeted on the clinical suspicion, would afterwards be tested in terms of correct and timely diagnosis. We expect that these results will help clarify the real role of ultrasound through the process of diagnosis and help giving a new insight into its correct placement in the management of inflammatory arthropathies.

AUTHOR CONTRIBUTIONS

GS, SC, GF, and AI conceived the study and supervised its conduction. SC performed the searches in the electronic databases. AA, ABa, ABo, AD, OD, CD, OE, EF, LI, AP, AZ, and GS performed the systematic literature review. GS drafted the manuscript. All authors revised critically the article, read and approved its final version for submission.

ACKNOWLEDGMENTS

The Authors would like to thank Cecilia Agnes, Irene Azzolin, Emanuela Bellis, Nicola Boffini Marco Canzoni, Marta Caprioli, Linda Carli, Francesco Cavatorta, Giovanni Ciancio, Giovanna Cuomo, Andrea Di Matteo, Ilaria Farina, Matteo Filippini, Valentina Foschi, Alessandra Gabba, Ariela Hoxha, Federica Martinis, Claudio Mastaglio, Augusta Ortolan, Simone Parisi, Marco Piras, Francesco Porta, Bernd Raffeiner, Roberta Ramonda, Daniela Rossi, Silvia Rossi, Crescenzio Scioscia, Palma Scolieri, Teodora Serban, Riccardo Terenzi, Giulia Tesei, Ilaria Tinazzi, Carmela Toscano, Carlo Venditti, and Gentiana Vukatana for contributing to the SLR.

REFERENCES

1. Smolen JS, Breedveld FC, Burmester GR, Bykerk V, Dougados M, Emery P, et al. Treating rheumatoid arthritis to target: 2014 update of the recommendations of an international task force. *Ann Rheum Dis.* (2016) 75:3–15. doi: 10.1136/annrheumdis-2015-207524
2. Aletaha D, Neogi T, Silman AJ, Funovits J, Felson DT, Bingham CO, et al. 2010 rheumatoid arthritis classification criteria: an American College of Rheumatology/European League Against Rheumatism collaborative initiative. *Ann Rheum Dis.* (2010) 69:1580–8. doi: 10.1136/ard.2010.138461
3. Mandl P, Navarro-Compan V, Terslev L, Aegerter P, van der Heijde D, D'Agostino MA, et al. EULAR recommendations for the use of imaging in the diagnosis and management of spondyloarthritis in clinical practice. *Ann Rheum Dis.* (2015) 74:1327–39. doi: 10.1136/annrheumdis-2014-206971
4. Colebatch AN, Edwards CJ, Østergaard M, van der Heijde D, Balint PV, D'Agostino M-A, et al. EULAR recommendations for the use of imaging of the joints in the clinical management of rheumatoid arthritis. *Ann Rheum Dis.* (2013) 72:804–14. doi: 10.1136/annrheumdis-2012-203158
5. Sakellariou G, Conaghan PG, Zhang W, Bijlsma JWJ, Boyesen P, D'Agostino MA, et al. EULAR recommendations for the use of imaging in the clinical management of peripheral joint osteoarthritis. *Ann Rheum Dis.* (2017) 76:1484–94. doi: 10.1136/annrheumdis-2016-210815
6. Matsos M, Harish S, Zia P, Ho Y, Chow A, Ioannidis G, et al. Ultrasound of the hands and feet for rheumatological disorders: influence on clinical diagnostic confidence and patient management. *Skeletal Radiol.* (2009) 38:1049–54. doi: 10.1007/s00256-009-0738-2
7. D'Agostino M-A, Saraux A, Chary-Valckenaere I, Marcelli C, Guis S, Gaudin P, et al. Can we improve the diagnosis of spondyloarthritis in patients with uncertain diagnosis? The EchoSpA prospective multicenter French cohort. *Joint Bone Spine Rev Rhum.* (2012) 79:586–90. doi: 10.1016/j.jbspin.2012.02.007
8. Dasgupta B, Cimmino MA, Maradit-Kremers H, Schmidt WA, Schirmer M, Salvarani C, et al. 2012 Provisional classification criteria for polymyalgia rheumatica: a European League Against Rheumatism/American College of Rheumatology collaborative initiative. *Ann Rheum Dis.* (2012) 71:484–92. doi: 10.1016/j.ymed.2012.09.009
9. Zabotti A, Bandinelli F, Batticciotto A, Scirè CA, Iagnocco A, Sakellariou G, et al. Musculoskeletal ultrasonography for psoriatic arthritis and psoriasis patients: a systematic literature review. *Rheumatology.* (2017) 56:1518–32. doi: 10.1093/rheumatology/kex179
10. Filippou G, Adinolfi A, Iagnocco A, Filippucci E, Cimmino M.A, Bertoldi I, et al. Ultrasound in the diagnosis of calcium pyrophosphate dihydrate deposition disease. a systematic literature review and a meta-analysis. *Osteoarthr Cartil.* (2016) 24:973–81. doi: 10.1016/j.joca.2016.01.136
11. Chen J, Liao M, Zhang H, Zhu D. Diagnostic accuracy of dual-energy CT and ultrasound in gouty arthritis: a systematic review. *Z Rheumatol.* (2017) 76:723–9. doi: 10.1007/s00393-016-0250-8
12. Lage-Hansen PR, Lindegaard H, Chrysidis S, Terslev L. The role of ultrasound in diagnosing rheumatoid arthritis, what do we know? an updated review. *Rheumatol Int.* (2017) 37:179–87. doi: 10.1007/s00296-016-3587-z
13. Mackie SL, Koduri G, Hill CL, Wakefield RJ, Hutchings A, Loy C, et al. Accuracy of musculoskeletal imaging for the diagnosis of polymyalgia rheumatica: systematic review. *RMD Open.* (2015) 1:e000100. doi: 10.1136/rmdopen-2015-000100
14. Filer A, De Pablo P, Allen G, Nightingale P, Jordan A, Jobanputra P, et al. Utility of ultrasound joint counts in the prediction of rheumatoid arthritis in patients with very early synovitis. *Ann Rheum Dis.* (2011) 70:500–7. doi: 10.1136/ard.2010.131573
15. Kawashiri SY, Suzuki T, Okada A, Yamasaki S, Tamai M, Nakamura H, et al. Musculoskeletal ultrasonography assists the diagnostic performance of the

2010 classification criteria for rheumatoid arthritis. *Mod Rheumatol.* (2013) 23:36–43. doi: 10.3109/s10165-012-0628-7

16. Nakagomi D, Ikeda K, Okubo A, Iwamoto T, Sanayama Y, Takahashi K, et al. Ultrasonographic assessment of synovitis improves the accuracy of 2010 american college of rheumatology/European league against rheumatism classification criteria for rheumatoid arthritis to predict development of a methotrexate-requiring disease. *Ann Rheum Dis.* (2013) 65:890–8.
17. Ji L, Deng X, Geng Y, Song Z, Zhang Z. The additional benefit of ultrasonography to 2010 ACR/EULAR classification criteria when diagnosing rheumatoid arthritis in the absence of anti-cyclic citrullinated peptide antibodies. *Clin Rheumatol.* (2017) 36:261–7. doi: 10.1007/s10067-016-3465-9
18. Minowa K, Ogasawara M, Murayama G, Gorai M, Yamada Y, Nemoto T, et al. Predictive grade of ultrasound synovitis for diagnosing rheumatoid arthritis in clinical practice and the possible difference between patients with and without seropositivity. *Mod Rheumatol.* (2015) 3:1–6. doi: 10.3109/14397595.2015.1069457
19. Broll M, Albrecht K, Tarner I, Müller-Ladner U, Strunk J. Sensitivity and specificity of ultrasonography and low-field magnetic resonance imaging for diagnosing arthritis. *Clin Exp Rheumatol.* (2012) 30:543–7.
20. Rezaei H, Torp-Pedersen S, Af Klint E, Backheden M, Kisten Y, Györi N, et al. Diagnostic utility of musculoskeletal ultrasound in patients with suspected arthritis–a probabilistic approach. *Arthritis Res Ther.* (2014) 16:448. doi: 10.1186/s13075-014-0448-6
21. Salaffi F, Ciapetti A, Gasparini S, Carotti M, Filippucci E, Grassi W. A clinical prediction rule combining routine assessment and power doppler ultrasonography for predicting progression to rheumatoid arthritis from early-onset undifferentiated arthritis. *Clin Exp Rheumatol.* (2010) 28:686–94.
22. Navalho M, Resende C, Rodrigues AM, Alberto Pereira DSJ, Fonseca JE, Campos J, et al. Bilateral evaluation of the hand and wrist in untreated early inflammatory arthritis: A comparative study of ultrasonography and magnetic resonance imaging. *J Rheumatol.* (2013) 40:1282–92. doi: 10.3899/jrheum.120713
23. Ozgul A, Yasar E, Arslan N, Balaban B, Taskaynatan MA, Tezel K, et al. The comparison of ultrasonographic and scintigraphic findings of early arthritis in revealing rheumatoid arthritis according to criteria of American College of Rheumatology. *Rheumatol Int.* (2009) 29:765–8. doi: 10.1007/s00296-008-0765-7
24. Platt PN, Pratt A. The predictive value of musculoskeletal ultrasound in unselected early arthritis clinic patients with polyarthralgia. *Rheumatology.* (2013) 52:i65.
25. Tămaş MM, Rednic N, Felea I, Rednic S. Ultrasound assessment for the rapid classification of early arthritis patients. *J Investig Med.* (2013) 61:1184–91. doi: 10.2310/JIM.0000000000000005
26. Macchioni P, Boiardi L, Catanoso M, Pazzola G, Salvarani C. Performance of the new 2012 EULAR/ACR classification criteria for polymyalgia rheumatica: Comparison with the previous criteria in a single-centre study. *Ann Rheum Dis.* (2014) 73:1190–3. doi: 10.1136/annrheumdis-2013-204167
27. Weigand S, Ehrenstein B, Fleck M, Hartung W. Joint involvement in patients with early polymyalgia rheumatica using high-resolution ultrasound and its contribution to the EULAR/ACR 2012 classification criteria for polymyalgia rheumatica. *J Rheumatol.* (2014) 41:730–4. doi: 10.3899/jrheum.130946
28. Zufferey P, Rebell C, Benaim C, Ziswiler HR, Dumusc A, So A. Ultrasound can be useful to predict an evolution towards rheumatoid arthritis in patients with inflammatory polyarthralgia without anticitrullinated antibodies. *Joint Bone Spine.* (2017) 84:299–303. doi: 10.1016/j.jbspin.2016.05.011
29. Gutierrez M, Filippucci E, Salaffi F, Di Geso L, Grassi W. Differential diagnosis between rheumatoid arthritis and psoriatic arthritis: the value of ultrasound findings at metacarpophalangeal joints level. *Ann Rheum Dis.* (2011) 70:1111–4. doi: 10.1136/ard.2010.147272
30. Iagnocco A, Spadaro A, Marchesoni A, Cauli A, de Lucia O, Gabba A, et al. Power doppler ultrasonographic evaluation of enthesitis in psoriatic arthritis. a multi-center study. *Joint Bone Spine.* (2012) 79:324–5. doi: 10.1016/j.jbspin.2011.10.005
31. Lin Z, Wang Y, Mei Y, Zhao Y, Zhang Z. High-Frequency ultrasound in the evaluation of psoriatic arthritis: a clinical study. *Am J Med Sci.* (2015) 350:42–6. doi: 10.1097/MAJ.0000000000000504
32. Melchiorre D, Calderazzi A, Maddali Bongi S, Cristofani R, Bazzichi L, Eligi C, et al. A comparison of ultrasonography and magnetic resonance imaging in the evaluation of temporomandibular joint involvement in rheumatoid arthritis and psoriatic arthritis. *Rheumatology.* (2003) 42:673–6. doi: 10.1093/rheumatology/keg181
33. Wiell C, Szkudlarek M, Hasselquist M, Moller JM, Vestergaard A, Norregaard J, et al. Ultrasonography, magnetic resonance imaging, radiography, and clinical assessment of inflammatory and destructive changes in fingers and toes of patients with psoriatic arthritis. *Arthritis Res Ther.* (2007) 9:R119. doi: 10.1186/ar2327
34. Falsetti P, Frediani B, Fioravanti A, Acciai C, Baldi F, Filippou G, et al. Sonographic study of calcaneal entheses in erosive osteoarthritis, nodal osteoarthritis, rheumatoid arthritis and psoriatic arthritis. *Scand J Rheumatol.* (2003) 32:229–34. doi: 10.1080/03009740310003721
35. Falsetti P, Frediani B, Filippou G, Acciai C, Baldi F, Storri L, et al. Enthesitis of proximal insertion of the deltoid in the course of seronegative spondyloarthritis. an atypical enthesitis that can mime impingement syndrome. *Scand J Rheumatol.* (2002) 31:158–62. doi: 10.1080/713798352
36. Fournié B, Margarit-Coll N, Champetier de Ribes TL, Zabraniecki L, Jouan A, Vincent V, et al. Extrasynovial ultrasound abnormalities in the psoriatic finger. Prospective comparative power-doppler study versus rheumatoid arthritis. *Joint Bone Spine.* (2006) 73:527–31. doi: 10.1016/j.jbspin.2006.01.019
37. Zabotti A, Salvin S, Quartuccio L, De Vita S. Differentiation between early rheumatoid and early psoriatic arthritis by the ultrasonographic study of the synovio-entheseal complex of the small joints of the hands. *Clin Exp Rheumatol.* (2016) 34:459–65.
38. Turner DE, Hyslop E, Barn R, McInnes IB, Steultjens MPM, Woodburn J. Metatarsophalangeal joint pain in psoriatic arthritis: a cross-sectional study. *Rheumatology.* (2014) 53:737–40. doi: 10.1093/rheumatology/ket435
39. Woodburn J, Hyslop E, Barn R, McInnes IB, Turner DE. Achilles tendon biomechanics in psoriatic arthritis patients with ultrasound proven enthesitis. *Scand J Rheumatol.* (2013) 42:299–302. doi: 10.3109/03009742.2012.747626
40. Eder L, Jayakar J, Thavaneswaran A, Haddad A, Chandran V, Salonen D, et al. Is the madrid sonographic enthesitis index useful for differentiating psoriatic arthritis from psoriasis alone and healthy controls? *J Rheumatol.* (2014) 41:466–72. doi: 10.3899/jrheum.130949
41. Ciancio G, Volpinari S, Fotinidi M, Furini F, Farina I, Bortoluzzi A, et al. Involvement of the inconstant bursa of the fifth metatarsophalangeal joint in psoriatic arthritis: a clinical and ultrasonographic study. *BioMed Res Int.* (2014) 2014:174841 doi: 10.1155/2014/174841
42. Bandinelli F, Prignano F, Bonciani D, Bartoli F, Collaku L, Candelieri A, et al. Ultrasound detects occult entheseal involvement in early psoriatic arthritis independently of clinical features and psoriasis severity. *Clin Exp Rheumatol.* (2013) 31:219–24.
43. Aydin SZ, Castillo-Gallego C, Ash ZR, Abignano G, Marzo-Ortega H, Wittmann M, et al. Potential use of optical coherence tomography and high-frequency ultrasound for the assessment of nail disease in psoriasis and psoriatic arthritis. *Dermatol Basel Switz.* (2013) 227:46–51. doi: 10.1159/000351702
44. Zayat AS, Ellegaard K, Conaghan PG, Terslev L, Hensor EM, Freeston JE, et al. The specificity of ultrasound-detected bone erosions for rheumatoid arthritis. *Ann Rheum Dis.* (2015) 745:897–903. doi: 10.1136/annrheumdis-2013-204864
45. Freeston JE, Coates LC, Helliwell PS, Hensor EM, Wakefield RJ, Emery P, et al. Is there subclinical enthesitis in early psoriatic arthritis? A clinical comparison with power doppler ultrasound. *Arthritis Care Res.* (2012) 64:1617–21. doi: 10.1002/acr.21733
46. Marchesoni A, de Lucia O, Rotunno L, de Marco G, Manara M. Entheseal power doppler ultrasonography: a comparison of psoriatic arthritis and fibromyalgia. *J Rheumatol.* (2012) 39:29–31. doi: 10.3899/jrheum.120238
47. Acquacalda E, Albert C, Montaudie H, Fontas E, Danre A, Roux CH, et al. Ultrasound study of entheses in psoriasis patients with or without musculoskeletal symptoms: a prospective study. *Joint Bone Spine.* (2015) 82:267–71. doi: 10.1016/j.jbspin.2015.01.016

48. Falcao S, de Miguel E, Castillo-Gallego C, Peiteado D, Branco J, Martín Mola E. Achilles enthesis ultrasound: the importance of the bursa in spondyloarthritis. *Clin Exp Rheumatol.* (2013) 31:422–7.
49. Ezzat Y, Gaber W, Abd ELRSF, Ezzat M, El Sayed M. Ultrasonographic evaluation of lower limb enthesis in patients with early spondyloarthropathies. *Egypt Rheumatol.* (2013) 35:29–35. doi: 10.1016/j.ejr.2012.09.004
50. Aydin SZ, Ash ZR, Tinazzi I, Castillo-Gallego C, Kwok C, Wilson C, et al. The link between enthesitis and arthritis in psoriatic arthritis: a switch to a vascular phenotype at insertions may play a role in arthritis development. *Ann Rheum Dis.* (2013) 72:992–5. doi: 10.1136/annrheumdis-2012-201617
51. Farouk HM, Mostafa AAA, Youssef SS, Elbeblawy MMS, Assaf NY, Elokda ESE. Value of entheseal ultrasonography and serum cartilage oligomeric matrix protein in the preclinical diagnosis of psoriatic arthritis. *Clin Med Insights Arthritis Musculoskelet Disord.* (2010) 3:7–14. doi: 10.4137/CMAMD.S4461
52. Groves C, Chandramohan M, Chew NS, Aslam T, Helliwell PS. Clinical examination, ultrasound and MRI imaging of the painful elbow in psoriatic arthritis and rheumatoid arthritis: which is better, ultrasound or MR, for imaging enthesitis? *Rheumatol Ther.* (2017) 4:71–84. doi: 10.1007/s40744-017-0053-7
53. De Simone C, Caldarola G, D'Agostino M, Carbone A, Guerriero C, Bonomo L, et al. Usefulness of ultrasound imaging in detecting psoriatic arthritis of fingers and toes in patients with psoriasis. *Clin Dev Immunol.* (2011) 2011:390726. doi: 10.1155/2011/390726
54. Aydin SZ, Castillo-Gallego C, Ash ZR, Marzo-Ortega H, Emery P, Wakefield RJ, et al. Ultrasonographic assessment of nail in psoriatic disease shows a link between onychopathy and distal interphalangeal joint extensor tendon enthesopathy. *Dermatology.* (2012) 225:231–5. doi: 10.1159/000343607
55. Mendonça JA. [Differences of spectral doppler in psoriatic arthritis and onychomycosis]. *Rev Bras Reumatol.* (2014) 54:490–3. doi: 10.1016/j.rbre.2014.03.028
56. Ruta S, Rosa J, Navarta DA, Saucedo C, Catoggio LJ, Monaco RG, et al. Ultrasound assessment of new onset bilateral painful shoulder in patients with polymyalgia rheumatica and rheumatoid arthritis. *Clin Rheumatol.* (2012) 31:1383–7. doi: 10.1007/s10067-012-2016-2
57. Cantini F, Salvarani C, Olivieri I, Niccoli L, Padula A, Macchioni L, et al. Shoulder ultrasonography in the diagnosis of polymyalgia rheumatica: a case-control study. *J Rheumatol.* (2001) 28:1049–55.
58. Cantini F, Niccoli L, Nannini C, Padula A, Olivieri I, Boiardi L, et al. Inflammatory changes of hip synovial structures in polymyalgia rheumatica. *Clin Exp Rheumatol.* (2005) 23:462–8.
59. Coari G, Paoletti F, Iagnocco A. Shoulder involvement in rheumatic diseases. sonographic findings. *J Rheumatol.* (1999) 26:668–73.
60. Lange U, Piegsa M, Teichmann J, Neeck G. Ultrasonography of the glenohumeral joints–a helpful instrument in differentiation in elderly onset rheumatoid arthritis and polymyalgia rheumatica. *Rheumatol Int.* (2000) 19:185–9. doi: 10.1007/s002960000051
61. Catay E, Ruta S, Rosa J, Navarta DA, Scolnik M, Garcia-Monaco R, et al. Knee effusion: Sensitivity and specificity of ultrasound for the identification of calcium pyrophosphate crystals. *Arthritis Rheum.* (2013) 65:S367.
62. Juge PA, Ottaviani S, Aubrun A, Palazzo E, Dieudé P. Sensitivity and reproducibility of ultrasonography in calcium pyrophosphate crystal deposition: a case-control study. *Ann Rheum Dis.* (2014) 73:492–509. doi: 10.1136/annrheumdis-2014-eular.3849
63. Ottaviani S, Juge PA, Aubrun A, Palazzo E, Dieudé P. Sensitivity and reproducibility of ultrasonography in calcium pyrophosphate crystal deposition in knee cartilage: a cross-sectional study. *J Rheumatol.* (2015) 42:1511–3. doi: 10.3899/jrheum.141067
64. Salcion A, Kozyreff-Meurice M, Richette P, Avenel G, Bisson-Vaivre A, Trouvin A.-P, et al. Assessment of the ultrasonography's efficiency as a diagnostic tool for calcium pyrophosphate crystal deposition disease. *Ann Rheum Dis.* (2015) 74:538. doi: 10.1136/annrheumdis-2015-eular.4964
65. Adinolfi A, Picerno V, Scanu A, Toscano C, Scirè C, Carrara G, et al. Diagnostic performance of the new omeract criteria for CPPD identification by us: correlation with synovial fluid analysis. *Ann Rheum Dis.* (2017) 2017:730–1. doi: 10.1136/annrheumdis-2017-eular.5164
66. Filippou G, Frediani B, Gallo A, Menza L, Falsetti P, Baldi F, et al. A 'new' technique for the diagnosis of chondrocalcinosis of the knee: sensitivity and specificity of high-frequency ultrasonography. *Ann Rheum Dis.* (2007) 66:1126–8. doi: 10.1136/ard.2007.069344
67. Ellabban AS, Kamel SR, Abo Omar HAS, El-Sherif AMH, Abdel-Magied RA. Ultrasonographic diagnosis of articular chondrocalcinosis. *Rheumatol Int.* (2012) 32:3863–8. doi: 10.1007/s00296-011-2320-1
68. Filippou G, Bozios P, Gambera D, Lorenzini S, Bertoldi I, Adinolfi A, et al. Ultrasound detection of calcium pyrophosphate dihydrate crystal deposits in menisci: a pilot *in vivo* and *ex vivo* study. *Ann Rheum Dis.* (2012) 71:1426–7. doi: 10.1136/annrheumdis-2011-201001
69. Forien M, Combier A, Gardette A, Palazzo E, Dieudé P, Ottaviani S. Comparison of ultrasonography and radiography of the wrist for diagnosis of calcium pyrophosphate deposition. *Joint Bone Spine.* (2018) 85:615–8. doi: 10.1016/j.jbspin.2017.09.006
70. Di Matteo A, Filippucci E, Salaffi F, Carotti M, Carboni D, Di Donato E, et al. Diagnostic accuracy of musculoskeletal ultrasound and conventional radiography in the assessment of the wrist triangular fibrocartilage complex in patients with definite diagnosis of calcium pyrophosphate dihydrate deposition disease. *Clin Exp Rheumatol.* (2017) 35:647–52.
71. Contant E, Ornetti P, Bohm A, Fortunet C, Maillefert JF. Interest of musculoskeletal ultrasound in the diagnosis of calcium pyrophosphate dihydrate deposition disease. *Ann Rheum Dis.* (2014) 73:775 doi: 10.1136/annrheumdis-2014-eular.3533
72. Lai KL, Chiu YM. Role of ultrasonography in diagnosing gouty arthritis. *J Med Ultrasound.* (2011) 19:7–13. doi: 10.1016/j.jmu.2011.01.003
73. Huppertz A, Hermann KGA, Diekhoff T, Wagner M, Hamm B, Schmidt WA. Systemic staging for urate crystal deposits with dual-energy CT and ultrasound in patients with suspected gout. *Rheumatol Int.* (2014) 34:763–71. doi: 10.1007/s00296-014-2979-1
74. Elsaman AM, Muhammad EMS, Pessler F. Sonographic findings in gouty arthritis: diagnostic value and association with disease duration. *Ultrasound Med Biol.* (2016) 42:1330–6. doi: 10.1016/j.ultrasmedbio.2016.01.014
75. Basaric MM, Radunovic G, Damjanov N, Perovic-Radak M. Sensitivity and specificity of ultrasound score for the diagnosis of gout. *Ann Rheum Dis.* (2016) 75:863–4. doi: 10.1136/annrheumdis-2016-eular.3750
76. Gruber M, Bodner G, Rath E, Supp G, Weber M, Schueller-Weidekamm C. Dual-energy computed tomography compared with ultrasound in the diagnosis of gout. *Rheumatol.* (2014) 53:173–9. doi: 10.1093/rheumatology/ket341
77. Pascal Z, Valcov R, Fabreguet I, Dumusc A, Omoumi P, So A. A prospective evaluation of ultrasound as a diagnostic tool in acute microcrystalline arthritis. *Arthritis Res Ther.* (2015) 17:188 doi: 10.1186/s13075-015-0701-7
78. Iagnocco A, Filippucci E, Ossandon A, Ciapetti A, Salaffi F, Basili S, et al. High resolution ultrasonography in detection of bone erosions in patients with hand osteoarthritis. *J Rheumatol.* (2005) 32:2381–3.
79. Keen HI, Lavie F, Wakefield RJ, D'Agostino MA, Berner Hammer H, Hensor EMA, et al. The development of a preliminary ultrasonographic scoring system for features of hand osteoarthritis. *Ann Rheum Dis.* (2008) 67:651–5. doi: 10.1136/ard.2007.077081
80. Koutroumpas AC, Alexiou IS, Vlychou M, Sakkas LI. Comparison between clinical and ultrasonographic assessment in patients with erosive osteoarthritis of the hands. *Clin Rheumatol.* (2010) 29:511–6. doi: 10.1007/s10067-009-1348-z
81. Hammer HB, Mathiessen A, Iagnocco A, Filippucci E, Gandjbakhch F, Kortekaas MC, et al. High reliability was found for ultrasound scoring of osteophytes in patients with hand osteoarthritis using an atlas as reference; an omeract initiative. *Arthritis Rheum.* (2013) 65:S728–9.
82. Vlychou M, Koutroumpas A, Malizos K, Sakkas LI. Ultrasonographic evidence of inflammation is frequent in hands of patients with erosive osteoarthritis. *Osteoarthr Cartil.* (2009) 17:1283–7. doi: 10.1016/j.joca.2009.04.020
83. Vlychou M, Koutroumpas A, Alexiou I, Fezoulidis I, Sakkas LI. High-resolution ultrasonography and 3.0 T magnetic resonance imaging in erosive and nodal hand osteoarthritis: high frequency of erosions in nodal osteoarthritis. *Clin Rheumatol.* (2013) 32:755–62. doi: 10.1007/s10067-013-2166-x

84. Wittoek R, Carron P, Verbruggen G. Structural and inflammatory sonographic findings in erosive and non-erosive osteoarthritis of the interphalangeal finger joints. *Ann Rheum Dis.* (2010) 69:2173–6. doi: 10.1136/ard.2010.128504
85. Wittoek R, Jans L, Lambrecht V, Carron P, Verstraete K, Verbruggen G. Reliability and construct validity of ultrasonography of soft tissue and destructive changes in erosive osteoarthritis of the interphalangeal finger joints: a comparison with MRI. *Ann Rheum Dis.* (2011) 70:278–83. doi: 10.1136/ard.2010.134932
86. Iagnocco A, Coari G. Usefulness of high resolution US in the evaluation of effusion in osteoarthritic first carpometacarpal joint. *Scand J Rheumatol.* (2000) 29:170–3. doi: 10.1080/030097400750002049
87. Akgul O, Guldeste Z, Ozgocmen S. The reliability of the clinical examination for detecting Baker's cyst in asymptomatic fossa. *Int J Rheum Dis.* (2014) 17:204–9. doi: 10.1111/1756-185X.12095
88. Chatzopoulos D, Moralidis E, Markou P, Makris V, Arsos G. Baker's cysts in knees with chronic osteoarthritic pain: a clinical, ultrasonographic, radiographic and scintigraphic evaluation. *Rheumatol Int.* (2008) 29:141–6. doi: 10.1007/s00296-008-0639-z
89. Eşen S, Akarirmak U, Aydin FY, Unalan H. Clinical evaluation during the acute exacerbation of knee osteoarthritis: the impact of diagnostic ultrasonography. *Rheumatol Int.* (2013) 33:711–7. doi: 10.1007/s00296-012-2441-1
90. Ike RW, Somers EC, Arnold EL, Arnold WJ. Ultrasound of the knee during voluntary quadriceps contraction: a technique for detecting otherwise occult effusions. *Arthritis Care Res.* (2010) 62:725–9. doi: 10.1002/acr.20047
91. Pendleton A, Millar A, O'Kane D, Wright GD, Taggart AJ. Can sonography be used to predict the response to intra-articular corticosteroid injection in primary osteoarthritis of the knee? *Scand J Rheumatol.* (2008) 37:395–7. doi: 10.1080/03009740802050738
92. Song IH, Althoff CE, Hermann KG, Scheel AK, Knetsch T, Burmester GR, et al. Contrast-enhanced ultrasound in monitoring the efficacy of a bradykinin receptor 2 antagonist in painful knee osteoarthritis compared with MRI. *Ann Rheum Dis.* (2009) 68:75–83. doi: 10.1136/ard.2007.080382
93. Yoon CH, Kim HS, Ju JH, Jee WH, Park SH, Kim HY. Validity of the sonographic longitudinal sagittal image for assessment of the cartilage thickness in the knee osteoarthritis. *Clin Rheumatol.* (2008) 27:1507–16. doi: 10.1007/s10067-008-0956-3
94. Okano T, Filippucci E, Carlo M.D, Draghessi A, Carotti M, Salaffi F, et al. Ultrasonographic evaluation of joint damage in knee osteoarthritis: Feature-specific comparisons with conventional radiography. *Rheumatol UK.* (2016) 55:2040–9. doi: 10.1093/rheumatology/kew304
95. Camerer M, Ehrenstein B, Hoffstetter P, Fleck M, Hartung W. High-resolution ultrasound of the midfoot: sonography is more sensitive than conventional radiography in detection of osteophytes and erosions in inflammatory and non-inflammatory joint disease. *Clin Rheumatol.* (2017) 36:2145–9. doi: 10.1007/s10067-017-3658-x
96. Mortada M, Zeid A, Abd El-Hamid Al-Toukhy M, Ezzeldin N, Elgawish M. Reliability of a proposed ultrasonographic grading scale for severity of primary knee osteoarthritis. *Clin Med Insights Arthritis Musculoskelet Disord.* (2016) 9:161–6. doi: 10.4137/CMAMD.S38141
97. Ellabban AS, Kamel SR, Omar HASA, El-Sherif AMH, Abdel-Magied RA. Ultrasonographic findings of Achilles tendon and plantar fascia in patients with calcium pyrophosphate deposition disease. *Clin Rheumatol.* (2012) 31:697–704. doi: 10.1007/s10067-011-1911-2
98. Ottaviani S. Ultrasonography in crystal-related diseases. *Rev Rhum Monogr.* (2015) 82:181–6. doi: 10.1016/j.monrhu.2015.04.005
99. Foldes K. Knee chondrocalcinosis: an ultrasonographic study of the hyalin cartilage. *Clin Imaging.* (2002) 26:194–6. doi: 10.1016/S0899-7071(01)00385-0
100. Falsetti P, Frediani B, Acciai C, Baldi F, Filippou G, Prada EP, et al. Ultrasonographic study of achilles tendon and plantar fascia in chondrocalcinosis. *J Rheumatol.* (2004) 31:2242–50.
101. Filippucci E, Gutierrez Riveros M, Georgescu D, Salaffi F, Grassi W. Hyaline cartilage involvement in patients with gout and calcium pyrophosphate deposition disease. *An ultrasound study. Osteoarthritis Cartilage.* (2009) 17:178–81. doi: 10.1016/j.joca.2008.06.003
102. Barskova VG, Kudaeva FM, Bozhieva LA, Smirnov AV, Volkov AV, Nasonov EL. Comparison of three imaging techniques in diagnosis of chondrocalcinosis of the knees in calcium pyrophosphate deposition disease. *Rheumatology.* (2013) 52:1090–4. doi: 10.1093/rheumatology/kes433
103. Gutierrez M, Di Geso L, Salaffi F, Carotti M, Girolimetti R, de Angelis R, et al. Ultrasound detection of cartilage calcification at knee level in calcium pyrophosphate deposition disease. *Arthritis Care Res.* (2014) 66:69–73. doi: 10.1002/acr.22190
104. Filippou G, Adinolfi A, Lorenzini S, Bertoldi I, Di Sabatino V, Picerno V, et al. Ultrasound versus X-rays versus synovial fluid analysis for the diagnosis of calcium pyrophosphate dihydrate deposition disease: Is it CPPD? *Arthritis Rheumatol.* (2014) 66:S77–8.
105. de Miguel E, Puig JG, Castillo C, Peiteado D, Torres RJ, Martín-Mola E. Diagnosis of gout in patients with asymptomatic hyperuricaemia: a pilot ultrasound study. *Ann Rheum Dis.* (2012) 71:157–8. doi: 10.1136/ard.2011.154997
106. Rettenbacher T, Ennemoser S, Weirich H, Ulmer H, Hartig F, Klotz W, et al. Diagnostic imaging of gout: comparison of high-resolution US versus conventional X-ray. *Eur Radiol.* (2008) 18:621–30. doi: 10.1007/s00330-007-0802-z
107. Naredo E, Uson J, Jiménez-Palop M, Martínez A, Vicente E, Brito E, et al. Ultrasound-detected musculoskeletal urate crystal deposition: which joints and what findings should be assessed for diagnosing gout? *Ann Rheum Dis.* (2014) 73:1522–8. doi: 10.1136/annrheumdis-2013-203487
108. Lamers-Karnebeek FBG, van Riel PLCM, Jansen TL. Additive value for ultrasonographic signal in a screening algorithm for patients presenting with acute mono-/oligoarthritis in whom gout is suspected. *Clin Rheumatol.* (2014) 33:555–9. doi: 10.1007/s10067-014-2505-6
109. Pattamapaspong N, Vuthiwong W, Kanthawang T, Louthrenoo W. Value of ultrasonography in the diagnosis of gout in patients presenting with acute arthritis. *Skeletal Radiol.* (2017) 46:759–67. doi: 10.1007/s00256-017-2611-z
110. Das S, Ghosh A, Ghosh P, Lahiri D, Sinhamahapatra P, Basu K. Sensitivity and specificity of ultrasonographic features of gout in intercritical and chronic phase. *Int J Rheum Dis.* (2017) 20:887–93. doi: 10.1111/1756-185X.12928

2

Comparison of the Effects of Cyclophosphamide and Mycophenolate Mofetil Treatment Against Immunoglobulin G4-Related Disease

Xuan Luo[1,2†], *Yu Peng*[1,2†], *Panpan Zhang*[1,2], *Jieqiong Li*[1,2], *Zheng Liu*[1,2], *Hui Lu*[1,2], *Xuan Zhang*[1,2], *Xiaofeng Zeng*[1,2], *Fengchun Zhang*[1,2], *Yunyun Fei*[1,2*] *and Wen Zhang*[1,2*]

[1] *Department of Rheumatology, Peking Union Medical College Hospital, Chinese Academy of Medical Sciences, Peking Union Medical College, Beijing, China,* [2] *National Clinical Research Center for Dermatologic and Immunologic Diseases (NCRC-DID), Key Laboratory of Ministry of Health, Beijing, China*

***Correspondence:**
Yunyun Fei
feiyunyun2013@hotmail.com
Wen Zhang
zhangwen91@sina.com

†These authors have contributed equally to this work

Background: Although there are multiple ways to manage immunoglobulin G4–related disease (IgG4-RD), including treatment with glucocorticoids, "steroid-sparing" immunosuppressive drugs, or biologic agents, few clinical trials on IgG4-RD have been conducted. This study aimed to compare the efficacy and safety of glucocorticoids (GCs) combined with cyclophosphamide (CYC) or mycophenolate mofetil (MMF) in IgG4-RD patients. This cohort study was registered at ClinicalTrials.gov (ID: NCT01670695).

Methods: This retrospective study included 155 IgG4-RD patients who received GCs with CYC or MMF at the Department of Rheumatology at Peking Union Medical College Hospital between January 2012 and July 2018. Propensity score matching (PSM) was conducted to match two groups of patients based on their baseline clinical characteristics. Treatment response, relapse rate, and drug safety were analyzed. The treatment response was evaluated based on complete response (CR), partial response (PR), and no change (NC), and the cumulative relapse rate and adverse events in each treatment group were compared using Kaplan–Meier curves and log-rank test, respectively.

Results: Of the 155 IgG4-RD patients, 90 were treated with GCs plus CYC (group I) and 65 with GCs plus MMF (group II). After propensity score–matched (PSM) analysis, 108 patients were selected (54 in each group), 49 of whom had "definite" IgG4-RD, 8 "probable" IgG4-RD, and 51 "possible" IgG4-RD. At the last follow-up, the total response in groups I and II was 98.15 and 96.3%, respectively, and within 12 months, the cumulative relapse rate in group II was significantly higher than that in group I (14.8 vs. 3.7%, $P = 0.046$). Recurrence occurred at the paranasal sinus, lacrimal glands, skin, lung, pancreas, and bile ducts, and the relapsed patients achieved remission after switching immunosuppressants or/and increasing the GC dose.

Conclusions: In IgG4-RD patients with internal organ involvement, GCs plus CYC or MMF are both effective with similar effects in disease response, while GCs plus CYC reduced the relapse rate better than GCs plus MMF.

Keywords: cyclophosphamide, efficacy, IgG4-related disease, mycophenolate mofetil, relapse, response

INTRODUCTION

Immunoglobulin G4–related disease (IgG4-RD) is a systemic fibroinflammatory condition that affects multiple organs including the pancreas, bile duct, lacrimal gland, salivary gland, thyroid, lung, liver, gastrointestinal tract, kidney, and retroperitoneum (1). It is characterized by tissue infiltration by IgG4-positive cells, and causes prominent pathological changes in most of the affected organs, including lymphoplasmacytic infiltration, storiform fibrosis, and obliterative phlebitis, as well as tumor-like lesions and even depletion (2).

Glucocorticoids (GCs) are the first-line therapy for achieving clinical remission in active or untreated IgG4-RD patients (3). Relapse occurred in about 50% patients with GC tapering or withdrawal (4), and long-term application of GCs may increase the risk of adverse reactions. Thus far, conventional immunosuppressants including azathioprine (AZA) (5), mycophenolate mofetil (MMF), 6-mercaptopurine (6-MP), methotrexate (MTX), tacrolimus, cyclophosphamide (CYC), and leflunomide (LEF) have been used in the treatment of patients with IgG4-RD (6, 7). Data from cohort and randomized controlled trial (RCT) studies show that IgG4-RD can be better controlled with GCs plus conventional immunosuppressants than with GC monotherapy (7–10). However, data comparing the efficacy and safety of combined treatment regimens in IgG4-RD are limited.

MMF, an immunomodulatory agent with antifibrotic effects, can be used for the treatment of IgG4-RD because of its ability to inhibit the transforming growth factor beta pathway (11). CYC is a bifunctional nonspecific cell cycle alkylating agent used for treating tumors, a variety of autoimmune diseases, and IgG4-RD. Our previous studies showed that GCs plus low-dose CYC or MMF can effectively reduce the relapse rate of IgG4-RD (4, 8, 9), but we could not identify which one was more effective in treating IgG4-RD and preventing clinical relapse. Therefore, in this study, we aimed to compare the efficacy of two regimens (GCs plus low-dose CYC or MMF) by retrospectively assessing the response rate, relapse rate, and side effects in eligible IgG4-RD patients who were treated with either of them.

METHODS

This prospective observational cohort study to investigate the disease course and treatment response of IgG4-RD patients was registered on ClinicalTrials.gov (ID: NCT01670695). From January 2012 to July 2018, consecutive patients treated with GCs plus CYC or MMF were retrospectively identified for this study. The study protocol was approved by the ethics board of Peking Union Medical College Hospital, and all study subjects provided written informed consent for study participation.

Inclusion and Exclusion Criteria

The inclusion criteria were as follows:

(1) 18 to 75 years of age.
(2) Agreement with the 2011 comprehensive diagnostic criteria for definite, probable, or possible IgG4-RD as follows: (1) characteristic diffuse/localized swelling, sclerosis, or inflammation affecting single or multiple organs; (2) elevated serum IgG4 concentrations (135 mg/dL); (3) increased number of lymphocytes, infiltrated IgG4+ plasma cells (IgG4+ cells/IgG-positive cells >40% and >10 IgG4+ plasma), and fibrosis. Patients who met criteria (1), (2), and (3) were diagnosed with definite IgG4-RD; those who met (1) and (3) were diagnosed with probable IgG4-RD; and those who met (1) and (2) were diagnosed with possible IgG4-RD (12).
(3) Presence of internal organ involvement.
(4) Use of GC and CYC or MMF for initial treatment and maintenance until the 12-month follow-up.
(5) Regularly followed up at months 1, 3, 6, and 12.

The exclusion criteria were as follows:

(1) Presenting only with IgG4-related dacryoadenitis and sialadenitis or lymphadenopathy of IgG4-RD.
(2) Serious infection.
(3) Presence of other rheumatic diseases.
(4) Presence of malignant diseases.
(5) Women with childbearing potential or currently planning a pregnancy.

Laboratory Tests, Imaging Studies, and Histological Examination

All patients underwent laboratory tests for complete blood count, erythrocyte sedimentation rate (ESR), hypersensitivity C-reactive protein (hs-CRP) levels, serum immunoglobulin, and IgG subclass concentrations, urinalysis, liver, and renal function tests; and at least one imaging examination, including ultrasonography, digital radiography (DR), computed tomography (CT), magnetic resonance imaging (MRI), or positron emission tomography/computed tomography (PET-CT). In total, 78 patients (72.22%) underwent CT scan, 24 (22.22%) underwent PET scan, 33 (30.56%) underwent MRI, and 49 (45.37%) underwent other imaging examinations, including ultrasound and DR. When necessary, tissue biopsies were analyzed and reviewed by pathologists using previously described methods (12), and laboratory tests and imaging studies were performed during the follow-up period.

TABLE 1 | Baseline characteristics before and after matching on the propensity score.

Variables	Before matching		*p*-value	After matching		*p*-value
	Group I (*N* = 90)	Group II (*N* = 65)		Group I (*N* = 54)	Group II (*N* = 54)	
Male, *N* (%)	68 (75.56%)	42 (64.62%)	0.14	37 (68.52%)	37 (68.52%)	1.00
Age at onset (years)	57.50 (52.00–63.75)	55.00 (48.00–62.00)	0.11	56.50 (9.94)	53.96 (12.22)	0.24
Allergy, *N* (%)	43 (47.78%)	34 (52.31%)	0.58	23 (42.59%)	29 (53.70%)	0.25
Biopsy, *N* (%)	46 (51.11%)	36 (55.38%)	0.60	31 (57.41%)	30 (55.56%)	0.44
Imaging examination						
CT scan	61 (67.78%)	48 (73.85%)	0.41	36 (66.67%)	42 (77.78%)	0.20
MRI	23 (25.56%)	18 (27.69%)	0.77	12 (22.22%)	12 (22.22%)	1.00
PET	28 (31.11%)	15 (23.08%)	0.27	19 (35.19%)	14 (25.93%)	0.30
Others	19 (21.11%)	18 (27.59%)	0.34	11 (20.37%)	14 (25.93%)	0.49
Definite IgG4-RD, *N* (%)	35 (38.89%)	30 (46.15%)	0.37	24 (44.44%)	25 (46.30%)	0.85
Probable IgG4-RD, *N* (%)	8 (8.89%)	4 (6.15%)	0.76	5 (9.26%)	3 (5.55%)	0.72
Possible IgG4-RD, *N* (%)	47 (52.22%)	31 (47.70%)	0.58	25 (46.30%)	26 (48.15)	0.85
Number of organs	4 (2–6)	4 (3–5.5)	0.13	4.00(2.75–6.00)	4.5 (3.00–6.00)	0.23
Multiorgan disease (≥3 organs), *N* (%)	46 (51.11%)	42 (64.62%)	0.09	30 (55.56%)	37 (68.52%)	0.17
Disease duration (months)	8.50 (3.00–36.00)	12.00 (5.00–36.00)	0.15	6.50 (3.00–24.00)	12.00 (2.00–36.00)	0.23
Organ involvements, *N* (%)						
Meninges	3 (3.33%)	0	0.27	0	0	–
Pituitary glands	3 (3.33%)	2 (3.08%)	1.00	1 (1.85%)	1 (1.85%)	1.00
Orbital lesion	6 (6.67%)	4 (6.15%)	0.90	4 (7.41%)	4 (7.41%)	1.00
Lacrimal glands	32 (35.56%)	25 (38.56%)	0.71	18 (33.33%)	22 (40.74%)	0.43
Parotid glands	20 (22.22%)	10 (15.38%)	0.29	10 (18.52%)	9 (16.67%)	0.80
Submandibular glands	37 (41.11%)	32 (49.23%)	0.32	24 (44.44%)	28 (51.85%)	0.44
Nasal cavity lesions and sinusitis	18 (20.00%)	23 (35.38%)	<0.05	12 (22.22%)	21 (38.89%)	0.06
Thyroid	3 (3.33%)	2 (3.08%)	1.00	2 (3.70%)	1 (1.85%)	1.00
Lung	32 (35.56%)	24 (36.92%)	0.86	22 (40.74%)	22 (40.74%)	1.00
Lymph nodes	34 (37.78%)	30 (46.15%)	0.30	23 (42.59%)	28 (51.85%)	0.34
Aorta and large blood vessels	18 (20.00%)	7 (10.77%)	0.12	10 (18.52%)	7 (12.96%)	0.43
Heart/pericardium	2 (2.22%)	2 (3.08%)	1.00	1 (1.85%)	2 (3.70%)	1.00
Retroperitoneal fibrosis	36 (40.00%)	13 (20.00%)	0.08	16 (29.63%)	13 (24.07%)	0.52
Sclerosing mediastinitis	10 (11.11%)	6 (9.23%)	0.70	7 (12.96%)	6 (11.11%)	0.77
Sclerosing mesenteritis	0	1(1.54%)	0.42	3 (5.56%)	2 (3.70%)	1.00
Pancreas	30 (33.33%)	42 (64.62%)	<0.01	27 (50.00%)	32 (59.26%)	0.33
Liver	3 (3.33%)	2 (3.08%)	1.00	2 (3.70%)	1 (1.85%)	1.00
Bile ducts	17 (18.89%)	23 (35.38%)	<0.05	16 (29.63%)	18 (33.33%)	0.68
Skin	5 (5.56%)	2 (3.08%)	0.70	4 (7.41%)	2 (3.70%)	0.68
Kidney	13 (13.33%)	7 (10.77%)	0.50	9 (16.67%)	7 (12.96%)	0.59
Prostate	17 (18.89%)	9 (13.85%)	0.41	8 (14.81%)	9 (16.67%)	0.79
Constitutional symptoms not attributable to involvement of a particular organ[a]	10 (11.11%)	4 (6.15%)	0.29	4 (7.41%)	4 (7.41%)	1.00
Other involvement: specify[b]	24 (26.67%)	18 (27.69%)	0.89	17 (31.48%)	11 (20.37%)	0.19
Serological						
Eosinophils (10^9/L)	2.60 (0.70–5.80)	2.50 (0.70–5.20)	0.69	3.2 (1.60–5.60)	2.45 (0.53–5.83)	0.23
C-reactive protein (mg/L)	3.51 (0.81–9.43)	3.53 (1.26–11.26)	0.66	4.40 (1.73–13.88)	2.48 (0.79–8.25)	0.13

(Continued)

TABLE 1 | Continued

Variables	Before matching		*p*-value	After matching		*p*-value
	Group I (*N* = 90)	Group II (*N* = 65)		Group I (*N* = 54)	Group II (*N* = 54)	
Erythrocyte sedimentation rate (mm/h)	32.50 (9.75–61.25)	23.00 (11.75–67.25)	0.73	32.00 (13.00–65.00)	24.50 (8.25–60.50)	0.43
IgE (KU/L)	180.00 (97.23–780.00)	263.00 (78.73–631.75)	0.18	327.00 (97.23–780.00)	206.00 (102.00–644.50)	0.57
IgG4 (mg/L)	5610.00 (2252.50–19,125.00)	11,000.00 (4190.00–19,300.00)	0.12	11,000 (4183.50–20,550.00)	7510 (2925.00–20,950.00)	0.59
IgG4-RD RI	11.63 ± 6.16	11.72 ± 5.06	0.70	12.28 ± 5.87	12.50 ± 4.90	0.65
Initial GC dose (mg/day)	42.69 ± 10.32	41.16 ± 8.37	0.18	41.13 ± 8.09	41.33 ± 10.89	0.54

[a] *Weight loss, fever, and fatigue caused by active IgG4-RD.*
[b] *Prostate, breast, gallbladder involvement, and others.*

Data Collection

Clinical features, laboratory results, imaging data, adverse events, and details of treatment protocol and disease relapse were evaluated at baseline and at 1, 3, 6, and 12 months after treatment or until relapse.

Assessment of Disease Activity and Definition of Clinical Response and Relapse

Disease activity per visit was assessed by the IgG4-RD responder index (RI), with a system score of 0–4 for each site/organ system (13). An IgG4-RD RI score ≥3 was used to identify patients with active disease (14).

Three categories of clinical response were defined: (1) complete response (CR), in which IgG4-RD RI <3 and declined ≥2 points after treatment; (2) partial response (PR), in which IgG4-RD RI declined ≥2 points after treatment but still remained ≥3, and if IgG4-RD RI was 3 at initial treatment a partial response was defined as a 1-point decline after treatment; and (3) no change (NC), in which there was no significant improvement in affected organs and clinical symptoms and change of IgG4-RD RI <2 points (8, 9, 15).

Relapse was defined as the recurrence of worsened/new disease manifestations or abnormality of organ-specific imaging findings despite treatment, with or without elevated serum IgG4 (8).

Statistical Analysis

Continuous variables are presented as mean ± standard deviation (SD), median, or interquartile range (IQR), and compared by *t*-test, whereas categorical variables were compared by the chi-square test, Fisher Exact test, or Mann–Whitney test. The Kaplan–Meier curves and log-rank test were used to calculate the cumulative relapse rate. Statistical analyses were performed using IBM SPSS statistics (Version 22.0, IBM, Armonk, NY, USA).

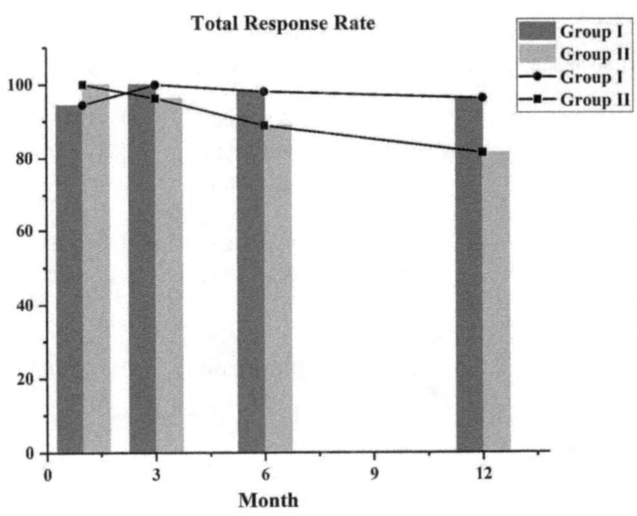

FIGURE 1 | The total response rates of two groups at 1, 3, 6, and 12 months.

RESULTS

Demographic and Baseline Features

From January 2012 to July 2018, 155 IgG4-RD patients who conformed to the inclusion criteria were selected. Among them, 90 were treated with GCs plus CYC (group I) and 65 were treated with GCs plus MMF (group II). Compared to group I, patients in group II had more paranasal sinus (35.38 vs. 20.00%, $p < 0.05$), pancreas (64.62 vs. 33.33%, $p < 0.01$), and bile duct (35.38 vs. 18.89%, $p < 0.05$) involvement.

To minimize the influence of confounders on the results of the study, we used 1:1 propensity score-matched (PSM) analysis to match group I patients with group II patients based on gender, age, involvement organs (meninges, pituitary gland, lacrimal glands, parotid glands, submandibular glands, nasal cavity lesions, thyroid, lungs, lymph nodes, aorta/large blood vessels, heart/pericardium, retroperitoneal fibrosis, sclerosing mediastinitis, sclerosing mesenteritis, pancreas, liver, bile ducts, kidney, and skin), and other involvement and constitutional symptoms not attributable to the involvement of a particular organ (weight loss, fever, and fatigue caused by active IgG4-RD). At the end of the analysis, 108 patients were selected (54 in each group), of whom 49 were diagnosed with definite IgG4-RD (group I vs. group II, 24 vs. 25), 8 with probable IgG4-RD (group I vs. group II, 5 vs. 3), and 51 with possible IgG4-RD (group I vs. group II, 25 vs. 26). In the post-match model, the differences of baseline characteristic between group I and group II was not statistically significance. All patients were treated with prednisone, which was gradually tapered down according to the individual's clinical response. The analyses indicated that the initial prednisone dosages were similar between the two groups (41.13 vs. 41.33 mg/day, respectively; $p = 0.54$).

TABLE 2 | Response rates of group I and group II.

Period (months)	Status, *N* (%)	Group I (*N* = 54)	Group II (*N* = 54)
1	CR	5 (9.26%)	2 (3.70%)
	PR	46 (85.19%)	52 (96.30%)
	NC	3 (5.56%)	0
	Relapse	0	0
3	CR	10 (18.52%)	7 (12.96%)
	PR	44 (81.48%)	45 (83.33%)
	NC	0	0
	Relapse	0	2 (3.70%)
6	CR	18 (33.33%)	17 (31.48%)
	PR	35 (64.82%)	33 (61.11%)
	NC	0	0
	Relapse	1 (1.85%)	4 (7.41%)
12	CR	30 (55.56%)	27 (50.00%)
	PR	23 (42.59%)	25 (46.30%)
	NC	0	0
	Relapse	1 (1.85%)	2 (3.70%)

CR, complete response; NC, no change; PR, partial response.

In group I, patients received CYC at a mean initial dose of 54.75 mg/day (oral, 50–100 mg/day). They maintained the initial dose for 3 months, after which it was reduced to 50 mg per day or every other day, consistent with previous treatment regimens (9). The mean cumulative dose of CYC over 12 months was 11.30 g. Patients in group II received MMF at a mean initial dose of 1,060 mg/day (1000–1500 mg/day), which was maintained for 6 months and decreased to 500–1000 mg/day for 6 months, consistent with previous reports (8, 16, 17). The baseline characteristics of the two groups before and after matching are summarized in **Table 1**.

Treatment Response

After using the PSM approach to control covariates, we compared the response rates of the two groups. The total response rates of the patients in the two groups are shown in **Figure 1**, and the majority of the patients achieved CR or PR. In the first month follow-up period, in group I, 46 patients achieved PR, 5 attained CR, and 3 did not respond to treatment (NC), and in group II, 2 attained CR and 52 achieved PR. After follow-up at 3 months, the 3 NC patients in group I achieved PR. In the third month follow-up period, the majority of patients in group I (10 achieved CR and 44 achieved PR) and group II (7 achieved CR and 45 achieved PR) had a good response. At the 6- and 12-month follow-up, the total response rates in group I were higher than those in group II, but there was no statistical difference between the two groups (**Table 2**).

The IgG4-RD RI and GC dose at each follow-up period are shown in **Figures 2A,B**. They both decreased over time, especially during the first 6 months of treatment, after which they stabilized. At the last follow-up period, IgG4-RD RI significantly declined in both groups, and the mean (SD) IgG4-RD RI decreased to 2.39 (2.10) in group I and 2.89 (1.76) in group II, with a mean decline of 80.54 and 76.88% of baseline level, respectively. Also, the GCs dose was reduced from the initial 41.13 to 7.95 mg/day in group I, and from 41.33 to 9.18 mg/day in group II, with no significant difference between both groups.

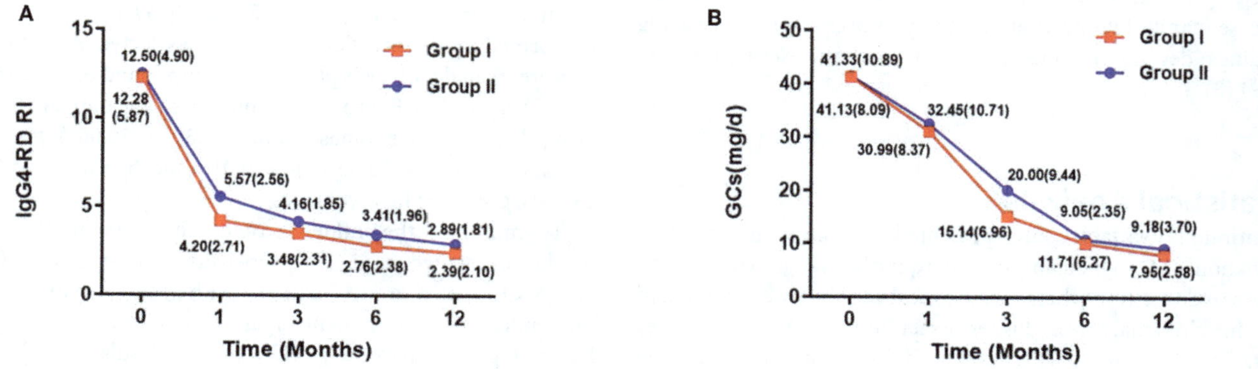

FIGURE 2 | IgG4-RD RI [mean (SD)] and GCs dose [mean (SD)] of two groups within follow-up time. **(A)** IgG4-RD RI evaluated during the follow-up period. **(B)** GC doses of each patient at baseline, and at 1, 3, 6, and 12 months. Doses of glucocorticoids are presented as means.

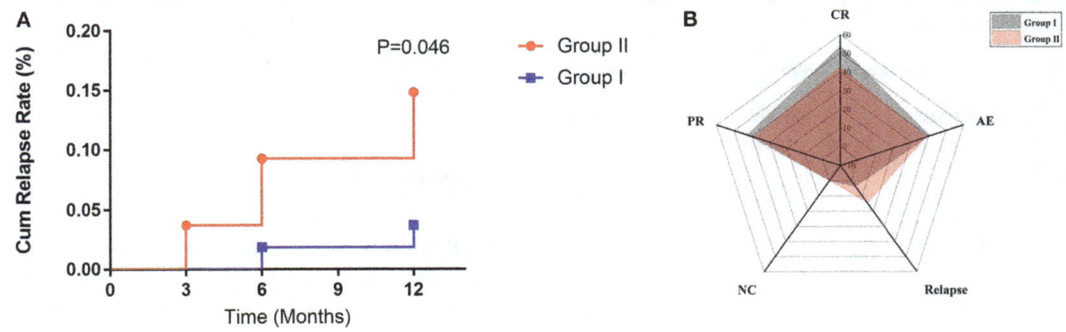

FIGURE 3 | (A) The relapse rate of two groups within follow-up time. **(B)** Radar map for evaluating the efficacy of two treatment regimens by response rate (CR, PR, and NC), relapse rate (RR), and adverse effect (AE).

TABLE 3 | Relapsed patients in Group I and Group II.

Patients	Group	Involvement organ	Relapsed organ	Time of relapse	Added treatment	Outcome
1	I	Aorta, retroperitoneal fibrosis, and pancreas	Pancreas	6	Increased GC dosage, changed CYC to MMF	PR
2	I	Submandibular glands, lymph nodes, retroperitoneal fibrosis, pancreas, and bile ducts	Lung	12	Increased GC dosage	PR
3	II	Aorta, retroperitoneal fibrosis, pancreas, and bile ducts	Skin and lung	3	GCs, MMF, and iguratimod	PR
4	II	Lacrimal glands, aorta, lymph nodes, lung, pancreas, and bile ducts	Lacrimal glands	3	Increased GC dosage, changed MMF to MTX	PR
5	II	Submandibular glands, lymph nodes, pancreas, lacrimal glands, and lung	Lacrimal glands	6	Increased GC and MMF dosage	PR
6	II	Submandibular glands, lymph nodes, pancreas, lacrimal glands, prostate, and lung	Lacrimal glands	6	Increased GC dosage and changed MMF to CYC	CR
7	II	Pancreas and bile ducts	Pancreas and bile ducts	6	Changed MMF to CYC	PR
8	II	Aorta, retroperitoneal fibrosis, and pancreas	Pancreas	6	Increased GC dosage	PR
9	II	Lacrimal gland, lung, and paranasal sinus	Lacrimal gland and paranasal sinus	12	Changed MMF to CYC	CR
10	II	Parotid glands and paranasal sinus	Paranasal sinus	12	Increased GC and MMF dosage	PR

CR, complete response; CYC, Cyclophosphamide; GC, glucocorticoid; MMF, Mycophenolate mofetil. MTX, methotrexate; PR, partial response.

Disease Relapse

In group I, 2 patients suffered relapse; one had a recurrence in the pancreas in the 6th month, which manifested as abdominal pain and the other had a worsened lung image on the 12th month with cough. In group II, 8 patients suffered relapse; 2 had recurrence on the skin, lung, and lacrimal glands at the 3rd month visit, 4 relapsed in the 6th month (lacrimal glands and pancreas), and 2 had recurrence in the 12th month (lacrimal glands and paranasal sinus). In group II, recurrence at the paranasal sinus, lacrimal glands, skin, lung, bile ducts, and pancreas accounted for 25, 50, 12.5, 12.5, 12.5, and 25%, respectively, with the lacrimal glands being the most vulnerable to recurrence. The cumulative recurrence rate in groups I and II was 3.7 and 14.8%, respectively, and group II had a higher relapse rate than group I ($p = 0.046$) (**Figure 3A**).

The follow-up data after retreatment in these 10 patients showed that they all achieved remission after the immunosuppressants were changes and/or the dose of GCs was increased according to their condition. In group I, for one patient, we increased the GCs dosage and replaced CYC with

TABLE 4 | Adverse events in response to glucocorticoid or immunosuppressant observed during treatment in two groups.

Adverse events	Number of patients		*p*-Value
	Group I	Group II	(*< 0.05)
Infection			
Upper respiratory tract infection	5	7	0.54
Pneumonia	0	2	0.50
Herpes zoster	2	1	1.00
Other	2	1	1.00
Glucose intolerance			
Newly diagnosed with diabetes mellitus	2	1	1.00
Aggravation of diabetes mellitus	2	3	1.00
Gastrointestinal reaction	6	5	0.75
Hematological system	1	0	1.00
Liver damage	1	0	1.00
Hemorrhagic cystitis	0	0	–
Other adverse reaction	0	0	–

MMF, whereas for the second patient, the GCs dosage was increased. Of the 8 relapsed patients in group II, the treatment was converted to GCs and CYC for 3, iguratimod was added for 1, GC dose was increased and MMF was replaced with MTX for 1, and previous regimens with increased dosages were maintained in 3 patients. The details of relapsed patients in group I and group II are shown in **Table 3**.

Adverse Effects

Table 4 shows the adverse effect (AEs) of therapy, with infections as the main adverse reaction caused by the two treatment regimens. In addition, a patient in group I developed persistent platelet reduction after treatment with GCs plus CYC, so CYC was replaced with MMF and the patient's platelet count was monitored. It was observed that the patient's platelet counts gradually returned to normal after CYC was replaced. Also, a 37-year-old female patient's treatment plan was changed to oral GCs plus MMF because she had amenorrhea and a gastrointestinal reaction after CYC treatment. For another patient in group I, CYC was replaced with MMF due to liver damage manifested as elevated transaminase after using CYC. In group II, MMF was discontinued in three patients or replaced with CYC due to recurrent infections. Other adverse reactions in group II were similar to those in group I, the majority of which were infections and gastrointestinal reactions. There was no significant difference in treatment-related side effects in the two groups.

Based on comprehensive assessment of disease response, relapse rate, and adverse reactions, it was suggested that GCs plus CYC had a better therapeutic effect than GCs plus MMF (**Figure 3B**).

DISCUSSION

Several immunosuppressants have been used as a steroid-sparing treatment for IgG4-RD, but there has been no head-to-head study comparing the efficacies between steroid-sparing drugs. In this retrospective cohort study, we aimed to explore the efficacies of GCs plus MMF therapy and GCs plus CTX and compare them in order to determine a better therapeutic strategy for IgG4-RD patients and prevent disease recurrence.

In this study, CYC and MMF were used because their efficacies in IgG4-RD had been proven in previous studies. In a recent study, CYC plus GCs yielded a lower relapse rate and higher response rate relative to GC monotherapy. Similar to the results of combined CYC regimens, a study from India showed clinical improvement in patients who were treated with GCs plus MMF, with no case of relapse within a median duration of 8 months. Furthermore, an RCT study from China reported that GCs plus MMF was more effective than GCs monotherapy.

In our study, IgG4-RD patients responded well to GCs plus CYC or MMF, and a majority of them experienced marked improvements within a month of treatment, which were manifested as improvement in the affected organs; reductions in the concentrations of serum ESR, CRP, IgG, and IgG4; as well as successful GC tapering. Both combined treatment regimens were efficient for IgG4-RD patients, having almost the same response rate during a year follow-up period. Comparing the ability of the two immunosuppressants to prevent flare by relapse rate, our results demonstrated that 10 patients (2 with CYC and 8 with MMF) relapsed, and relapse occurred earlier and more frequently in those receiving MMF than CYC (14.8 vs. 3.7%). Additionally, patients receiving CYC had less cumulative GCs than those receiving MMF, indicating that the steroid-sparing effect of CYC is superior to that of MMF. Therefore, the combined treatment with CYC decreased organ recurrence and maintained disease remission much better than combined treatment with MMF. Therefore, it was suggested that a low-dose CYC combination treatment regimen might be a better choice than low-dose MMF therapy in IgG4-RD patients with multiple organ involvement.

In a recent RCT study that enrolled IgG4-RD patients with multiple organ involvement, it was pointed out that lacrimal glands and paranasal sinus were most susceptible to recurrence in patients receiving low-dose MMF plus GCs (8). However, in a prospective cohort study of combined CYC treatment for IgG4-RD, it was observed that no patient experienced recurrence of superficial organs such as lacrimal glands and paranasal sinuses in the group receiving GCs plus CYC (9). In the present study, the relapse of patients in group II was more likely due to recurrence in the lacrimal glands (4/8, 50.00%) and paranasal sinus (2/8, 25.00%), and the other relapsed organs including the pancreas and lung were similar to those in group I. In accordance with the results obtained from this study, it is necessary to find other more efficient treatments for lacrimal glands and paranasal sinus involvement.

Regarding safety issues, since low doses of CYC and MMF were applied in this study, both drugs were well tolerated, and this is consistent with previous IgG4-RD studies. The main adverse reactions in the CYC or MMF groups were infections and gastrointestinal reactions, and they did not differ between both groups (**Table 4**). Previous studies observed that the incidence of severe infection significantly increased in the Asian population compared with those of other races when MMF at 3 g/day was used in the treatment of lupus nephritis (16, 17). Based on our clinical experience, patients over 60 years of age showed vulnerability to MMF of more than 1.5 g per day, with an increased risk of opportunistic infection, while most IgG4-RD patients are older than 60 years old. In the CYC group, two patients had drug-induced liver damage and persistent reduction in platelets, respectively, but the symptoms disappeared after CYC was discontinued. When CYC is used, it is applied only in patients with internal organ involvement. We carefully monitored short-term and long-term side effects of CYC, and strictly controlled the cumulative dose for every patient, although in our experience in treating systemic rheumatic diseases, such as systemic lupus erythematosus and systemic vasculitis, Chinese patients tolerate CYC much better than patients reported from Western countries.

So far, this is the first study to compare the effects of different immunosuppressive agents in IgG4-RD, although there are some limitations. Since the study is a retrospective cohort study, unknown variables might affect the results, leaving room for potential bias such as adverse effects that were as retrieved from the patients' hospital records. However, the results are quite reliable because there were no statistically significant differences in the baseline characteristics between the two groups.

In conclusion, most IgG4-RD patients had a good response to both treatment regimens, but GCs plus CYC had a lower rate of relapse within a year than GCs plus MMF. This suggests that GCs plus CYC might be a more effective treatment option for IgG4-RD patients with internal organ involvement. However, larger prospective and RCT studies are required to understand the role of CYC and MMF in IgG4-RD.

AUTHOR CONTRIBUTIONS

XL and YP designed the research, analyzed data, and wrote the manuscript. PZ, ZL, JL, and HL collected and analyzed data and revised the manuscript. XZh, FZ, and XZe optimized the research and proofread the paper. YF and WZ designed the study and wrote the manuscript. All authors contributed to the article and approved the submitted version.

REFERENCES

1. Umehara H, Okazaki K, Masaki Y, Kawano M, Yamamoto M, Saeki T, et al. A novel clinical entity, igG4-related disease (IgG4RD): general concept and details. *Modern Rheumatol.* (2012) 22:1–14. doi: 10.3109/s10165-011-0508-6
2. Sekiguchi H, Horie R, Kanai M, Suzuki R, Yi ES, Ryu JH. IgG4-Related disease: retrospective analysis of one hundred sixty-Six patients. *Arthr Rheumatol.* (2016) 68:2290–9. doi: 10.1002/art.39686
3. Khosroshahi A, Wallace ZS, Crowe JL, Akamizu T, Azumi A, Carruthers MN, et al. International consensus guidance statement on the management and treatment of igG4-Related disease. *Arthr Rheumatol.* (2015) 67:1688–99. doi: 10.1002/art.39132
4. Hart PA, Kamisawa T, Brugge WR, Chung JB, Culver EL, Czako L, et al. Long-term outcomes of autoimmune pancreatitis: a multicentre, international analysis. *Gut.* (2013) 62:1771–6. doi: 10.1136/gutjnl-2012-303617
5. Venetsanopoulou A, Tzioufas A. 58-year-old patient with IgG4-related thoracic aortitis. *Mediterr J Rheumatol.* (2016) 27:191–3. doi: 10.31138/mjr.27.4.191
6. Brito-Zeron P, Bosch X, Ramos-Casals M, Stone JH. IgG4-related disease: advances in the diagnosis and treatment. *Best Pract Res Clin Rheumatol.* (2016) 30:261–78. doi: 10.1016/j.berh.2016.07.003
7. Wang Y, Zhao Z, Gao D, Wang H, Liao S, Dong C, et al. Additive effect of leflunomide and glucocorticoids compared with glucocorticoids monotherapy in preventing relapse of igG4-related disease: a randomized clinical trial. *Sem Arthr Rheum.* (2020) doi: 10.1016/j.semarthrit.2020.01.010
8. Yunyun F, Yu P, Panpan Z, Xia Z, Linyi P, Jiaxin Z, et al. Efficacy and safety of low dose mycophenolate mofetil treatment for immunoglobulin g4-related disease: a randomized clinical trial. *Rheumatology.* (2018) 58:52–60. doi: 10.1093/rheumatology/key227
9. Yunyun F, Yu C, Panpan Z, Hua C, Di W, Lidan Z, et al. Efficacy of cyclophosphamide treatment for immunoglobulin g4-related disease with addition of glucocorticoids. *Sci Rep.* (2017) 7:6195. doi: 10.1038/s41598-017-06520-5
10. Wang L, Zhang P, Wang M, Feng R, Lai Y, Peng L, et al. Failure of remission induction by glucocorticoids alone or in combination with immunosuppressive agents in igG4-related disease: a prospective study of 215 patients. *Arthr Res Ther.* (2018) 20:65. doi: 10.1186/s13075-018-1567-2
11. Roos N, Poulalhon N, Farge D, Madelaine I, Mauviel A, Verrecchia F. *In vitro* evidence for a direct antifibrotic role of the immunosuppressive drug mycophenolate mofetil. *J Pharmacol Exp Ther.* (2007) 321:583–9. doi: 10.1124/jpet.106.117051
12. Umehara H, Okazaki K, Masaki Y, Kawano M, Yamamoto M, Saeki T, et al. Comprehensive diagnostic criteria for igG4-related disease (IgG4-RD), 2011. *Moder Rheumatol.* (2012) 22:21–30. doi: 10.3109/s10165-011-0571-z
13. Carruthers MN, Topazian MD, Khosroshahi A, Witzig TE, Wallace ZS, Hart PA, et al. Rituximab for igG4-related disease: a prospective, open-label trial. *Ann Rheum Dis.* (2015) 74:1171–7. doi: 10.1136/annrheumdis-2014-206605
14. Wallace ZS, Mattoo H, Carruthers M, Mahajan VS, Della Torre E, Lee H, et al. Plasmablasts as a biomarker for igG4-related disease, independent of serum igG4 concentrations. *Ann Rheum Dis.* (2015) 74:190–5. doi: 10.1136/annrheumdis-2014-205233

15. Campochiaro C, Ramirez GA, Bozzolo EP, Lanzillotta M, Berti A, Baldissera E, et al. IgG4-related disease in italy: clinical features and outcomes of a large cohort of patients. *Scand J Rheum.* (2016) 45:135–45. doi: 10.3109/03009742.2015.1055796
16. An Y, Zhou Y, Bi L, Liu B, Wang H, Lin J, et al. Combined immunosuppressive treatment (CIST) in lupus nephritis: a multicenter, randomized controlled study. *Clin Rheumatol.* (2019) 38:1047–54. doi: 10.1007/s10067-018-4368-8
17. Appel GB, Contreras G, Dooley MA, Ginzler EM, Isenberg D, Jayne D, et al. Mycophenolate mofetil versus cyclophosphamide for induction treatment of lupus nephritis. *J Am Soc Nephrol.* (2009) 20:1103–12. doi: 10.1681/ASN.2008101028

3

Power Doppler Ultrasound Assessment of A1 Pulley: A New Target of Inflammation in Psoriatic Arthritis?

Gianluca Smerilli[1*†], *Edoardo Cipolletta*[1†], *Marco Di Carlo*[1†], *Andrea Di Matteo*[1,2†], *Walter Grassi*[1] *and Emilio Filippucci*[1†]

[1] *Rheumatology Unit, Department of Clinical and Molecular Sciences, Polytechnic University of Marche, "Carlo Urbani" Hospital, Jesi, Ancona, Italy,* [2] *Leeds Institute of Rheumatic and Musculoskeletal Medicine, University of Leeds, Leeds, United Kingdom*

Correspondence:
Gianluca Smerilli
smerilli.gianluca@gmail.com

†*ORCID:*
Gianluca Smerilli
orcid.org/0000-0002-3972-4458
Edoardo Cipolletta
orcid.org/0000-0002-6881-8197
Marco Di Carlo
orcid.org/0000-0002-0906-4647
Andrea Di Matteo
orcid.org/0000-0003-0867-7051
Emilio Filippucci
orcid.org/0000-0002-7251-7784

Objective: To determine the prevalence of grey scale and power Doppler (PD) ultrasound (US) features of A1 pulley inflammation in a cohort of psoriatic arthritis (PsA) patients compared with rheumatoid arthritis (RA) patients.

Methods: Sixty patients (30 with PsA and 30 with RA) were consecutively enrolled. The main clinimetric indexes were recorded, and US assessment of A1 pulleys from second to fifth fingers bilaterally was carried out. The presence of A1 pulley inflammation, defined as PD signal within a thickened pulley, was registered.

Results: A1 pulley inflammation was found in 15 of 240 fingers (6.3%) of eight PsA patients (26.7%) and in one of 240 fingers (0.4%) of one RA patient (3.3%) ($p < 0.01$ and $p = 0.03$, respectively). Seven of eight PsA patients (88%) with at least one inflamed A1 pulley had a moderate/high disease activity score. The regression linear analysis ($R^2 = 0.36$, adjusted $R^2 = 0.31$) showed that A1 pulley inflammation was correlated with Disease Activity Index for Psoriatic Arthritis (DAPSA) ($\beta = 0.43$, $p = 0.03$).

Conclusion: US A1 pulley inflammation appears to be relatively common at patient level in PsA, seems to be a characteristic feature of PsA compared to RA, and correlates with DAPSA.

Keywords: ultrasonography, psoriatic arthritis, rheumatoid arthritis, diagnostic imaging, annular pulley

INTRODUCTION

Finger flexor tendons and their surrounding synovial sheaths are located in osteofibrous channels, which are composed by the palmar aspect of the phalanges and metacarpal heads and by the digital fibrous tendon sheaths made by the digital pulleys (1). These structures are divided into annular pulleys (A1–A5) and cruciform pulleys, and their main function is to stabilize the tendons during finger flexion (1).

While feasibility of high-frequency ultrasound (US) assessment of annular pulleys has been well documented (2, 3), cruciform pulleys are not easily depictable with US because of their small size (3).

A1 pulley thickening has been recognized having a key role in the pathogenesis of "trigger finger," and US has proven to be useful in depicting this morphostructural abnormality (4).

In 2015, a magnetic resonance imaging (MRI) study turned the attention to the annular pulleys, demonstrating that these are common targets of inflammation in psoriatic arthritis (PsA) patients with dactylitis (5). Since then, two US studies evaluated the thickness of annular pulleys in chronic arthropathies, and both concluded that this is increased in PsA patients compared to rheumatoid arthritis (RA) patients and healthy subjects (6, 7). A possible link between A1 pulley thickening and dactylitis through a "deep Koebner" phenomenon was hypothesized because of the correlation between this finding and previous dactylitis (7). In a case report, inflammatory involvement of annular pulleys was depicted by US in a PsA patient (8), and power Doppler (PD) enhancement of annular pulleys was found in active psoriatic dactylitis (9). Moreover, in a very recent article, MRI signs of inflammatory involvement of annular pulleys were more often encountered in a small cohort of PsA patients compared to RA patients and healthy controls (10).

Thus, we believe that PD US potential in the assessment of A1 pulley involvement in PsA has not been adequately investigated yet.

The main aim of the present study was to determine the prevalence of PD US findings indicative of A1 pulley inflammation in PsA patients and in controls with RA.

MATERIALS AND METHODS

Patients

Consecutive patients with PsA according to the Classification Criteria for Psoriatic Arthritis criteria (11) and controls with RA fulfilling the American College of Rheumatology/European League Against Rheumatism (ACR/EULAR) criteria (12) were enrolled at the Rheumatology Unit of "Carlo Urbani" Hospital, in Jesi (Ancona, Italy). Patients younger than 18 years were excluded.

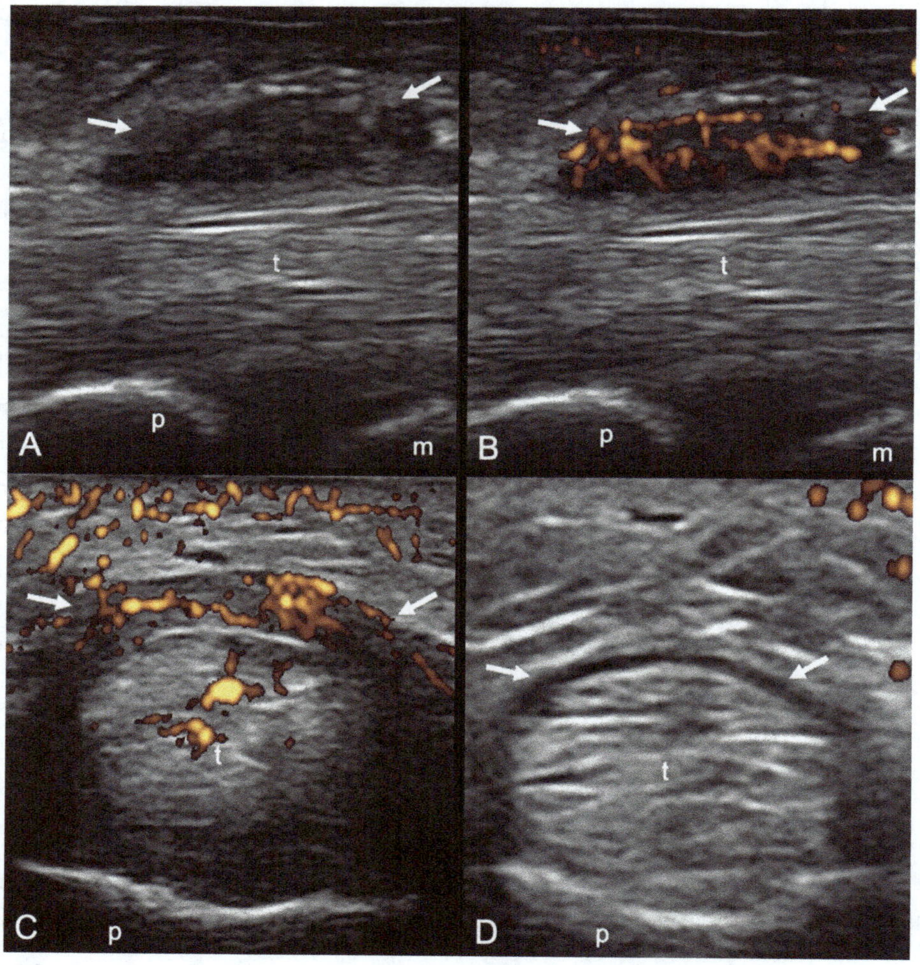

FIGURE 1 | Psoriatic arthritis. Longitudinal **(A,B)** and transverse **(C,D)** scans of the annular pulley A1 using a 22-MHz probe. In **(A,B)** a markedly thickened and inflamed A1 pulley (arrows) is depicted without and with power Doppler mode, respectively. In **(C,D)** a right–left comparison of the A1 pulley (arrows) of the third finger of another patient is illustrated. Note the thickening of the inflamed pulley and the presence of power Doppler within it in **(C)** compared to **(D)**. In **(C)** concomitant intratendinous power Doppler signal can be appreciated. m, metacarpal head; p, proximal phalanx; t, finger flexor tendons.

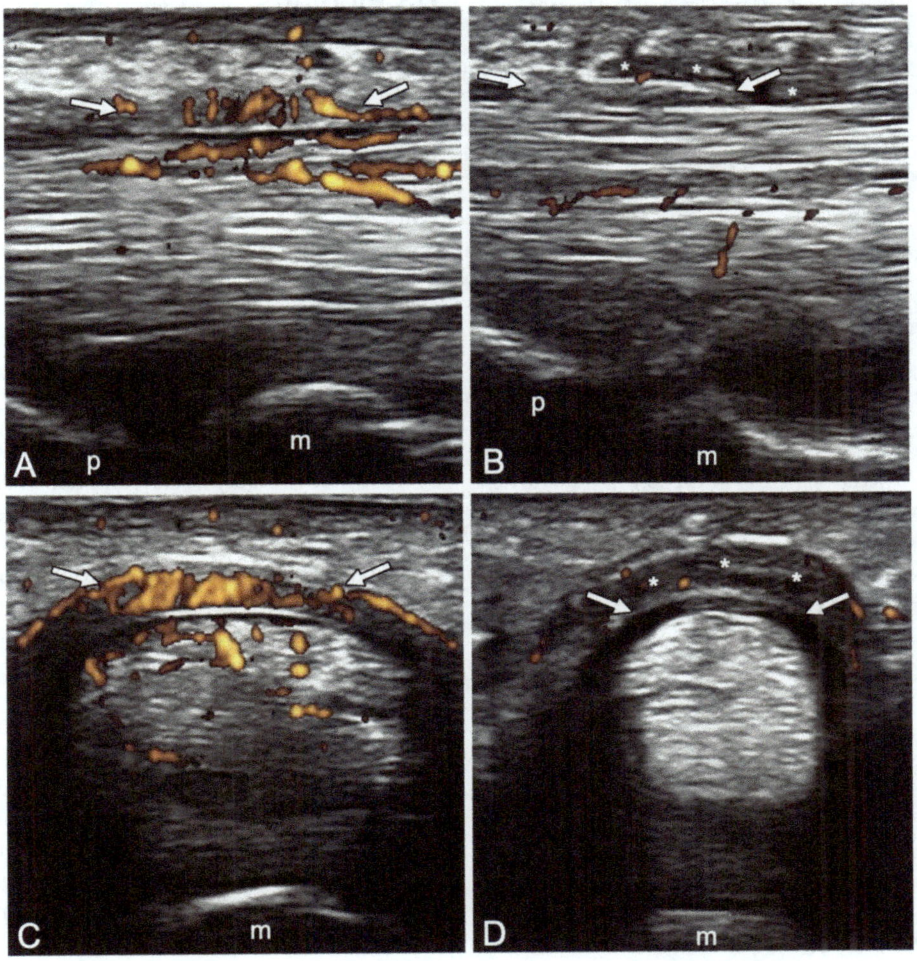

FIGURE 2 | Longitudinal **(A,B)** and transverse **(C,D)** scans of the annular pulley A1 using a 22-MHz probe in psoriatic arthritis **(A,C)** and rheumatoid arthritis **(B,D)** patients. In **(A,C)**, A1 pulley (arrows) inflammation is depicted (power Doppler signal inside a thickened pulley). Power Doppler signal is also noticeable within the superficial flexor tendon in the portion closest to the pulley. In **(B,D)**, A1 pulley (arrows) is not inflamed. The presence of synovial proliferation in the tendon sheath spilling over the normal pulley is shown (asterisks), representing a potential diagnostic pitfall. m, metacarpal head; p, proximal phalanx.

The study was conducted in accordance with the Helsinki Declaration and was approved by the local ethics committee. All patients signed informed consent.

Clinical Examination

A rheumatologist (E.C.) recorded for each patient the presence of "trigger finger", current or previous dactylitis (second to fifth fingers bilaterally), and tenderness in the A1 pulley region (second to fifth fingers bilaterally). The main clinimetric indexes (Disease Activity Index for PSoriatic Arthritis [DAPSA] in PsA patients and 28-joint Disease Activity Score [DAS28-C reactive protein (CRP)] in RA patients) were calculated.

Disease activity was interpreted according to the following cutoff values: DAPSA >28 and DAS28 >5.1 correspond to high disease activity, 28 ≥ DAPSA > 14 and 5.1 ≥ DAS28 ≥ 3.2 to moderate disease activity, 14 ≥ DAPSA > 4 and 3.2 > DAS28 ≥ 2.6 to low disease activity, and DAPSA ≤4 and DAS28 <2.6 to a remission status.

US Assessment

On the same day, another rheumatologist (G.S.) blinded to clinical data performed all the US examinations using a MyLabClassC (Esaote, Genova, Italy) equipped with a 10- to 22-MHz linear transducer. Patients were asked not to talk about their clinical condition with the sonographer.

A1 pulley from second to fifth fingers were assessed bilaterally adopting longitudinal and transverse scans as indicated by the 2017 EULAR standardized procedures for US imaging in rheumatology (13). The following pathological US findings were recorded: inflammation of the pulley (defined as the presence of PD signal within a thickened pulley) and tenosynovitis of the digital flexor tendons at finger level according to OMERACT definition (14). Thickening of the pulley was defined comparing the assessed structure with the adjacent and contralateral fingers (2). Particular attention was paid to the correct distinction between inflammatory involvement of the A1 pulley and tenosynovitis of flexor tendons (**Figures 1**, **2**). A thorough US examination with dynamic

TABLE 1 | Demographic and clinical characteristics of PsA and RA patients.

	PsA ($n = 30$)	RA ($n = 30$)
Age, mean ± SD (years)	58.6 ± 10.8	58.5 ± 13.6
Female/male	14/16	23/7
BMI, mean ± SD (kg/m^2)	25.9 ± 2.9	25.0 ± 5.4
R/L dominant hand	27/3	30/0
Trigger fingers (%)	2 (6.7)	2 (6.7)
Previous hand dactylitis (%)	8 (26.6)	0 (0)
Current hand dactylitis (%)	1 (3.3)	0 (0)
WORKING CONDITION		
Blue collar workers (%)	16 (53.3)	7 (23.3)
White collar workers (%)	5 (16.7)	5 (16.7)
Retired/unoccupied (%)	9 (30.0)	18 (60.0)
DISEASE ACTIVITY		
Disease duration, mean ± SD (years)	7.5 ± 10.1	6.0 ± 7.3
Disease activity (DAPSA/DAS28), mean ± SD	14.2 ± 11.2	3.4 ± 1.3
Remission/low disease activity	16 (53.3)	16 (53.3)
Moderate/high disease activity	14 (46.7)	14 (46.7)
TREATMENT		
cDMARDs (%)	13 (43.3)	17 (56.7)
bDMARDs (%)	17 (56.7)	8 (26.7)
Steroid (%)	2 (6.7)	13 (43.3)

bDMARDs, biologic disease-modifying antirheumatic drugs; BMI, body mass index; cDMARDs, conventional disease-modifying antirheumatic drugs; DAPSA, Disease Activity in PSoriatic Arthritis score; DAS28, Disease Activity Score in 28 joints for rheumatoid arthritis; L, left; PsA, psoriatic arthritis; R, right; RA, rheumatoid arthritis; SD, standard deviation.

assessment during passive finger flexion and extension was conducted to distinguish the pulley, which stays still, from the tendons and the tenosynovial proliferation, which move with the finger.

Statistical Analysis

The association between the sonographic findings and clinical–demographic data was tested using Cramer's *V* (*V*), point-biserial correlation (Rpb), and Spearman correlation coefficient (*R*). Stepwise linear regression analysis was performed to define predictive values of A1 pulley inflammation. DAPSA was used as the dependent variable, whereas independent variables were the presence of pulley inflammation and the presence of tenosynovitis. Statistical analysis was performed using SPSS (Chicago, IL, USA).

RESULTS

Sixty patients were enrolled in this cross-sectional and monocentric study: 30 with PsA and 30 with RA. **Table 1** reports the demographic and clinical characteristics of PsA and RA patients.

Tenderness of the volar side of the metacarpophalangeal joint was reported in 28 fingers (11.7%) of 13 PsA patients (43.3%) and in 13 fingers (4.6%) of six RA patients (20.0%).

US Findings

Inflammation of A1 pulley was found in 15 of 240 fingers (6.3%) of eight PsA patients (26.7%) and in one of 240 fingers (0.4%) of one RA patient (3.3%) ($p < 0.01$ and $p = 0.03$, respectively). Inflammation of A1 pulley in the absence of tenosynovitis was reported in six A1 pulleys (2.5%) of six PsA patients (20.0%).

No significant difference was reported regarding the prevalence of flexor finger flexor tendons between PsA [22 fingers (9.2%) in 10 PsA patients (33.3%)] and RA patients [21 fingers (8.8%) in six RA patients (20.0%)] ($p = 1.0$ and $p = 0.24$, respectively).

Correlation Between Demographic, Clinical, and Sonographic Data

Both pulley inflammation and tenosynovitis were correlated with DAPSA (Rpb = 0.56, $p < 0.01$, and Rpb = 0.48, $p < 0.01$). In fact, seven of eight PsA patients (88%) with at least one inflamed A1 pulley had a moderate/high disease activity score.

The regression linear analysis ($R^2 = 0.36$, adjusted $R^2 = 0.31$) showed that A1 pulley inflammation was predictive of higher DAPSA scores ($\beta = 0.43$, $p = 0.03$), whereas tenosynovitis did not reach statistical significance ($\beta = 0.25$, $p = 0.18$).

Both A1 pulley inflammation and flexor tendons tenosynovitis were associated with tenderness ($V = 0.55$, $p < 0.01$, and $V = 0.38$, $p < 0.01$).

No significant association was reported between A1 pulley inflammation and past or current episodes of dactylitis ($p = 0.09$). However, the only current dactylitis assessed showed A1 pulley inflammation. No significant correlations were found between A1 pulley inflammation and other demographic variables.

No significant association was found between the presence of at least one inflamed A1 pulley and working condition ($p = 0.84$).

DISCUSSION

The identification of the pathophysiological processes underlying the inflammatory involvement of periarticular structures during PsA is still a fascinating area of research, and US is capable of providing a clear depiction of finger pathology in PsA (15–19).

Annular pulleys are functional entheses, being subjected to very high shear stress provoked by continuous friction with adjacent tendons (7). The repetitive microtrauma makes them an ideal target for PsA inflammation, which can often be triggered mechanically. On the other hand, RA has a predilection for synovial structures; thus, we hypothesized that A1 pulley could be relatively spared.

To the best of our knowledge, this is the first study that compared PD US findings indicative of inflammation at A1 pulley level in PsA and RA patients. As expected, inflammation of A1 pulley was relatively common in PsA patients, whereas it was found in only one of 240 RA fingers examined. Moreover, the only inflamed A1 pulley in RA was found in a clinically diagnosed trigger finger and may therefore not be a RA manifestation in that patient. Indeed, an increased PD signal within the pulley has been described in trigger finger (4). However, according to our preliminary data, A1 pulley inflammation is only rarely associated with trigger finger symptoms in PsA [one of 15 (6.6%)].

This finding, in our PsA cohort, was correlated with a higher disease activity (DAPSA), and this is an interesting aspect to be explored in future research.

The link between pulleys involvement and psoriatic dactylitis is currently a topic of growing interest. In fact, pulleys are thicker in fingers previously affected by dactylitis, and recently PD signal within pulleys has been found to be common in dactylitic fingers, with a prevalence reaching 51% for A1 pulley (7, 9). The absence of a clear correlation in our cohort between A1 pulley inflammation and previous dactylitis raises an interesting question about the chronological relationship of pulley inflammation with dactylitis, and a prospective study may shed light on this possibly crucial pathogenetic moment.

The main limitations of our study were the small number of patients assessed and the fact that we only assessed A1 pulley. Another limitation of our study was that the two groups were not matched for working condition. However, no significant association was found between the presence of A1 pulley inflammation and working condition at patient level, and five of nine patients (55.5%) with at least one A1 pulley inflamed were not blue collar workers.

One of the limitations acknowledged by the authors in a recent article (9) was that the presence digital flexor tendons tenosynovitis could be misinterpreted as pulley inflammation. However, high-frequency US probes allow an excellent anatomical resolution of small structures such as A1 pulley, and a detailed and dynamic US examination with longitudinal and transverse scans allows distinguishing tenosynovitis from inflammation of the pulley with great accuracy, avoiding this potential pitfall.

To summarize, in the present pilot study, we found that A1 pulley inflammatory involvement is not uncommon in PsA at patient level, seems to be a characteristic feature of PsA compared to RA, and correlates with disease activity.

ETHICS STATEMENT

The studies involving human participants were reviewed and approved by CERM MARCHE. The patients/participants provided their written informed consent to participate in this study.

AUTHOR CONTRIBUTIONS

GS, EC, and EF substantially contributed to study conception and design, acquisition of data, and analysis and interpretation of data. MD substantially contributed to acquisition of data, and analysis and interpretation of data. WG and AD substantially contributed to study conception and design. All the authors revised the paper and approved the final version of the article to be published.

REFERENCES

1. Doyle JR. Anatomy of the finger flexor tendon sheath and pulley system. *J Hand Surg Am.* (1988) 13:473–84. doi: 10.1016/S0363-5023(88) 80082-0
2. Bianchi S, Martinoli C, de Gautard R, Gaignot C. Ultrasound of the digital flexor system: Normal and pathological findings. *J Ultrasound.* (2007) 10:85–92. doi: 10.1016/j.jus.2007.03.002
3. Boutry N, Titécat M, Demondion X, Glaude E, Fontaine C, Cotten A. High-frequency ultrasonographic examination of the finger pulley system. *J Ultrasound Med.* (2005) 24:1333–9. doi: 10.7863/jum.2005.24.10.1333
4. Guerini H, Pessis E, Theumann N, Le Quintrec JS, Campagna R, Chevrot A, et al. Sonographic appearance of trigger fingers. *J Ultrasound Med.* (2008) 27:1407–13. doi: 10.7863/jum.2008.27.10.1407
5. Tan AL, Fukuba E, Halliday NA, Tanner SF, Emery P, McGonagle D. High-resolution MRI assessment of dactylitis in psoriatic arthritis shows flexor tendon pulley and sheath-related enthesitis. *Ann Rheum Dis.* (2015) 74:185–9. doi: 10.1136/annrheumdis-2014-205839
6. Furlan A, Stramare R. The thickening of flexor tendons pulleys: a useful ultrasonographical sign in the diagnosis of psoriatic arthritis. *J Ultrasound.* (2018) 21:309–14. doi: 10.1007/s40477-018-0325-2
7. Tinazzi I, McGonagle D, Aydin SZ, Chessa D, Marchetta A, Macchioni P. "Deep Koebner" phenomenon of the flexor tendon-associated accessory pulleys as a novel factor in tenosynovitis and dactylitis in psoriatic arthritis. *Ann Rheum Dis.* (2018) 77:922–5. doi: 10.1136/annrheumdis-2017-212681
8. Zabotti A, Idolazzi L, Batticciotto A, De Lucia O, Scirè CA, Tinazzi I, et al. Enthesitis of the hands in psoriatic arthritis: an ultrasonographic perspective. *Med Ultrason.* (2017) 19:438–43. doi: 10.11152/mu-1172
9. Tinazzi I, McGonagle D, Macchioni P, Aydin SZ. Power Doppler enhancement of accessory pulleys confirming disease localization in psoriatic dactylitis. *Rheumatology (Oxford).* (2019). doi: 10.1093/rheumatology/kez549
10. Abrar DB, Schleich C, Nebelung S, Frenken M, Radke KL, Vordenbäumen S, et al. High-resolution MRI of flexor tendon pulleys using a 16-channel hand coil: disease detection and differentiation of psoriatic and rheumatoid arthritis. *Arthritis Res Ther.* (2020) 22:40. doi: 10.1186/s13075-020-2135-0
11. Taylor W, Gladman D, Helliwell P, Marchesoni A, Mease P, Mielants H. Classification criteria for psoriatic arthritis: development of new criteria from a large international study. *Arthritis Rheum.* (2006) 54:2665–73. doi: 10.1002/art.21972
12. Aletaha D, Neogi T, Silman AJ, Funovits J, Felson DT, Bingham CO 3rd, et al. Rheumatoid arthritis classification criteria: an American College of Rheumatology/European League against Rheumatism collaborative initiative. *Arthritis Rheum.* (2010) 62:2569–81. doi: 10.1136/ard.2010.138461
13. Möller I, Janta I, Backhaus M, Ohrndorf S, Bong DA, Martinoli C, et al. The 2017 EULAR standardised procedures for ultrasound imaging in rheumatology. *Ann Rheum Dis.* (2017) 76:1974–79.
14. Naredo E, D'Agostino MA, Wakefield RJ, Möller I, Balint PV, Filippucci E, et al. Reliability of a consensus-based ultrasound score for tenosynovitis in rheumatoid arthritis. *Ann Rheum Dis.* (2013) 72:1328–34. doi: 10.1136/annrheumdis-2012-202092
15. Tinazzi I, McGonagle D, Zabotti A, Chessa D, Marchetta A, Macchioni P. Comprehensive evaluation of finger flexor tendon

entheseal soft tissue and bone changes by ultrasound can differentiate psoriatic arthritis and rheumatoid arthritis. *Clin Exp Rheumatol.* (2018) 36:785–90.

16. Delle Sedie A, Riente L. Psoriatic arthritis: what ultrasound can provide us. *Clin Exp Rheumatol.* (2015) 33(5 Suppl 93):S60–5.
17. Ficjan A, Husic R, Gretler J, Lackner A, Graninger WB, Gutierrez M, et al. Ultrasound composite scores for the assessment of inflammatory and structural pathologies in Psoriatic Arthritis (PsASon-Score). *Arthritis Res Ther.* (2014) 16:476. doi: 10.1186/s13075-014-0476-2
18. Lackner A, Duftner C, Ficjan A, Gretler J, Hermann J, Husic R, et al. The association of clinical parameters and ultrasound verified inflammation with patients' and physicians' global assessments in psoriatic arthritis. *Semin Arthritis Rheum.* (2016) 46:183–9. doi: 10.1016/j.semarthrit.2016.05.010
19. Zabotti A, Mandl P, Zampogna G, Dejaco C, Iagnocco A. One year in review 2018: ultrasonography in rheumatoid arthritis and psoriatic arthritis. *Clin Exp Rheumatol.* (2018) 36:519–25. doi: 10.1136/annrheumdis-2017-211585

4

Chinese Herbal Formula Huayu-Qiangshen-Tongbi Decoction Compared With Leflunomide in Combination With Methotrexate in Patients With Active Rheumatoid Arthritis

Jiaqi Wu[1†], Xianghong Chen[1†], Yuan Lv[2], Kaixin Gao[2], Zehao Liu[3], Yue Zhao[1], Xiumin Chen[1,2,4], Xiaohong He[1], Yongliang Chu[1], Xiaodong Wu[1], Aihua Ou[1], Zehuai Wen[1], Jianyong Zhang[5], Jianhong Peng[6], Zhisheng Huang[7], Per-Johan Jakobsson[8], Qingchun Huang[1] and Runyue Huang[1,2,4*]*

[1] The Second Affiliated Hospital of Guangzhou University of Chinese Medicine (Guangdong Provincial Hospital of Chinese Medicine), Guangzhou, China, [2] Second Clinical Medical College, Guangzhou University of Chinese Medicine, Guangzhou, China, [3] Ruikang Hospital Affiliated to Guangxi University of Chinese Medicine, Guangxi, China, [4] Guangdong Provincial Key Laboratory of Clinical Research on Traditional Chinese Medicine Syndrome, and State Key Laboratory of Dampness Syndrome of Chinese Medicine, The Second Affiliated Hospital of Guangzhou University of Chinese Medicine, Guangzhou, China, [5] Shenzhen Hospital of Traditional Chinese Medicine, Shenzhen, China, [6] Dongguan Hospital of Traditional Chinese Medicine, Dongguan, China, [7] Guangzhou Hospital of Integrated Traditional Chinese and Western Medicine, Huadu, China, [8] Rheumatology Unit, Department of Medicine Solna, Karolinska Institutet, Karolinska University Hospital, Stockholm, Sweden

***Correspondence:**
Qingchun Huang
qch1963@163.com
Runyue Huang
ryhuang@gzucm.edu.cn

†These authors have contributed equally to this work

Background: Traditional Chinese Medicine is complementary and an alternative to modern medicine. The combination therapies of herbal products with disease-modifying anti-rheumatic drugs are gradually and widely adopted in the management of rheumatoid arthritis (RA) in China.

Purpose: To evaluate the efficacy and safety of Huayu-Qiangshen-Tongbi (HQT) decoction, a Chinese medicine formula, combined with methotrexate (MTX) in the treatment of patients with active RA, in comparison with the combination therapy of MTX with leflunomide (LEF).

Methods: This pilot study was a monocenter, open-label, randomized controlled trial with two parallel arms. Ninety patients with active RA were randomly allocated to receive either HQT at a dose of 250 ml twice daily or LEF at a dose of 20 mg once daily, and all participants received MTX at a dose of 10–15 mg once weekly. The primary efficacy endpoint was the proportion of patients who achieved a 20% improvement in the American College of Rheumatology criteria (ACR20) after a 24-week treatment.

Results: 84.4% (76/90) patients completed the 24-week observation. In the intention-to-treat analysis, the percentage values of patients achieving the ACR20 response criteria were 72.1% (31/43) in MTX + HQT group and 74.4% (32/43) in MTX + LEF group ($p = 0.808$). No significant difference was observed in other parameters, including ACR50, ACR70, clinical disease activity index good responses, European League Against Rheumatism good response, remission rate, and low disease activity rate. The results of the per-protocol analysis showed consistency with those of the intention-to-treat analysis. The mean change from baseline at week 24 for the van der Heijde modified total sharp score had no significant difference between two groups (3.59 $\pm$ 4.75 and 1.34 $\pm$ 8.67 in the MTX + HQT group and MTX + LEF group, respectively, $p = 0.613$). The frequency of adverse events was similar in both groups (11 cases in the MTX + HQT and 17 cases in the MTX + LEF, $p > 0.05$).

Conclusions: In patients with active RA, treatment with the combination of HQT and MTX was associated with improvement in signs, symptoms, and physical function. With a beneficial clinical response and acceptable tolerability, HQT or other Chinese medicine formula may be a good therapeutic option in combination with MTX for RA treatment.

Trial registration: Chinese Clinical Trails Registry, ChiCTR-INR-16009031, Registered on 15th August 2016, http://www.chictr.org.cn/enindex.aspx.

Keywords: combination therapy, Chinese medical formula, Huayu-Qiangshen-Tongbi decoction, randomized controlled clinical trial, pilot study

INTRODUCTION

Rheumatoid arthritis (RA) is a common autoimmune musculoskeletal disease affecting the joints primarily, leads to structural damage including cartilage destruction and bone erosion, and brings about extra-articular harm such as cardiovascular, pulmonary, and psychological disorders (1). Disease-modifying anti-rheumatic drugs (DMARDs) are the principal choice of first-line treatments for patients with RA, among which methotrexate (MTX) is well-established as an anchor drug for both treatment and research (2). However, not all patients receiving MTX monotherapy achieved low disease activity (LDA) or clinical remission (3). Over the last two decades, the treatment of RA has been transformed, and today, in patients with insufficient response to MTX monotherapy, combination with biological DMARDs or other conventional synthetic DMARDs (csDMARDs) is an international consensus of RA therapeutic strategy (2). Although new effective treatment regimens increased the clinical response rate of achieving full or long-lasting remission, a substantial number of RA patients did not respond to the current therapeutic strategies and even suffered from adverse effects (AEs) caused by long-term treatments, such as gastrointestinal toxicity, hepatotoxicity, bone marrow suppression, tuberculosis, and infection (2, 4). Previous researches reported that the use of prednisone and certain biological DMARDs increased the risk of tuberculosis and other opportunistic infections occurring in RA patients (4–6). Due to the development of advance effects, a portion of RA patients did not benefit from these combination therapeutic regimens and discontinued the treatment (7, 8). Therefore, there is still a considerable unmet need in RA treatment, and an application of new effective and safe treatment strategies should now be the priority of research efforts.

Traditional Chinese medicine (TCM), such as herbal products and acupuncture, has been widely practiced in clinics for over thousands of years in China and has found to be effective in treating many types of diseases, such as RA. Several Chinese medical herbs and their formulas, extracts, active ingredients, and even single compounds have been used for the RA treatment. Their clinical efficacy against RA and the safety have been evidenced by clinical practices and clinical trials in RA patients (9–12). Huayu-Qiangshen-Tongbi decoction (HQT) is a Chinese medical formula used in RA treatment in Guangdong Provincial Hospital of Chinese Medicine, which is composed of the following natural materials: the root and rhizoma of *Salvia miltiorrhiza* Bunge (Danshen), the rhizoma of *Dioscorea nipponica* Makino (Chuanshanlong), the root of *Astragalus membranaceus* (Huangqi), the root of *Paeonia tacti lora Pall* (Baishao), the root, stem, and leaf of *Saussurea involucrata* (Kar. et Kir.) Sch.-Bip (Tianshanxuelian), the bark of *Eucommia ulmoides* Oliver (Duzhong), the root and rhizoma of *Davallia mariesii* Moore ex Bak (Gusuibu), the root of *Dipsacus asperoides* C. Y. Cheng et T. M. Ai (Chuanxuduan), the earthnut of Chinese Foxglove (Shudi), and the root and rhizoma of *Glycyrrhiza*

Abbreviations: ACR, American College of Rheumatology criteria; ACR, American College of Rheumatology; ANOVA, analysis of variance; cDAIs, clinical disease activity index good responses; csDMARDs, conventional synthetic DMARDs; DAS28-CRP, 28-joint disease activity score based on C-reactive protein; DMARDs, disease-modifying antirheumatic drugs; EULAR, European League against rheumatism; ESR, erythrocyte sedimentation; HQT, Huayu-Qiangshen-Tongbi decoction; HAQ, Health Assessment Questionnaire; ITT, intention-to-treat; JSN, joint space narrowing; LDA, low disease activity; LEF, Leflunomide; mTSS, van der Heijde modified total sharp score; MTX, methotrexate; NSAIDs, Nonsteroidal anti-inflammatory drugs; PaGADA, physician's or patient's assessment of global health status; PhGADA, patient's assessment of global health status; PP, per-protocol; RA, rheumatoid arthritis; RCT, randomized controlled trial; RF, rheumatoid factor; TB, tuberculosis; TCM, Traditional Chinese medicine.

uralensis (Gancao). In our hospital, HQT has been used for RA management with the combination of csDMARDs, especially the MTX. Notably, we had undertaken a retrospective record review to evaluate the clinical response and AEs of the combination therapy of HQT and MTX in 2019. The result of the retrospective study showed that HQT combined with MTX had favorable therapeutic effects in improving the overall symptoms of RA patients with good tolerance (13). HQT may function as a kind of DMARDs, which can be used as an alternative or add-on treatment against RA. The purpose of this study is to determine the efficacy and safety of HQT in combination with MTX by performing an investigator-initiated, 24-week prospective, randomized clinical study, which might provide basic data and evidence for a further undergoing multicenter, double-blinded, randomized, placebo-controlled trial.

METHODS

Study Design

This pilot study was a 24-week, monocenter, open-label, randomized controlled trial, which was conducted in the Second Affiliated Hospital of Guangzhou University of Chinese Medicine (Guangdong Provincial Hospital of Chinese Medicine) between August 2016 and September 2018. All the participants were provided written informed consent, and the protocol was first approved by the Medical Ethics Committee of the Second Affiliated Hospital of Guangzhou University of Chinese Medicine (B2016-076-01) and subsequently registered with the World Health Organization clinical trial registry (no. ChiCTR-INR-16009031).

Patients

All participants were recruited from an outpatient rheumatology clinic at the Second Affiliated Hospital of Guangzhou University of Chinese Medicine (Guangdong Provincial Hospital of Chinese Medicine) in Guangzhou, China. Individuals with RA were all screened in clinics based on the inclusion and exclusion criteria, which are described later. If the eligibility criteria were met, the patients would be asked if they were interested in participating in the trial. The trial coordinator contacted participants to explain the requirements and purpose of the study, and the informed consent was completed as well.

Inclusion/Exclusion Criteria

Participants should meet the following criteria in this study: (1) aged between 18 and 65 years; (2) diagnosed with RA based on the diagnostic criteria of 1987 American College of Rheumatology (ACR) (14) or the 2009 ACR criteria (15); (3) were in functional class I, II, or III (according to the 1987 American Rheumatism Association classification standard) (14); (5) Chinese medicine inclusion criteria: with a syndrome pattern including wind and damp stagnation, cold and damp stagnation, hot and damp stagnation, phlegm and stasis stagnation, and deficiency of kidney and liver (criteria of Chinese medicine symptoms assessment is shown in **Appendix 1**); (5) the 28-joint disease activity score (DAS) based on C-reactive protein (DAS28-CRP) score > 3.2 (16); (6) received a stable dose of non-steroidal anti-inflammatory drug (NSAID) during the 4 weeks before screening, or did not take NSAIDs before screening for at least 1 week; (7) did not take DMARDs (including biological DMARDs and csDMARDs) before screening during the 4 weeks; the patients who received DMARDs must have a period of DMARD washout that lasted for at least 4 weeks before the trial; (8) if patients took corticosteroids such as prednisone, the dose should be $\leq$ 10 mg, and they must have already taken more than 4 weeks before starting this study; and (9) agreed to participate in the trial and signed a form of informed consent.

Patients were excluded from this trial if they: (1) had a history of another autoimmune rheumatic disease, Sjögren's syndrome or systemic lupus erythematosus for instance; with joint swelling because of osteoarthritis, trauma, septic arthritis, or crystal arthritis; recent, current, or chronic infection, for example, the infection with hepatitis B or hepatitis C; evidence of any extents of *Mycobacterium tuberculosis* infection; (2) had other severe disorders, such as hematopoietic, brain, lung, or cardiovascular diseases; (3) had a hemoglobin level of <90 g/L, a platelet count of $<100 \times 10^9$/L, or a white cell count of $<3.0 \times 10^9$/L; (4) had an estimated glomerular filtration rate of $\leq$40 ml/min (evaluated by Cockcroft and Gault method); (5) with a alanine aminotransferase or aspartate aminotransferase level > 1.5 times the upper normal limit; (6) had a gastritis or active gastroduodenal ulcer induced by the long-term treatment of NSAIDs; (7) were hypersensitive to medication used in the trial; (8) had participated in any other trials within 4 weeks at the time of screening; (9) women currently pregnant or who were planning on becoming pregnant during the study period; and (10) patients with mental disease.

Interventions

Eligible patients were allocated to receive either HQT (orally, twice per day, 250 ml for each time, 30 min after meals) or LEF (20 mg once daily) for 24 successive weeks. All the patients took MTX orally once a week, starting with 10 mg and increasing to 12.5 or 15 mg after a 4-week treatment. The ingredients and cooking method of HQT are shown in **Table 1**. The result observed from high-performance liquid chromatography analysis of HQT decoction is shown in **Appendix 2**. Patients were allowed to continue to receive NSAIDs and/or stable dosage of oral glucocorticoid (5–10 mg per day, prednisolone or equivalent) if the patients suffered intolerable pain (patient's assessment of pain $\geq$40 mm), folic acid, bone protection drugs such as alendronate and calcium/vitamin D, and antacids during the trial. Patients could withdraw from the trial at any time if they were not satisfied with the clinical response.

Outcomes and Measurements

Primary Outcomes

Patients were assessed concerning the outcomes and clinical parameters at baseline on weeks 4, 12, and 24 by different trained evaluators who did not know the treatments in the trial. The primary outcome was the patient's proportion achieving an ACR response of at least 20% (ACR20) at 24 weeks, according to the ACR criteria (17). To be considered as an ACR20 responder, a

TABLE 1 | Main components of HQT.

Pinyin Name	Latin Name	Doses
Danshen	*Salvia miltiorrhiza* Bunge	20 g
Chuanshanlong	*Dioscorea nipponica* Makino	30 g
Huangqi	*Astragalus membranaceus*	30 g
Baishao	*Paeonia tacti lora* Pall	20 g
Tianshanxuelian	*Saussurea involucrata* (Kar. et Kir.) Sch.-Bip	3 g
Duzhong	*Eucommia ulmoides* Oliver	20 g
Gusuibu	*Davallia mariesii* Moore ex Bak	20 g
Chuanxuduan	*Dipsacus asperoides* C. Y. Cheng et T. M. Ai	15 g
Shudi	Chinese Foxglove	15 g
Gancao	*Glycyrrhiza uralensis*	10 g

HQT, Huayu-Qiangshen-Tongbi decoction. The decoction was made in the following manner: (1) Put the herbals and the right amount of cold water in the casserole, and soak the herbals in the cold water for 30 min. (2) Add 1,200 ml of cold water in the casserole, heat to boiling, and boil for 40 min, then filter the decoction two times; (3) Add 800 ml of hot water to the casserole with the boiled herbs together, boil for 30 min, and then filter the decoction two times; (4) Mix the decoctions together twice in 1 day, 250 ml for each time.

patient should achieve ≥20% improvement in both tender and swollen joints (28 tender and 28 swollen joints were evaluated) and ≥20% improvement in following three or more parameters: the patient's assessment of pain on a visual analog scale (0–100 mm), the physician's or patient's assessment of global health status (PaGADA/PhGADA, 0–100 mm), the patient's assessment of function with a modified version of the Health Assessment Questionnaire (HAQ, scores are based on an overall mean score ranging from the highest within each group), and the serum level of CRP or erythrocyte sedimentation (ESR).

Secondary Outcomes

Secondary efficacy measures were the proportion of patients with 50 or 70% improvement, ACR50 or ACR70, at week 24, the clinical disease activity index (cDAI) good response, European League Against Rheumatism (EULAR) good and moderate responses, clinical remission, and LDA. The criteria of EULAR response were evaluated based on the individual amount of change in the DAS as well as the achieved DAS (low, moderate, or high). Moderate EULAR responses were a decrease (improvement) of >0.6 and ≤1.2 and a DAS <5.1, whereas good responses are a reduction of >1.2 and a DAS <2.6 (18). A good response for cDAI was defined when achieving ≥50% improvement or a cDAI ≤2.8 (19). The extent of disease activity was assessed based on the DAS in DAS28-CRP as remission (<2.6) and LDA (<3.2) (16).

The following clinical and laboratory indexes were also assessed: the 28-joint tender joint count, 28-joint swollen joint count, morning stiffness duration, the patient's assessment of pain on a visual analog scale, PaGADA, PhGADA, CRP, ESR, rheumatoid factor (RF), HAQ score, and DAS28-CRP. Radiographs of the hands (including wrists) were performed at the screening visit and after 24-week treatment. Radiographs of the hands (including wrists) were evaluated by the van der Heijde modified total sharp score (mTSS), which was utilized to assess radiographic joint damage progression (20) taken at baseline and after 24 weeks in the trial. Sixteen and 15 areas were included for the evaluation of erosions and joint space narrowing (JSN) in hands and wrists. The maximum score of erosion was 160, and the maximum JSN score was 120. The sum of the earlier mentioned scores (maximum 280) was the mTSS. All radiographs in the trial were scored centrally in chronological order by a professional while blinded reader.

Safety Outcomes

Measurement of safety was evaluated by patient-expressed AEs, physical examinations, and laboratory investigations, which included a routine blood test, urine analysis, renal function, and liver function. These evaluations were undertaken at each visit during the period of treatment (baseline, 4, 12, and 24 weeks). Chest X-ray examinations and electrocardiography were conducted at the screening visit and after 24-week treatment. Hepatotoxicity was defined by the abnormal increase of the hepatic enzyme level. Hematological adverse events were assessed by the changes in hematologic characteristics, such as anemia (hemoglobin < 90 g/L), leukopenia (<3.5 × 10^9/L), and thrombocytopenia (<100 × 10^9/L).

Sample Size

Due to the lack of previous similar trials and pilot studies to consult, the sample size of this pilot study was set as 45 cases in each group.

Randomization and Blinding

An independent statistician performed randomization. SAS 9.2 software (SAS Institute Inc., Cary, USA) was used to generate the randomization sequence. Participants were randomly assigned at a 1:1 ratio by a randomization system to the MTX + HQT group or the MTX + LEF group. Blinding and placebo tables were not available for this investigator-initiated clinical trial, and the allocation sequence was not concealed from both the researchers and participants.

Statistical Analysis

SPSS17.0 and GraphPad Prism 7 statistical software packages were used to establish the database by an independent statistician who was blinded to the group allocation. The full analysis set evaluated baseline data, and the efficacy in the two groups was assessed by both intent-to-treat (ITT) analysis and per-protocol (PP) analysis. The ITT analysis included participants who received at least 4 weeks of treatment, whereas the PP analysis only included the patients who finished 24-week treatment. The data from the patients who withdrew from the trial prematurely were considered missing, and these data were calculated using the last observation when performing the ITT analysis. Safety set analysis was used to assess the safety of two treatments, including all patients who received treatment once.

Baseline characteristics of participants were reported as the mean ± standard deviation or as numbers with corresponding percentages for categorical variables. To determine the differences in baseline characteristics between two groups, the independent *t*-tests were used for normally distributed variables, chi-square tests for categorical variables, and Mann–Whitney

U-tests for non-normally distributed variables. Analysis of the primary endpoint (the ACR20) and some secondary efficacy endpoints (the numeration data) was analyzed by using a chi-square test or Fisher's exact test, whereas the measurement data of secondary endpoints were detected by one-way repeated measures ANOVA of the mean values from baseline to weeks 4, 12, and 24 for each group. Missing values were replaced using the last observation. All statistical tests were two-sided, which were performed at the $p < 0.05$ significance level.

RESULTS

Characteristics of the Sample

Totally, 107 active RA patients were screened in this trial. Among these participants 90 patients were eligible to be enrolled in this trial based on inclusion criteria. All of them were randomly assigned to the two groups: MTX + HQT ($n = 45$) and MTX + LEF ($n = 45$). The percentages of patients who did not finish the 24-week treatment were 13.3% in the MTX + HQT group and 17.8% in the MTX + LEF group. There were four and three patients in the MTX + HQT group and MTX + LEF group, respectively, excluded from the PP set for the protocol violation. Additionally, because of the adverse events, there were two patients in the MTX + HQT group and five patients in the MTX + LEF group who discontinued treatment (**Figure 1**).

There were no statistically significant differences in age, sex, demographics, or patient clinical characteristics between the two groups ($p > 0.05$). Demographics and clinical characteristics at baseline of patients with active RA are shown in **Table 2**. Patients received MTX at a dose of 11.84 ± 1.46 mg/week in the MTX + HQT group and 10.56 ± 1.14 mg/week in the MTX + LEF group. Concomitant medication evaluation was also performed to compare the two groups during the trial. There was no statistically significant difference in the proportion of the patients who used glucocorticoids, NSAIDs, antacids, folic acid, or calcitriol/calcium ($p > 0.05$). Besides, the mean values of the glucocorticoid doses in patients each day were 5.17 ± 0.93 mg in the MTX + HQT group and 5.0 ± 0.0 mg in the MTX + LEF group. The major concomitant medications in this study of the two groups are shown in **Table 2**. Furthermore, 85.6% (77/90) participants had a period of DMARD washout that lasted for at least 4 weeks before participating in this trial. Of them, 82.2% (37/45) participants were in the MTX + HQT group, and 88.9% (40/45) participants were in the MTX + LEF group; the rest of the participants, 17.8% (8/45) in the MTX + HQT group and 11.1% (5/45) in the MTX + LEF group, had never taken DMARDs. No significant difference between the two groups was observed in the rate of receiving DMARDs treatment before participating in this trial ($p > 0.05$).

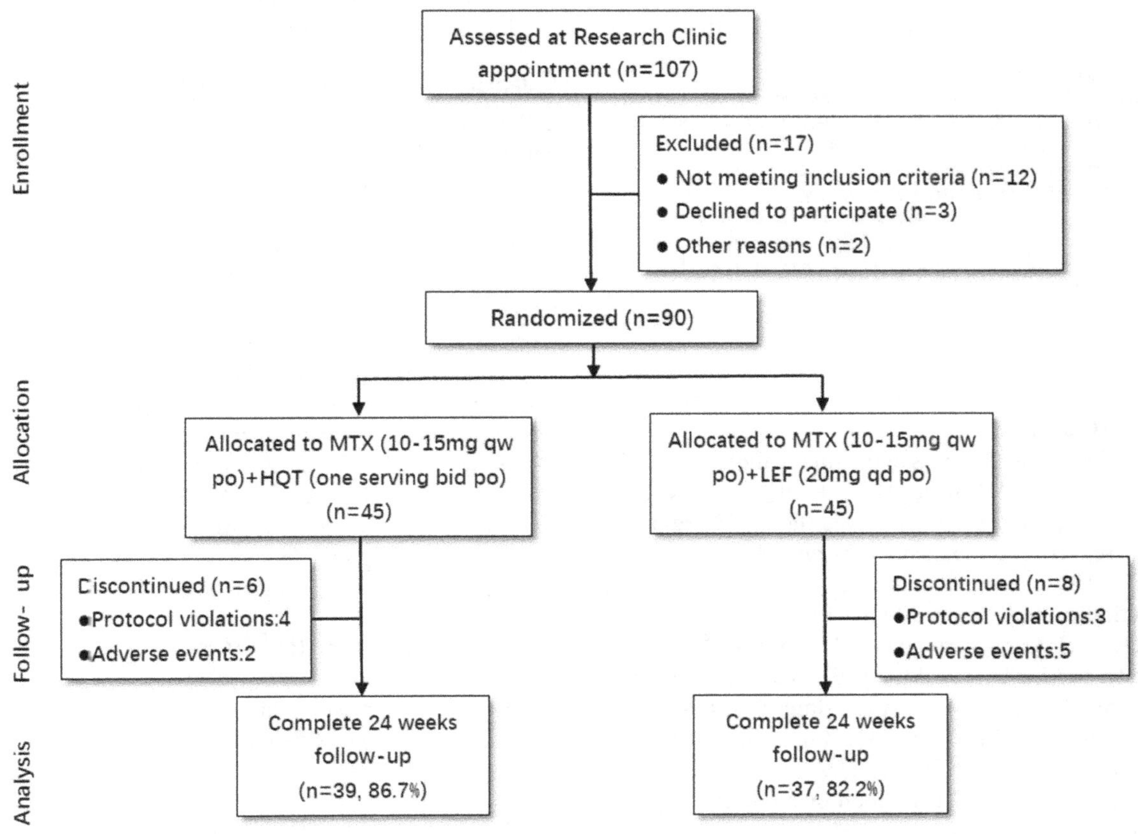

FIGURE 1 | Participant flow through the trial.

TABLE 2 | Demographic and characteristics data of RA patients at baseline in FAS.

Characteristics	MTX + HQT (*n* = 45)	MTX + LEF (*n* = 45)	*P*
Age (SD), years	51.67 (9.92)	47.56 (11.40)	0.099
Female, *n* (%)	35.00 (77.80)	31.00 (68.90)	0.340
Disease duration (SD), months	41.82 (45.93)	33.90 (36.53)	0.783
TJC (SD), *n*	8.62 (5.09)	9.20(6.15)	0.948
SJC (SD), *n*	6.29 (4.19)	4.67(3.02)	0.053
Patient's assessment of pain (SD), mm	65.09 (16.40)	59.78(20.17)	0.183
PhGADA† (SD), mm	61.11 (14.81)	56.33(18.84)	0.246
PaGADA† (SD), mm	62.00 (18.17)	57.56(20.47)	0.295
Morning stiffness (SD), min	47.11 (32.80)	53.89 (50.56)	0.798
HAQ, mean ± SD	0.65 (0.56)	0.92 (0.67)	0.063
hs-CRP (SD), mg/L	17.72 (19.10)	27.62 (35.15)	0.161
ESR (SD), mm/h	60.09 (27.29)	55.64 (31.39)	0.368
RF# (SD), U/ml	216.15 (298.88)	180.89 (194.82)	0.812
Anti-CCP#, positive rate	86.05% (37/43)	87.80% (36/41)	0.811
DAS28-CRP	6.02 (1.81)	5.97 (2.17)	0.620
cDAI (SD)	27.22 (8.98)	25.12 (10.06)	0.284
Concomitant treatments			
NSAIDs, *n* (%)	43 (95.6%)	44 (97.8%)	1.000
Glucocorticoid oral, *n* (%)	29 (64.4%)	27 (60.0%)	0.664
Folic acid tablet, *n* (%)	41 (91.1%)	44 (97.8%)	0.357
Calcitriol/calcium carbonate, *n* (%)	37 (82.2%)	43 (95.6%)	0.094
Antacids, *n* (%)	40 (88.9%)	42 (93.3%)	0.711

Data are presented as the mean (SD) or n (%).
FAS, full analysis set; TJC, tender joint count; SJC, swollen joint count; PhGADA, physician's global assessment of disease activity; PaGADA, patient's global assessment of disease activity; HAQ, Health Assessment Questionnaire; CRP, C-reactive protein; ESR, erythrocyte sedimentation rate; RF, rheumatoid factor; anti-CCP, anti-cyclic citrullinated peptide antibody; DAS28-CRP, 28-joint disease activity score- C-reactive protein; cDAI, clinical disease activity index; NSAIDs, non-steroidal anti-inflammatory drugs.
RF# was measured by immunonephelometric with a cutoff value of 20 U/ml. Anti-CCP# was measured using a commercially available second-generation ELISA kit (Abbott, USA) with a cutoff value of 25 U/ml.
†Measured on a 100-mm visual analog scale; the upper limit of normal for CRP is 0–6 mg/L.

Clinical Efficacy

In the ITT analyses after 24 weeks of treatment, there were 72.1% (31/43) and 74.4% (32/43) in the MTX + HQT and the MTX + LEF groups, respectively, who achieved the ACR20 response. Although there were more patients achieving ACR20 response in the MTX + HQT group, as compared with the MTX + LEF group, statistically, there was no difference ($p = 0.808$, **Figure 2**). ACR50, ACR70, cDAI good responses, EULAR good response, remission rate, and LDA rates of the patients at each evaluation point in the MTX + HQT group were similar to those in the MTX + LEF group (ACR50: 60.5 [26/43] vs. 60.5% (26/43); ACR70: 30.2 [13/43] vs. 30.2% [13/43]; cDAI good response: 76.7 [33/43] vs. 72.1% [31/43]; EULAR good or moderate response: 86.0 [37/43] vs. 86.0% [37/43]; EULAR good response: 51.2 [22/43] vs. 62.8% [27/43]; remission rate: 34.9 [15/43] vs. 48.8% [21/43]; LDA rate: 55.8 [24/43] vs. 67.4% [29/43]) (**Figure 2**). There was no appreciable difference between the two groups in those response rates mentioned earlier ($p > 0.05$).

In both groups, improvements in clinical symptoms (28-joint tender joint count, 28-joint swollen joint count, patient's assessment of pain, PaGADA, PhGADA, and morning stiffness duration), disease activity (DAS28-CRP), laboratory investigations (ESR, CRP, and RF), health status, and quality-of-life outcome (HAQ) were observed as early as week 4 and maintained through week 24 ($p < 0.05$). Overall, no clear differences were found between the two therapeutic regimens ($p > 0.05$). The clinical symptoms and laboratory investigations in the two groups at each point are shown in **Table 3**.

Additionally, we performed a PP analysis of the data from the patients who finished the 24-week treatment. At 24 weeks, ACR20 responses were attained in 76.9% (30/39) patients who received MTX and HQT and 75.7% (28/37) patients who received MTX and LEF, and no statistical significance was observed between the two groups ($p > 0.05$). The result of the PP analysis was in agreement with those found in the ITT analysis. Similar results of statistical analyses were seen for ACR50, ACR70, EULAR good response, cDAI good response, clinical remission, and LDA rate at week 24 in the PP analysis (**Figure 3**). A full list of the mean (standard deviation) on clinical symptoms and laboratory investigations at each point is provided in **Appendix 3**. After treatment, the clinical symptoms, laboratory investigations, HAQ score, and DAS were significantly improved compared with those before ($p < 0.05$). No statistical significance was observed in the improvement of those measures from baseline to week 24 between the two groups ($p > 0.05$).

Evaluation of the Radiographic Joint Damage

After 24-week treatment, 82.2% (37/45) of the patients in the MTX + HQT group provide the reports of radiographs at the two evaluation points and 71.1% (32/45) of the patients in the MTX + LEF group. Mean change values from baseline at week 24 were 3.59 ± 4.75 and 1.34 ± 8.67 with mTSS, 1.24 ± 2.39 and 0.63 ± 3.78 with JSN scores, 2.35 ± 2.96 and 0.72 ± 5.48 with erosions scores in the MTX + HQT and MTX + LEF groups, respectively; no significant differences were found between the two groups ($p > 0.05$). Comparing with the baseline, mTSS and erosions scores resulted in significant differences in the patients treated with two different treatment regimens at week 24 ($p < 0.05$), so as the JSN score in the MTX + HQT group ($p < 0.05$), whereas no significant differences of JSN score were observed in the MTX + LEF group ($p > 0.05$). Radiographs of the hands (including wrists) assessed by mTSS are shown in **Table 4**.

Safety and Tolerability

Safety evaluation was performed in the safety set analysis; all adverse events reported in this trial are listed in **Table 5**. In total, 28 patients (31.1%) experienced one or more adverse events (11 cases in the MTX + HQT group and 17 cases in the MTX + LEF group). The most common adverse events related to MTX + HQT were gastrointestinal discomfort, and all of the participants alleviated quickly and continued our trial after treatment with an antacid, although hepatic dysfunction, and gastrointestinal

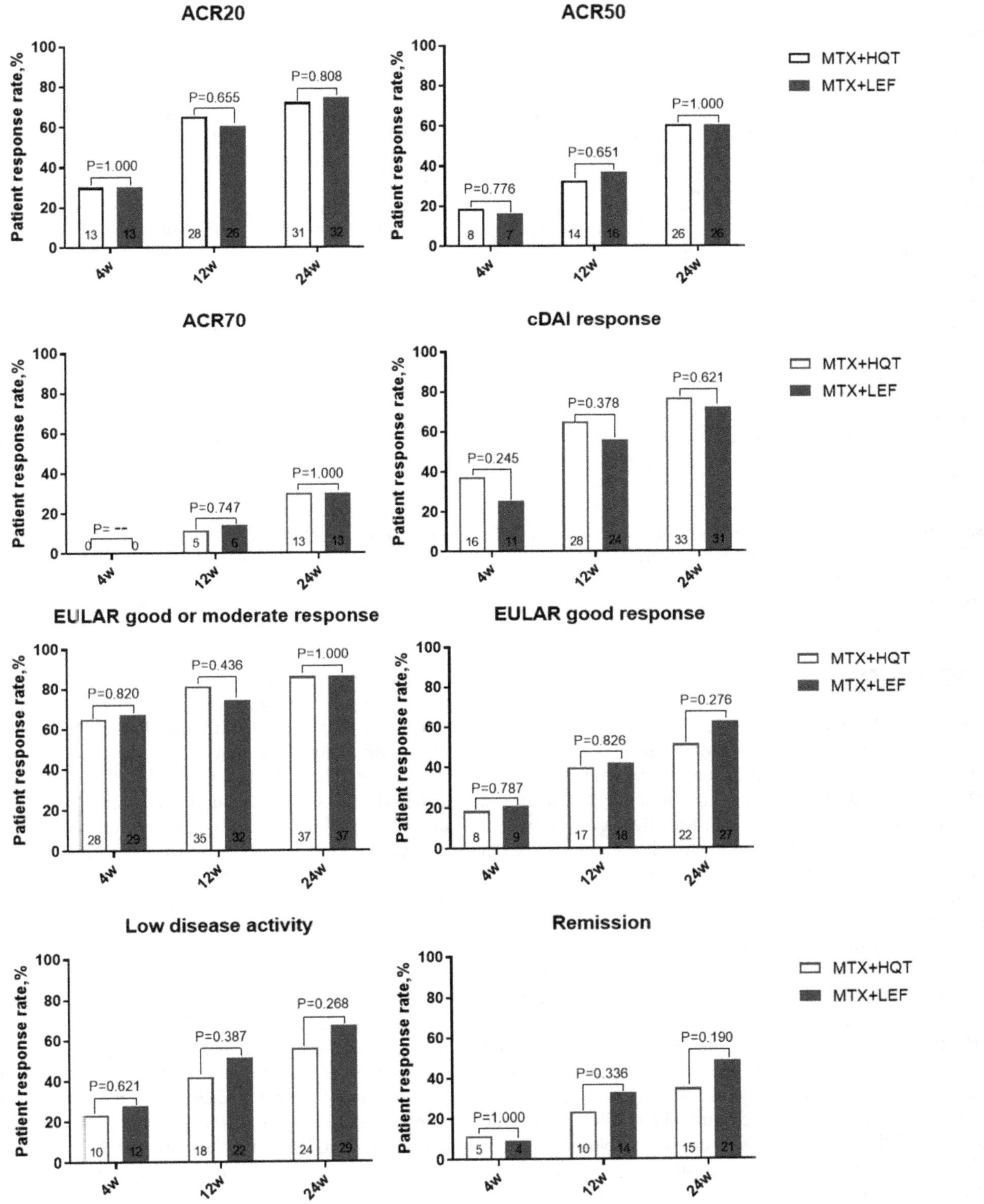

FIGURE 2 | Over time measurements of primary and secondary efficacy endpoints in the ITT analysis. A comparison between two combination treatments was performed by using the chi-square test or Fisher's exact test. ACR, American College of Rheumatology; cDAI, clinical disease activity index; EULAR, European League Against Rheumatism; ITT, intention-to-treat.

TABLE 3 | Clinical and laboratory measures of the two groups at each visit in the ITT analysis.

Measures	MTX + HQT				MTX + LEF			
	0W	4W	12W	24W	0W	4W	12W	24W
TJC, *n*	8.40 (5.10)	6.47 (4.86)	4.72 (3.53)	3.56 (4.04)	8.98 (5.92)	6.36 (5.19)	4.77 (5.02)	3.32 (5.01)
SJC, *n*	6.33 (4.28)	4.05 (3.37)	2.00 (2.40)	1.81 (3.81)	4.61 (3.03)	2.91 (2.87)	1.89 (2.53)	1.07 (1.89)
Patient's assessment of pain, mm†	65.09 (16.75)	45.81 (17.89)	30.35 (20.66)	23.44 (18.20)	60.00 (20.35)	42.45 (22.35)	29.91 (21.30)	21.48 (19.55)
PaGADA, mm†	61.86 (18.55)	39.70 (20.52)	29.53 (19.75)	19.95 (17.47)	58.18 (20.26)	44.32 (22.45)	29.32 (20.95)	20.80 (20.17)
PhGADA, mm†	61.16 (15.15)	40.81 (20.18)	28.60 (18.85)	20.70 (16.53)	56.25 (19.05)	43.18 (20.88)	30.57 (21.41)	21.25 (19.68)
Morning stiffness, min	47.91 (33.35)	26.98 (28.10)	17.84 (32.62)	19.30 (49.07)	54.20 (51.01)	35.00 (41.81)	14.55 (18.48)	11.50 (22.49)
CRP, mg/L	18.42 (19.25)	14.36 (19.21)	12.50 (15.38)	11.52 (18.39)	27.16 (35.78)	15.07 (25.27)	18.12 (55.57)	10.13 (16.96)
ESR, mm/h	60.70 (26.44)	55.05 (27.41)	51.81 (31.30)	46.91 (27.69)	54.43 (30.79)	51.95 (32.14)	44.12 (29.49)	42.09 (28.45)
RF, U/ml	204.14 (283.21)	157.91 (222.86)	153.38 (224.95)	222.09 (437.13)	182.05 (196.06)	182.21 (246.89)	123.59 (202.98)	113.37 (149.13)
HAQ	0.64 (0.57)	0.43 (0.45)	0.38 (0.53)	0.26 (0.46)	0.91 (0.68)	0.59 (0.63)	0.44 (0.56)	0.31 (0.57)
DAS28-CRP	5.98 (1.85)	4.73 (2.08)	3.69 (1.60)	3.21 (1.77)	5. 90 (2.09)	4.47 (2.04)	3.64 (2.09)	2.98 (2.05)

**Values are the mean (SD).*
TJC, tender joint count; SJC, swollen joint count; PaGADA, patient's global assessment of disease activity; PhGADA, physician's global assessment of disease activity; HAQ, Health Assessment Questionnaire; ESR, erythrocyte sedimentation rate, CRP, C-reactive protein; RF, rheumatoid factor; DAS28, 28-joint disease activity score.
†Measured on a 100-mm visual analog scale.

discomfort were the most common adverse events with MTX + LEF, and five patients withdrew from the trial (four patients for hepatic dysfunction and one for hypertension). There was no statistical significance between the two groups in the incidences of all adverse events ($p > 0.05$).

DISCUSSION

Over thousands of years, TCM has been beneficial to many patients in China. Nowadays, TCM is regarded as a basic or complementary therapy for RA patients, and, therefore, a variety of TCM herbs have been used in the clinic for RA treatment. The anti-inflammatory and antiarthritic activities of many TCM herbs have been validated in arthritic models and also tested in clinical trials in patients with RA (10, 19, 21). Thus, Chinese herbals may also function as DMARDs, which could be used as an alternative or basic treatment for RA patients.

In TCM theory, RA belongs to "Bi" disease, which is a group of disorders with symptoms and signs similar to arthritis or other rheumatism defined in Western medicine (22–24). The development of "Bi" syndrome is due to an evil spirit, the pathogeny of TCM, including wind, cold, and wet that invade the human body and lead to poor circulation of Qi and blood, so-called "blood stasis" (23, 25, 26). Based on years of clinical experience and observation, "removing blood stasis" theory of TCM and the use of blood-activating herbs had efficacy in relieving clinical symptoms, signs, and indicators of inflammatory activity in RA patients (27). HQT is a Chinese herbal formula, and it is prepared for treating RA by activating blood circulation, dissipating blood stasis, and dispelling pathogenic wind, cold, and wet.

During the 24-week trial, the treatment with MTX + HQT resulted in significant improvement in clinical signs and symptoms of RA, including joint pain, joint swelling, morning stiffness duration, and measures of quality-of-life outcome, as well as in many inflammatory indicators, such as CRP, ESR, and the autoantibody RF. Comparing with MTX + LEF (a recommended therapy for refractory RA) (28–30), MTX + HQT led to a similar improvement in terms of patients achieving ACR20, ACR50, ACR70, cDAI, LDA, and remission responses and to moderate or good improvement in DAS28-CRP. In this pilot study, the combinational therapy of HQT with MTX effectively and safely alleviated symptoms and signs of patients with active RA. It is well-known that the destruction of smaller joints more frequently attacks the RA patients and that radiographs of both hands and feet are the most popular standard to evaluate structural changes, which is regarded as one of the criteria for assessing therapeutic efficacy (31). After 24-week treatment, both groups had higher mTSS than before treatment. However, X-ray analyses in our study showed no statistical difference in terms of mTSS between the two groups in the progression of radiographic joint damage. We considered that increasing mTSS might be in association with the high proportion (60.9%) of patients with disease duration of 2 years or more who enrolled in radiographic analyses set.

Our trial showed for the first time that MTX combined with Chinese herbal formula is equivalently effective as MTX combined with LEF in active RA patients. Previous studies have shown that herbal medicine monotherapy or combination therapy has efficacy in relieving clinical symptoms, signs, and indicators of inflammatory activity for RA patients (12, 32). According to previous pharmacological studies, the herbals in HQT formula are proven to have a variety of pharmacological effects, such as anti-inflammatory properties, analgesia, and immune suppression (33, 34), supporting the clinical efficacy of HQT in RA treatment. The root and rhizoma of *S. miltiorrhiza* Bunge (Danshen) and the rhizoma of *D. nipponica* Makino (Chuanshanlong) are the most important components of HQT. Previous pharmacological studies have demonstrated that *S. miltiorrhiza* injection could inhibit the proliferation of

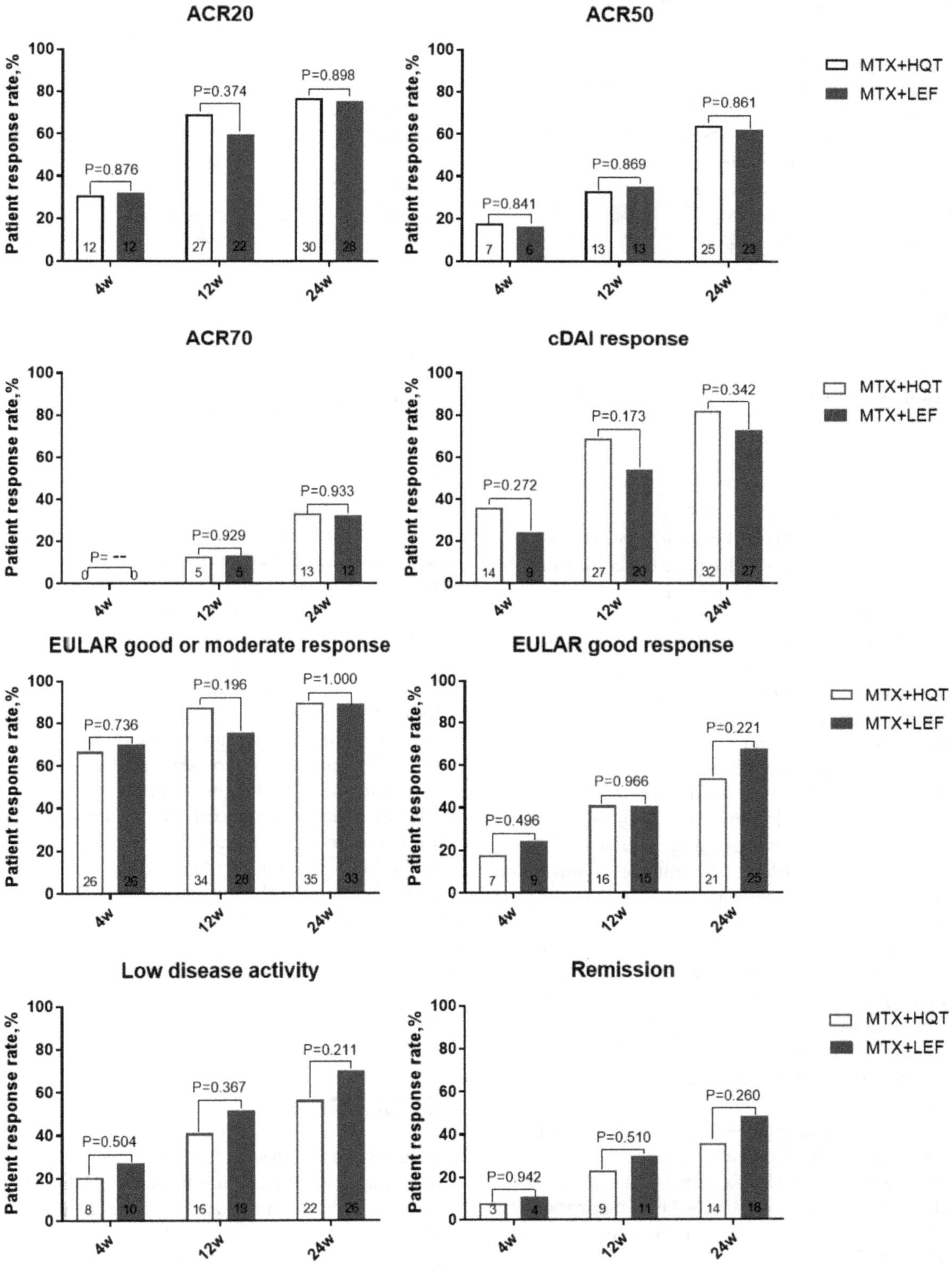

FIGURE 3 | Over time measurements of primary and secondary efficacy endpoints in the PPS analysis. A comparison between two combination treatments was performed by using the chi-square test or Fisher's exact test. ACR, American College of Rheumatology; cDAI, clinical disease activity index; EULAR, European League Against Rheumatism; PPS, per-protocol set.

TABLE 4 | Mean (SD) in the van der Heijde modified total sharp score (mTSS) in the two groups.

Joint damage	MTX + HQT (N = 37)	MTX + LEF (N = 32)	P (between groups)
mTSS			
Baseline, mean (SD)	50.92 (53.66)	36.44 (32.46)	0.736
Week 24, mean (SD)	54.51 (55.80)	37.78 (31.70)	0.613
P value (within the group)	<0.01	0.013	
JSN SCORE			
Baseline, mean (SD)	23.92 (25.46)	15.47 (14.87)	0.535
Week 24, mean (SD)	25.16 (26.33)	16.09 (14.35)	0.413
P value (within the group)	0.002	0.132	
EROSION SCORE			
Baseline, mean (SD)	27.00 (30.33)	20.97 (19.53)	0.928
Week 24, mean (SD)	29.35 (31.60)	21.69 (19.35)	0.814
P-value (within the group)	<0.01	0.017	

mTSS, the van der Heijde modified total sharp score; JSN, joint space narrowing; SD, standard deviation.

TABLE 5 | Summary of adverse events in the safety analysis set.

Adverse events	MTX + HQT (n = 45)	MTX + LEF (n = 45)	P
All	11 (24.4%)	17 (37.8%)	
ALT/AST elevation	0 (0%)	4 (8.9%)	0.117
Gastrointestinal reactions	9 (20.0%)	10 (22.2%)	0.796
Rash	1 (2.2%)	1 (2.2%)	1.000
Atrial fibrillation	1 (2.2%)	0 (0%)	1.000
Leukopenia	0 (0%)	1 (2.2%)	1.000
Hypertension	0 (0%)	1 (2.2%)	1.000

Data are presented as n (%).
ALT, alanine aminotransferase; AST, aspartate aminotransferase.

fibroblast-like synoviocytes obtained from RA patients (35, 36). Also, tanshinone VI, an abietane diterpene extracted from the root of *S. miltiorrhiza* Bunge, could improve bone loss by inhibiting osteoclastic bone resorption through inhibition of nuclear factor-κB and receptor activator of nuclear factor kappa-κ ligand pathways (37). Diosgenin, a major alkaloid monomer from the rhizoma of *D. nipponica* Makino, has a variety of pharmacological effects to relieve pain, reduce inflammation, regulate cytokine expression, and inhibit the proliferation of fibroblast-like synoviocytes, and, therefore, it has been frequently used to treat RA (38, 39). Many pharmacological studies reported that *D. mariesii* Moore ex Bak (Gusuibu), *D. asperoides* C. Y. Cheng et T. M. Ai (Chuanxuduan), and *E. ulmoides* Oliver (Duzhong) hold the potentials to prevent osteoporosis and inflammation associated with arthritis (40–42). Our previous study demonstrated that the combined therapy of HQT and MTX could significantly improve the clinical symptoms of RA patients with good tolerance (13). Furthermore, many experimental studies showed that the active ingredients of the other six herbs in HQT also exert anti-arthritic effects in both *in vivo* and *in vitro* models (43–47). Pieces of evidence from these pharmacological or mechanism studies support the clinical efficacy of MTX + HQT observed in our trial.

In our current study, all AEs were predominantly mild or moderate, with a low incidence rate. Gastrointestinal reactions and liver abnormalities were AEs. Reported AEs suggested that the most significant safety issue of MTX + LEF combination was potential liver toxicity, which was undoubtedly consistent with the real situation of LEF usage in RA treatment (48). In our study, liver abnormalities occurred in 8.9% of the MTX + LEF, which was lower than those reported in several other RCTs in RA (28, 29). The result of the previous study found that the incidence of alanine aminotransferase/aspartate aminotransferase elevations increased ∼ 2–5 folds in the combination of MTX and LEF, which depended on the dosages of MTX (48). In our study, we used the low dose of MTX (10–12.5 mg/week), reflecting the standard of the Chinses recommendations for the management of RA currently, which might be one of the reasons for the low rate of adverse events that occurred in our trial. Besides, more than 90% of patients in our trial received folic acid, which had the efficacy of lessening toxicity without altering efficacy during long-term treatment with MTX for RA (49).

Several critical factors in the course of analyzing the observational data should be considered in this work. Firstly, this trial was an open-label, monocenter, clinical trial, and the treating physicians and patients were not blinded to medication. To make an objective assessment of the efficacy and safety of the MTX + HQT combination therapy, the clinical outcomes were assessed and analyzed by evaluators and statisticians who were unaware of the therapy. However, a completely objective assessment needs to be verified in a multicenter, double-blind RCT in the future. Secondly, it was a 24-week observation trial, which may not be sufficient to show the long-term benefit of the MTX + HQT combination therapy, especially the radiographic progression. Thirdly, this trial did not compare the HQT in monotherapy with the MTX or another csDMARD in monotherapy, so the clinical efficacy of HQT itself cannot be evaluated or compared directly. Finally, due to a lack of similar clinical studies and pilot studies to reference, the sample size and the hypothesis test type (non-inferiority trial, equivalence trial, or superiority trial) in the design of this pilot study could not be pre-estimated accurately. However, the result of this pilot study can be the basic data and reference for further study.

CONCLUSION

This pilot study was the first time to evaluate the effect and safety of HQT, a Chinese medicine formula, combined with MTX, comparing with the combination of MTX and LEF. The results of this analysis indicate that the therapeutic regimen of HQT combined with MTX provides a potentially beneficial clinical response with acceptable tolerability for treating patients with active RA, which implies that HQT or other Chinese medicine formula may be a good therapeutic option in combination with MTX for RA treatment. However, it should be stressed that interpretations of the efficacy data are limited by the shortcoming mentioned earlier. A multicentric, double-blinded, preferably placebo-controlled, as well as with a longer follow-up, RCT is motivated to definitively establish the efficacy and safety of the HQT + MTX combination therapy and even the HQT in monotherapy.

ETHICS STATEMENT

The studies involving human participants were reviewed and approved by The Medical Ethics Committee of the Second Affiliated Hospital of Guangzhou University of Chinese Medicine (B2016-076-01). The patients/participants provided their written informed consent to participate in this study.

AUTHOR CONTRIBUTIONS

XiaC, YL, YZ, XiuC, YC, XW, ZW, P-JJ, QH, and RH: design and conception. JW, KG, AO, ZL, YL, YZ, and XiuC: acquisition, analysis, and interpretation. JZ, JP, ZH, XiuC, JW, KG, QH, and RH: major contributors in writing the manuscript. All authors read and approved the final manuscript. All authors contributed to the study design and review before submission according to their interests and scientific expertise.

FUNDING

This study was supported by Key-Area Research and Development Program of Guangdong Province (No. 2020B1111100010), National Natural Science Foundation of China (Nos. 81774218, 81804041), the Key Research Project of Guangzhou University of Chinese Medicine (No. XK2019021), the Clinical Research Project of Guangdong Provincial Hospital of Chinese Medicine (Nos. YN10101906, YN2018ZD06), the Science and Technology Planning Project of Guangdong Province (No. 2017B030314166), the Guangzhou Science and Technology Innovation Committee Project (No. 201710010076), the Natural Science Foundation of Guangdong Province (No. 2017KT1805), and the Guangdong Provincial Key Laboratory Project of Chinese Medicine (Nos. 2017B030314166, 2018B030322012).

ACKNOWLEDGMENTS

We thank Dr. Maojie Wang for his suggestions on this manuscript.

REFERENCES

1. Mcinnes IB, Schett G. The pathogenesis of rheumatoid arthritis. *N Engl J Med.* (2011) 365:2205–19. doi: 10.1056/NEJMra1004965
2. Sepriano A, Kerschbaumer A, Smolen JS, Van Der Heijde D, Dougados M, Van Vollenhoven R, et al. Safety of synthetic and biological DMARDs: a systematic literature review informing the 2019 update of the EULAR recommendations for the management of rheumatoid arthritis. *Ann Rheum Dis.* (2020) 7:760–70. doi: 10.1136/annrheumdis-2019-216653
3. Chatzidionysiou K, Sfikakis PP. Low rates of remission with methotrexate monotherapy in rheumatoid arthritis: review of randomized controlled trials could point towards a paradigm shift. *RMD Open.* (2019) 5:e000993. doi: 10.1136/rmdopen-2019-000993
4. Badavanis G, Pasmatzi E, Monastirli A, Tsambaos D. Biologic agents in systemic dermatotherapy: cutaneous and systemic side effects. *Curr Drug Saf.* (2017) 12:76–94. doi: 10.2174/1574886312666170518124014
5. Jick SS, Lieberman ES, Rahman MU, Choi HK. Glucocorticoid use, other associated factors, ad the risk of tuberculosis. *Arthritis Rheum.* (2006) 55:19–26. doi: 10.1002/art.21705
6. Novosad SA, Winthrop KL. Beyond tumor necrosis factor inhibition: the expanding pipeline of biologic therapies for inflammatory diseases and their associated infectious sequelae. *Clin Infect Dis.* (2014) 58:1587–98. doi: 10.1093/cid/ciu104
7. Du Pan SM, Dehler S, Ciurea A, Ziswiler HR, Gabay C, Finckh A, et al. Comparison of drug retention rates and causes of drug discontinuation between anti-tumor necrosis factor agents in rheumatoid arthritis. *Arthritis Rheum.* (2009) 61:560–8. doi: 10.1002/art.24463
8. Cohen SB, Czeloth N, Lee E, Klimiuk PA, Peter N, et al. Long-term safety, efficacy, and immunogenicity of adalimumab biosimilar BI 695501 and adalimumab reference product in patients with moderately-to-severely active rheumatoid arthritis: results from a phase 3b extension study (VOLTAIRE-RAext). *Expert Opin Biol Ther.* (2019) 19:1097–105. doi: 10.1080/14712598.2019.1645114
9. Lu MC, Livneh H, Chiu LM, Lai NS, Yeh CC, Tsai TY. A survey of traditional Chinese medicine use among rheumatoid arthritis patients: a claims data-based cohort study. *Clin Rheumatol.* (2019) 38:1393–400. doi: 10.1007/s10067-018-04425-w
10. Huang RY, Pan HD, Wu JQ, Zhou H, Li ZG, Qiu P, et al. Comparison of combination therapy with methotrexate and sinomenine or leflunomide for active rheumatoid arthritis: A randomized controlled clinical trial. *Phytomedicine.* (2019) 57:403–10. doi: 10.1016/j.phymed.2018.12.030
11. Chen XM, Wu JQ, Huang QC, Zhang JY, Pen JH, Huang ZS, et al. Systematic review and meta-analysis of the efficacy and safety of Biqi capsule in rheumatoid patients arthritis. *Exp Ther Med.* (2018) 15:5221–30. doi: 10.3892/etm.2018.6121
12. He YT, Ou AH, Yang XB, Chen W, Fu LY, Lu AP, et al. Traditional Chinese medicine versus western medicine as used in China in the management of rheumatoid arthritis: a randomized, single-blind, 24-week study. *Rheumatol Int.* (2014) 34:1647–55. doi: 10.1007/s00296-014-3010-6
13. Lv Y, Chen XH, Huang RY, Zhao Y, Wu JQ, Chen XM, et al. Clinical analysis of chinese medicine compound huayu-qiangshen-tongbi decoction combined with Methotrexate for the treatment of chinese patients with rheumatoid arthritis: a retrospective study. *Zhongguo Zhong Xi Yi Jie He Za Zhi.* (2019) 39:547–52.
14. Arnett FC, Edworthy SM, Bloch DA, Mcshane DJ, Fries JF, Cooper NS, et al. The American rheumatism association 1987 revised criteria for the classification of rheumatoid arthritis. *Arthritis Rheum.* (1988) 31:315–24. doi: 10.1002/art.1780310302
15. Aletaha D, Neogi T, Silman AJ, Funovits J, Felson DT, Bingham CO, et al. 2010 Rheumatoid arthritis classification criteria: an American College of Rheumatology/European League Against Rheumatism collaborative initiative. *Arthritis Rheum.* (2010) 62:2569–81. doi: 10.1002/art.27584
16. Madsen OR. Is DAS28-CRP with three and four variables interchangeable in individual patients selected for biological treatment in daily clinical practice? *Clin Rheumatol.* (2011) 30:1577–82. doi: 10.1007/s10067-011-1847-6

17. Felson DT, Anderson JJ, Boers M, Bombardier C, Furst D, Goldsmith C, et al. American college of rheumatology. Preliminary definition of improvement in rheumatoid arthritis. *Arthritis Rheum.* (1995) 38:727–35. doi: 10.1002/art.1780380602
18. Fransen J, Van Riel PL. The disease activity score and the EULAR response criteria. *Rheum Dis Clin North Am.* (2009) 35:745–57. doi: 10.1016/j.rdc.2009.10.001
19. Lv QW, Zhang W, Shi Q, Zheng WJ, Li X, Chen H, et al. Comparison of *Tripterygium wilfordii* hook F with methotrexate in the treatment of active rheumatoid arthritis (TRIFRA): a randomised, controlled clinical trial. *Ann Rheum Dis.* (2015) 74:1078–86. doi: 10.1136/annrheumdis-2013-204807
20. Van Der Heijde D. How to read radiographs according to the Sharp/van der Heijde method. *J Rheumatol.* (2000) 27:261–3. doi: 10.1097/00002281-200007000-00005
21. Venkatesha SH, Rajaiah R, Berman BM, Moudgil KD. Immunomodulation of autoimmune arthritis by herbal CAM. *Evid Based Complement Alternat Med.* (2011) 2011:986797. doi: 10.1155/2011/986797
22. Zhang C, Jiang M, Lu AP. Evidence-based Chinese medicine for rheumatoid arthritis. *J Tradit Chin Med.* (2011) 31:152–7. doi: 10.1016/S0254-6272(11)60031-9
23. Lo LC, Chen CY, Chiang JY, Cheng TL, Lin HJ, Chang HH. Tongue diagnosis of traditional Chinese medicine for rheumatoid arthritis. *Afr J Tradit Complement Altern Med.* (2013) 10:360–9. doi: 10.4314/ajtcam.v10i5.24
24. Wang M, Chen G, Lu C, Xiao C, Li L, Niu X, et al. Rheumatoid arthritis with deficiency pattern in traditional Chinese medicine shows correlation with cold and hot patterns in gene expression profiles. *Evid Based Complement Alternat Med.* (2013) 2013:248650. doi: 10.1155/2013/248650
25. Zhou X, Zhou Z, Jin M, Wang H, Wu M, Gu Q, et al. Intermediate and late rheumatoid arthritis treated by tonifying the kidney, resolving phlegm and removing blood stasis. *J Tradit Chin Med.* (2000) 20:87–92.
26. Chu YL, Jiang YQ, Sun SL, Zheng BL, Xiong WS, Li WJ, et al. The differential profiles of long non-coding RNAs between rheumatoid arthritis and gouty arthritis. *Discov Med.* (2017) 24:133–46.
27. Huang QC, Chu YL, He XH, Huang RY. Regulatory roles of compound danshen in the downstream path of cyclooxygenases in rheumatoid arthritis patients' synovium. *Zhongguo Zhong Xi Yi Jie He Za Zhi.* (2013) 33:1416–9.
28. Antony T, Jose VM, Paul BJ, Thomas T. Efficacy and safety of leflunomide alone and in combination with methotrexate in the treatment of refractory rheumatoid arthritis. *Indian J Med Sci.* (2006) 60:318–26. doi: 10.4103/0019-5359.26608
29. Londono J, Santos AM, Santos PI, Cubidez MF, Guzman C, Valle-Onate R. Therapeutic efficacy and safety of methotrexate + leflunomide in Colombian patients with active rheumatoid arthritis refractory to conventional treatment. *Rev Bras Reumatol.* (2012) 52:837–45. doi: 10.1590/S0482-50042012000600003
30. Hodkinson B, Magomero KR, Tikly M. Combination leflunomide and methotrexate in refractory rheumatoid arthritis: a biologic sparing approach. *Ther Adv Musculoskelet Dis.* (2016) 8:172–9. doi: 10.1177/1759720X16664324
31. Fransen J, Van Riel PL. Outcome measures in inflammatory rheumatic diseases. *Arthritis Res Ther.* (2009) 11:244. doi: 10.1186/ar2745
32. Lee S, Cho Y, Kim J, Kang JW, Yoon GY, Lee JH, et al. The efficacy and safety of the herbal medicine geonchildan for patients with active rheumatoid arthritis: study protocol for a randomized, double-blind, placebo-controlled, parallel pilot trial. *Trials.* (2018) 19:471. doi: 10.1186/s13063-018-2849-3
33. Wang Z, Lin HH, Linghu K, Huang RY, Li G, Zuo H, et al. Novel compound-target interactions prediction for the herbal formula hua-yu-qiang-shen-tong-bi-fang. *Chem Pharm Bull.* (2019) 67:778–85. doi: 10.1248/cpb.c18-00808
34. Wang Z, Linghu KG, Hu Y, Zuo H, Yi H, Xiong SH, et al. Deciphering the pharmacological mechanisms of the huayu-qiangshen-tongbi formula through integrating network pharmacology and *in vitro* pharmacological investigation. *Front Pharmacol.* (2019) 10:1065. doi: 10.3389/fphar.2019.01065
35. Liu QS, Zhu XC, Li JA, Xing Y, Jiang H, Zhang J, et al. Effects of danshen injection on the proliferation of rheumatoid arthritis fibroblast-like synoviocytes cultured with human serum. *Zhongguo Zhong Xi Yi Jie He Za Zhi.* (2013) 33:674–8.
36. Jie L, Du H, Huang Q, Wei S, Huang R, Sun W. Tanshinone IIA induces apoptosis in fibroblast-like synoviocytes in rheumatoid arthritis via blockade of the cell cycle in the G2/M phase and a mitochondrial pathway. *Biol Pharm Bull.* (2014) 37:1366–72. doi: 10.1248/bpb.b14-00301
37. Nicolin V, Dal Piaz F, Nori SL, Narducci P, De Tommasi N. Inhibition of bone resorption by Tanshinone VI isolated from Salvia miltiorrhiza Bunge. *Eur J Histochem.* (2010) 54:e21. doi: 10.4081/ejh.2010.e21
38. Liagre B, Vergne-Salle P, Corbiere C, Charissoux JL, Beneytout JL. Diosgenin, a plant steroid, induces apoptosis in human rheumatoid arthritis synoviocytes with cyclooxygenase-2 overexpression. *Arthritis Res Ther.* (2004) 6:R373–83. doi: 10.1186/ar1199
39. Liagre B, Leger DY, Vergne-Salle P, Beneytout JL. MAP kinase subtypes and Akt regulate diosgenin-induced apoptosis of rheumatoid synovial cells in association with COX-2 expression and prostanoid production. *Int J Mol Med.* (2007) 19:113–22. doi: 10.3892/ijmm.19.1.113
40. Jung HW, Jung JK, Son KH, Lee DH, Kang TM, Kim YS, et al. Inhibitory effects of the root extract of Dipsacus asperoides C.Y. Cheng et al. T.M.Ai on collagen-induced arthritis in mice. *J Ethnopharmacol.* (2012) 139:98–103. doi: 10.1016/j.jep.2011.10.020
41. Lin TH, Yang RS, Wang KC, Lu DH, Liou HC, Ma Y, et al. Ethanol extracts of fresh *Davallia formosana* (WL1101) inhibit osteoclast differentiation by suppressing RANKL-induced nuclear factorkappa B activation. *Evid Based Complement Alternat Med.* (2013) 2013:647189. doi: 10.1155/2013/647189
42. Wang JY, Yuan Y, Chen XJ, Fu SG, Zhang L, Hong YL, et al. Extract from Eucommia ulmoides Oliv. ameliorates arthritis via regulation of inflammation, synoviocyte proliferation and osteoclastogenesis in vitro and in vivo. *J Ethnopharmacol.* (2016) 194:609–16. doi: 10.1016/j.jep.2016.10.038
43. Jiang JB, Qiu JD, Yang LH, He JP, Smith GW, Li HQ. Therapeutic effects of astragalus polysaccharides on inflammation and synovial apoptosis in rats with adjuvant-induced arthritis. *Int J Rheum Dis.* (2010) 13:396–405. doi: 10.1111/j.1756-185X.2010.01555.x
44. Zhou J, Xu G, Yan J, Li K, Bai Z, Cheng W, et al. Rehmannia glutinosa (Gaertn.) DC polysaccharide ameliorates hyperglycemia, hyperlipemia and vascular inflammation in streptozotocin-induced diabetic mice. *J Ethnopharmacol.* (2015) 164:229–38. doi: 10.1016/j.jep.2015.02.026
45. Xu M, Guo Q, Wang S, Wang N, Wei L, Wang J. Anti-rheumatoid arthritic effects of *Saussurea involucrata* on type II collagen-induced arthritis in rats. *Food Funct.* (2016) 7:763–70. doi: 10.1039/C5FO00603A
46. Luo J, Song WJ, Xu Y, Chen GY, Hu Q, Tao QW. Benefits and safety of tripterygium glycosides and total glucosides of paeony for rheumatoid arthritis: an overview of systematic reviews. *Chin J Integr Med.* (2019) 25:696–703. doi: 10.1007/s11655-019-3221-5
47. Zhai KF, Duan H, Cui CY, Cao YY, Si JL, Yang HJ, et al. Liquiritin from glycyrrhiza uralensis attenuating rheumatoid arthritis via reducing inflammation, suppressing angiogenesis, and inhibiting MAPK signaling pathway. *J Agric Food Chem.* (2019) 67:2856–64. doi: 10.1021/acs.jafc.9b00185
48. Curtis JR, Beukelman T, Onofrei A, Cassell S, Greenberg JD, Kavanaugh A, et al. Elevated liver enzyme tests among patients with rheumatoid arthritis or psoriatic arthritis treated with methotrexate and/or leflunomide. *Ann Rheum Dis.* (2010) 69:43–7. doi: 10.1136/ard.2008.101378
49. Shea B, Swinden MV, Ghogomu ET, Ortiz Z, Katchamart W, Rader T, et al. Folic acid and folinic acid for reducing side effects in patients receiving methotrexate for rheumatoid arthritis. *J Rheumatol.* (2014) 41:1049–60. doi: 10.3899/jrheum.130738

5

Whole-Body Magnetic Resonance Imaging Assessment of Joint Inflammation in Rheumatoid Arthritis—Agreement With Ultrasonography and Clinical Evaluation

Sin Ngai Ng [1,2], *Mette B. Axelsen* [1], *Mikkel Østergaard* [1,3], *Susanne Juhl Pedersen* [1], *Iris Eshed* [4], *Merete L. Hetland* [1,3], *Jakob M. Møller* [3,5] *and Lene Terslev* [1,3*]

[1] Copenhagen Center for Arthritis Research, Center for Rheumatology and Spine Diseases, Rigshospitalet, Glostrup, Denmark, [2] Department of Medicine, Queen Elizabeth Hospital, Kowloon, Hong Kong, [3] Department of Clinical Medicine, Faculty of Health Sciences, University of Copenhagen, Copenhagen, Denmark, [4] Department of Diagnostic Imaging, Sheba Medical Center, Tel Giborim Affiliated With Tel Aviv University, Tel Aviv, Israel, [5] Department of Radiology, Herlev-Gentofte Hospital, Copenhagen, Denmark

***Correspondence:**
Lene Terslev
terslev@dadlnet.dk;
lene.terslev.01@regionh.dk

Objective: To compare joint inflammation seen by whole-body magnetic resonance imaging (WBMRI), with "whole-body" ultrasound and clinical assessments, in patients with active rheumatoid arthritis (RA) before and during tumor necrosis factor-inhibitor (TNF-I, adalimumab) treatment.

Methods: In 18 patients with RA, clinical assessment for joint tenderness and swelling, WBMRI, and ultrasound were obtained at baseline and week 16. Wrist, metacarpophalangeal (MCP) and proximal interphalangeal (PIP), elbow (except for WBMRI), shoulder, knee, ankle, and metatarsophalangeal joints were examined. Joint inflammation was defined by WBMRI as the presence of synovitis and/or osteitis and by ultrasound as gray-scale synovial hypertrophy grade >2 and/or color Doppler grade >1. On patient level, agreement was assessed by Spearman correlation coefficients (rho) for sum scores for 28 joints (i.e., wrists, MCPs, PIPs, elbows, shoulders, and knees) between clinical examination (DAS28CRP), ultrasound (US28), and WBMRI (WBMRI26; elbows not included). On joint level, agreement on inflammation between WBMRI, ultrasound, and clinical findings was calculated with Cohen's kappa (κ).

Results: At patient level, WBMRI26 and US28 sum scores showed good correlation (rho = 0.72; $p < 0.01$) at baseline, but not at follow-up (rho = 0.25; $p = 0.41$). At joint level, moderate agreement was seen for hand joints (κ = 0.41–0.44); for other joints κ < 0.40. No correlation with DAS28CRP was seen. No statistically significant correlations were observed between changes in WBMRI26, US28, and DAS28CRP during treatment.

Conclusions: WBMRI and ultrasound joint inflammation sum scores at patient level showed good agreement in clinically active RA patients before TNF-I initiation, whereas agreement was poorer at joint level, and after treatment.

Keywords: ultrasound, WBMRI, rheumatoid arhtritis, inflammation, agreement

INTRODUCTION

Suppression of joint inflammation is essential in modern management of rheumatoid arthritis (RA) and is a key element in clinical trials (1, 2) and is traditionally assessed by clinical joint examination, but magnetic resonance imaging (MRI) and ultrasound have been demonstrated to be more sensitive than clinical assessment for detecting joint involvement (3–6) and have been shown to be sensitive to change during treatment with TNF inhibitors (7–10). While, conventional MRI is limited to assessing one or a few joint regions per examination whole-body (WB) MRI has been introduced as a potential method for accurately assessing joint inflammation in the entire body in one session, covering both axial and peripheral joints. Its potential use for monitoring disease activity has been indicated in studies demonstrating a decrease in inflammation scores after biologic treatment in RA (11, 12), psoriatic arthritis (13), and axial spondyloarthritis (14); however, the sensitivity has not been assessed.

Ultrasound can assess multiple joints in one session and several studies have shown that ultrasound has good agreement with conventional MRI for detecting synovitis (3, 4) and is, consequently, a well-suited comparator for the ability of WBMRI for detecting joint inflammation.

The aim of the current study was to assess the agreement between WBMRI findings of joint inflammation with "whole-body" ultrasound joint inflammation and clinical joint assessment and the ability to assess change during treatment with adalimumab in a cohort of clinically active RA patients.

METHODS

Study Design

The current study was undertaken as a sub-study related to an investigator-initiated clinical trial (EudraCT number NCT01029613), of 37 patients with clinically active (DAS28CRP>3.2) RA, fulfilling the 1987 American College of Rheumatology classification criteria for RA (15) with the aim to use WBMRI to visualize inflammation and structural lesions during treatment with Adalimumab (see Axelsen et al. (11) for details). The patients had to be naïve to biological therapy and initiated treatment with adalimumab 40 mg sub-cutaneous every other week. The patients were not allowed to receive glucocorticoids or any synthetic Disease Modifying antirheumatic Drugs other than methotrexate from 4 weeks before inclusion and throughout the study. The patients included in the main study were invited to participate in the sub-study and 19 of these patients accepted to participate. However, one patient were subsequently excluded due technical problems with the baseline WBMRI.

At each clinical visit bilateral wrist, metacarpophalangeal joints (MCPs) 1–5, proximal interphalangeal joints (PIPs) 1–5, elbow, shoulder and knee joints, ankles, and metatarsal-phalangeal joints (MTPs) 1–5 were assessed for swelling and tenderness. Visual analog scale (VAS, 0–100 mm) assessments of pain and patients and physician's global assessment, Health Assessment Questionnaire (HAQ), and C-reactive protein (CRP) were determined, and the DAS28CRP was calculated. The ultrasound examination was performed prior to the WBMRI with an average of 2 days in between. The clinical examination, the ultrasound examination, and WBMRI were performed at baseline before initiation of treatment and at week 16.

All the patients were seen by the same clinician throughout the study. At 16 weeks, the clinical response was evaluated applying the EULAR response criteria.

The study was approved by the local ethical committee and the Danish Medicines Agency, following the Helsinki Declaration and the Good Clinical Practice guidelines.

MRI Methodology

All WBMRI scans were performed in the same 3T MRI unit (Achieva, Philips, Best, the Netherlands). Short tau inversion recovery (STIR) and pre-contrast T1-weighted spin-echo images were obtained for six imaging stations, assessing the following anatomical areas: cervical spine, shoulder/thoracic spine, lumbar spine, hips/hands, knees, and feet. The field of view was 470 × 253–287 mm, slice thickness 3 mm for hips/hands and feet, while 5 mm for the other locations. The T1-weighted sequences of hips/hands and feet were repeated after intravenous gadolinium-contrast injection (16).

Joints within the field of view, were read and scored separately for the presence/absence of synovitis and bone marrow edema (BME), respectively, using the validated OMERACT definitions developed for conventional MRI (17).

The examined joints included 26 of the 28 peripheral joints used in DAS28 (elbows were not examined by WBMRI as they were outside the field of view). In addition, ankles metatarsophalangeal joint 1–5 were examined bilaterally. MRI synovitis and BME were separately scored as present/absent (0–1) applying the aforementioned OMERACT definitions and an WBMRI joint inflammation score (range 0–2) was calculated per joint. To assess the inflammation at patient level the score per joint was used for calculating total WBMRI scores per patient (WBMRI26; range 0–52) by summing up the joint score in 26 joints. At joint level, joint inflammation was considered present if either synovitis or BME was present.

The WBMRIs were evaluated by one experienced WBMRI radiologist (IE), who was blinded to time point, clinical and biochemical data. Average duration of the WBMRI examination was 60 min and with similar average duration for evaluation and scoring the WBMRI.

Ultrasound Methodology

All ultrasound examinations were performed with a General Electric Logiq 9 ultrasound machine equipped with a high-frequency linear probe ML 6–15 MHz. Doppler setting was adjusted for slow flow according to published recommendations (18). The examined joints were the same as for MRI plus the elbows.

Applying the validated OMERACT definition for synovitis (19) all joints were scored using a semi-quantitative score (0–3) for gray scale (GS) and color Doppler (CD) (20). Each component (GS and CD, respectively) was scored separately and subsequently converted to a binary score (presence/absence,

0–1, as follows: positive GS synovitis was defined as a score >2, and positive CD was defined as a score >*1*. Based on these binary scores for GS synovitis and CD an ultrasound joint inflammation score (range 0–2) was calculated per joint, and to assess the inflammation on patient level the joint scores for 28 joints were added to calculate a total US inflammation score per patient (US28 score; range 0–56). At joint level, joint inflammation was considered present if either GS synovitis (>2) or CD (>1) was present. All ultrasound examinations were performed by one experienced sonographer (LT) blinded to clinical and biochemical data, but not to time point. Each ultrasound examination and scoring of the joints for joint inflammation lasted ~60 min.

Assessment of Agreement at Joint Level

At joint level, the agreement between WBMRI and ultrasound was evaluated using presence vs absence of joint inflammation for the wrists, MCP and PIP 1–5, elbows, shoulders, knees, ankles, and MTP 1–5. In addition, the agreement between clinical SJ and TJ and WBMRI and ultrasound, respectively, was assessed on data from baseline and week16 follow-up, i.e., data from both baseline and follow-up were pooled and analyzed together.

Assessment of Agreement at Patient Level

To assess the total inflammatory burden at patient level, composite scores were established including only the joints necessary to establish DAS28CRP (wrists, MCP, and PIP1–5, elbows, shoulders, knees). For clinical assessment a DAS28CRP were calculated and 28 tender (TJC28) and 28 swollen (SJC28) joint counts. For ultrasound and MRI the US28 and MRI26 (described above) were used. The correlation between US28 and WBMRI26 and with DAS28CRP was assessed as were the correlation to TJC28 and SJC28.

Statistics

Agreement between clinical assessment, ultrasound, and WBMRI at joint level was assessed with Cohen's kappa (κ) where κ values 0–0.20 indicates slight, 0.21–0.40 fair, 0.41–0.60 moderate, 0.61–0.80 substantial, and 0.81–1 perfect agreement) (21). Percentages of observed agreement (i.e., percentage of observations that obtained the same score) were also calculated. At patient level, sum scores were compared using the Spearman correlation analyses (rho). $P < 0.05$ was considered statistically significant. Statistical analyses were performed by IBM SPSS program version 20.0 (SPSS Incorporated, Chicago, USA).

RESULTS

Clinical Characteristics

Baseline characteristics are shown in **Table 1**. Eighteen patients were included in the study; 89% women, median age 54.4 years (range 26–73), and median disease duration 4.5 years (range 1–28). Thirteen patients were seen at 16 week-follow-up, whereas 5 were lost to follow up due to lack of treatment effect (2 patients), side effects to medication (1 patient), fracture (1 patient), and patient's cancellation of ultrasound appointment (1 patient).

TABLE 1 | Patient characteristics at baseline and follow up.

n	Baseline	Week 16
	18 patients	**13 patients**
Gender (female) (%)	89%	85%
Age (years)	54.5 (26–73)	55 (29–73)
Disease duration	4.5 (1–28)	5.5 (1–28)
DAS28 CRP (mg/dl)	4.52 (3.48–6.66)	3.26 (1.97–4.76)
Tender joint count (0–28)	6.5 (2–19)	3 (0–11)
Swollen Joint (0–28)	5.5 (1–13)	1 (0–5)
WBMRI26 inflammation (0–52)	8 (0–26)	5 (1–21)
US28 inflammation (0–56)	4 (0–29)	3 (0–26)

Values are median (range) if not otherwise indicated. N, number of patients; WBMRI26, whole body magnetic resonance imaging sum score for 26 joints; US28, ultrasound sum score for 28 joints.

Overall, the cohort had low inflammatory activity at baseline at patient level by both US28 and WBMRI26 with a median (range) US28 score of 4 (0–29) and a WBMRI26 score of 8 (0–26).

Correlation at Patient Level at Baseline and Follow-Up

The correlation between WBMRI26 and US28 was good at baseline (rho = 0.78; $p < 0.01$), while there was no correlation at 16 weeks (rho = 0.25; $p = 0.41$). Neither WBMRI26 nor US28 correlated with DAS28CRP at baseline (rho = 0.05, $p = 0.86$, and rho = −0.28, $p = 0.26$, respectively) or at week 16 (rho = 0.13, $p = 0.67$; rho = −0.26, $p = 0.39$, respectively).

WBMRI26 did not correlate with TJC28 at baseline (rho = −0.24, $p = 0.34$) nor at week 16 (rho = 0.39, $p = 0.19$). No correlation was found with SJC28 at baseline (rho = 0.37, $p = 0.13$) nor at week 16 (rho = −0.07, $p = 0.83$).

US28 had a negative correlation with TJC28 at baseline and week 16 (rho = −0.53, $p = 0.02$ and rho = −0.36, $p = 0.23$) and no correlation was found for SJC28 at baseline (rho = 0.42, $p = 0.09$) nor at week 16 (rho = 0.23, $p = 0.46$).

Agreement at Joint Level

In the pooled joint analysis, a moderate agreement was found between WBMRI and ultrasound for the wrist, MCP and PIP joints (κ = 0.41, 0.41, and 0.44, respectively)—**Figure 1**, whereas the agreement was fair-poor for other joints (κ < 0.40), **Table 2**.

The agreement between WBMRI and clinical TJ and SJ was fair-poor with κ < 0.40 for all joints (**Table 2**).

The agreement between ultrasound and clinical SJC in shoulders was moderate (κ = 0.48), while fair-poor (κ < 0.40) for other joints. Poor agreement was found with TJC (κ < 0.23).

The percent agreement between WBMRI and ultrasound was generally low for ankle, MTP, and knee joints (30, 59, and 6%, respectively) and high for shoulder, MCP, and PIP joints (80, 70, and 76%, respectively).

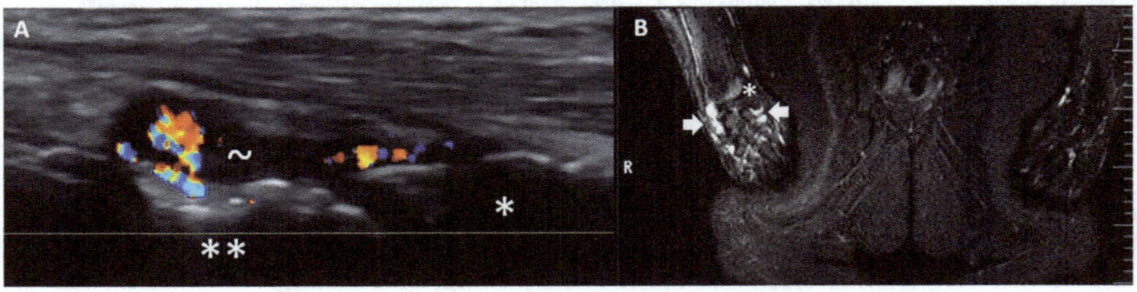

FIGURE 1 | Inflammatory activity in the right (R) wrist as shown by ultrasound **(A)** and WBMRI (STIR) **(B)**. * = radius, ** = schaphoid bone, ~ = synovial hypertrophy with Doppler activity, white thick arrows = high signal intensity in the wrist compatible with inflammation.

TABLE 2 | Agreement between ultrasound, WBMRI, and clinical evaluation at joint level.

Sites	**Ultrasound inflammation**			**MRI inflammation**	
Kappa *P*-value % agreement *N*	**MRI inflammation**	**Clinically tender joints**	**Clinically swollen joints**	**Clinically tender joints**	**Clinically swollen joints**
Shoulders	0.20	0.10	0.48	0.08	0.05
	0.01	0.247	0.000	0.504	0.485
	80%	81%	97%	67%	72%
	59	59	59	64	64
Elbows	–	0.08	0.37	–	–
		0.514	0.000		
		76%	90%		
		59	59		
Wrists	0.41	0.26	0.13	0.14	−0.01
	0.000	0.037	0.309	0.163	0.908
	69%	64%	57%	52%	42%
	59	61	61	62	62
MCP1–5 joints	0.41	0.10	0.27	0.06	0.07
	0.001	0.362	0.026	0.645	0.955
	70%	52%	62%	54%	51%
	60	61	61	63	63
PIP1–5 joints	0.44	0.22	0.30	0.33	0.36
	0.001	0.067	0.019	0.007	0.003
	76%	62%	74%	67%	74%
	58	61	61	61	61
Knees	0.12	0.15	0.13	0.15	0.07
	0.298	0.198	0.309	0.223	0.433
	61%	69%	80%	60%	58%
	57	59	59	60	60
Ankles	−0.06	0.10	0.18	0.16	0.07
	0.246	0.325	0.110	0.092	0.395
	30%	68%	76%	52%	40%
	61	59	59	62	62
MTP1–5 joints	0.11	0.01	−0.12	0.08	0.08
	0.265	0.918	0.259	0.418	0.102
	59%	53%	41%	63%	35%
	61	59	59	62	62

Values are kappa (1st row), p-values for kappa statistic (2nd row), Percent agreement (3rd row) and number on observations (n, 4th row).

WBMRI, whole body magnetic resonance imaging; MCP, metacarpophalangeal; PIP, proximal interphalangeal; MTP, metatarsophalangeal.

Correlation Between Changes During Treatment

After 16 weeks of treatment, median DAS28CRP had decreased from median 4.52 to 3.26, the tender joint count from 7 to 3 and the swollen joint count from 6 to 1, WBMRI26 from 8 to 5 and US28 from 4 to 3—showing a numerical decline for all parameters (**Table 1**). Six patients (46%) had achieved a good EULAR response, and 7 patients (54%) a moderate response.

The change in WBMRI26 during treatment did not correlate with the change in US28 (rho = 0.38; p = 0.21). Neither WBMRI26 nor US28 correlated with the change in DAS28CRP (rho = −0.07, p = 0.82 and rho = 0.10, p = 0.76, respectively).

DISCUSSION

This study is the first study to compare whole body assessment of joint inflammation as detected by both WBMRI and ultrasound in clinically active RA patients initiating a biological Disease Modifying anti-rheumatic Drug (DMARD) due to persistent elevated DAS28CRP despite conventional DMARD treatment. We found a good correlation between WBMRI26 and US28 at baseline at patient level, while the agreement at joint level was moderate for the hands and poor for the other joints. Both modalities correlated poorly with the DAS28CRP and clinical joint evaluation.

The strong correlation between WBMRI26 and US28 at baseline (at patient level) combined with the moderate-poor correlation at joint level suggest that ultrasound and MRI both provide measures of the overall inflammatory burden, but take different aspects into account. This could be explained by very different image acquisitions techniques, e.g., ultrasound cannot visualize bone marrow edema. The lack of correlation between the two imaging modalities for changes during treatment and at week 16 may partly be explained by the low level of inflammation in a small patient cohort, particular at follow-up, leaving a narrow disease severity spectrum, which will give small variations in the detected joint inflammation between the two modalities a larger impact on the correlation coefficient. Another contributing factor may be the overall low degree of peripheral inflammation by imaging in the cohort, even at baseline, and hence a lesser potential to improve during treatment.

With the ability to assess multiple joints in a single session ultrasound appeared a well-suited comparator to WBMRI for peripheral inflammatory changes in RA patients. Previous studies comparing conventional MRI and ultrasound have reported a relatively good agreement for synovitis in small peripheral joints (3, 4), i.e., a better agreement than in the present study. When obtaining WBMRI, more anatomical areas are scanned than by conventional MRI and to shorten the imaging time, the image slices are typically thicker and in-plane resolution reduced compared with conventional MRI. Together with the lack of dedicated receiver coils larger voxels and less optimal positioning the image quality is generally lower as compared to conventional MRI with the same field strength. As an example, the hand will at conventional MRI be positioned in a dedicated hand coil in the isocenter of the MRI unit, where the magnetic field is most homogenous, while during WBMRI the hand will have no specific coil and will be positioned below the buttocks, more distant from the isocenter of the magnet. This probably contributed to the observed lower agreement on the individual joint level. It should be emphasized, that the image quality has markedly improved since the study was performed in 2012 and is still undergoing continuous improvements which may positively influence the agreement in the future. Another factor that could have impaired the concordance at joint level is the fact that ultrasound cannot visualize bone marrow edema.

In our study, WBMRI and ultrasound sum scores did not correlate with DAS28CRP at baseline nor at follow-up and the agreement with clinical examination at joint level was generally poor. This is in line with previous studies (22, 23) and may be related to the lower sensitivity of clinical examination for synovitis as compared to ultrasound and MRI (3–6). Furthermore, joint inflammation by imaging was not an inclusion criterion. The low number of patients and the low degree of peripheral inflammation in the investigated cohort may also have contributed to the contra-intuitive findings such as the negative correlation between ultrasound and TJC. WBMRI has the potential, with technical improvements, to become a well-suited tool for clinical trials but is currently not suggested as a clinical tool due to generally lower availability and delay in information to the clinician about the inflammatory status as compared to ultrasound examination.

In conclusion, WBMRI and ultrasound showed good correlation for joint inflammation at patient level indicating that WBMRI is a potential tool for assessing the overall inflammatory burden in RA patients. Further studies implementing recent technical improvements in WBMRI, are needed.

ETHICS STATEMENT

The studies involving human participants were reviewed and approved by De Videnskabsetiske Komiteer, Kongens Vænge 2, 3400 Hilleroed, Denmark and the Danish Medicines Agency (EudraCT number NCT01029613). The patients/participants provided their written informed consent to participate in this study.

AUTHOR CONTRIBUTIONS

SN has performed data analysis and interpretation and written the manuscript. MA has conducted patient examination, performed data analysis and corrected the proof. MØ has performed data analysis, read WBMRIs, and written the manuscript. SP has performed data interpretation, read WBMRIs, and contributed to the manuscript. IE has read all the WBMRI images and contributed to the manuscript. MH conducted patient examination, contributed to the manuscript. JM has performed all the WBMRIs and contributed to the manuscript. LT has performed all the ultrasound examinations, performed data analysis, and written the manuscript. All authors contributed to the article and approved the submitted version.

ACKNOWLEDGMENTS

The authors acknowledge AbbVie A/S Denmark for providing financial support for this investigator-initiated study and for adalimumab during the study period. AbbVie A/S Denmark was not involved in study set-up, data collection, analysis or interpretation, and had no influence on the publication of data.

REFERENCES

1. Smolen JS, Aletaha D, Bijlsma JW, Breedveld FC, Boumpas D, Burmester G, et al. T2T Expert Committee. Treating rheumatoid arthritis to target: recommendations of an international task force. *Ann Rheum Dis.* (2010) 69:631–7. doi: 10.1136/ard.2009.123919
2. Haavardsholm EA, Aga AB, Olsen IC, Lillegraven S, Hammer HB, Uhlig T, et al. Ultrasound in management of rheumatoid arthritis: ARCTIC randomised controlled strategy trial. *BMJ.* (2016) 354:i4205. doi: 10.1136/bmj.i4205
3. Terslev L, Torp-Pedersen S, Savnik A, von der Recke P, Qvistgaard E, Danneskiold-Samsøe B, et al. Doppler ultrasound and magnetic resonance imaging of synovial inflammation of the hand in rheumatoid arthritis: a comparative study. *Arthritis Rheum.* (2003) 48:2434–41. doi: 10.1002/art.11245
4. Szkudlarek M, Klarlund M, Narvestad E, Court-Payen M, Strandberg C, Jensen KE, et al. Ultrasonography of the metacarpophalangeal and proximal interphalangeal joints in rheumatoid arthritis: a comparison with magnetic resonance imaging, conventional radiography and clinical examination. *Arthritis Res Ther.* (2006) 8:R52. doi: 10.1186/ar1904

5. Conaghan PG, Emery P, Østergaard M, Keystone EC, Genovese MC, Hsia EC, Xu W, et al. Assessment by MRI of inflammation and damage in rheumatoid arthritis patients with methotrexate inadequate response receiving golimumab: results of the GO-FORWARD trial. *Ann Rheum Dis.* (2011) 70:1968–74. doi: 10.1136/ard.2010.146068
6. Wakefield RJ, Green MJ, Marzo-Ortega H, Conaghan PG, Gibbon WW, McGonagle D, et al. Should oligoarthritis be reclassified? Ultrasound reveals a high prevalence of subclinical disease. *Ann Rheum Dis.* (2004) 63:382–5. doi: 10.1136/ard.2003.007062
7. Filippucci E, Iagnocco A, Salaffi F, Cerioni A, Valesini G, Grassi W. Power Doppler sonography monitoring of synovial perfusion at the wrist joints in patients with rheumatoid arthritis treated with adalimumab. *Ann Rheum Dis.* (2006) 65:1433–7. doi: 10.1136/ard.2005.044628
8. Hammer HB, Kvien TK. Ultrasonography shows significant improvement in wrist and ankle tenosynovitis in rheumatoid arthritis patients treated with adalimumab. *Scand J Rheumatol.* (2011) 40:178–82. doi: 10.3109/03009742.2010.517549
9. Døhn UM, Ejbjerg B, Boonen A, Hetland ML, Hansen MS, Knudsen LS, et al. No overall progression and occasional repair of erosions despite persistent inflammation in adalimumab-treated rheumatoid arthritis patients: results from a longitudinal comparative MRI, ultrasonography, CT and radiography study. *Ann Rheum Dis.* (2011) 70:252–8. doi: 10.1136/ard.2009.123729
10. Østergaard M, Emery P, Conaghan PG, Fleischmann R, Hsia EC, Xu W, Rahman MU.Significant improvement in synovitis, osteitis, and bone erosion following golimumab and methotrexate combination therapy as compared with methotrexate alone: a magnetic resonance imaging study of 318 methotrexate-naive rheumatoid arthritis patients. *Arthritis Rheum.* (2011). 63:3712–22. doi: 10.1002/art.30592
11. Axelsen MB, Eshed I, Østergaard M, Hetland ML, Møller JM, Jensen DV, et al. Monitoring total-body inflammation and damage in joints and entheses: the first follow-up study of whole-body magnetic resonance imaging in rheumatoid arthritis. *Scand J Rheumatol.* (2017) 46:253–62. doi: 10.1080/03009742.2016.1231338
12. Kono M, Kamishima T, Yasuda S, Sakamoto K, Abe S, Noguchi A, et al. Effectiveness of whole-body magnetic resonance imaging for the efficacy of biologic anti-rheumatic drugs in patients with rheumatoid arthritis: a retrospective pilot study. *Mod Rheumatol.* (2017) 27:953–60. doi: 10.1080/14397595.2016.1276425
13. De Marco G, Helliwell P, McGonagle D, Emery P, Coates LC, Hensor EMA, et al. The GOLMePsA study protocol: an investigator-initiated, double-blind, parallel-group, randomised, controlled trial of GOLimumab and methotrexate versus methotrexate in early diagnosed psoriatic arthritis using clinical and whole body MRI outcomes. *BMC Musculoskelet Disord.* (2017) 18:1–13. doi: 10.1186/s12891-017-1659-1
14. Krabbe S, Østergaard M, Eshed I, Sørensen IJ, Jensen B, Møller JM, et al. Whole-body magnetic resonance imaging in axial spondyloarthritis: reduction of sacroiliac, spinal, and entheseal inflammation in a placebo-controlled trial of adalimumab. *J Rheumatol.* (2018) 45:621–9. doi: 10.3899/jrheum.170408
15. Arnett FC, Edworthy SM, Bloch DA, McShane DJ, Fries JF, Cooper NS, et al. The American Rheumatism Association 1987 revised criteria for the classification of rheumatoid arthritis. *Arthritis Rheum.* (1988) 31:315–24. doi: 10.1002/art.1780310302
16. Poggenborg RP, Eshed I, Østergaard M, Sørensen IJ, Møller JM, Madsen OR, et al. Enthesitis in patients with psoriatic arthritis, axial spondyloarthritis and healthy subjects assessed by 'head-to-toe' whole-body MRI and clinical examination. *Ann Rheum Dis.* (2015) 74:823–9. doi: 10.1136/annrheumdis-2013-204239
17. Østergaard M, Peterfy C, Conaghan P, McQueen F, Bird P, Ejbjerg B, et al. OMERACT rheumatoid arthritis magnetic resonance imaging studies. Core set of MRI acquisitions, joint pathology definitions, and the OMERACT RA-MRI scoring system. *J Rheumatol.* (2003) 30:1385–6.
18. Torp-Pedersen S, Terslev L. Settings and artefacts relevant in colour/power Doppler ultrasound in rheumatology. *Ann Rheum Dis.* (2008) 67:143–9. doi: 10.1136/ard.2007.078451
19. Wakefield RJ, Balint PV, Szkudlarek M, Filippucci E, Backhaus M, D'Agostino MA, et al. Musculoskeletal ultrasound including definitions for ultrasonographic pathology. *J Rheumatol.* (2005) 32:2485–7.
20. Szkudlarek M, Court-Payen M, Jacobsen S, Klarlund M, Thomsen HS, Østergaard M. Interobserver agreement in ultrasonography of the finger and toe joints in rheumatoid arthritis. *Arthritis Rheum.* (2003) 48:955–62. doi: 10.1002/art.10877
21. Landis JR, Koch G. The measurement of observer agreement for categorical data. *Biometrics.* (1977) 33:159–74. doi: 10.2307/2529310
22. Gandjbakhch F, Haavardsholm EA, Conaghan PG, Ejbjerg B, Foltz V, Brown AK, et al. Determining a magnetic resonance imaging inflammatory activity acceptable state without subsequent radiographic progression in rheumatoid arthritis: Results from a followup MRI Study of 254 patients in clinical remission or low disease activity. *J Rheumatol.* (2014) 41:398–406. doi: 10.3899/jrheum.131088
23. Brown AK, Conaghan PG, Karim Z, Quinn MA, Ikeda K, Peterfy CG, et al. An explanation for the apparent dissociation between clinical remission and continued structural deterioration in rheumatoid arthritis. *Arthritis Rheum.* (2008) 58:2958–67. doi: 10.1002/art.23945

6

The Link Between Autonomic Nervous System and Rheumatoid Arthritis: From Bench to Bedside

Francesca Ingegnoli[1,2*†], *Massimiliano Buoli*[3,4†], *Flavia Antonucci*[5†], *Lavinia Agra Coletto*[1,2†], *Cecilia Maria Esposito*[3,4†] *and Roberto Caporali*[1,2†]

[1] *Division of Clinical Rheumatology, Gaetano Pini Hospital, Milan, Italy,* [2] *Department of Clinical Sciences and Community Health, Research Center for Adult and Pediatric Rheumatic Diseases, Università degli Studi di Milano, Milan, Italy,* [3] *Department of Neurosciences and Mental Health, Fondazione Istituto di Ricovero e Cura a Carattere Scientifico (IRCCS) Ca'Granda Ospedale Maggiore Policlinico, Milan, Italy,* [4] *Department of Pathophysiology and Transplantation, Università degli Studi di Milano, Milan, Italy,* [5] *Department of Medical Biotechnology and Translational Medicine (BIOMETRA), Università degli Studi di Milano, Milan, Italy*

Correspondence:
Francesca Ingegnoli
francesca.ingegnoli@unimi.it
orcid.org/0000-0002-6727-1273

† These authors have contributed equally to this work

Neuronal stimulation is an emerging field of research focused on the management and treatment of various diseases through the reestablishment of physiological homeostasis. Electrical vagus nerve stimulation has recently been proposed as a revolutionary therapeutic option for rheumatoid arthritis (RA) in combination with or even as a replacement for conventional and biological drugs. In the past few years, disruption of the autonomic system has been linked to RA onset and activity. Novel research on the link between the autonomic nervous system and the immune system (immune-autonomics) has paved the way for the development of innovative RA management strategies. Clinical evidence supports this approach. Cardiovascular involvement, in terms of reduced baroreflex sensitivity and heart rate variability-derived indices, and mood disorders, common comorbidities in patients with RA, have been linked to autonomic nervous system dysfunction, which in turn is influenced by increased levels of circulating pro-inflammatory cytokines. This narrative review provides an overview of the autonomic nervous system and RA connection, discussing most of the common cardiac and mental health-related RA comorbidities and their potential relationships to systemic and joint inflammation.

Keywords: vagus nerve, central nervous system, autonomic nervous system, mood disorder, rheumatoid arthritis, depression, therapy

INTRODUCTION

Rheumatoid arthritis (RA) is a chronic autoimmune inflammatory disease leading to progressive joint damage and associated with vascular, metabolic, and psychological comorbidities. RA is considered to pose a major global public health challenge, as its overall prevalence and incidence rates are increasing worldwide (1). Fundamentally, it is of paramount importance to reduce the future burden of this disease through the pursuit of innovative RA treatments that are driven mainly by increasing knowledge of its pathophysiology. An emergent field in this context is the study of autonomic nervous system (ANS) imbalance observed in association with many immune-mediated inflammatory diseases, comprising RA, systemic lupus erythematosus, systemic sclerosis, and inflammatory bowel diseases (2–4). The immune system and ANS can express and respond to numerous common regulatory molecules (e.g., glucocorticoids, cytokines, neuropeptides, and neurotransmitters), which constitute the molecular basis of a complex bidirectional response

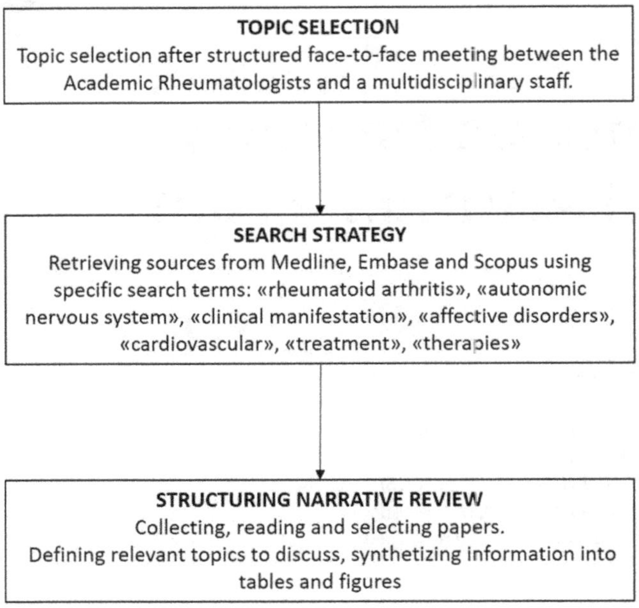

FIGURE 1 | The flow diagram of the narrative review process.

to homeostasis perturbations induced by infection or inflammation. These findings have led to an innovative research field in RA focused on the emerging concept of "immuno-autonomics," reflecting the anatomical and functional linkage of the immune system to the nervous system (5). With the understanding of the relevance of this connection, we may consider if and where the ANS is disrupted in RA and hence which therapeutic implications might be relevant. Whether ANS impairment is the result of chronic inflammation or a primitive alteration that affects immune system functioning, disease onset, and severity remains to be established. In this narrative review (**Figure 1**) (6), we discuss and review the ongoing progress in this field, focusing mainly on current knowledge of the potential connections between ANS and the pathogenesis and clinical manifestations of RA. We then consider the potential innovative therapeutic prospects that target this pathway.

RELEVANCE OF THE AUTONOMIC NERVOUS SYSTEM TO THE PATHOGENESIS OF RHEUMATOID ARTHRITIS

The ANS operates through visceral reflex arcs mediated by cholinergic and catecholaminergic signaling (**Figure 2**). Communication between the ANS and the immune system occurs in two main ways: (i) via direct innervation of the lymphoid organs by the efferent sympathetic nervous system (SNS) [postganglionic noradrenergic fibers innervate the bone marrow, thymus, spleen, and lymph nodes by liberating noradrenaline (NA), neuropeptides (substance P, somatostatin, vasoactive intestinal peptide, and neuropeptide Y), neurokinins, and opioids whose receptors are expressed on immune cells] and (ii) by indirect humoral action mediated by NA (liberated into the bloodstream after medullary activation by the SNS) and steroids [due to activation of the hypothalamic–pituitary–adrenal (HPA) axis neuroendocrine response] (7, 8).

Via beta-2 adrenergic receptors, NA inhibits lymphocyte proliferation, the release of pro-inflammatory cytokines [interleukin (IL)-2, IL-12, interferon gamma, and tumor necrosis factor (TNF)-α], chemotaxis, the activity of natural killer cells and T lymphocytes, and the production of antibodies by B cells. It also stimulates anti-inflammatory cytokines (IL-4, IL-5, and IL-10). Not only postganglionic fibers but also lymphocytes can release NA and acetylcholine, thereby regulating some immune functions in autocrine and paracrine ways (7, 8).

Conversely, the immune system is capable of communicating with the nervous system, mainly via HPA axis activation by pro-inflammatory cytokines and afferent vagal fibers. Neurons express pattern recognition receptors, including toll-like and cytokine receptors (e.g., TNF-R and type 1 IL-1 receptors) (9, 10). This dialog extends beyond the HPA axis; cytokines also directly influence the cerebral cortex and primitive brain (the limbic system, brain stem, and hypothalamus). Cerebral manifestations such as fever, illness, attention deficit, anorexia, and disrupted interaction with external stimuli are examples of their effects during the acute phase of immune activation. In efforts to discern the physiology and pathology of RA, the identification of specific reflexes and pathways is fundamental. A "cholinergic anti-inflammatory pathway," named after its principal mediator acetylcholine, has been described; its identification has led to the understanding of the "inflammatory reflex" (11). This neural circuit, like other visceral reflex arcs, includes afferent and efferent arms. Vagus afferent fibers are activated peripherally by products of inflammation and then the signal travels to the nucleus tractus solitarius; once the stimulus has been relayed and integrated by other nuclei in the brain stem or hypothalamus (e.g., the rostral ventrolateral medulla and locus coeruleus) (12, 13), the efferent signal leaves the nucleus ambiguus and dorsal motor nucleus and travels back through the vagus nerve until it reaches the celiac ganglia (13, 14). There, preganglionic cholinergic fibers form synapses with adrenergic interneurons, whose splenic fibers end up in the white pulp of the spleen and interact, via NA release, with beta-2 adrenergic receptors of a specific T cell subset. The latter is distinguished by the expression of choline acetyltransferase and when activated induces acetylcholine biosynthesis and release, which in turn stimulates macrophages of the red pulp binding alpha-7 subunit of nicotinic acetylcholine receptors (α7nAChRs) toward an anti-inflammatory immune response (15, 16). The anti-inflammatory signal may bypass the vagus efferent fibers, traveling from the preganglionic fibers of the sympathetic chain directly to the interneurons of the celiac ganglia.

Thus, under basal conditions, the vagus nerve senses the precise location of nascent inflammation and rapidly tonically dampens the overactivation of the innate immune response (17). As the major regulator of the peripheral nervous system (PNS), the vagus modulates inflammation in many anatomical regions, comprising the liver (14), heart (18), pancreas (19), and gastrointestinal tract (20, 21).

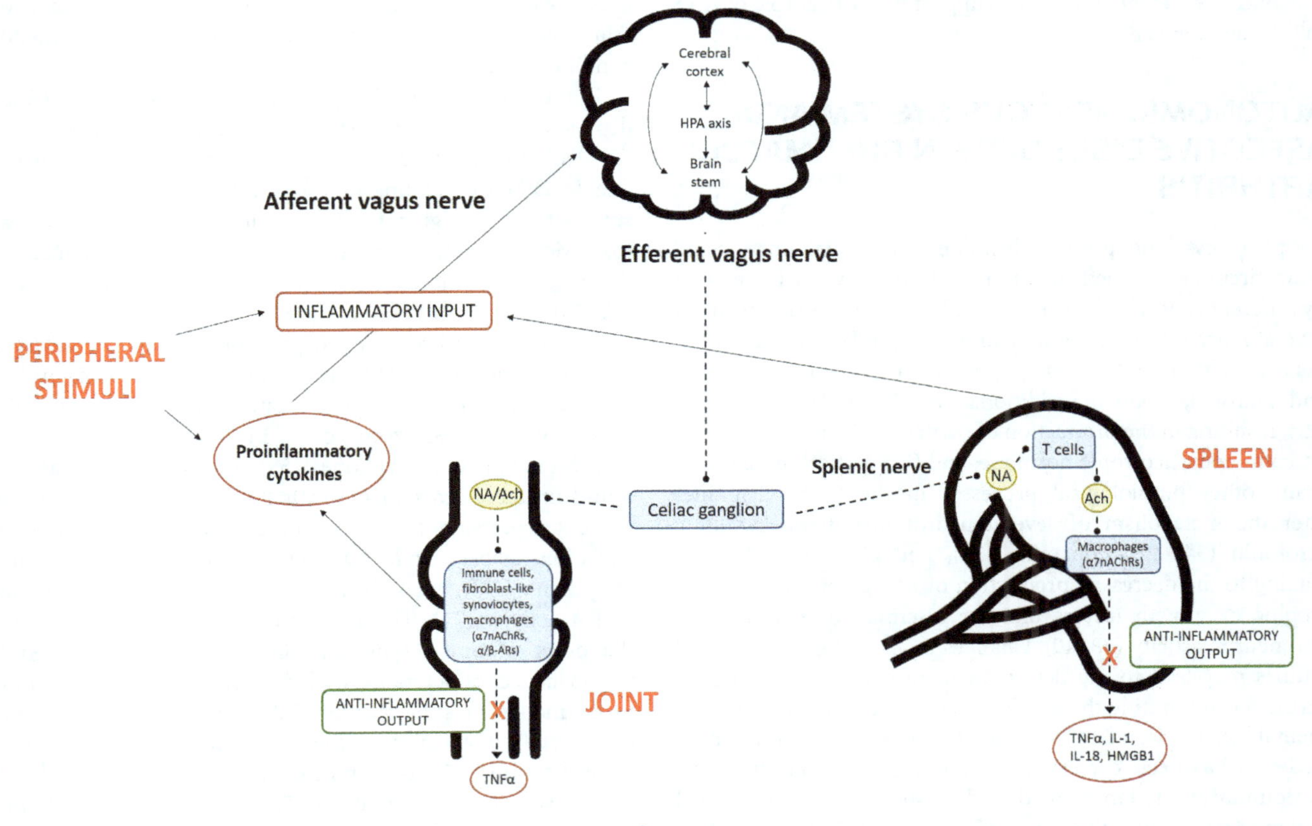

FIGURE 2 | Overview of the inflammatory reflex in rheumatoid arthritis (RA). The central nervous system (CNS) detects peripheral inflammation through the afferent vagus nerve and pro-inflammatory cytokines. The signals act at different levels via (i) activation of the hypothalamic–pituitary–adrenal (HPA) axis, which reduces inflammation; (ii) the cerebral cortex; and (iii) nuclei in the brain stem. The efferent branch of the vagus nerve is activated via the activation of alpha-7 subunit of nicotinic acetylcholine receptors (α7nAChRs) on macrophages, resulting in decreased cytokine production. This mechanism is called the "cholinergic anti-inflammatory pathway." The combination of inflammation in peripheral tissues, signaling of this information to the brain, and the subsequent efferent neuronal response comprises the "inflammatory reflex." The activation of α7nAChRs on macrophages can occur locally in the RA joint or in the spleen. The sympathetic fibers of the splenic nerve are activated in the celiac ganglion, leading to noradrenaline (NA) production in the spleen. NA binds to α/β-adrenergic receptors (α/β-ARs) on choline acetyltransferase-positive T cells, which then produce the anti-inflammatory parasympathetic neurotransmitter acetylcholine (Ach), in turn activating α7nAChRs and leading to the reduced production of pro-inflammatory cytokines. In the joint, the activation of a7nAChRs on fibroblast-like synoviocytes or other immune cells also reduces cytokine production. TNF, tumor necrosis factor; IL, interleukin; HMGB1, high mobility group box 1.

The establishment and maintenance of a chronic response involves humoral neuroendocrine mechanisms. This cooperation not only affects innate immunity but also modulates cell trafficking and the lymphoid architecture, ultimately leading to the regulation of humoral immunity and possibly the prevention of T cell-mediated tissue damage (22, 23).

Autonomic imbalance seems to be an early finding, rather than the result of chronic inflammation, in patients with RA. In a prospective cohort study, in which ANS activity was assessed using a validated method via the measurement of subjects' resting heart rate (HR) and heart rate variability (HRV), individuals at risk of RA who subsequently developed arthritis had significantly higher resting HRs than healthy subjects (24). This finding is in agreement with those from other studies, which reflect reduced PNS activity and hence an impaired inflammatory reflex, in patients with RA (25, 26). The early impairment of the PNS in RA, even before the fulfillment of the disease classification criteria (27), is consistent with the correlation between increased inflammatory status and decreased parasympathetic activity observed in healthy subjects in large observational studies (28–30). In detail, levels of inflammatory markers [C-reactive protein (CRP) and IL-6] are inversely related to HRV in young adults (29), and circulating TNF level is an independent predictor of depressed HRV (31), reinforcing the concept of a complex dialog between immunity and the ANS.

As the PNS and SNS work together, we would expect the SNS to be less active when the PNS is impaired. Contrary to this expectation, the SNS has been found to be overactive in patients with RA and high NA levels (25), rendering comprehension of its pathogenetic role difficult (32). One explanation could involve a difference in intracellular signaling (5). Splenic beta-2 adrenergic receptors usually promote a T helper (Th) 2 and T regulatory (Treg) response via G-coupled proteins and protein kinase A pathways. However, the scenario in which the SNS seems to be chronically activated may entail the downregulation of beta-2 adrenergic receptors and a shift toward Th1 and/or Th17 immune responses via mitogen-activated protein kinase pathways (5).

Collectively taken, these data support the critical role of ANS in RA pathogenic network.

AUTONOMIC NERVOUS SYSTEM AND AFFECTIVE DISORDERS IN RHEUMATOID ARTHRITIS

Peripheral cytokines profoundly influence neuronal function and brain circuitry. As briefly mentioned above, they reach the brain by different routes and, once there, affect brain function through several mechanisms. They may directly stimulate (i) the central nervous system (CNS) cell population (microglia, astrocytes, and neurons), producing additional cytokines (33); (ii) the HPA axis, resulting in the production of corticotropin-releasing factor and adrenocorticotropic hormone; and (iii) cortisol, influencing many other physiological processes in the CNS. Cytokines alter the metabolism of several neurotransmitters, including serotonin (34, 35), dopamine (35), and glutamate (36, 37), leading to the decreased production of norepinephrine and the trophic or growth factors that are essential for neurogenesis and neuroplasticity (38–40). Changes in all of these factors and amines may lead to the development of psychiatric disorders, further corroborating the link between cytokine increments and mental health. In many studies, the continuous elevation of IL levels has been correlated with impairments in structures profoundly affected in mood disorders, such as the hippocampal region (41, 42) and other areas of the brain (43–45), as well as changes in functional connectivity (46, 47).

In the CIA model, researchers observed exacerbated symptomatology in association with greater cytokine production in mice lacking α7nAChR, suggesting that nicotinic receptor expression is relevant in RA and that the activation of these receptors would have beneficial effects. Interestingly, cholinergic agonists suppressed inflammatory cytokine production in RA whole blood cultures (48). Choline acetyltransferase expression was observed in fibroblast-like synoviocytes and mononuclear cells in RA and osteoarthritis synovial biopsy samples, suggesting that local acetylcholine production contributes to the regulation of joint inflammation by the aforementioned "cholinergic anti-inflammatory pathway" (49). Although the activation of α7nAChR leads to control of the degree of inflammation, the effects of this receptor's action on central neurons, brain functionality, and related cognitive behaviors have not been examined. In general, results indicate that (i) muscarinic agonist administration, (ii) electrical vagus nerve stimulation (VNS) to activate preganglionic parasympathetic nerves, and (iii) treatment with nAChR agonists can all act systemically (although not necessarily identically) to reduce the production of inflammatory cytokines (presumably mostly by macrophages).

Abundant data support associations between autoimmune diseases and psychiatric disorders, with immune activation identified as the common core feature (50, 51). The prominence of psychiatric comorbidities, including major depressive disorder (MDD), bipolar disorder, and anxiety disorders (ADs), in the presence of autoimmune diseases such as RA supports the theory that affective disorders can be considered to be inflammatory conditions (52).

From an epidemiological point of view, concomitant RA and depression has been reported in 6.8–66.2% of patients (53–62). Risk factors for MDD onset in patients with RA include female sex (63, 64), unmarried status, the lack of sufficient social support (65), a high rate of disability (66), and chronic pain (67). Moreover, the presence of depressive symptoms increases the risk of suicide in subjects, and especially women, with RA (68).

In most described cases, depression appears secondary to RA development (69–72). Several pathogenetic mechanisms have been proposed to explain this association. From a neurobiological perspective, reduced expression of BDNF, but not serum levels of pro-inflammatory cytokines (59) or TNF-α (57), has been found in depressed patients with RA with respect to subjects without depression. In contrast, other studies have documented a relationship between MDD and the inflammatory state, defined by plasma CRP levels (73) or indirectly via clinical indices of RA activity (74). The implication of over-inflammation in the onset of mood symptoms in RA is also supported by the evidence of alterations in the micro-structure of brain white matter in subjects with RA and comorbid depression as a result of vasculitis, ischemic brain lesions, and dots of demyelination (75). In contrast, one study failed to identify shared genetic vulnerability to RA and MDD (76). From a psychological perspective, the RA self-schema construct seems to predict the onset of depression. Interpersonal conflicts seem to increase the risk of depression in patients with RA. Vulnerability to depressive symptoms in patients with RA appears to be related to functional disabilities (59, 77–79) and pain (78, 80–82) caused by the disease, although some researchers failed to find an association between RA activity or severity and depression (56, 81, 83).

Comorbid depression increases social impairment (84, 85) and disability (86) in patients with RA. Functional capacity seems to be more compromised in women than in men with concomitant RA and MDD (63). The occurrence of depression in patients with RA worsens the subjective sensation of pain (87–90), thereby encouraging the abuse of analgesic compounds (91, 92). After all, the association between depression and pain sensitivity is already known within the framework of fibromyalgia (93). Of note, the presence of depressive symptoms in musculoskeletal pathologies even reach 81.8% as reported in a recent study (94), where a correlation between the severity of depressive symptoms and fibromyalgia was also identified. Although most studies have focused on the effects of RA on mental health, some authors have hypothesized conversely that depression directly influences RA activity and the number of compromised joints (95–97). In addition, comorbid depression in patients with RA favors the onset of medical complications such as atherosclerosis (98) and myocardial infarction (99), resulting in increased lethality (100, 101). Depressive symptoms also may prevent patients' treatment adherence, thereby worsening the prognosis of RA (96, 102).

Taken as a whole, these data indicate that depression worsens the quality of life (90, 103) and general health status (104) of subjects with RA.

Depression is often underestimated in patients with RA, delaying its proper management (94, 105). The treatment of depressive symptoms seems to ameliorate the clinical symptoms of RA (106), although some data contradict the existence of this effect (107). Antidepressants demonstrated to be effective in cases of RA-MDD comorbidity include dothiepin (108) and sertraline (109), eventually combined with cognitive behavioral treatment (107). Non-pharmacological strategies, including yoga, mindfulness meditation, and emotion regulation therapy, have been shown to significantly ameliorate mood symptoms and inflammatory status in patients with RA (110, 111). Finally, immunomodulating drugs, such as anti-TNF-α drugs (105, 112), anti-IL-6 monoclonal antibodies (113), and other biologics (114), appear to ameliorate anxiety and depressive symptoms in patients with RA. Of note, in line with the autonomic dysfunctions already mentioned for RA, VNS was proposed as a treatment for depression in the light of its anti-inflammatory effect (115). This convergence of the efficacy of VNS both for RA and depression opens up extremely promising therapeutic prospective for the treatment of subjects suffering from RA and mood symptoms (116).

ADs have the common psychopathological nucleus of anxiety and partly shared neurobiological abnormalities. They include panic disorder, social phobia (SP) (also known as social anxiety disorder), and generalized anxiety disorder (GAD). Their prevalence in RA ranges from 13 to 70% (53, 55, 65, 78, 117–119) with higher incidence and prevalence compared to the general population (120). Anxious states often occur concomitantly with depressive symptoms (54, 65). SP seems to be more common in individuals with RA than in those with other autoimmune conditions (121, 122). ADs are considered to be a risk factor for the future development of RA (120) and appear to negatively affect its course, worsening functional disabilities (78, 90, 123) and quality of life (90, 103, 124, 125) and changing pain perceptions (82, 89, 126). Moreover, psychological stress and anxiety symptoms were reported to be the most frequent causes of joint symptom exacerbation (127). In support of these clinical data, patients with RA and anxiety were found to have higher serum levels of IL-17 than those without AD (128).

Some authors have hypothesized that ADs in patients with RA are triggered by psychosocial factors, such as pronounced neuroticism, a lower educational level, and poor social support (69). According to this explanation, RA-associated disability in case of AD comorbidity is attributable more to psychological factors implicated in all chronic diseases than to the worsening of symptoms as a result of an increased pro-inflammatory state (129).

Proper AD treatment in patients with RA is essential to prevent functional decline (130) and poor adherence to treatment (131). Some drugs prescribed for RA, such as anti-TNF-α medications, seem to have beneficial effects on anxiety symptoms (112), and their discontinuation is related to the worsening of anxiety (132).

AUTONOMIC NERVOUS SYSTEM AND CARDIOVASCULAR MANIFESTATIONS IN RHEUMATOID ARTHRITIS

Cardiovascular autonomic dysfunction in RA has been investigated by measuring heart rate (HR) and heart rate variability (HRV) (24). The link between the cardiovascular system and ANS imbalance in RA could partly explain the well-documented augmented cardiovascular disease and RA-related mortality, not fully justified by traditional risk factors.

It is well known how chronic inflammation influences the development of cardiovascular disease (CVD) by promoting atherosclerosis, myocardial remodeling, and insulin resistance and by modifying lipid levels and function and oxidative stress (133). Furthermore, multimodality imaging is useful to identify high-risk patients who benefit from preventive strategies or treatment intervention (134); the link between brain and heart damage in RA has been documented by magnetic resonance imaging (135).

Fundamentally, we have limited understanding of the mechanisms underpinning the connections between ANS and CVD. An extensive assessment of ANS by means of HR, cardiac/sympathetic baroreflex, and muscle sympathetic nerve activity (MSNA) was carried out in 30 RA patients (normo- and hypertensive) matched with a control group. Regardless the presence of hypertension, HR and sympathetic activity were increased and cardiac baroreflex sensitivity was reduced in RA patients, while sympathetic baroreflex sensitivity was preserved. Moreover, these findings were correlated with pain (VAS) and inflammation (CPR). Hence, a heightened sympathetic outflow was confirmed along with a reduced arterial baroreflex control of the heart both linked directly to RA symptoms, excluding the bias hypertension, a common cardiovascular risk factor (136).

Although data suggest that ANS imbalance is detrimental for cardiovascular disease, including cardiac arrhythmias, hypertension (137), and increased mortality (138, 139), breaking through the original trigger of this vicious circle with ultimate damage of the cardiovascular system is particularly difficult. Moreover, patients with RA without clinical cardiovascular disease have reduced left ventricular systolic function assessed by global longitudinal strain by speckle-tracking echocardiography, and it is related with disease activity (140).

Another study showed how a reduced coronary microvascular perfusion in RA patients, in terms of subendocardial viability ratio, associates with markers of disease activity and classical CVD risk factors, including heart rate. This reinforces the hypothesis that inflammation, by the stimulation of ANS, may impair myocardial perfusion (141).

Finally, according to previous literature, the evidence of cardiovascular autonomic dysfunction might be used to identify patients with RA who respond better to TNF inhibitors (25, 142). In particular, a low parasympathetic outflow and a high sympathetic outflow were associated with a poor anti-TNF response, making HRV a promising useful predictor of outcome, with great benefits for overall costs and quality-adjusted life-years (QALYs) (143).

TABLE 1 | Targeting vagus nerve by electrical stimulation in rheumatoid arthritis.

Clinical trial	Study population	Device and regimen	Primary endpoint	Safety data	Length
Koopman 2016 (151)	17 active RA (7 naïve to bDMARDs and 10 bDMARDs failure) Open label	Cyberonics device around the cervical vagus nerve; implantation under general anesthesia. Day 0–28 daily stimulation with escalating intensity	DAS28-CRP at week 6 (baseline 6.05 ± 0.18 at day −21 vs. 4.16 ± 0.39 at day 42, $p < 0.001$)	No serious adverse events, mild/moderate events associated with implanting device	12 weeks
Addorisio 2019 (152)	9 active RA Randomized cross-over	Non-invasive vibrotactile auricular stimulation Stimulation twice daily for 2 days	DAS28-CRP at week 1 (baseline 4.19 ± 0.33 vs. 2.79 ± 0.21 at day 7, $p < 0.01$)	No adverse events	1 week
Marsal 2020* (153)	30 active RA Open label	Non-invasive vibrotactile auricular stimulation Data on regimen stimulation not available	DAS28-CRP at week 12–1.40 ($p < 0.01$)	1 device superficial skin abrasion resolved without intervention	12 weeks
Genovese 2020 (154)	14 active RA with insufficient response ≧ 2 b/tsDMARDs Stage 1 open label; stage 2 randomized, multicentre, sham-controlled trial	Miniaturized VNS device implanted on the left cervical vagus nerve	Safety and tolerability of the implantation surgical procedure, device and the active treatment	Horner's syndrome, procedural pain, contact dermatitis, vocal cord paralysis. All adverse events were related to the surgical procedure and resolved without permanent clinically significant sequelae	12 weeks

*RA, rheumatoid arthritis; DAS, disease activity score; CRP, C-reactive protein; bDMARD, biological disease-modifying anti-rheumatic drug; tsDMARDS, targeted synthetic DMARDs; VNS, vagus nerve stimulation. *Results only available from the congress abstract.*

Furthermore, cardiovascular autonomic imbalance associates with comorbidities including depressive and anxiety disturbances compared to healthy controls (144). Finally, looking at a therapeutic prospective, non-pharmacological intervention such as exercise training, given its well-known benefits on cardiovascular autonomic function, might help restore ANS imbalance, increasing vagal-related indices in RA with consequent potential benefit on pain and inflammation (145). Likewise, ANS imbalance could be partially restored by optimizing pain management (146).

IMPLICATIONS FOR TREATMENT AND FUTURE PERSPECTIVES

Altered ANS parameters have been associated with increased Disease Activity Score-28 (DAS-28), CRP, and erythrocyte sedimentation rate (25, 147). Seropositive RA patients are more prone to ANS dysfunction and more likely to experience the amelioration of cardiovascular autonomic neuropathy when treated with synthetic and biologic disease-modifying antirheumatic drugs (DMARDS) than seronegative patients with RA (148, 149). Thus, seropositivity, along with disease activity and pro-inflammatory cytokine levels, is predictive of autonomic dysfunction (150). Moreover, in patients with RA and ankylosing spondylitis, HRV was shown to predict the clinical response to anti-TNF therapy; specifically, patients with more vagal activity responded better to this treatment (142). Biologic, and to a lesser extent synthetic, DMARDs significantly improved autonomic neuropathy, including all of its parasympathetic, sympathetic, and sudomotor components, in patients with RA and ankylosing spondylitis (148).

Multiple strategies can be used to achieve these goals. VNS can dampen inflammation early in a discrete and localized manner. Administration of the specific agonist of splenic α7nAChR acts on downstream of the pathway. Antagonization of the SNS is a possible alternative that should be explored. As shown in **Table 1**, four clinical trials examining VNS have been published (151–154), and one of these has been presented at the last EULAR e-congress (153). As they involved the use of different devices, modalities, timing, and stimulation sites, comparison of their results is (152) not feasible, but the researchers observed significant and rapid declines in the production of pro-inflammatory cytokines such as TNF-α, IL-6, and IL-1b after VNS in patients with epilepsy, those with RA, and healthy subjects (151, 152). In the first trial, VNS was performed directly via an electronic device (Cyberonics) implanted under general anesthesia. Three helical coiled cuffs around the vagus nerve and a lead were then tunneled subcutaneously from the neck and connected to a pulse generator placed in a subcutaneous pocket on the chest wall (151). The only adverse events reported were mild/moderate and related to the surgical implanting approach. In the most recent trial, a MicroRegulator device was implanted on the left cervical vagus nerve. The device was well tolerated without adverse events. The sample size was small, but VNS reduced disease activity in 50% of the highly drug refractory RA patients (154). In the other two trials, a non-invasive device consisting of a hand-held probe with a tip producing radial displacement in a circular pattern at the probe was used. Transcutaneous auricular VNS consisted of the application of electrical signals to the cutaneous territory supplied by the auricular branch of the vagus nerve at the cymba concha (152, 153). In all trials, disease activity was rapidly attenuated after VNS in patients with active RA (biologic-naïve subjects and those for whom multiple treatments had failed).

Considering the consistent percentage of patients who do not respond at all to the available drugs or have unsatisfactory responses, have gradual loss of responsiveness over time, or have drug-related adverse events, a non-pharmacological approach such as bioelectronics might be a useful further tool in the successful expansion of the therapeutic armamentarium of RA.

Bioelectronic medicine, based on neuromodulation of the nervous system restoring organ and immune system function, is a new potential tantalizing and promising field. In particular, the use of non-invasive devices has lesser adverse effects than drugs and has greater treatment adherence. Naturally, the therapeutic potential of immuno-autonomics has been further demonstrated, and the optimal neurostimulation parameters to achieve and maintain significant clinical changes are still unknown.

CONCLUSION

The innovative view of the ANS and RA axis described here allows for the development of new strategies for RA management. The ANS influences key aspects of joint pathophysiology and may be a target of novel therapeutic approaches. The emergence of immuno-autonomics and encouraging results of clinical trials could have extraordinary implications for RA monitoring and treatment. Further research in this field will be useful to understand the full potential of therapeutic models based on the brain–joint axis, with the integration of different findings.

AUTHOR CONTRIBUTIONS

All authors listed have made a substantial, direct and intellectual contribution to the work, and approved it for publication.

REFERENCES

1. Safiri S, Kolahi AA, Hoy D, Smith E, Bettampadi D, Mansournia MA, et al. Global, regional and national burden of rheumatoid arthritis 1990-2017: a systematic analysis of the Global Burden of Disease study 2017. *Ann Rheum Dis.* (2019) 78:1463–71. doi: 10.1136/annrheumdis-2019-215920
2. Cao X, Aballay A. Neural inhibition of dopaminergic signaling enhances immunity in a cell-non-autonomous manner. *Curr Biol.* (2016) 26:2398. doi: 10.1016/j.cub.2016.08.046
3. Aydemir M, Yazisiz V, Basarici I, Avci AB, Erbasan F, Belgi A, et al. Cardiac autonomic profile in rheumatoid arthritis and systemic lupus erythematosus. *Lupus.* (2010) 19:255–61. doi: 10.1177/0961203309351540
4. Stojanovich L, Milovanovich B, de Luka SR, Popovich-Kuzmanovich D, Bisenich V, Djukanovich B, et al. Cardiovascular autonomic dysfunction in systemic lupus, rheumatoid arthritis, primary Sjogren syndrome and other autoimmune diseases. *Lupus.* (2007) 16:181–5. doi: 10.1177/0961203306076223
5. Taylor PC, Holman AJ. Rheumatoid arthritis and the emergence of immuno-autonomics. *Rheumatology.* (2019) 58:2079–80. doi: 10.1093/rheumatology/key225
6. Gasparyan AY, Ayvazyan L, Blackmore H, Kitas GD. Writing a narrative biomedical review: considerations for authors, peer reviewers, and editors. *Rheumatol Int.* (2011) 31:1409–17. doi: 10.1007/s00296-011-1999-3
7. Rosas-Ballina M, Olofsson PS, Ochani M, Valdes-Ferrer SI, Levine YA, Reardon C, et al. Acetylcholine-synthesizing T cells relay neural signals in a vagus nerve circuit. *Science.* (2011) 334:98–101. doi: 10.1126/science.1209985
8. Kawashima K, Fujii T, Moriwaki Y, Misawa H. Critical roles of acetylcholine and the muscarinic and nicotinic acetylcholine receptors in the regulation of immune function. *Life Sci.* (2012) 91:1027–32. doi: 10.1016/j.lfs.2012.05.006
9. Wong CH, Jenne CN, Lee WY, Leger C, Kubes P. Functional innervation of hepatic iNKT cells is immunosuppressive following stroke. *Science.* (2011) 334:101–5. doi: 10.1126/science.1210301
10. Li M, Shi J, Tang JR, Chen D, Ai B, Chen J, et al. Effects of complete Freund's adjuvant on immunohistochemical distribution of IL-1beta and IL-1R I in neurons and glia cells of dorsal root ganglion. *Acta Pharmacol Sin.* (2005) 26:192–8. doi: 10.1111/j.1745-7254.2005.00522.x
11. Tracey KJ. The inflammatory reflex. *Nature.* (2002) 420:853–9. doi: 10.1038/nature01321
12. Pavlov VA, Wang H, Czura CJ, Friedman SG, Tracey KJ. The cholinergic anti-inflammatory pathway: a missing link in neuroimmunomodulation. *Mol Med.* (2003) 9:125–34. doi: 10.1007/BF03402177
13. Berthoud HR, Neuhuber WL. Functional and chemical anatomy of the afferent vagal system. *Auton Neurosci.* (2000) 85:1–17. doi: 10.1016/S1566-0702(00)00215-0
14. Borovikova LV, Ivanova S, Zhang M, Yang H, Botchkina GI, Watkins LR, et al. Vagus nerve stimulation attenuates the systemic inflammatory response to endotoxin. *Nature.* (2000) 405:458–62. doi: 10.1038/35013070
15. Wang H, Yu M, Ochani M, Amella CA, Tanovic M, Susarla S, et al. Nicotinic acetylcholine receptor alpha7 subunit is an essential regulator of inflammation. *Nature.* (2003) 421:384–8. doi: 10.1038/nature01339
16. Wang H, Liao H, Ochani M, Justiniani M, Lin X, Yang L, et al. Cholinergic agonists inhibit HMGB1 release and improve survival in experimental sepsis. *Nat Med.* (2004) 10:1216–21. doi: 10.1038/nm1124
17. Rosas-Ballina M, Goldstein RS, Gallowitsch-Puerta M, Yang L, Valdes-Ferrer SI, Patel NB, et al. The selective alpha7 agonist GTS-21 attenuates cytokine production in human whole blood and human monocytes activated by ligands for TLR2, TLR3, TLR4, TLR9, and RAGE. *Mol Med.* (2009) 15:195–202. doi: 10.2119/molmed.2009.00039
18. Bernik TR, Friedman SG, Ochani M, DiRaimo R, Ulloa L, Yang H, et al. Pharmacological stimulation of the cholinergic antiinflammatory pathway. *J Exp Med.* (2002) 195:781–8. doi: 10.1084/jem.20011714
19. van Westerloo DJ, Giebelen IA, Florquin S, Bruno MJ, Larosa GJ, Ulloa L, et al. The vagus nerve and nicotinic receptors modulate experimental pancreatitis severity in mice. *Gastroenterology.* (2006) 130:1822–30. doi: 10.1053/j.gastro.2006.02.022
20. Ghia JE, Blennerhassett P, Collins SM. Vagus nerve integrity and experimental colitis. *Am J Physiol Gastrointest Liver Physiol.* (2007) 293:G560–7. doi: 10.1152/ajpgi.00098.2007
21. Ghia JE, Blennerhassett P, Kumar-Ondiveeran H, Verdu EF, Collins SM. The vagus nerve: a tonic inhibitory influence associated with inflammatory bowel disease in a murine model. *Gastroenterology.* (2006) 131:1122–30. doi: 10.1053/j.gastro.2006.08.016
22. Nakai A, Hayano Y, Furuta F, Noda M, Suzuki K. Control of lymphocyte egress from lymph nodes through beta2-adrenergic receptors. *J Exp Med.* (2014) 211:2583–98. doi: 10.1084/jem.20141132

23. Mina-Osorio P, Rosas-Ballina M, Valdes-Ferrer SI, Al-Abed Y, Tracey KJ, Diamond B. Neural signaling in the spleen controls B-cell responses to blood-borne antigen. *Mol Med.* (2012) 18:618–27. doi: 10.2119/molmed.2012.00027
24. Koopman FA, Tang MW, Vermeij J, de Hair MJ, Choi IY, Vervoordeldonk MJ, et al. Autonomic dysfunction precedes development of rheumatoid arthritis: a prospective cohort study. *EBioMedicine.* (2016) 6:231–7. doi: 10.1016/j.ebiom.2016.02.029
25. Adlan AM, Lip GY, Paton JF, Kitas GD, Fisher JP. Autonomic function and rheumatoid arthritis: a systematic review. *Semin Arthrit Rheum.* (2014) 44:283–304. doi: 10.1016/j.semarthrit.2014.06.003
26. Koopman FA, Stoof SP, Straub RH, Van Maanen MA, Vervoordeldonk MJ, Tak PP. Restoring the balance of the autonomic nervous system as an innovative approach to the treatment of rheumatoid arthritis. *Mol Med.* (2011) 17:937–48. doi: 10.2119/molmed.2011.00065
27. Koopman FA, van Maanen MA, Vervoordeldonk MJ, Tak PP. Balancing the autonomic nervous system to reduce inflammation in rheumatoid arthritis. *J Intern Med.* (2017) 282:64–75. doi: 10.1111/joim.12626
28. Sajadieh A, Nielsen OW, Rasmussen V, Hein HO, Abedini S, Hansen JF. Increased heart rate and reduced heart-rate variability are associated with subclinical inflammation in middle-aged and elderly subjects with no apparent heart disease. *Eur Heart J.* (2004) 25:363–70. doi: 10.1016/j.ehj.2003.12.003
29. Sloan RP, McCreath H, Tracey KJ, Sidney S, Liu K, Seeman T. RR interval variability is inversely related to inflammatory markers: the CARDIA study. *Mol Med.* (2007) 13:178–84. doi: 10.2119/2006-00112.Sloan
30. Thayer JF, Fischer JE. Heart rate variability, overnight urinary norepinephrine and C-reactive protein: evidence for the cholinergic anti-inflammatory pathway in healthy human adults. *J Intern Med.* (2009) 265:439–47. doi: 10.1111/j.1365-2796.2008.02023.x
31. Malave HA, Taylor AA, Nattama J, Deswal A, Mann DL. Circulating levels of tumor necrosis factor correlate with indexes of depressed heart rate variability: a study in patients with mild-to-moderate heart failure. *Chest.* (2003) 123:716–24. doi: 10.1378/chest.123.3.716
32. Vlcek M, Rovensky J, Blazicek P, Radikova Z, Penesova A, Kerlik J, et al. Sympathetic nervous system response to orthostatic stress in female patients with rheumatoid arthritis. *Ann N Y Acad Sci.* (2008) 1148:556–61. doi: 10.1196/annals.1410.026
33. Loggia ML, Chonde DB, Akeju O, Arabasz G, Catana C, Edwards RR, et al. Evidence for brain glial activation in chronic pain patients. *Brain.* (2015) 138(Pt 3):604–15. doi: 10.1093/brain/awu377
34. Capuron L, Ravaud A, Neveu PJ, Miller AH, Maes M, Dantzer R. Association between decreased serum tryptophan concentrations and depressive symptoms in cancer patients undergoing cytokine therapy. *Mol Psychiatry.* (2002) 7:468–73. doi: 10.1038/sj.mp.4000995
35. Capuron L, Miller AH. Cytokines and psychopathology: lessons from interferon-alpha. *Biol Psychiatry.* (2004) 56:819–24. doi: 10.1016/j.biopsych.2004.02.009
36. Haydon PG, Carmignoto G. Astrocyte control of synaptic transmission and neurovascular coupling. *Physiol Rev.* (2006) 86:1009–31. doi: 10.1152/physrev.00049.2005
37. Yang X, Yang HB, Xie QJ, Liu XH, Hu XD. Peripheral inflammation increased the synaptic expression of NMDA receptors in spinal dorsal horn. *Pain.* (2009) 144:162–9. doi: 10.1016/j.pain.2009.04.005
38. Hayley S, Poulter MO, Merali Z, Anisman H. The pathogenesis of clinical depression: stressor- and cytokine-induced alterations of neuroplasticity. *Neuroscience.* (2005) 135:659–78. doi: 10.1016/j.neuroscience.2005.03.051
39. Barrientos RM, Sprunger DB, Campeau S, Watkins LR, Rudy JW, Maier SF. BDNF mRNA expression in rat hippocampus following contextual learning is blocked by intrahippocampal IL-1beta administration. *J Neuroimmunol.* (2004) 155:119–26. doi: 10.1016/j.jneuroim.2004.06.009
40. Duman RS, Monteggia LM. A neurotrophic model for stress-related mood disorders. *Biol Psychiatry.* (2006) 59:1116–27. doi: 10.1016/j.biopsych.2006.02.013
41. Marsland AL, Gianaros PJ, Abramowitch SM, Manuck SB, Hariri AR. Interleukin-6 covaries inversely with hippocampal grey matter volume in middle-aged adults. *Biol Psychiatry.* (2008) 64:484–90. doi: 10.1016/j.biopsych.2008.04.016
42. Zimmerman G, Shaltiel G, Barbash S, Cohen J, Gasho CJ, Shenhar-Tsarfaty S, et al. Post-traumatic anxiety associates with failure of the innate immune receptor TLR9 to evade the pro-inflammatory NFkappaB pathway. *Transl Psychiatry.* (2012) 2:e78. doi: 10.1038/tp.2012.4
43. Wartolowska K, Hough MG, Jenkinson M, Andersson J, Wordsworth BP, Tracey I. Structural changes of the brain in rheumatoid arthritis. *Arthritis Rheum.* (2012) 64:371–9. doi: 10.1002/art.33326
44. Chang L, Shoptaw S, Normand J. Brain abnormalities in HIV and stimulant users: interventions and prevention. *J Food Drug Anal.* (2013) 21:S7–9. doi: 10.1016/j.jfda.2013.09.021
45. Li Q, Cheung C, Wei R, Cheung V, Hui ES, You Y, et al. Voxel-based analysis of postnatal white matter microstructure in mice exposed to immune challenge in early or late pregnancy. *Neuroimage.* (2010) 52:1–8. doi: 10.1016/j.neuroimage.2010.04.015
46. Baliki MN, Geha PY, Apkarian AV, Chialvo DR. Beyond feeling: chronic pain hurts the brain, disrupting the default-mode network dynamics. *J Neurosci.* (2008) 28:1398–403. doi: 10.1523/JNEUROSCI.4123-07.2008
47. Napadow V, Kim J, Clauw DJ, Harris RE. Decreased intrinsic brain connectivity is associated with reduced clinical pain in fibromyalgia. *Arthritis Rheum.* (2012) 64:2398–403. doi: 10.1002/art.34412
48. Bruchfeld A, Goldstein RS, Chavan S, Patel NB, Rosas-Ballina M, Kohn N, et al. Whole blood cytokine attenuation by cholinergic agonists *ex vivo* and relationship to vagus nerve activity in rheumatoid arthritis. *J Intern Med.* (2010) 268:94–101. doi: 10.1111/j.1365-2796.2010.02226.x
49. Grimsholm O, Rantapaa-Dahlqvist S, Dalen T, Forsgren S. Unexpected finding of a marked non-neuronal cholinergic system in human knee joint synovial tissue. *Neurosci Lett.* (2008) 442:128–33. doi: 10.1016/j.neulet.2008.06.082
50. Bennett FC, Molofsky AV. The immune system and psychiatric disease: a basic science perspective. *Clin Exp Immunol.* (2019) 197:294–307. doi: 10.1111/cei.13334
51. Jeppesen R, Benros ME. Autoimmune diseases and psychotic disorders. *Front Psychiatry.* (2019) 10:131. doi: 10.3389/fpsyt.2019.00131
52. Bauer ME, Teixeira AL. Inflammation in psychiatric disorders: what comes first? *Ann N Y Acad Sci.* (2019) 1437:57–67. doi: 10.1111/nyas.13712
53. el-Miedany YM, el-Rasheed AH. Is anxiety a more common disorder than depression in rheumatoid arthritis? *Joint Bone Spine.* (2002) 69:300–6. doi: 10.1016/S1297-319X(02)00368-8
54. VanDyke MM, Parker JC, Smarr KL, Hewett JE, Johnson GE, Slaughter JR, et al. Anxiety in rheumatoid arthritis. *Arthritis Rheum.* (2004) 51:408–12. doi: 10.1002/art.20474
55. Covic T, Cumming SR, Pallant JF, Manolios N, Emery P, Conaghan PG, et al. Depression and anxiety in patients with rheumatoid arthritis: prevalence rates based on a comparison of the Depression, Anxiety and Stress Scale (DASS) and the hospital, Anxiety and Depression Scale (HADS). *BMC Psychiatry.* (2012) 12:6. doi: 10.1186/1471-244X-12-6
56. Sato E, Nishimura K, Nakajima A, Okamoto H, Shinozaki M, Inoue E, et al. Major depressive disorder in patients with rheumatoid arthritis. *Mod Rheumatol.* (2013) 23:237–44. doi: 10.3109/s10165-012-0643-8
57. Uguz F, Kucuk A, Aydogan S, Arslan S, Kurt HG, Toker A, et al. Is major depression associated with serum levels of tumor necrosis factor-alpha in patients with rheumatoid arthritis? *J Psychosom Res.* (2015) 79:530–2. doi: 10.1016/j.jpsychores.2015.09.011
58. Katz P, Margaretten M, Trupin L, Schmajuk G, Yazdany J, Yelin E. Role of sleep disturbance, depression, obesity, and physical inactivity in fatigue in rheumatoid arthritis. *Arthritis Care Res.* (2016) 68:81–90. doi: 10.1002/acr.22577
59. Cheon YH, Lee SG, Kim M, Kim HO, Sun Suh Y, Park KS, et al. The association of disease activity, pro-inflammatory cytokines, and neurotrophic factors with depression in patients with rheumatoid arthritis. *Brain Behav Immun.* (2018) 73:274–81. doi: 10.1016/j.bbi.2018.05.012
60. Kwiatkowska B, Klak A, Raciborski F, Maslinska M. The prevalence of depression and insomnia symptoms among patients with rheumatoid arthritis and osteoarthritis in Poland: a case control study. *Psychol Health Med.* (2019) 24:333–43. doi: 10.1080/13548506.2018.1529325
61. Milic V, Grujic M, Barisic J, Marinkovic-Eric J, Duisin D, Cirkovic A, et al. Personality, depression and anxiety in primary Sjogren's syndrome

- Association with sociodemographic factors and comorbidity. *PLoS ONE.* (2019) 14:e0210466. doi: 10.1371/journal.pone.0210466

62. Nichter B, Norman S, Haller M, Pietrzak RH. Physical health burden of PTSD, depression, and their comorbidity in the U.S. veteran population: morbidity, functioning, and disability. *J Psychosom Res.* (2019) 124:109744. doi: 10.1016/j.jpsychores.2019.109744
63. Aurrecoechea E, Llorca Diaz J, Diez Lizuain ML, McGwin G Jr, Calvo-Alen J. Gender-associated comorbidities in rheumatoid arthritis and their impact on outcome: data from GENIRA. *Rheumatol Int.* (2017) 37:479–85. doi: 10.1007/s00296-016-3628-7
64. Hsieh MC, Hsu CW, Lu MC, Koo M. Increased risks of psychiatric disorders in patients with primary Sjogren's syndrome-a secondary cohort analysis of nationwide, population-based health claim data. *Clin Rheumatol.* (2019) 38:3195–203. doi: 10.1007/s10067-019-04705-z
65. Lok EY, Mok CC, Cheng CW, Cheung EF. Prevalence and determinants of psychiatric disorders in patients with rheumatoid arthritis. *Psychosomatics.* (2010) 51:338-e8. doi: 10.1176/appi.psy.51.4.338
66. Khongsaengdao B, Louthrenoo W, Srisurapanont M. Depression in Thai patients with rheumatoid arthritis. *J Med Assoc Thai.* (2000) 83:743–7.
67. Katon WJ, Buchwald DS, Simon GE, Russo JE, Mease PJ. Psychiatric illness in patients with chronic fatigue and those with rheumatoid arthritis. *J Gen Int Med.* (1991) 6:277–85. doi: 10.1007/BF02597420
68. Timonen M, Viilo K, Hakko H, Sarkioja T, Ylikulju M, Meyer-Rochow VB, et al. Suicides in persons suffering from rheumatoid arthritis. *Rheumatology.* (2003) 42:287–91. doi: 10.1093/rheumatology/keg082
69. Evers AW, Kraaimaat FW, Geenen R, Jacobs JW, Bijlsma JW. Longterm predictors of anxiety and depressed mood in early rheumatoid arthritis: a 3 and 5 year followup. *J Rheumatol.* (2002) 29:2327–36.
70. Covic T, Adamson B, Spencer D, Howe G. A biopsychosocial model of pain and depression in rheumatoid arthritis: a 12-month longitudinal study. *Rheumatology.* (2003) 42:1287–94. doi: 10.1093/rheumatology/keg369
71. Wang SL, Chang CH, Hu LY, Tsai SJ, Yang AC, You ZH. Risk of developing depressive disorders following rheumatoid arthritis: a nationwide population-based study. *PLoS ONE.* (2014) 9:e107791. doi: 10.1371/journal.pone.0107791
72. Ryu E, Chamberlain AM, Pendegraft RS, Petterson TM, Bobo WV, Pathak J. Quantifying the impact of chronic conditions on a diagnosis of major depressive disorder in adults: a cohort study using linked electronic medical records. *BMC Psychiatry.* (2016) 16:114. doi: 10.1186/s12888-016-0821-x
73. Kojima M, Kojima T, Suzuki S, Oguchi T, Oba M, Tsuchiya H, et al. Depression, inflammation, and pain in patients with rheumatoid arthritis. *Arthritis Rheum.* (2009) 61:1018–24. doi: 10.1002/art.24647
74. Kuriya B, Joshi R, Movahedi M, Rampakakis E, Sampalis JS, Bombardier C, et al. High disease activity is associated with self-reported depression and predicts persistent depression in early rheumatoid arthritis: results from the ontario best practices research initiative. *J Rheumatol.* (2018) 45:1101–8. doi: 10.3899/jrheum.171195
75. Hamed SA, Selim ZI, Elattar AM, Elserogy YM, Ahmed EA, Mohamed HO. Assessment of biocorrelates for brain involvement in female patients with rheumatoid arthritis. *Clin Rheumatol.* (2012) 31:123–32. doi: 10.1007/s10067-011-1795-1
76. Tylee DS, Sun J, Hess JL, Tahir MA, Sharma E, Malik R, et al. Genetic correlations among psychiatric and immune-related phenotypes based on genome-wide association data. *Am J Med Genet Part B Neuropsychiatr Genet.* (2018) 177:641–57. doi: 10.1002/ajmg.b.32652
77. Doeglas DM, Suurmeijer TP, van den Heuvel WJ, Krol B, van Rijswijk MH, van Leeuwen MA, et al. Functional ability, social support, and depression in rheumatoid arthritis. *Qual Life Res.* (2004) 13:1053–65. doi: 10.1023/B:QURE.0000031339.04589.63
78. Zyrianova Y, Kelly BD, Gallagher C, McCarthy C, Molloy MG, Sheehan J, et al. Depression and anxiety in rheumatoid arthritis: the role of perceived social support. *Ir J Med Sci.* (2006) 175:32–6. doi: 10.1007/BF03167946
79. Zagar I, Delimar V, Pap M, Peric D, Laktasic Zerjavic N, Peric P. Prevalence and correlation of depressive symptoms with functional scores, therapy and disease activity among croatian patients with rheumatoid arthritis: a preliminary study. *Psychiatr Danub.* (2018) 30:452–8. doi: 10.24869/psyd.2018.452
80. Cakirbay H, Bilici M, Kavakci O, Cebi A, Guler M, Tan U. Sleep quality and immune functions in rheumatoid arthritis patients with and without major depression. *Int J Neurosci.* (2004) 114:245–56. doi: 10.1080/00207450490269471
81. Melikoglu MA, Melikoglu M. The relationship between disease activity and depression in patients with Behcet disease and rheumatoid arthritis. *Rheumatol Int.* (2010) 30:941–6. doi: 10.1007/s00296-009-1080-7
82. Ryan S, McGuire B. Psychological predictors of pain severity, pain interference, depression, and anxiety in rheumatoid arthritis patients with chronic pain. *Br J Health Psychol.* (2016) 21:336–50. doi: 10.1111/bjhp.12171
83. Santos EF, Duarte CM, Ferreira RO, Pinto AM, Geenen R, da Silva JP. Multifactorial explanatory model of depression in patients with rheumatoid arthritis: a structural equation approach. *Clin Exp Rheumatol.* (2019) 37:641–8.
84. Dickens C, Jackson J, Tomenson B, Hay E, Creed F. Association of depression and rheumatoid arthritis. *Psychosomatics.* (2003) 44:209–15. doi: 10.1176/appi.psy.44.3.209
85. Mok CC, Lok EY, Cheung EF. Concurrent psychiatric disorders are associated with significantly poorer quality of life in patients with rheumatoid arthritis. *Scand J Rheumatol.* (2012) 41:253–9. doi: 10.3109/03009742.2012.664648
86. Soosova MS, Macejova Z, Zamboriova M, Dimunova L. Anxiety and depression in Slovak patients with rheumatoid arthritis. *J Ment Health.* (2017) 26:21–7. doi: 10.1080/09638237.2016.1244719
87. Garip Y, Eser F, Bodur H. Comorbidities in Turkish patients with rheumatoid arthritis: association with the health-related quality of life in terms of disease activity, functional and radiological status, severity of pain, and social and emotional functioning. *Acta Reumatol Port.* (2016) 41:344–9.
88. Zautra AJ, Parrish BP, Van Puymbroeck CM, Tennen H, Davis MC, Reich JW, et al. Depression history, stress, and pain in rheumatoid arthritis patients. *J Behav Med.* (2007) 30:187–97. doi: 10.1007/s10865-007-9097-4
89. Rogers HL, Brotherton HT, de Luis A, Olivera-Plaza SL, Cordoba-Patino AF, Pena-Altamar ML. Depressive symptoms are independently associated with pain perception in Colombians with rheumatoid arthritis. *Acta Reumatol Port.* (2015) 40:40–9.
90. Piccinni A, Maser JD, Bazzichi L, Rucci P, Vivarelli L, Del Debbio A, et al. Clinical significance of lifetime mood and panic-agoraphobic spectrum symptoms on quality of life of patients with rheumatoid arthritis. *Compr Psychiatry.* (2006) 47:201–8. doi: 10.1016/j.comppsych.2005.08.002
91. Jobski K, Kollhorst B, Garbe E, Schink T. The risk of ischemic cardio- and cerebrovascular events associated with oxycodone-naloxone and other extended-release high-potency opioids: a nested case-control study. *Drug Saf.* (2017) 40:505–15. doi: 10.1007/s40264-017-0511-8
92. Lee YC, Kremer J, Guan H, Greenberg J, Solomon DH. Chronic opioid use in rheumatoid arthritis: prevalence and predictors. *Arthritis Rheumatol.* (2019) 71:670–7. doi: 10.1002/art.40789
93. Dunne FJ, Dunne CA. Fibromyalgia syndrome and depression: common pathways. *Br J Hosp Med.* (2012) 73:211–7. doi: 10.12968/hmed.2012.73.4.211
94. Ingegnoli F, Schioppo T, Ubiali T, Ostuzzi S, Bollati V, Buoli M, et al. Patient perception of depressive symptoms in rheumatic diseases: a cross-sectional survey. *J Clin Rheumatol.* (2020). doi: 10.1097/RHU.0000000000001564. [Epub ahead of print].
95. Irwin MR, Olmstead R, Carrillo C, Sadeghi N, Fitzgerald JD, Ranganath VK, et al. Sleep loss exacerbates fatigue, depression, and pain in rheumatoid arthritis. *Sleep.* (2012) 35:537–43. doi: 10.5665/sleep.1742
96. Cabrera-Marroquin R, Contreras-Yanez I, Alcocer-Castillejos N, Pascual-Ramos V. Major depressive episodes are associated with poor concordance with therapy in rheumatoid arthritis patients: the impact on disease outcomes. *Clin Exp Rheumatol.* (2014) 32:904–13.
97. Euesden J, Matcham F, Hotopf M, Steer S, Cope AP, Lewis CM, et al. The relationship between mental health, disease severity, and genetic risk for depression in early rheumatoid arthritis. *Psychosom Med.* (2017) 79:638–45. doi: 10.1097/PSY.0000000000000462
98. Liu YL, Szklo M, Davidson KW, Bathon JM, Giles JT. Differential association of psychosocial comorbidities with subclinical atherosclerosis in rheumatoid arthritis. *Arthritis Care Res.* (2015) 67:1335–44. doi: 10.1002/acr.22635

99. Scherrer JF, Virgo KS, Zeringue A, Bucholz KK, Jacob T, Johnson RG, et al. Depression increases risk of incident myocardial infarction among Veterans Administration patients with rheumatoid arthritis. *Gen Hosp Psychiatry.* (2009) 31:353–9. doi: 10.1016/j.genhosppsych.2009.04.001

100. Marrie RA, Walld R, Bolton JM, Sareen J, Patten SB, Singer A, et al. Psychiatric comorbidity increases mortality in immune-mediated inflammatory diseases. *Gen Hosp Psychiatry.* (2018) 53:65–72. doi: 10.1016/j.genhosppsych.2018.06.001

101. Nikiphorou E, de Lusignan S, Mallen C, Roberts J, Khavandi K, Bedarida G, et al. Prognostic value of comorbidity indices and lung diseases in early rheumatoid arthritis: a UK population-based study. *Rheumatology.* (2020) 59:1296–305. doi: 10.1093/rheumatology/kez409

102. Brandstetter S, Riedelbeck G, Steinmann M, Loss J, Ehrenstein B, Apfelbacher C. Depression moderates the associations between beliefs about medicines and medication adherence in patients with rheumatoid arthritis: cross-sectional study. *J Health Psychol.* (2018) 23:1185–95. doi: 10.1177/1359105316646440

103. Savka S. Improved quality of life of patients with rheumatoid arthritis and nonpsychotic mental disorders. *Wiad Lek.* (2019) 72:47–51. doi: 10.36740/WLek201901109

104. Smarr KL, Parker JC, Kosciulek JF, Buchholz JL, Multon KD, Hewett JE, et al. Implications of depression in rheumatoid arthritis: do subtypes really matter? *Arthritis Care Res.* (2000) 13:23–32. doi: 10.1002/1529-0131(200002)13:1<23::AID-ART5>3.0.CO;2-W

105. Hider SL, Tanveer W, Brownfield A, Mattey DL, Packham JC. Depression in RA patients treated with anti-TNF is common and under-recognized in the rheumatology clinic. *Rheumatology.* (2009) 48:1152–4. doi: 10.1093/rheumatology/kep170

106. Hewlett S, Ambler N, Almeida C, Cliss A, Hammond A, Kitchen K, et al. Self-management of fatigue in rheumatoid arthritis: a randomised controlled trial of group cognitive-behavioural therapy. *Ann. Rheum Dis.* (2011) 70:1060–7. doi: 10.1136/ard.2010.144691

107. Parker JC, Smarr KL, Slaughter JR, Johnston SK, Priesmeyer ML, Hanson KD, et al. Management of depression in rheumatoid arthritis: a combined pharmacologic and cognitive-behavioral approach. *Arthritis Rheum.* (2003) 49:766–77. doi: 10.1002/art.11459

108. Dhavale HS, Gawande S, Bhagat V, Durge V, Londhe V, Kini S, et al. Evaluation of efficacy and tolerability of dothiepin hydrochloride in the management of major depression in patients suffering from rheumatoid arthritis. *J Indian Med Assoc.* (2005) 103:291–4.

109. Slaughter JR, Parker JC, Martens MP, Smarr KL, Hewett JE. Clinical outcomes following a trial of sertraline in rheumatoid arthritis. *Psychosomatics.* (2002) 43:36–41. doi: 10.1176/appi.psy.43.1.36

110. Zautra AJ, Davis MC, Reich JW, Nicassario P, Tennen H, Finan P, et al. Comparison of cognitive behavioral and mindfulness meditation interventions on adaptation to rheumatoid arthritis for patients with and without history of recurrent depression. *J Consult Clin Psychol.* (2008) 76:408–21. doi: 10.1037/0022-006X.76.3.408

111. Gautam S, Tolahunase M, Kumar U, Dada R. Impact of yoga based mind-body intervention on systemic inflammatory markers and co-morbid depression in active Rheumatoid arthritis patients: a randomized controlled trial. *Restor Neurol Neurosci.* (2019) 37:41–59. doi: 10.3233/RNN-1 80875

112. Uguz F, Akman C, Kucuksarac S, Tufekci O. Anti-tumor necrosis factor-alpha therapy is associated with less frequent mood and anxiety disorders in patients with rheumatoid arthritis. *Psychiatry Clin Neurosci.* (2009) 63:50–5. doi: 10.1111/j.1440-1819.2008.01905.x

113. Sun Y, Wang D, Salvadore G, Hsu B, Curran M, Casper C, et al. The effects of interleukin-6 neutralizing antibodies on symptoms of depressed mood and anhedonia in patients with rheumatoid arthritis and multicentric Castleman's disease. *Brain Behav Immun.* (2017) 66:156–64. doi: 10.1016/j.bbi.2017.06.014

114. Genty M, Combe B, Kostine M, Ardouin E, Morel J, Lukas C. Improvement of fatigue in patients with rheumatoid arthritis treated with biologics: relationship with sleep disorders, depression and clinical efficacy. A prospective, multicentre study. *Clin Exp Rheumatol.* (2017) 35:85–92.

115. Bottomley JM, LeReun C, Diamantopoulos A, Mitchell S, Gaynes BN. Vagus nerve stimulation (VNS) therapy in patients with treatment resistant depression: a systematic review and meta-analysis. *Compr Psychiatry.* (2019) 98:152156. doi: 10.1016/j.comppsych.2019.152156

116. Johnson RL, Wilson CG. A review of vagus nerve stimulation as a therapeutic intervention. *J Inflamm Res.* (2018) 11:203–13. doi: 10.2147/JIR.S163248

117. Isik A, Koca SS, Ozturk A, Mermi O. Anxiety and depression in patients with rheumatoid arthritis. *Clin Rheumatol.* (2007) 26:872–8. doi: 10.1007/s10067-006-0407-y

118. Lisitsyna TA, Veltishchev DY, Seravina OF, Kovalevskaya OB, Starovoytova MN, Desinova OV, et al. Comparative analysis of anxiety-depressive spectrum disorders in patients with rheumatic diseases. *Ter Arkh.* (2018) 90:30–7. doi: 10.26442/terarkh201890530-37

119. Hassan AA, Nasr MH, Mohamed AL, Kamal AM, Elmoghazy AD. Psychological affection in rheumatoid arthritis patients in relation to disease activity. *Medicine.* (2019) 98:e15373. doi: 10.1097/MD.0000000000015373

120. Marrie RA, Walld R, Bolton JM, Sareen J, Walker JR, Patten SB, et al. Rising incidence of psychiatric disorders before diagnosis of immune-mediated inflammatory disease. *Epidemiol Psychiatr Sci.* (2019) 28:333–42. doi: 10.1017/S2045796017000579

121. Watad A, Bragazzi NL, Adawi M, Aljadeff G, Amital H, Comaneshter D, et al. Anxiety disorder among rheumatoid arthritis patients: insights from real-life data. *J Affect Disord.* (2017) 213:30–4. doi: 10.1016/j.jad.2017.02.007

122. Reinhorn IM, Bernstein CN, Graff LA, Patten SB, Sareen J, Fisk JD, et al. Social phobia in immune-mediated inflammatory diseases. *J Psychosom Res.* (2020) 128:109890. doi: 10.1016/j.jpsychores.2019.109890

123. Stebbings S, Herbison P, Doyle TC, Treharne GJ, Highton J. A comparison of fatigue correlates in rheumatoid arthritis and osteoarthritis: disparity in associations with disability, anxiety and sleep disturbance. *Rheumatology.* (2010) 49:361–7. doi: 10.1093/rheumatology/kep367

124. Mangelli L, Gribbin N, Buchi S, Allard S, Sensky T. Psychological well-being in rheumatoid arthritis: relationship to 'disease' variables and affective disturbance. *Psychother Psychosom.* (2002) 71:112–6. doi: 10.1159/000049354

125. Karimi S, Yarmohammadian MH, Shokri A, Mottaghi P, Qolipour K, Kordi A, et al. Predictors and effective factors on quality of life among Iranian patients with rheumatoid arthritis. *Mater Sociomed.* (2013) 25:158–62. doi: 10.5455/msm.2013.25.158-162

126. Esen SA, Karabulut Y, Esen I, Atmis V. Effects of the Disease Characteristics and the treatment on psychological status in patients with rheumatoid arthritis and ankylosing spondylitis. *Curr Rheumatol Rev.* (2018) 14:271–8. doi: 10.2174/1573397113666170728123518

127. Yilmaz V, Umay E, Gundogdu I, Karaahmet ZO, Ozturk AE. Rheumatoid arthritis: are psychological factors effective in disease flare? *Eur J Rheumatol.* (2017) 4:127–32. doi: 10.5152/eurjrheum.2017.16100

128. Liu Y, Ho RC, Mak A. The role of interleukin (IL)-17 in anxiety and depression of patients with rheumatoid arthritis. *Int J Rheum Dis.* (2012) 15:183–7. doi: 10.1111/j.1756-185X.2011.01673.x

129. Murphy H, Dickens C, Creed F, Bernstein R. Depression, illness perception and coping in rheumatoid arthritis. *J Psychosom Res.* (1999) 46:155–64. doi: 10.1016/S0022-3999(98)00073-7

130. Whitehouse CE, Fisk JD, Bernstein CN, Berrigan LI, Bolton JM, Graff LA, et al. Comorbid anxiety, depression, and cognition in MS and other immune-mediated disorders. *Neurology.* (2019) 93:1081–2. doi: 10.1212/WNL.0000000000006854

131. Adina TS, Mihaela-Simona S, Lucia CP, Stefan Cristian D, Maria B, Lili BA, et al. The influence of socio-demographic factors, lifestyle and psychiatric indicators on adherence to treatment of patients with rheumatoid arthritis: a cross-sectional study. *Medicina.* (2020) 56:178–192. doi: 10.3390/medicina56040178

132. Mattey DL, Dawes PT, Hassell AB, Brownfield A, Packham JC. Effect of psychological distress on continuation of anti-tumor necrosis factor therapy in patients with rheumatoid arthritis. *J Rheumatol.* (2010) 37:2021–4. doi: 10.3899/jrheum.100050

133. Urman A, Taklalsingh N, Sorrento C, McFarlane IM. Inflammation beyond the joints: rheumatoid arthritis and cardiovascular disease. *Scifed J Cardiol.* (2018) 2:1000019.

134. Mavrogeni S, Dimitroulas T, Sfikakis PP, Kitas GD. Heart involvement in rheumatoid arthritis: multimodality imaging and the emerging role of cardiac magnetic resonance. *Semin Arthritis Rheum.* (2013) 43:314–24. doi: 10.1016/j.semarthrit.2013.05.001

135. Markousis-Mavrogenis G, Koutsogeorgopoulou L, Dimitroulas T, Katsifis G, Vartela V, Mitsikostas D, et al. Is there a brain/heart interaction in rheumatoid arthritis and seronegative spondyloartropathies? A combined brain/heart magnetic resonance imaging reveals the answer. *Curr Rheumatol Rep.* (2020) 22:39. doi: 10.1007/s11926-020-00922-7
136. Adlan AM, Paton JF, Lip GY, Kitas GD, Fisher JP. Increased sympathetic nerve activity and reduced cardiac baroreflex sensitivity in rheumatoid arthritis. *J Physiol.* (2017) 595:967–81. doi: 10.1113/JP272944
137. Fisher JP, Paton JF. The sympathetic nervous system and blood pressure in humans: implications for hypertension. *J Hum Hypertens.* (2012) 26:463–75. doi: 10.1038/jhh.2011.66
138. Barretto AC, Santos AC, Munhoz R, Rondon MU, Franco FG, Trombetta IC, et al. Increased muscle sympathetic nerve activity predicts mortality in heart failure patients. *Int J Cardiol.* (2009) 135:302–7. doi: 10.1016/j.ijcard.2008.03.056
139. Panoulas VF, Toms TE, Douglas KM, Sandoo A, Metsios GS, Stavropoulos-Kalinoglou A, et al. Prolonged QTc interval predicts all-cause mortality in patients with rheumatoid arthritis: an association driven by high inflammatory burden. *Rheumatology.* (2014) 53:131–7. doi: 10.1093/rheumatology/ket338
140. Hanvivadhanakul P, Buakhamsri A. Disease activity is associated with LV dysfunction in rheumatoid arthritis patients without clinical cardiovascular disease. *Adv Rheumatol.* (2019) 59:56. doi: 10.1186/s42358-019-0100-x
141. Sandoo A, Protogerou AD, Hodson J, Smith JP, Zampeli E, Sfikakis PP, et al. The role of inflammation, the autonomic nervous system and classical cardiovascular disease risk factors on subendocardial viability ratio in patients with RA: a cross-sectional and longitudinal study. *Arthritis Res Ther.* (2012) 14:R258. doi: 10.1186/ar4103
142. Holman AJ, Ng E. Heart rate variability predicts anti-tumor necrosis factor therapy response for inflammatory arthritis. *Auton Neurosci.* (2008) 143:58–67. doi: 10.1016/j.autneu.2008.05.005
143. Zimmermann M, Vodicka E, Holman AJ, Garrison LP, Jr. Heart rate variability testing: could it change spending for rheumatoid arthritis patients in the United States? An exploratory economic analysis. *J Med Econ.* (2018) 21:712–20. doi: 10.1080/13696998.2018.1470519
144. Hu MX, Milaneschi Y, Lamers F, Nolte IM, Snieder H, Dolan CV, et al. The association of depression and anxiety with cardiac autonomic activity: the role of confounding effects of antidepressants. *Depress Anxiety.* (2019) 36:1163–72. doi: 10.1002/da.22966
145. Pecanha T, Lima AH. Inflammation and cardiovascular autonomic dysfunction in rheumatoid arthritis: a bidirectional pathway leading to cardiovascular disease. *J Physiol.* (2017) 595:1025–6. doi: 10.1113/JP273649
146. Fazalbhoy A, Birznieks I, Macefield VG. Individual differences in the cardiovascular responses to tonic muscle pain: parallel increases or decreases in muscle sympathetic nerve activity, blood pressure and heart rate. *Exp Physiol.* (2012) 97:1084–92. doi: 10.1113/expphysiol.2012.066191
147. Lazzerini PE, Acampa M, Capecchi PL, Hammoud M, Maffei S, Bisogno S, et al. Association between high sensitivity C-reactive protein, heart rate variability and corrected QT interval in patients with chronic inflammatory arthritis. *Eur J Intern Med.* (2013) 24:368–74. doi: 10.1016/j.ejim.2013.02.009
148. Syngle A, Verma I, Krishan P, Garg N, Syngle V. Disease-modifying anti-rheumatic drugs improve autonomic neuropathy in arthritis: DIANA study. *Clin Rheumatol.* (2015) 34:1233–41. doi: 10.1007/s10067-014-2716-x
149. Sandhu V, Allen SC. The effects of age, seropositivity and disease duration on autonomic cardiovascular reflexes in patients with rheumatoid arthritis. *Int J Clin Pract.* (2004) 58:740–5. doi: 10.1111/j.1368-5031.2004.00210.x
150. Syngle V, Syngle A, Garg N, Krishan P, Verma I. Predictors of autonomic neuropathy in rheumatoid arthritis. *Auton Neurosci.* (2016) 201:54–9. doi: 10.1016/j.autneu.2016.07.008
151. Koopman FA, Chavan SS, Miljko S, Grazio S, Sokolovic S, Schuurman PR, et al. Vagus nerve stimulation inhibits cytokine production and attenuates disease severity in rheumatoid arthritis. *Proc Natl Acad Sci USA.* (2016) 113:8284–9. doi: 10.1073/pnas.1605635113
152. Addorisio ME, Imperato GH, de Vos AF, Forti S, Goldstein RS, Pavlov VA, et al. Investigational treatment of rheumatoid arthritis with a vibrotactile device applied to the external ear. *Bioelectron Med.* (2019) 5:4. doi: 10.1186/s42234-019-0020-4
153. Marsal S, Corominas H, Lopez Lasanta M, Reina-Sanz D, Perez-Garcia C, Borrell Paños H, et al. Pilot clinical study of a non-invasive auricular vagus nerve stimulation device in patients with rheumatoid arthritis. *Ann Rheum Dis.* (2020) 79:999. doi: 10.1136/annrheumdis-2020-eular.3315
154. Genovese MC, Gaylis NB, Sikes D, Kivitz A, Horowitz DL, Peterfy C, et al. Safety and efficacy of neurostimulation with a miniaturised vagus nerve stimulation device in patients with multidrug-refractory rheumatoid arthritis: a two-stage multicentre, randomised pilot study. *Lancet Rheumatol.* (2020) 2:e527–38. doi: 10.1016/S2665-9913(20)30172-7

7

Magnetic Resonance Imaging of Enthesitis in Spondyloarthritis, Including Psoriatic Arthritis

Ashish J. Mathew[1,2,3,4*] *and Mikkel Østergaard*[1,2]

[1] Copenhagen Center for Arthritis Research (COPECARE), Center for Rheumatology and Spine Diseases, Glostrup, Denmark, [2] Department of Clinical Medicine, Faculty of Health and Medical Sciences, University of Copenhagen, Copenhagen, Denmark, [3] Clinical Immunology and Rheumatology, Christian Medical College, Vellore, India, [4] Centre for Prognosis Studies in the Rheumatic Diseases, Krembil Research Institute, University Health Network, University of Toronto, Toronto, ON, Canada

***Correspondence:**
Ashish J. Mathew
ashishjacobmathew@gmail.com

Enthesitis, inflammation at the attachment sites of tendons, ligaments, fascia, and joint capsules to bones plays a critical role in the pathogenesis of spondyloarthritis (SpA), including psoriatic arthritis (PsA). Magnetic resonance imaging (MRI) has aided in a better understanding of pathophysiology, early diagnosis, prognostication, therapeutic outcomes, and follow up of enthesitis. The concept of enthesitis as a focal insertional pathology has transformed over the past decade, with the help of MRI, to a more widespread entity involving both bone and surrounding soft tissues. The utility of MRI in the differential diagnosis of suspected enthesitis has recently been explored. With the emergence of the treat-to-target concept, and a domain-based approach in the management of SpA, objective and sensitive monitoring of response to targeted therapy becomes prudent. Properties like high sensitivity, ability to image intra-osseous pathology along with surrounding structures exemplify the utility of MRI technology. Considering the lack of a comprehensive, validated MRI score the Outcome Measures in Rheumatology (OMERACT) MRI in Arthritis Working Group, informed by a systematic literature review, developed the first international, consensus-based MRI-scoring system, combined with MRI definitions of pathologies for enthesitis in patients with spondyloarthritis (SpA) and PsA. An atlas with representative images of each grade of the scoring system was subsequently developed by the group to aid readers interested in using the heel enthesitis MRI scoring system (HEMRIS). The HEMRIS can find utility in clinical trials targeting enthesitis as the primary outcome. MRI also finds value for global assessment of the total burden of enthesitis. The concept of whole-body MRI (WBMRI), enabling visualization of entheses throughout the body using a single image is relatively new. The MRI whole-body score for inflammation in peripheral joints and entheses (MRI-WIPE) is a promising scoring system, which is undergoing further testing in clinical trials and longitudinal cohorts evaluating global measures of inflammation at entheses. This review discusses the role of MRI in diagnosis and monitoring of enthesitis in SpA and PsA, along with recent advances in the field, based on published literature.

Keywords: magnetic resonance imaging (MRI), enthesitis, spondyloarthritis, psoriatic arthritis, inflammation

INTRODUCTION

The entheses are insertion sites of tendon, ligament, fascia, or joint capsule into bone. Enthesopathy refers to involvement of entheses due to trauma, degeneration, or in pathological conditions including metabolic syndrome, endocrine disorders, and inflammatory arthritis (1). Inflammation at the entheseal sites, enthesitis plays a cardinal role in the pathophysiology of spondyloarthritis (SpA), including psoriatic arthritis (PsA) (2). Initially thought to be just a focal insertional site, enthesis is better known currently as being part of an "enthesis organ," with intricate immune-pathogenetic relationship with synovium, substantiated by McGonagle and colleagues as the concept of synovio-entheseal complex (3). Biomechanical stress induced micro-injuries in the synovio-entheseal complex lead to a cascade of inflammatory process in the adjoining fibrocartilage, bursae, synovium, and trabecular bone by interleukin (IL)-23 from macrophages, dendritic cells and innate lymphoid cells—type 3 (ILC3) (4).

The prevalence of enthesitis in SpA, including PsA from various studies has been reported to be 13.6–35%, with Achilles tendon, plantar fascia, and lateral epicondyle insertion being the most common sites (5, 6). Presence of enthesitis has shown to be associated with higher disease activity, disability and incapacity to work ultimately leading to poor quality of life (6–8). Clinical enthesitis measures including the Leeds enthesitis index (LEI), the Spondyloarthritis Research Consortium of Canada (SPARCC) enthesitis index and the Maastricht Ankylosing Spondylitis Enthesitis Score (MASES) offer poor reliability and sensitivity compared to advanced imaging techniques like ultrasound and magnetic resonance imaging (MRI) (9, 10).

By providing sensitive visualization of the extent of disease, MRI and ultrasound (US) in patients with PsA have shown utility in diagnosis, prognostication, and monitoring of treatment response. (11) The European League Against Rheumatism (EULAR) recommendations for the use of imaging in SpA, built on research-based evidence and expert opinion highlight the role of MRI in diagnosis and monitoring peripheral enthesitis, acknowledging the need for further research to optimize the use of imaging in clinical practice (12).

This review aims at elucidating the role of magnetic resonance imaging (MRI) in better understanding of enthesitis in SpA, including PsA, highlighting the recent advances in this field.

HOW HAS MRI CONTRIBUTED TO THE UNDERSTANDING OF PATHOGENESIS OF ENTHESITIS IN SPA?

Based on their structure and location two types of entheses have been described - fibrous and fibrocartilaginous, with the latter being affected more commonly in SpA (13, 14). MRI, with its potential to visualize both soft tissue and intra-osseous abnormalities has fostered our understanding of the entheseal organ concept by demonstrating extension of enthesitis to adjacent bone and surrounding structures, including fibrocartilage, bursa, fat pad and deeper fascia (15, 16). McGonagle and colleagues described the correlation of HLA-B27 with the degree of MRI bone marrow edema surrounding the entheses in patients with SpA, compared to those with mechanically induced disease (17). The close link between enthesitis and synovitis in swollen peripheral joints, as demonstrated by MRI studies in PsA and SpA has invoked the possibility of enthesitis inciting an inflammatory response within the closely located synovial tissue (18, 19). This augments the hypothesis that enthesitis is a critical lesion in SpA.

The importance of enthesitis in explaining the relationship between the nail and distal interphalangeal joint disease in PsA was studied by Tan et al. using high-resolution MRI and histology, comparing patients with osteoarthritis (OA) and PsA. The MRI inflammation observed over the entire nail bed region was shown to be anatomically associated with an enthesitis organ apparatus, providing a novel explanation for distal interphalangeal joint (DIP) arthritis in PsA patients with nail involvement (20). Yet another study from the same group applying high resolution MRI to explore flexor tenosynovitis in PsA patients with dactylitis observed microscopic enthesitis in miniature pulleys around the flexor tendon, explaining the tenosynovitis, and also the concept of enthesitis in PsA (21). In a recent study Abrar et al. compared high resolution MRI of hands using a 3 T scanner and dedicated 16-channel hand coil in patients with PsA, rheumatoid arthritis (RA) and healthy controls. Compared to the other groups, PsA patients had significantly thicker A1 and A2 flexor tendon pulleys. This study corroborates the role of enthesitis in the pathogenesis of SpA (22).

UTILITY OF MRI IN THE DIAGNOSIS OF ENTHESITIS IN SPA

Given the avascular nature of the entheses at bony attachment sites and low density of vessels in the surrounding ligaments and tendons, diagnosis of enthesitis with imaging can be demanding (14). MRI has the unique advantage of identifying peri-entheseal inflammation with adjacent bone marrow edema, potentially facilitating early diagnosis in SpA (23) (**Figures 1a–d**). Fat-suppressed MRI with or without gadolinium enhancement is the most sensitive method of visualizing active enthesitis (24, 25). The European Society of Musculoskeletal Imaging (ESSR) arthritis subcommittee for the use of MRI has suggested specific sequences based on the area to be examined for inflammatory changes (26). The OMERACT MRI in enthesitis initiative proposes T1weighted post gadolinium sequence for entheseal soft tissue inflammation, STIR/T2weighted fat suppressed sequence for entheseal osteitis, and T1 weighted pre-gadolinium sequence for entheseal structural changes (27). MRI is useful in diagnosing enthesitis in the appendicular and axial skeleton. Bone marrow edema (BME) in PsA is often located close to the entheses, as compared to capsular attachments and subchondral areas in RA and OA, respectively (28).

An MRI and power doppler ultrasound (PDUS) study at the heel region compared SpA patients with current heel pain and those with no pain or past history of heel pain. MRI

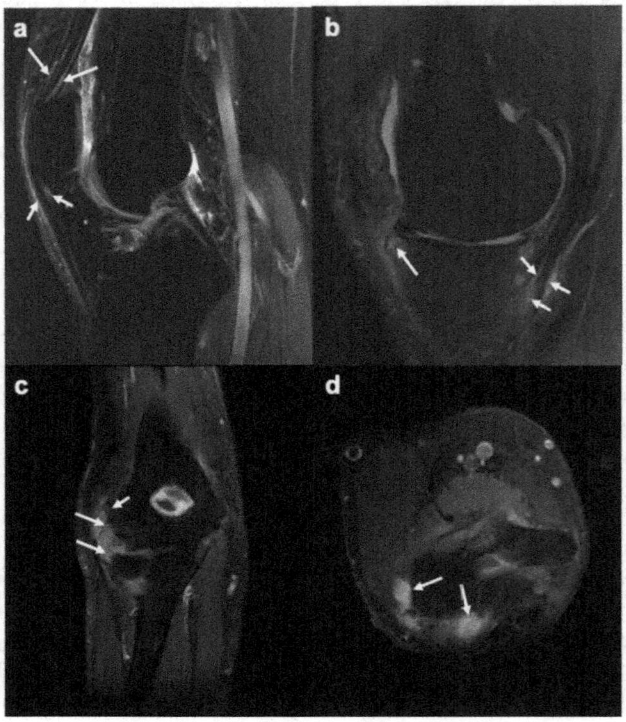

FIGURE 1 | MR images of the knee and elbow depicting enthesitis. **(a)** Sagittal STIR image of the knee showing soft tissue high signal intensity (intra- and peritendinous) at the insertions of the quadriceps tendon (long arrows) and the patellar ligament (short arrows) at the patella, suggesting enthesitis. **(b)** Sagittal T2-weighted fat suppressed image of the knee showing high signal intensity (intra- and peritendinous) in the soft tissues of the pes anserine (short arrows), indicating pes anserine enthesitis, as well as bone marrow edema (long arrows) close to the insertion of the medial patellar retinaculum at medial tibial plateau. **(c,d)** Coronal (c) and axial (d) STIR images of the elbow showing bone marrow edema (mild, short arrow) and soft tissue high signal intensity (long arrows) at the common extensor tendon insertion at the lateral epicondyle, indicating enthesitis. Images courtesy of Professor Iris Eshed, Sackler School of Medicine, Tel Aviv University, Tel Aviv, Israel.

lesions considered to depict early injury included Achilles tendon (tendonitis) or aponeurosis hypersignal, peri-tendon or peri-aponeurosis hypersignal, retrocalcaneal bursitis, inferior or posterior BME, and thickening of the tendon, and those depicting chronic injury included enthesophytes and bone erosions. MRI pathologies of enthesitis were noted in 81% of SpA patients with current heel pain, compared to 56% of SpA patients without heel pain or with history of heel pain. Intra- or peri-aponeurosis MRI signal abnormalities were the most useful features, while only BME in calcaneum was specific to distinguish patients with SpA from controls (29). A similar study including SpA patients with heel or ankle pain compared high-field and low-field MRI to evaluate the hindfoot. Retrocalcaneal bursitis and plantar fasciitis were the commonest lesions in this study, which inferred an acceptable diagnostic quality for both the units (30). Enthesitis of the rotator cuff, with intense acromial BME at the deltoid origin is described as a highly specific feature of ankylosing spondylitis (AS) (31). According to a recent study erosive changes at the heel entheses seem to be more frequent in peripheral SpA patients compared to non-SpA individuals with painful heels or knees (32).

High resolution MRI with specialized "microscopy coils" have been used for detecting enthesitis at insertions of flexor and extensor tendons to the phalanges. Tan et al. investigated the microanatomic basis for localization of hand disease at the DIP joints in patients with PsA and OA using a high-resolution MRI. More severe changes at the DIP joint entheseal insertions, and marked extracapsular enhancement were noted in patients with PsA as compared to those with OA (33). Another MRI study comparing small joints of hands in RA and SpA patients demonstrated enthesitis and extracapsular changes adjacent to synovial joints more commonly in the latter (34).

MRI is the imaging method of choice for diagnosing axial enthesitis. The revised definition of MRI enthesitis in sacroiliac joints of patients with SpA excludes the inter-osseous soft tissues in the ligamentary portion of the SI joint (35). Pelvic enthesitis on MRI of sacroiliac joints is highly specific for the diagnosis of SpA, and the specificity increases with the number of sites with enthesitis. Enthesitis at the iliac crest and retroarticular ligaments have high positive predictive value for diagnosis of SpA (36). Spinal enthesitis may be seen on spine MRIs as increased signal intensity over inter-spinal ligaments extending between the transverse or spinous processes, supra-spinal ligaments and osteitis of adjacent bone marrow in the spinous process on short tau inversion recovery (STIR) images, T2-weighted fat-suppressed images and contrast enhanced T1-weighted fat-suppressed images (37). The vertebral corners (or edges) are often inflamed in axial SpA and PsA, and this finding represents enthesitis at the insertions of the anterior and posterior longitudinal ligaments (38) (**Figures 2a–f**).

Conventional MRI methods generally allow assessment of only one or few selected areas of the human body. Enthesitis in SpA, especially PsA can be widespread, and capturing the extent of disease can be challenging using conventional MRIs (39). Whole-body MRI (WBMRI), with recent technical advancements allows visualization of the entire body in one imaging session. WBMRI may, in the future clinical practice aid in diagnosis of early forms of SpA, enabling evaluation of both axial and peripheral entheses and joints. (40–42) Readability and reproducibility of WBMRI were high in spine and SI joints, but lower in the peripheral joints in earlier studies (43). However, a more recent study has found good reliability in peripheral entheses too (41). Poggenborg et al. investigated the ability of WBMRI to assess axial and peripheral enthesitis in patients with PsA and axial SpA, and observed moderate agreement between clinical examination and WBMRI. The most frequent sites of enthesitis included greater femoral trochanter, supraspinatus and Achilles tendon insertions (10). Weckbach et al. reported enthesitis in 68% of the hip regions among 30 patients with PsA using WBMRI (44). Althoff et al. compared MRI findings in patients with radiographic and non-radiographic axial SpA (nr-axSpA) using WBMRI. Enthesitis, mostly multilocular was significantly more in the SpA group as compared to the nr-axSpA group (45). Weber et al., assessed inflammation at the anterior chest wall using WBMRI in 122 patients, and reported

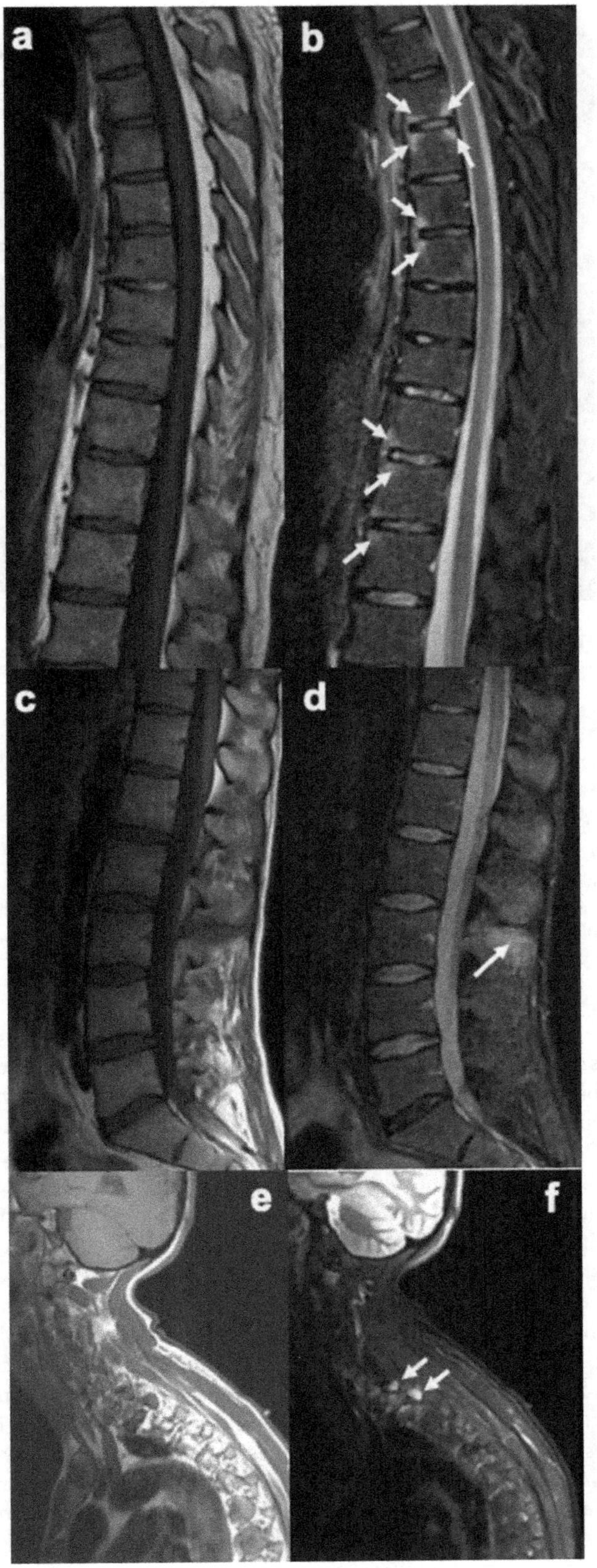

FIGURE 2 | Sagittal MR images of the spine, showing enthesitis at different locations (T1-weighted images on the left, short tau inversion recovery (STIR) *(Continued)*

FIGURE 2 | images on the right). **(a,b)** Several anterior and posterior corner inflammatory lesions (arrows) are seen in the thoracic spine, representing enthesitis at the insertion of the anterior and posterior longitudinal ligaments. **(c,d)** Bone marrow edema is seen at several spinous processes, particularly at the L3 spinous process (arrow), representing enthesitis. **(e,f)** Bone marrow edema is seen in two upper thoracic transverse processes (arrows), representing enthesitis. Images are from University of Copenhagen, Denmark.

inflammation in 49.5 and 25.9% of patients with SpA and nr-axSpA, respectively as opposed to 26% by clinical assessment using the Maastricht Ankylosing Spondylitis Enthesitis Score (MASES) (46). Though fairly sensitive in its diagnostic capacity, further studies are warranted to demonstrate the ability of MRI in distinguishing inflammatory enthesitis from other forms.

ROLE OF MRI IN MONITORING INFLAMMATORY AND STRUCTURAL ENTHESITIS IN SPA AND PSA

Monitoring of disease progression and treatment response is dependent on the responsiveness of the applied measure. MRI has found utility in following up patients with SpA and PsA on treatment. Marzo-Ortega et al., determining the efficacy of etanercept on axial and peripheral entheseal lesions in patients with SpA using MRIs noted improvement or regression in 86% of MRI detected entheseal lesions between baseline and 6 months (47). A similar study by the same group ascertained the efficacy of anakinra on spinal enthesitis in patients with active ankylosing spondylitis (AS) using MRI. There was complete regression or improvement in 23 of the 38 regions of enthesitis (61%) determined by MRI at baseline following 3 months of treatment (48).

Karpitschka et al. demonstrated significant reduction in enthesitis using WBMRI with gadolinium enhancement at week 52 in patients with active AS being treated with etanercept. MRI enthesitis lesions showed reduction during therapy by 94% at week 52 (49). In an investigator initiated randomized controlled trial of adalimumab in patients with axSpA, Krabbe et al. demonstrated the resolution of inflammation at multiple entheseal sites. A higher frequency of clinical resolution was observed in the joints which were tender with MRI inflammation compared to those which were tender without MRI inflammation. This supports the utility of MRI in differentiating inflammatory from non-inflammatory causes of tenderness in patients with SpA (50). Another randomized, double-blind, placebo-controlled trial on adalimumab investigated the responsiveness of WBMRI in axial and peripheral joints and entheses in patients with axSpA. The authors could demonstrate significant reductions in the WBMRI enthesis inflammation index after 6 weeks of adalimumab therapy. The WBMRI total inflammation index, covering both axial and peripheral joints and entheses, could also distinguish treatment from placebo groups (51). Further development and validation of WBMRI inflammation index may be efficacious in assessing responsiveness to treatment of the global entheseal inflammatory burden in future clinical trials.

EVIDENCE ON MRI ENTHESITIS IN PROGNOSTICATION OF SPA AND PSA

Existence of a pre-clinical phase in PsA characterized by nonspecific arthralgias, stiffness and fatigue has been established in a prospective cohort study (52). Ultrasound studies have noted baseline sonographic evidence of enthesitis being associated with future development of clinical PsA (53, 54). MRI may aid in detection of the pre-clinical phase of PsA. However, there is scarcity of MRI studies on this topic. Whether pre-clinical MRI enthesitis can predict subsequent development of PsA remains to be established. Enthesitis presumably precedes synovitis in SpA and PsA (3, 55). Peri-entheseal BME at the tibial plateau and bony attachments of patellar tendon and posterior cruciate ligament, detected by McGonagle et al. in SpA and PsA patients with knee swelling of recent onset, indicates subclinical enthesitis near the swollen joint and suggests enthesitis as the primary lesion (18). Emad et al. studied the entheseal changes at knee joints in patients with psoriasis and SpA, including axSpA, inflammatory bowel disease (IBD) and PsA. Subclinical enthesitis was noted in patients with psoriasis and IBD. The authors concluded that enthesitis at the knee joint may be an early and pathognomonic MRI finding in patients with SpA (56). Erdem et al. determined MRI changes of foot in psoriasis patients with no clinical arthritis and healthy controls. Achilles tendonitis and retrocalcaneal bursitis were observed in more than half of the psoriasis patients, with none in the healthy control group having similar findings (57).

These studies, although with significant limitations did provide insight into the possibility of MRI enthesitis being the initial subclinical pathology in SpA. In a recent study Simon et al., scanning psoriasis patients without clinical arthritis from a longitudinal cohort have established the role of structural enthesitis at the 2nd and 3rd metacarpophalangeal joints of the dominant hand in prediction of PsA (58). Another study evaluating MRI inflammation in the hand joints of patients with psoriasis without PsA and healthy controls noted a 55.5% likelihood of developing PsA in psoriasis patients with arthralgia and evidence of MRI synovitis. This observation should, nevertheless be interpreted in the background of a 29.6% conversion rate to PsA in this cohort within the short follow up period of 1 year. Moreover, osteitis, periarticular inflammation and tenosynovitis were comparable in psoriasis patients and controls (59).

HOW HAVE CLINICAL TRIALS APPLIED MRI FOR ASSESSING ENTHESITIS?

With the advent of treat-to-target strategies in SpA and domain specific treatment approach in PsA, a subset of future clinical trials with novel molecules are expected to focus on enthesitis as their primary outcome (60–62). Inclusion of enthesitis as a core domain by the outcome measures in rheumatology (OMERACT) PsA group warrants its assessment in all clinical trials and observational studies (63). MRI, despite being an objective and sensitive adjunct to clinical examination for monitoring response of enthesitis to therapy, has not been employed in clinical trials distinctly. One of the early placebo-controlled, randomized clinical trials of etanercept to determine its efficacy in patients with refractory heel enthesitis used MRI as an adjunct to clinical examination. No statistically significant differences were noted between the placebo and etanercept groups among the 19 patients who presented with positive MRI heel enthesitis, defined by BME at calcaneus insertions of Achilles tendon and plantar fascia (64). The ACHILLES trial is a randomized, quadruple-blind study (NCT02771210) evaluating the efficacy of secukinumab in resolution of Achilles tendon enthesitis in patients with active PsA and axSpA in which MRI is applied as a secondary outcome measure. The recruitment of this trial has been completed and the results are awaited (65).

Improvement in overall enthesitis in the body, as assessed by WBMRI, have been studied in few clinical trials. A randomized clinical trial compared etanercept and sulphasalazine on active bony inflammation in patients with early axSpA using WBMRI.

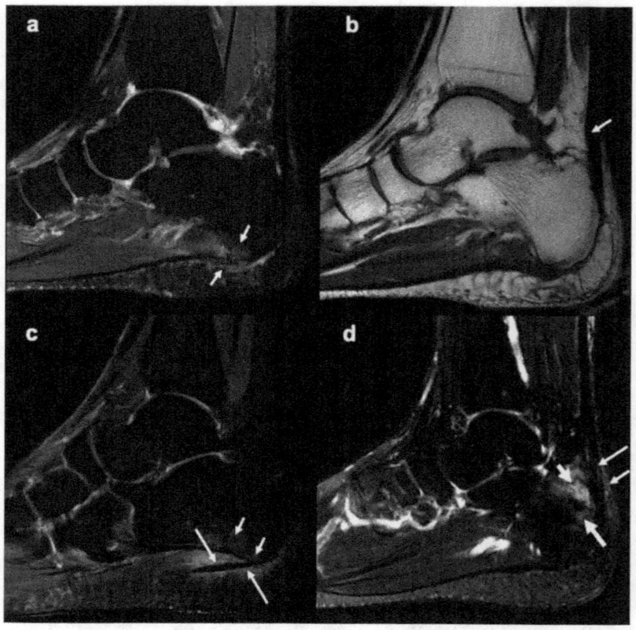

FIGURE 3 | Sagittal MR images of the heel region depicting enthesitis at Achilles tendon and plantar fascia attachments. **(a)** STIR image showing bone marrow edema at the plantar fascia insertion to the calcaneum, intrafascia high signal intensity and perifascia high signal intensity. **(b)** Corresponding T1-weighted image showing probable mild thickening of a part of the Achilles tendon (arrow). **(c)** STIR image showing bone marrow edema (short arrows) close to the plantar fascia insertion to calcaneum and severe perifascia high signal intensity (long arrows). **(d)** STIR image showing bone marrow edema (long thick arrow) at the Achilles tendon insertion to calcaneum, intratendonous (long thin arrow) and, peritendonous (short thin arrow) high signal intensity, as well as retrocalcaneal bursitis (short thick arrow). **(a,b)** Courtesy of Professor Iris Eshed, Sackler School of Medicine, Tel Aviv University, Tel Aviv, Israel. **(c,d)** have been taken from the OMERACT MRI heel enthesitis exercises (27, 80).

Reduction of peripheral enthesitis on MRI was a secondary endpoint. The authors demonstrated a 58% reduction in MRI enthesitis in patients on etanercept at week 48, as compared to no reduction in the comparator arm (66). Another randomized, placebo-controlled trial to investigate efficacy of adalimumab on WBMRI indices of inflammation at entheses in patients with axSpA demonstrated significant reduction of both BME and soft tissue indices in the treatment group compared to placebo at week 6 (51).

For MRI assessment of enthesitis in clinical trials, it is recommended to apply validated assessment methods, such as the OMERACT MRI scoring systems (27, 41). More studies are needed to validate and optimize the existing MRI outcome measures. Different aspects of validity, including criterion validity (comparison with gold standard reference, such as histopathology) and discriminant validity (reproducibility and sensitivity to change) should preferably be investigated.

UTILITY OF MRI IN ENTHESITIS IN JUVENILE ARTHRITIS

Active enthesitis and arthritis in patients with enthesitis related arthritis (ERA) at baseline has been reported to predict sacroiliitis at follow up (67). Enthesitis detected by MRI of the pelvis has been described as a specific finding in juvenile spondyloarthritis (68). Herregods et al. determined the diagnostic value of enthesitis on pelvic MRIs in patients with ERA, and noted high correlation between pelvic enthesitis and sacroiliitis (69). WBMRI is increasingly being used in the pediatric population to determine the overall inflammatory and structural burden of synovitis and enthesitis (70). Enthesitis has been included in the inflammatory MRI components of the recently developed OMERACT juvenile idiopathic arthritis MRI score (71).

LIMITATIONS OF IMAGING ENTHESITIS IN SPA AND PSA USING MRI

Notwithstanding all these benefits, MRI has certain limitations which curtails its application in routine clinical settings. Practical impediments for clinical practice like cost, referrals to specialist facilities, and some contraindications, such as claustrophobia, pacemakers, or certain metal implants, cannot be overlooked. The avascular nature and limited water accumulation in structures that make up the entheses contribute to technical difficulties, with MR signals often being low (72). A major limitation with MRI enthesitis until recently was the lack of a comprehensive, generally accepted, validated scoring system with proper definition of pathologies to be scored, which can be applied uniformly in all clinical trials and longitudinal observational studies. Most scoring methods and lesions adapted in studies of MRI enthesitis display poor content and construct validity, and lack responsiveness (73).

Limitations with WBMRI include the examination time, low resolution of images and attainable spatial resolution compared to conventional MRI (74, 75). The total scan time for WBMRI, including peripheral and axial joints, and entheses is generally around 60 min (41, 43). Patients with active arthritis may find it challenging to remain stationary in the same position for long periods of time, which may result in motion artifacts. Image resolution with current acquisition techniques could be compromised, especially in the distal small joints. With advances in technology these limitations could be addressed to a great extent. Experience of the reader also plays a pivotal role with WBMRI. Reliability among experienced readers has been shown to be good, while poorer among less experienced ones (41).

For use in clinical trials, however, MRI has the major advantage of allowing fully standardized image acquisition across all study sites, storage of the entire examination for later review and centralized reading. This makes MRI the ideal method for objective assessment of entheseal inflammation in future clinical trials.

RECENT ADVANCES IN THE FIELD OF MRI ENTHESITIS IN SPA

Expected advancements countering the technical shortcomings of MRI in imaging entheses have recently been reported. Diffusion-weighted imaging (DWI), known to have a high signal to noise ratio has been analyzed as an encouraging alternative to STIR and T2 weighted fat suppressed sequences for sacroiliac joint assessment (76–78). Lecouvet et al. compared the diagnostic accuracy of DWI and STIR sequences in WBMRI of SpA patients. DWI was found to offer higher sensitivity for detection of inflammatory lesions compared to STIR sequences, and to differentiate inflammatory from degenerative changes (78). Ultrashort echo time (UTE) sequences have been explored for better visualization of entheses. Chen et al. demonstrated higher resolution of enthesis at the Achilles tendon in healthy volunteers and patients with PsA using three-dimensional UTE-cones sequences, compared to gradient recalled echo (GRE) and fast spine echo (FSE) sequences. The authors stressed the utility of this sequence in morphological and quantitative evaluation of enthesitis in PsA patients (79). The same group recently explored the MRI morphology of Achilles tendons and entheses using high resolution MRI UTE sequences, and described its utility as biomarkers of biomechanical degradation of entheses in SpA (80).

The OMERACT MRI in arthritis Working Group, informed by a systematic review has developed consensus-based definitions and reader rules for enthesitis in patients with SpA and PsA. Through a series of multi-reader scoring exercises focusing on the heel region using an intuitive web-based image platform and data entry the group developed the OMERACT heel enthesitis in MRI scoring system (HEMRIS). HEMRIS exhibited good reliability and responsiveness among trained readers (27). This was followed by an atlas of the OMERACT HEMRIS, with detailed definitions and reader rules (**Box 1**), which could be used as a guide while scoring Achilles tendon and plantar fascia enthesitis (**Figures 3a–d**) in future clinical trials and longitudinal studies using MRI (81). Applying a similar methodology the group also developed a WBMRI scoring system (MRI-WIPE) for

BOX 1 | OMERACT HEMRIS recommendations for MRI acquisition, definitions and scoring of inflammatory and structural pathologies at the entheses (Adapted from Box 1, Mathew et al. (81)).

A. Core set of basic MRI sequences and imaging planes
MRI studies that intend to assess inflammatory and structural changes at entheses should include at least the following sequences:

- Short tau inversion recovery (STIR)/T2-weighted fat suppressed (T2wFS) images or, alternatively, gadolinium-enhanced T1-weighted fat suppressed images
- T1-weighted images without contrast injection (not mandatory if only inflammation is being assessed)

Suggested imaging planes for the heel region:

- Achilles tendon—Sagittal and preferably also axial
- Plantar fascia—Sagittal and preferably also coronal

B. Definitions and grades of inflammatory and structural pathologies at the Achilles tendon insertion and the plantar fascia insertion to the calcaneum
(Adapted from **Box 1**, Mathew et al. (81))
1. Intratendon/intrafascia hypersignal (STIR/T2FS)
Definition
Signal characteristics consistent with increased water content/inflammation within the tendon/fascia, close to its insertion[¥].
Grades
0: No intratendon/intrafascia hypersignal. ∗
1: Minimal intratendon/intrafascia hypersignal spots ∗ (≤25% of the tendon volume).
2: Moderate intratendon/intrafascia hypersignal ∗ (>25% and ≤50% of the tendon volume).
3: Severe intratendon/intrafascia hypersignal ∗ (>50% of the tendon volume).
¥ For Achilles tendon: From the tendon insertion up to 2 cm proximal to the posterosuperior corner of calcaneum on all the available images. For Plantar fascia: From the fascia insertion up to 2 cm proximal to the anterior margin of the plantar tuberosity on all the available images.
2. Peritendon/perifascia hypersignal (STIR/T2FS)
Definition
Signal characteristics consistent with increased water content/inflammation in the soft tissues surrounding the tendon or fascia, close to its insertion.
Grades
0: No hypersignal. ∗
1: Minimal[†] (or mild) focal hypersignal. ∗
2: Moderate[†] hypersignal. ∗
3: Severe[†] hypersignal. ∗
† *By comparison with reference images (see Mathew et al. (81))*
∗ For Achilles tendon: From tendon insertion up to 2 cm proximal to the posterosuperior corner of calcaneum. For Plantar fascia: From fascia insertion up to 2 cm proximal to the anterior margin of the plantar tuberosity on all the available images.
3. Achilles tendon/plantar fascia calcaneal bone marrow edema
Definition
Bone marrow edema (BME) should be assessed in the bone from the entheseal insertion to a depth of 1 cm on all available images.
Grades:
The scale is 0-3, based on the proportion of bone with edema, compared to the "assessed bone volume", judged on all available images:
0: no edema.
1: 1–33% of the bone is edematous (i.e. BME occupying 1–33% of the assessed bone volume).
2: 34–66% of the bone is edematous.
3: 67–100% of the bone is edematous.
If the lesion is judged borderline, i.e., 1 vs. 2 or 2 vs. 3, lesion intensity may be considered. For example, if a lesion is borderline between 1 (mild) and 2 (moderate), it may be scored 1 (mild) if not judged intense. Similarly, if a lesion is borderline between 2 (moderate), and 3 (severe), it may be scored 3 (severe) if judged intense.
4. Retrocalcaneal bursitis (only relevant at Achilles tendon insertion)
Definition
Signal characteristics consistent with increased water content/inflammation in an above-normal sized bursa.
Grades
0: No hypersignal or maximal diameter of hyper-signal in the shorter of two perpendicular dimensions to be <0.25 cm.
1: Maximal diameter of hypersignal in the shorter of two perpendicular dimensions to be ≥0.25 cm to <0.5 cm.
2: Maximal diameter of hypersignal in the shorter of two perpendicular dimensions to be 0.5 cm to <1.0 cm.
3: Maximal diameter of hypersignal in the shorter of two perpendicular dimensions to be ≥1.0 cm.
5. Tendon/fascia thickening
Definition
Abnormal thickening of the tendon/fascia close to its insertion. ∗
Grades
0: None.
1: Mild.[†] ∗
2: Moderate.[†] ∗
3: Severe.[†] ∗
† *By comparison with reference images (see Mathew et al. (81))*

BOX 1 | Continued

∗ For Achilles tendon: Maximally 2 cm proximal from the postero-superior corner of calcaneum. For plantar fascia: Maximally 2 cm proximal to the anterior margin of the plantar tuberosity.

6. Achilles tendon/plantar fascia calcaneal enthesophyte

Definition

Abnormal bone formation at the insertion of tendon/fascia into the bone

Grades

0: None.
1: Small.†
2: Medium-sized.†
3: Large.†

† *By comparison with reference images (see Mathew et al. (81))*

7. Achilles tendon/plantar fascia calcaneal bone erosion

Definition

A sharply marginated bone lesion, with typical signal characteristics and a visible cortical break, located close to the tendon/fascia insertion.

Grades

0: None.
1: Small.†
2: Medium-sized.†
3: Large.†

† *By comparison with reference images (see Mathew et al. (81))*

peripheral arthritis and enthesitis, which depicted good reliability among the experienced readers (41, 42).

FUTURE PERSPECTIVES

Technical Advancements

New and potentially better MRI sequences have been described in SpA, but they need validation in longitudinal studies and clinical trials, applying novel and established MRI enthesitis measures in the same studies, to document validity and additional value as outcome measures. Also, their utility in assessing axial and peripheral entheses, and differentiating inflammatory from degenerative and other causes of enthesitis needs to be appraised in larger number of patients. The UTE sequence in high resolution MRI may help in better understanding of pathogenesis of different forms of enthesitis. There seems to be a window of opportunity in patients with SpA and PsA wherein early diagnosis and prompt initiation of therapy will be key in curtailing long-term damage (82). The utility of pre-clinical enthesitis visualized by MRI in prognostication of future PsA or SpA needs validation.

Refinement and Further Validation of MRI Scoring Systems

The recently developed MRI enthesitis indices should be further tested in clinical trials. Refinements may further improve their utility. Development of detailed MRI scoring systems for other regions than the heel may be relevant, even though it seems likely that clinical trials aiming to document the effect of a new drug on enthesitis will choose either a detailed evaluation of the most common region, like the heel, or an overall measure of enthesitis in the entire body, by WBMRI. Image resolution in WBMRI needs further enhancement for better visualization of peripheral entheses. The OMERACT MRI in arthritis Working Group is currently endeavoring on a modular approach in WBMRI to assess the overall inflammation burden at individual sites, thus further validating the WIPE-MRI scoring system. Based on the definitions laid out by the Working Group scoring systems for other regions need to be developed.

Role of MRI in Disease Prediction and Interception

In the transition phase toward the development of PsA, a subclinical phase with soluble biomarkers and imaging findings but no clinical sign is well recognized (83). Longitudinal studies with high-resolution MRI of hand or foot at baseline in psoriasis patients at risk of developing PsA are warranted to further validate the role of imaging in predicting PsA. For instance, WBMRI could be utilized in quantification of the global inflammatory burden of enthesitis in psoriasis patients at risk of developing PsA, and it could be investigated if this overall enthesitis burden is closely related with future development of PsA in the "at risk" patients.

Effect of treatment strategies to impede the development of PsA in psoriasis patients at risk may also be estimated. In the Interception in very early PsA (IVEPSA) study, MRI was used to assess inflammatory and structural changes in the joints at baseline and 24 weeks following secukinumab therapy (84). Most of the intervention studies with this objective focus on imaging synovitis in the hand joints. Nevertheless, technical advancements and validated scoring systems like the HEMRIS and WIPE-MRI can pave the way for harnessing MRI enthesitis as an outcome in future clinical trials targeting disease interception.

CONCLUSION

MRI has aided in understanding the pathogenesis, assessment of inflammatory and structural pathologies, monitoring, and prognostication of enthesitis in patients with SpA, including PsA. There is robust evidence for MRI as an adjunct to clinical examination in the assessment and follow up of enthesitis. Having a sound knowledge of its strengths and weaknesses, as compared to other imaging modalities, will facilitate optimal application of MRI in clinical trials, longitudinal studies and clinical practice.

AUTHOR'S NOTE

All the figures in this manuscript are unpublished, and original. These figures are based on the "MRI definitions of key entheseal pathologies" as described by the OMERACT MRI in arthritis Working Group in Table 1 of Mathew et al. (27).

AUTHOR CONTRIBUTIONS

AM prepared the first draft of the manuscript, and MØ critically reviewed and modified the manuscript. All authors contributed to the article and approved the submitted version.

ACKNOWLEDGMENTS

The authors would like to acknowledge Professor Iris Eshed, Sackler School of Medicine, Tel Aviv University, Tel Aviv, Israel for kindly providing images for **Figures 1, 3**.

REFERENCES

1. Benjamin M, McGonagle D. The enthesis organ concept and its relevance to the spondyloarthropathies. *Adv Exp Med Biol.* (2009) 649:57–70. doi: 10.1007/978-1-4419-0298-6_4
2. Schett G, Lories RJ, D'Agostino MA, Elewaut D, Kirkham B, Soriano ER, et al. Enthesitis: from pathophysiology to treatment. *Nat Rev Rheumatol.* (2017) 13:731–41. doi: 10.1038/nrrheum.2017.188
3. McGonagle D, Lories RJU, Tan AL, Benjamin M. The concept of a 'synovio-entheseal complex' and its implications for understanding joint inflammation and damage in psoriatic arthritis and beyond. *Arthritis Rheum.* (2007) 56:2482–91. doi: 10.1002/art.22758
4. McGonagle D, Stockwin L, Isaacs J, Emery P. An enthesitis based model for the pathogenesis of spondyloarthropathy, additive effects of microbial adjuvant and biomechanical factors at disease sites. *J Rheumatol.* (2001) 28:2155–59.
5. de Winter JJ, van Mens LJ, van der Heijde D, Landewé R, Baeten DL. Prevalence of peripheral and extra-articular disease in ankylosing spondylitis versus non-radiographic axial spondyloarthritis: a meta-analysis. *Arthritis Res Ther.* (2016) 18:196. doi: 10.1186/s13075-016-1093-z
6. Polachek A, Li S, Chandran V, Gladman DD. Clinical enthesitis in a prospective longitudinal psoriatic arthritis cohort: incidence, prevalence, characteristics and outcome. *Arthritis Care Res (Hoboken).* (2017) 69:1685–91. doi: 10.1002/acr.23174
7. Carneiro S, Bortoluzzo A, Gonçalves C, da Silva JAB, Ximenes AC, Bertolo M, et al. Effect of enthesitis on 1505. Brazilian patients with spondyloarthritis. *J Rheumatol.* (2013) 40:1719–25. doi: 10.3899/jrheum.121145
8. Rezvani A, Bodur H, Ataman S, Kaya T, Bugdayci DS, Demir SE, et al. Correlations among enthesitis, clinical, radiographic and quality of life parameters in patients with ankylosing spondylitis. *Mod Rheumatol.* (2014) 24:651–56. doi: 10.3109/14397595.2013.850182
9. Bakewell C, Aydin SZ, Ranganath VK, Eder L, Kaeley GS. Imaging techniques: options for the diagnosis and monitoring of treatment of enthesitis in psoriatic arthritis. *J Rheumatol.* (2019). doi: 10.3899/jrheum.190512. [Epub ahead of print].
10. Poggenborg RP, Eshed I, Østergaard M, Sørensen IJ, Møller JM, Madsen OR, et al. Enthesitis in patients with psoriatic arthritis, axial spondyloarthritis and healthy subjects assessed by 'head-to-toe'whole body MRI and clinical examination. *Ann Rheum Dis.* (2015) 74:823–29. doi: 10.1136/annrheumdis-2013-204239
11. Baraliakos X, Conaghan PG, D'Agostino MA, Maksymowych W, Naredo E, Østergaard M, et al. Imaging in rheumatoid arthritis, psoriatic arthritis, axial spondyloarthritis, and osteoarthritis: an international viewpoint on the current knowledge and future research priorities. *Eur J Rheumatol.* (2019) 6:38–47. doi: 10.5152/eurjrheum.2018.18121
12. Mandl P, Navarro-Compán V, Terslev L, Aegerter P, van der Heijde D, D'Agostino MA, et al. EULAR recommendations for the use of imaging in the diagnosis and management of spondyloarthritis in clinical practice. *Ann Rheum Dis.* (2015) 74:1327–39. doi: 10.1136/annrheumdis-2014-206971
13. Rufai A, Ralphs JR, Benjamin M. Structure and histopathology of the insertional region of the human Achilles tendon. *J Orthop Res.* (1995) 13:585–93. doi: 10.1002/jor.1100130414
14. Benjamin M, McGonagle D. The anatomical basis for disease localisation in seronegative spondyloarthropathy at entheses and related sites. *J Anat.* (2001) 199:503–26. doi: 10.1046/j.1469-7580.2001.19950503.x
15. Benjamin M, Moriggl B, Brenner E, Emery P, McGonagle D, Redman S. The 'enthesitis organ' concept: why enthesopathies may not present as focal insertional disorders. *Arthritis Rheum.* (2004) 50:3306–13. doi: 10.1002/art.20566
16. McGonagle D. Imaging the joint and enthesis: insights into pathogenesis of psoriatic arthritis. *Ann Rheum Dis.* (2005) 64(Suppl II):ii58-ii60. doi: 10.1136/ard.2004.034264
17. McGonagle D, Marzo-Ortega H, O'Connor P, Gibbon W, Pease C, Reece R, et al. The role of biomechanical factors and HLA-B27 in magnetic resonance imaging-determined bone changes in plantar fascia enthesopathy. *Arthritis Rheum.* (2002) 46:489–93. doi: 10.1002/art.10125
18. McGonagle D, Gibbon W, O'Connor P, Green M, Pease C, Emery P. Characteristic magnetic resonance imaging entheseal changes in knee synovitis in spondyloarthropathy. *Arthritis Rheum.* (1998) 41:694–700. doi: 10.1002/1529-0131(199804)41:4<694::AID-ART17>3.0.CO;2-#
19. McGonagle D, Gibbon W, Emery P. Classification of inflammatory arthritis by enthesitis. *Lancet.* (1998) 352:1137–40. doi: 10.1016/S0140-6736(97)12004-9
20. Tan AL, Benjamin M, Toumi H, Grainger AJ, Tanner SF, Emery P, et al. The relationship between the extensor tendon enthesis and the nail in distal interphalangeal joint disease in psoriatic arthritis - a high-resolution MRI and histological study. *Rheumatology.* (2007) 46:253–56. doi: 10.1093/rheumatology/kel214
21. Tan AL, Fukuba E, Halliday NA, Tanner SF, Emery P, McGonagle D. High-resolution MRI assessment of dactylitis in psoriatic arthritis shows flexor tendon pulley and sheath-related enthesitis. *Ann Rheum Dis.* (2015) 74:185–89. doi: 10.1136/annrheumdis-2014-205839
22. Abrar DB, Schleich C, Nebelung S, Frenken M, Radke KL, Vordenbäumen S, et al. High-resolution MRI of flexor tendon pulleys using a 16-channel hand coil: disease detection and differentiation of psoriatic and rheumatoid arthritis. *Arthritis Res Ther.* (2020) 22:40. doi: 10.1186/s13075-020-2135-0
23. Mathew AJ, Coates LC, Danda D, Conaghan PG. Psoriatic arthritis: lessons from imaging studies and implications for therapy. *Exp Rev Clin Immunol.* (2017) 13:133–42. doi: 10.1080/1744666X.2016.1215245

24. Watad A, Eshed I, McGonaghle D. Lessons learned from imaging of enthesitis in psoriatic arthritis. *IMAJ.* (2017) 19:703–07.
25. Eshed I, Bollow M, McGonagle DG, Tan AL, Althoff CE, Asbach P, et al. MRI of enthesitis of the appendicular skeleton in spondyloarthritis. *Ann Rheum Dis.* (2007) 66:1553–59. doi: 10.1136/ard.2007.070243
26. Sudol-Szopinska I, Jurik AG, Eshed I, Lennart J, Grainger A, Østergaard M, et al. Recommendations of the ESSR arthritis subcommittee for the use of magnetic resonance imaging in musculoskeletal rheumatic diseases. *Semin Musculoskelet Radiol.* (2015) 19:396–411. doi: 10.1055/s-0035-1564696
27. Mathew AJ, Krabbe S, Eshed I, Gandjbakhch F, Bird P, Pedersen SJ, et al. The OMERACT MRI in enthesitis initiatives: definitions of key pathologies, suggested MRI sequences, and a novel heel enthesitis scoring system. *J Rheumatol.* (2019) 46:1232–38. doi: 10.3899/jrheum.181093
28. Poggenborg RP, Terslev L, Pedersen SJ, Østergaard M. Recent advances in imaging in psoriatic arthritis. *Ther Adv Musculoskel Dis.* (2011) 3:43–53. doi: 10.1177/1759720X10394031
29. Feydy A, Lavie-Brion M-C, Gossec L, Laive F, Guerini H, Nguyen C, et al. Comparative study of MRI and power Doppler ultrasonography of the heel in patients with spondyloarthritis with and without heel pain and in controls. *Ann Rheum Dis.* (2012) 71:498–503. doi: 10.1136/annrheumdis-2011-200336
30. Eshed I, Althoff CE, Feist E, Minden K, Schink T, Hamm B, et al. Magnetic resonance imaging of hindfoot involvement in patients with spondyloarthritides: comparison of low-field and high-field strength units. *Eur J Radiol.* (2008) 65:140–47. doi: 10.1016/j.ejrad.2007.03.009
31. Lambert RGW, Dhillon SS, Jhangri GS, Sacks J, Sacks H, Wong B, et al. High prevalence of symptomatic enthesopathy of the shoulder in ankylosing spondylitis: deltoid origin involvement constitutes a hallmark of disease. *Arthritis Rheum.* (2004) 51:681–90. doi: 10.1002/art.20681
32. Baraliakos X, Kiltz U, Appel H, Dybowski F, Igelmann M, Kalthoff L, et al. Chronic but not inflammatory changes at the Achilles' tendon differentiate patients with peripheral spondyloarthritis from other diagnoses - results from a prospective clinical trial. *RMD Open.* (2017) 3:e000541. doi: 10.1136/rmdopen-2017-000541
33. Tan AL, Grainger AJ, Tanner SF, Emery P, McGonagle D. A high-resolution magnetic resonance imaging study of distal interphalangeal joint arthropathy in psoriatic arthritis and osteoarthritis. Are they same? *Arthritis Rheumatol.* (2006) 54:1328–33. doi: 10.1002/art.21736
34. Jevtic V, Watt I, Rozman B, Kos-Golja M, Demsar F, Jarh O. Distinctive radiological features of small hand joints in rheumatoid arthritis and seronegative spondyloarthritis demonstrated by contrast-enhanced (Gd-DTPA) magnetic resonance imaging. *Skeletal Radiol.* (1995) 24:351–55. doi: 10.1007/BF00197064
35. Maksymowych WP, Lambert RGW, Østergaard M, Pedersen SJ, Machado PM, Weber U, et al. MRI lesions in the sacroiliac joints of patients with spondyloarthritis: an update of definitions and validation by the ASAS MRI working group. *Ann Rheum Dis.* (2019) 78:1550–58. doi: 10.1136/annrheumdis-2019-215589
36. Jans L, van Langenhove C, Van Praet L, Carron P, Elewaut D, van den Bosch F, et al. Diagnostic value of pelvic enthesitis on MRI of the sacroiliac joints in spondyloarthritis. *Eur Radiol.* (2014) 24:866–71. doi: 10.1007/s00330-013-3074-9
37. Hermann K-G A, Althoff CE, Schneider U, Zühlsdorf S, Lembcke A, Hamm B, et al. Spinal changes in patients with spondyloarthritis: comparison of MR imaging and radiographic appearances. *Radiographics.* (2005) 25:559–70. doi: 10.1148/rg.253045117
38. Lambert RGW, Pedersen SJ, Maksymowych WP, Chiowchanwisawakit P, Østergaard M. Active inflammatory lesions detected by magnetic resonance imaging in the spine of patients with spondyloarthritis - definitions, assessment system, and reference imaging set. *J Rheumatol.* (2009) 36 Suppl 84:3–17. doi: 10.3899/jrheum.090616
39. Eder L, Aydin SZ, Kaeley GS, Maksymowych WP, Østergaard M. Options for assessing joints and entheses in psoriatic arthritis by ultrasonography and magnetic resonance imaging: How to move forward. *J Rheumatol Suppl.* (2018) 94:44–7. doi: 10.3899/jrheum.180140
40. Mager A-K, Althoff CE, Sieper J, Hamm B, Hermann K-GA. Role of whole-body magnetic resonance imaging in diagnosing early spondyloarthritis. *Eur J Radiol.* (2009) 71:182–88. doi: 10.1016/j.ejrad.2009.04.051
41. Krabbe S, Eshed I, Gandjbakhch F, Pedersen SJ, Bird P, Mathew AJ, et al. Development and validation of an OMERACT MRI whole-body score for inflammation in peripheral joints and entheses in inflammatory arthritis (MRI-WIPE). *J Rheumatol.* (2019) 46:1215–21. doi: 10.3899/jrheum.181084
42. Østergaard M, Eshed I, Althoff CE, Poggenborg RP, Diekhoff T, Krabbe S, et al. Whole-body magnetic resonance imaging in inflammatory arthritis: systematic literature review and first steps toward standardization and an OMERACT scoring system. *J Rheumatol.* (2017) 44:1699–705. doi: 10.3899/jrheum.161114
43. Poggenborg RP, Pedersen SJ, Eshed I, Sørensen IJ, Møller JM, Madsen OR, et al. Head-to-toe whole-body MRI in psoriatic arthritis, axial spondyloarthritis and healthy subjects: first steps towards global inflammation and damage scores of peripheral and axial joints. *Rheumatology.* (2015) 54:1039–40. doi: 10.1093/rheumatology/keu439
44. Weckbach S, Schewe S, Michaely HJ, Steffinger D, Reiser MF, Glaser C. Whole-body MR imaging in psoriatic arthritis: additional value of therapeutic decision. *Eur J Radiol.* (2011) 77:149–55. doi: 10.1016/j.ejrad.2009.06.020
45. Althoff CE, Sieper J, Song I-H, Haibel H, Weiß A, Diekhoff T, et al. Active inflammation and structural change in early active axial spondyloarthritis as detected by whole-body MRI. *Ann Rheum Dis.* (2013) 72:967–73. doi: 10.1136/annrheumdis-2012-201545
46. Weber U, Lambert RGW, Rufibach K, Maksymowych WP, Hodler J, Zejden A, et al. Anterior chest wall inflammation by whole-body magnetic resonance imaging in patients with spondyloarthritis: lack of association between clinical and imaging findings in a cross-sectional study. *Arthritis Res Ther.* (2012) 14:R3. doi: 10.1186/ar3551
47. Marzo-Ortega H, McGonagle D, O'Connor P, Emery P. Efficacy of etanercept in the treatment of the entheseal pathology in resistant spondyloarthropathy. *Arthritis Rheum.* (2001) 44:2112–17. doi: 10.1002/1529-0131(200109)44:9<2112::AID-ART363>3.0.CO;2-H
48. Tan AL, Marzo-Ortega H, O'Connor P, Fraser A, Emery P, McGonagle D. Efficacy of anakinra in active ankylosing spondylitis: a clinical and magnetic resonance imaging study. *Ann Rheum Dis.* (2004) 63:1041–45. doi: 10.1136/ard.2004.020800
49. Karpitschka M, Godau-Kellner P, Kellner H, Horng A, Theisen D, Glaser C, et al. Assessment of therapeutic response in ankylosing spondylitis patients undergoing anti-tumour necrosis factor therapy by whole-body magnetic resonance imaging. *Eur Radiol.* (2013) 23:1773–84. doi: 10.1007/s00330-013-2794-1
50. Krabbe S, Eshed I, Sørensen IJ, Jensen B, Møller JM, Balding L, et al. Whole-body magnetic resonance imaging inflammation in peripheral joints and entheses in axial spondyloarthritis: distribution and changes during adalimumab treatment. *J Rheumatol.* (2020) 47:50–8. doi: 10.3899/jrheum.181159
51. Krabbe S, Østergaard M, Eshed I, Sørensen IJ, Jensen B, Møller JM, et al. Whole-body magnetic resonance imaging in axial spondyloarthritis: reduction of sacroiliac, spinal and entheseal inflammation in a placebo-controlled trial of adalimumab. *J Rheumatol.* (2018) 45:621–29. doi: 10.3899/jrheum.170408
52. Eder L, Polachek A, Rosen CF, Chandran V, Cook R, Gladman DD. The development of psoriatic arthritis in patients with psoriasis is preceded by a period of nospecific musculoskeletal symptoms. A prospective cohort study. *Arthritis Rheumatol.* (2017) 69:622–29. doi: 10.1002/art.39973
53. Zabotti A, McGonagle DG, Giovannini I, Errichetti E, Zuliani F, Zanetti A, et al. Transition phase towards psoriatic arthritis: clinical and ultrasonographic characterization of psoriatic arthralgia. *RMD Open.* (2019) 5:e001067. doi: 10.1136/rmdopen-2019-001067
54. Elnady B, El Shaarawy NK, Dawoud NM, Elkhouly T, Desouky DE, El Shafey EN, et al. Subclinical synovitis and enthesitis in psoriasis patients and controls by ultrasonography in Saudi Arabia: incidence of psoriatic arthritis during two years. *Clin Rheumatol.* (2019) 38:1627–35. doi: 10.1007/s10067-019-04445-0
55. Takata T, Takahashi A, Taniguchi Y, Terada Y, Sano S. Detection of asymptomatic enthesitis in psoriasis patients: an onset of psoriatic arthritis? *J Dermatol.* (2016) 43:650–54. doi: 10.1111/1346-8138.13212
56. Emad Y, Ragab Y, Bassyouni I, Moawayh O, Fawzy M, Saad A, et al. Enthesitis and related changes in knees in seronegative spondyloarthropathies and skin psoriasis: magnetic resonance imaging case-control study. *J Rheumatol.* (2010) 37:1709–17. doi: 10.3899/jrheum.100068

57. Erdem CZ, Tekin NS, Sarikaya S, Erdem LO, Gulec S. MR imaging features of foot involvement in patients with psoriasis. *Eur J Radiol.* (2008) 67:521–25. doi: 10.1016/j.ejrad.2007.08.005
58. Simon D, Tascilar K, Kleyer A, Bayat S, Kampylafka E, Sokolova M, et al. Structural enthesitis lesions in patients with psoriasis are associated with an increased risk of progression to psoriatic arthritis. *Arthritis Rheumatol.* (2020). doi: 10.1002/art.41239. [Epub ahead of print].
59. Faustini F, Simon D, Oliveira I, Kleyer A, Haschka J, Englbrecht M, et al. Subclinical joint inflammation in patients with psoriasis without concomitant psoriatic arthritis: a cross-sectional and longitudinal analysis. *Ann Rheum Dis.* (2016) 75:2068–74. doi: 10.1136/annrheumdis-2015-208821
60. Smolen JS, Schöls M, Braun J, Dougados M, FitzGerald O, Gladman DD, et al. Treating axial spondyloarthritis and peripheral spondyloarthritis, especially psoriatic arthritis, to target: 2017 update of recommendations by an international task force. *Ann Rheum Dis.* (2018) 77:3–17. doi: 10.1136/annrheumdis-2017-211734corr1
61. Coates LC, Kavanaugh A, Mease PJ, Soriano ER, Laura Acosta-Felquer M, Armstrong AW, et al. Group for research and assessment of psoriasis and psoriatic arthritis 2015 treatment recommendations for psoriatic arthritis. *Arthritis Rheumatol.* (2016) 68:1060–71. doi: 10.1002/art.39573
62. Gossec L, Smolen JS, Ramiro S, de Wit M, Cutolo M, Dougados M, et al. European league against rheumatism (EULAR) recommendations for the management of psoriatic arthritis with pharmacological therapies: 2015 update. *Ann Rheum Dis.* (2016) 75:499–510. doi: 10.1136/annrheumdis-2015-208337
63. Orbai AM, de Wit M, Mease PJ, Callis Duffin K, Elmamoun M, Tillet W, et al. Updataing the psoriatic arthritis (PsA) core domain set: a report from the PsA workshop at OMERACT (2016). *J Rheumatol.* (2017) 44:1522–28. doi: 10.3899/jrheum.160904
64. Dougados M, Combe B, Braun J, Landewè R, Sibilia J, Cantagrel A, et al. A randomised, multicentre, double-blind, placebo-controlled trial of etanercept in adults with refractory heel enthesitis in spondyloarthritis: the HEEL trial. *Ann Rheum Dis.* (2010) 69:1430–35. doi: 10.1136/ard.2009.121533
65. ClinicalTrials.gov. *Study of Efficacy and Safety of Secukinumab in Psoriatic Arthritis and Axial Spondyloarthritis Patients With Active Enthesitis Including One Achilles Tendon Site (ACHILLES).* Available online at: https://clinicaltrials.gov/ct2/show/record/NCT02771210?term=NCT02771210&rank=1
66. Song IH, Hermann KG, Haibel H, Althoff CE, Listing J, Burmester GR, et al. Effects of etanercept versus sulfasalazine in early axial spondyloarthritis on active inflammatory lesions as detected by whole-body MRI (ESTHER): a 48-week randomised controlled trial. *Ann Rheum Dis.* (2011) 70:590–96. doi: 10.1136/ard.2010.139667
67. Pagnini I, Savelli S, Matucci-Cerinic M, Fonda C, Cimaz R, Simonini G. Early predictors of juvenile sacroiliitis in enthesitis-related arthritis. *J Rheumatol.* (2010) 37:2395–401. doi: 10.3899/jrheum.100090
68. Lin C, MacKenzie JD, Courtier JL, Gu JT, Milojevic D. Magnetic resonance imaging findings in juvenile spondyloarthropathy and effects of treatment observed on subsequent imaging. *Pediatr Rheumatol Online J.* (2014) 12:25. doi: 10.1186/1546-0096-12-25
69. Herregods N, Dehoorne J, Pattyn E, Jaremko JL, Baraliakos X, Elewaut D, et al. Diagnostic value of pelvic enthesitis on MRI of the sacroiliac joints in enthesitis related arthritis. *Pedatr Rheumatol Online J.* (2015) 13:46. doi: 10.1186/s12969-015-0045-5
70. Panwar J, Patel H, Tolend M, Akikusa J, Herregods N, Highmore K, et al. Toward developing a semiquantitative whole body-MRI scoring for juvenile idiopathic arthritis: critical appraisal of the state of the art, challenges, and opportunities. *Acad Radiol.* (2020). doi: 10.1016/j.acra.2020.01.022. [Epub ahead of print].
71. Otobo TM, Conaghan PG, Maksymowych WP, van der Heijde D, Weiss P, Sudol-Szopinska I, et al. Preliminary definitions for sacroiliac joint pathologies in the OMERACT juvenile idiopathic arthritis MRI score (OMERACT JAMRIS-SIJ). *J Rheumatol.* (2019) 46:1192–97. doi: 10.3899/jrheum.181115
72. Kehl AS, Corr M, Weisman MH. Enthesitis: new insights into pathogenesis, diagnostic modalities, and treatment. *Arthritis Rheumatol.* (2016) 68:312–22. doi: 10.1002/art.39458
73. Mathew AJ, Krabbe S, Kirubakaran R, Barr AJ, Conaghan PG, Bird P, et al. Utility of magnetic resonance imaging (MRI) in diagnosing and monitoring enthesitis in patients with spondyloarthritis: a systametic literature review. *J Rheumatol.* (2019) 46:1207–14. doi: 10.3899/jrheum.181083
74. Østergaard M, Eder L, Christiansen SN, Kaeley GS. Imaging in the diagnosis and management of peripheral psoriatic arthritis - the clinical utility of magnetic resonance imaging and ultrasonography. *Best Pract Res Clin Rheumatol.* (2016) 30:624–37. doi: 10.1016/j.berh.2016.08.012
75. Kwee TC. Can whole-body MRI replace (18)F-fluorodeoxyglucose PET/CT? *Lancet Oncol.* (2014) 15:243–44. doi: 10.1016/S1470-20451470037-3
76. Gezmis E, Donmez FY, Agildere M. Diagnosis of early sacroiliitis in seronegative spondyloarthropathies by DWI and correlation of clinical and laboratory findings with ADC values. *Eur J Radiol.* (2013) 82:2316–21. doi: 10.1016/j.ejrad.2013.08.032
77. Vendhan K, Bray TJ, Atkinson D, Punwani S, Fisher C, Sen D, et al. A diffusion-based quantification technique for assessment of sacroiliitis in adolescents with enthesitis-related arthritis. *Br J Radiol.* (2016) 89:20150775. doi: 10.1259/bjr.20150775
78. Lecouvet FE, Maren NV, Collette L, Michoux N, Triqueneaux P, Stoenoiu M, et al. Whole-body MRI in spondyloarthritis (SpA): preliminary results suggest that DWI outperforms STIR for lesion detection. *Eur Radiol.* (2018) 28:4163–73. doi: 10.1007/s00330-018-5377-3
79. Chen B, Zhao Y, Cheng X, Ma Y, Chang EY, Kavanaugh A, et al. Three-dimensional ultrashort echo time cones (3D UTE-Cones) magnetic resonance imaging of entheses and tendons. *Magn Reson Imaging.* (2018) 49:4–9. doi: 10.1016/j.mri.2017.12.034
80. Chen B, Cheng X, Dorthe EW, Zhao Y, D'Lima D, Bydder GM, et al. Evaluation of normal cadaveric achilles tendon and enthesis with ultrashort echo time (UTE) magnetic resonance imaging and indentation testing. *NMR Biomed.* (2019) 32:e4034. doi: 10.1002/nbm.4034
81. Mathew AJ, Krabbe S, Eshed I, Lambert RGW, Laredo JD, Maksymowych WP, et al. Atlas of the OMERACT heel enthesitis MRI scoring system (HEMRIS). *RMD Open.* (2020) 6:e001150. doi: 10.1136/rmdopen-2019-001150
82. Haroon M, Gallagher P, Fitzgerald O. Diagnostic delay of more than 6 months contributes to poor radiographic and functional outcome in psoriatic arthritis. *Ann Rheum Dis.* (2015) 74:1045–50. doi: 10.1136/annrheumdis-2013-204858
83. Scher JU, Ogdie A, Merola JF, Ritchlin C. Preventing psoriatic arthritis: focusing on patients with psoriasis at increased risk of transition. *Nat Rev Rheumatol.* (2019) 15:153–56. doi: 10.1038/s41584-019-0175-0
84. Kampylafka E, Simon D, d'Oliveira I, Linz C, Lerchen V, Englbrecht M, et al. Disease interception with interleukin-17 inhibition in high-risk psoriasis patients with subclinical joint inflammation - data from the prospective IVEPSA study. *Arthritis Res Ther.* (2019) 21:178. doi: 10.1186/s13075-019-1957-0

8

Fast-Track Ultrasound Clinic for the Diagnosis of Giant Cell Arteritis Changes the Prognosis of the Disease but Not the Risk of Future Relapse

Sara Monti[1,2*], *Alice Bartoletti*[1], *Elisa Bellis*[1], *Paolo Delvino*[1,2] *and Carlomaurizio Montecucco*[1]

[1] *Rheumatology Department, IRCCS Policlinico S. Matteo Foundation, University of Pavia, Pavia, Italy,* [2] *PhD in Experimental Medicine, University of Pavia, Pavia, Italy*

***Correspondence:**
Sara Monti
sara.saramonti@gmail.com

Background: Color Duplex sonography (CDS) of temporal arteries and large vessels (LV) is a recently validated diagnostic methodology for Giant Cell Arteritis (GCA). CDS combined with a fast-track approach (FTA) has improved the early diagnosis of the disease.

Objectives: To assess FTA effects on the prevention of permanent visual loss (PVL), relapse and late complications of GCA compared to conventional practice. To assess the impact of COVID-19 pandemic on outcomes of GCA patients assessed with FTA.

Methods: GCA patients diagnosed up to June 2020 at the Rheumatology Department, University of Pavia, were included. FTA was implemented since October 2016. FTA consists in the referral within 1 working day of a suspected GCA case to an expert rheumatologist who performs clinical evaluation and CDS.

Results: One hundred sixty patients were recruited [female 120 (75%), mean age 72.4 ± 8.2 years]. Sixty-three (39.4%) evaluated with FTA, 97 (60.6%) with conventional approach. FTA patients were older (75.1 ± 7.6 vs. 70.6 ± 8.2 years old; $p < 0.001$). Median follow-up duration was shorter in the FTA group compared to the conventional one (0.9 vs. 5.0 years; $p < 0.001$). There was no difference between the two cohorts regarding major vessel district involvement (LV-GCA 17.5% vs. 22.7%; $p = 0.4$). PVL occurred in 8 (12.7%) FTA patients and 26 (26.8%) conventional ones ($p = 0.03$). The relative risk of blindness in the conventional group was 2.11 (95% C.I. 1.02–4.36; $P = 0.04$) as compared to FTA. Median symptom latency of patients experiencing PVL was higher in the conventional group (23 days IQR 12–96 vs. 7 days IQR 4–10, $p = 0.02$). During COVID-19 there was a significant increase in the occurrence of PVL (40%) including bilateral blindness despite a regularly operating FTA clinic. Cumulative incidence of relapses and time to first relapse did not change after FTA introduction ($P = 0.2$). No difference in late complications (stenosis/aneurysms) was detected.

Conclusions: FTA including CDS evaluation contributed to a substantial reduction of PVL in GCA by shortening the time to diagnosis and treatment initiation. Relapse rate did not change upon FTA introduction, highlighting the need for better disease activity monitoring and treatment strategies optimization based on risk stratification that would predict the occurrence of relapse during glucocorticoid de-escalation.

Keywords: giant cell arteritis, sonography, ultrasoud, fast-track, permanent visual loss, large vessel vasculitis

INTRODUCTION

Giant Cell Arteritis (GCA) is the most prevalent primary systemic vasculitis (1). GCA typically affects the aorta and its major branches, even though medium and small-sized arteries may be targeted as well (2). Indeed, permanent visual loss (PVL), one of the most feared complications of GCA, results from damage to ophthalmic, retinal or ciliary arteries (3). Other clinical manifestations include headache, jaw or tongue claudication, scalp tenderness and polymyalgia rheumatica (PMR). Sometimes the picture is protean with increased inflammatory markers, fever and weight loss and it may get underdiagnosed. The heavy morbidity burden of GCA is due to its rather late onset (usually occurring over the age of 50 years old) and the occurrence of PVL in approximately 20% patients, usually at the very beginning of the disease. Treatment with high-dose glucocorticoids (GC) should be promptly initiated when the disease is suspected to prevent PVL. The clinical spectrum of GCA also comprises large vessel complications such as thoracic and abdominal aortic aneurysm or dissection, which can increase the risk of mortality (2, 4).

Strategies for early GCA diagnosis have been implemented in the last decade in order to reduce the occurrence of blindness. Color-duplex sonography (CDS) of temporal arteries (TAs) and large extra-cranial vessels (LVs) has been recently recognized as a first-line diagnostic tool for patients with suspected GCA in centers with the adequate expertise in the technique. A fast track approach (FTA), incorporating CDS has been associated with a significant reduction of PVL in two retrospective studies (5, 6). However, some patients still manifest with PVL as the very first symptom of this disease.

The role of imaging, including CDS, as a prognostic tool and in the follow-up of patients with GCA including the detection of relapses is still controversial (7).

OBJECTIVES

The aim of this study is to assess the role of FTA on PVL prevention and long-term relapse risk and outcome of patients with GCA, comparing the FTA outcomes with conventional practice while taking into-account the influence of the severe acute respiratory syndrome coronavirus-2 (SARS-CoV-2) pandemic on the FTA activity.

METHODS

The present study included patients who were diagnosed with GCA between January 1st, 2005 and June 30th, 2020 at the Rheumatology Department of IRCCS Fondazione Policlinico San Matteo hospital in Pavia, Italy.

The study has been approved by the Institutional Review Board of the University of Pavia and patients consented to their data use.

FTA was implemented since October 1st, 2016. FTA consists in the referral within one working day of a suspected GCA case to an expert rheumatologist, who performs the clinical examination and CDS of temporal and axillary arteries. Other anatomical sites (e.g., facial arteries, occipital arteries, carotid arteries) could be assessed according to the patient's clinical picture. Patients can be referred to the FTA from the general practitioner or other Departments. Patients enrolled after October 2016 were considered FTA if they received a rheumatologist's evaluation within one working day after the first medical contact. Patients assessed as part of the FTA between March 1st and June 30th 2020 during the coronavirus 2019 (COVID-19) pandemic were analyzed separately. Patients assessed prior to October 2016 were included in the conventional practice group (no-FTA).

The diagnosis of GCA was confirmed by the expert rheumatologist on the basis of typical symptoms, data on inflammatory markers, and imaging (CDS, ^{18}FDG PET-CT) or temporal artery biopsy (TAB) findings. Since the FTA implementation, the same rheumatologist (S.M.) performed the clinical and ultrasonographic assessment.

Clinical manifestations at disease onset, laboratory tests, date of symptoms onset, date of diagnosis, comorbidities, information on treatment, and follow-up, including relapses were extracted from the clinical records and recorded on an electronic database. Data were extracted retrospectively for the conventional cohort. FTA patients were assessed prospectively since diagnosis. Treatment followed current recommendations for both cohorts including high-dose GC (1 mg/kg/day; maximum 60 mg/day) maintained for 1 month and then tapered while monitoring disease activity. In patients with recent onset of ischaemic visual symptoms i.v. methylprednisolone was prescribed for the first 3 days (1 g/day). Adjunctive immunosuppressive treatment (most frequently Methotrexate or Tocilizumab) were prescribed to relapsing patients (8, 9). PVL was defined by the complete or partial visual impairment caused by vasculitic damage of the visual pathway [e.g., anterior ischaemic optic neuropathy (AION); posterior ischaemic optic neuropathy

(PION)] confirmed after ophthalmologic assessment. Symptom latency was calculated as the time interval between the onset of the first symptom attributable to GCA (e.g., date of headache or other cranial symptoms onset, girdle inflammatory pain onset, systemic symptoms onset) and the diagnosis. Large-vessel GCA (LV-GCA) was defined as the presence of extra-cranial LV involvement (e.g., aortic, axillary arteries) detected by imaging (most frequently CDS and/or ^{18}FDG PET-CT) with or without temporal artery involvement. Relapse was defined as the reoccurrence of symptoms and signs of GCA, with or without elevation of the inflammatory markers, with the need to increase the dosage of GC or to add or increase the dose of another immunosuppressive drug. Disease complications during follow-up are defined by the occurrence of stenosis or aneurysms/dissections and/or ischaemic complications.

Ultrasonographic Assessment

CDS was performed by the same rheumatologist experienced in vascular ultrasound for the assessment of large vessel vasculitis (S.M.). Patients were assessed with the MyLab Seven Esaote ultrasound machine with a high-frequency (18–6 MHz) linear transducer. Focus was set at 5 mm for temporal arteries and 3 cm for axillary arteries. A Doppler frequency of 10 MHz was applied. Pulse repetition frequency (PRF) was set at 2–3 KHz for temporal artery, and at 3–4 KHz for axillary arteries. A low wall filter was selected to allow the identification of low velocity flow. The color box was adjusted to obtain an angle steer correction ≤ 60 degrees.

The common, parietal, and frontal branches of each temporal artery and the axillary arteries in longitudinal and transverse plans were assessed at each visit. The presence of a halo was defined according to the accepted definitions as a homogenous, hypoechoic wall thickening, well-delineated toward the luminal side, visible both in longitudinal and transverse planes, most commonly concentric in transverse scans (10). The compression sign was applied in transverse views to confirm the findings (11). CDS was defined as positive if displaying a halo at the level of at least one branch of the temporal artery or at least one axillary artery. Intima-media thickness was measured at the site of maximum thickness on longitudinal plans.

Statistical Analysis

Categorical variables were presented as numbers and percentages. Continuous variables were displayed as means with standard deviation (S.D.) if normally distributed or as medians with interquartile range (IQR) in case of non-normal distribution. Ratios were presented with 95% confidence intervals (C.I.). For comparison between groups, the independent-samples t-test for continuous variables and the chi-squared test for categorical variables were applied. For non-parametric numerical variables, the Wilcoxon signed-rank test was used. Statistical analysis was performed the software RStudio (R version 3.6.3 2020-02-29, Copyright © 2020 The R Foundation for Statistical Computing). $P < 0.05$ were considered to be significant.

RESULTS

Baseline Assessment

One-hundred and sixty patients were recruited, 120 were females (75%), the mean age at diagnosis was 72.4 ± 8.2 years. Sixty-three (39.4%) were evaluated with FTA, while 97 (60.6%) underwent the conventional approach.

FTA patients were older (75.1 ± 7.6 vs. 70.6 ± 8.2 years old; $p < 0.001$). At the time of diagnosis, a larger percentage of comorbidity-free patients was observed in the non-FTA group (16.7 vs. 3.8%; $P = 0.02$). Nevertheless, major cardiovascular comorbidities like coronary artery disease, dyslipidaemia, diabetes, stroke, peripheral artery disease and hypertension were similar between the two cohorts ($P > 0.05$) except for heart failure (1.0% conventional vs. 7.5% FTA; $P = 0.03$). Overall, 19.4% (ranging 15.5–25%) of patients with newly diagnosed GCA had a previous diagnosis of polymyalgia rheumatica.

FTA contributed to shorten the time to diagnosis (62 days IQR 20–122 in the conventional cohort vs. 33 days IQR 15–83 in the FTA cohort; $P = 0.035$) (**Table 1**), especially for cranial GCA patients (61 days IQR 15–107 vs. 30 days IQR 13–53; $P = 0.007$). Of note, among patients with PVL the duration of symptoms (since the onset of the first symptom attributable to GCA) before receiving a diagnosis of GCA was higher in the conventional group (23 days IQR 12–96 vs. 7 days IQR 4–10; $P = 0.02$).

There was no difference between FTA and the conventional group regarding major vessel district involvement (cranial GCA 82.5 vs. 77.3%, respectively; $P = 0.4$). The clinical presentation was similar between the two groups: the frequency of PMR, headache, amaurosis fugax, jaw claudication and fever did not change between the two cohorts ($P > 0.05$). Some symptoms were more frequently recorded in the FTA group compared to the conventional practice: weight loss (30.2 vs. 13.4%; $P = 0.01$), tongue claudication (11.1 vs. 1.0%; $P = 0.004$) and scalp tenderness (20.6 vs. 5.2%; $P = 0.003$). PVL occurred in 8 (12.7%) patients in the FTA group compared to 26 (26.8%) in the conventional one ($P = 0.03$). The relative risk of blindness in the conventional group was 2.11 (95% C.I. 1.02–4.36; $P = 0.04$) as compared to FTA. The overall occurrence of ischaemic manifestations of GCA (AION, PION and cerebrovascular accidents) was higher in the non-FTA cohort (28.9 vs. 12.7; $P = 0.02$) (**Table 2**). The relationship between symptoms latency in the whole cohort and visual outcomes, and visual survival over time are shown in **Supplementary Figures 1, 2**.

Forty-four (45.4%) patients of the conventional cohort underwent TAB, with 25 (56.8%) samples were compatible with GCA at the histological examination. TAB was performed in 3 patients of the new cohort, two of them without signs of active vasculitis and one with a sampling error. TAB sensitivity was 53.2% (95% C.I. 38.1–67.9%).

Within the FTA group, all 63 (100.0%) were evaluated with CDS at the time of diagnosis, 52 of them having specific ultrasound findings of GCA (**Figures 1, 2**), yielding a sensitivity of 82.5% (95% C.I. 70.9–91.0%). Thirty-one (49.2%) had bilateral halo at CDS. Forty-three presented with halo sign exclusively at temporal arteries, 4 had only axillary artery halos, 5 had both districts involved. Temporal artery abnormalities at the

TABLE 1 | Clinical features of the cohort at baseline.

	Total ($N = 160$)	Conventional ($N = 97$)	FTA ($n = 63$)	*P*-value
Age at diagnosis, mean (S.D.), years	72.4 (8.2)	70.6 (8.2)	75.1 (7.6)	<0.001
Female, *n* (%)	120 (75)	77 (79.4)	43 (68.3)	0.1
Previous PMR, *n* (%)	31 (19.4)	15 (15.5)	16 (25.4)	0.1
Symptom latency, median (IQR), days	46 (15–101)	62 (20–122)	33 (15–83)	0.04
Symptoms latency of patients with PVL, median (IQR), days	14 (8–65)	23 (12–96)	7 (4–10)	0.02
Comorbidities				
Coronary heart disease	15 (10.1)	9 (9.4)	6 (11.3)	0.7
Dyslipidaemia	30 (20.1)	18 (18.8)	12 (22.6)	0.6
Diabetes mellitus	18 (12.1)	14 (14.6)	4 (7.5)	0.2
Stroke	14 (9.4)	11 (11.5)	3 (5.7)	0.2
Peripheral artery disease	7 (4.7)	5 (5.2)	2 (3.8)	0.2
Hypertension	85 (57.0)	53 (55.2)	32 (60.4)	0.5
Heart failure	5 (3.4)	1 (1.0)	4 (7.5)	0.03
Other comorbidities	102 (68.5)	73 (76.0)	39 (73.6)	0.7
No comorbidities	18 (12.1)	16 (16.7)	2 (3.8)	0.02

TABLE 2 | Clinical picture at the time of diagnosis in the two cohorts: conventional approach (No FTA) vs. FTA.

	No FTA ($N = 97$)	FTA ($N = 63$)	*P*-value
Symptoms at diagnosis			
Constitutional (fever or weight loss), *n* (%)	36 (37.1)	28 (44.4)	0.4
Fever ≥ 38°C (≥100.4 F), *n* (%)	32 (33.0)	17 (27.0)	0.4
Weight loss ≥2 kg, *n* (%)	13 (13.4)	19 (30.2)	0.01
Any cranial symptom, *n* (%)	88 (90.7)	53 (84.1)	0.2
Any ocular symptom, *n* (%)	37 (38.1)	17 (27.0)	0.1
Permanent visual loss, *n* (%)	26 (26.8)	8 (12.7)	0.03
Amaurosis fugax, *n* (%)	14 (14.4)	7 (11.1)	0.5
Diplopia, *n* (%)	4 (4.1)	1 (1.6)	0.4
Jaw claudication, *n* (%)	33 (34.0)	29 (46.0)	0.1
Tongue claudication, *n* (%)	1 (1.0)	7 (11.1)	0.004
Scalp tenderness, *n* (%)	5 (5.2)	13 (20.6)	0.003
Headache, *n* (%)	77 (79.4)	45 (71.4)	0.3
PMR, *n* (%)	48 (49.5)	32 (50.7)	0.9
Increased ESR/CRP, *n* (%)	79 (90.8)	59 (96.7)	0.2
ESR (mm/h), median (IQR)	82 (48–102)	78 (63–96)	0.5
CRP (mg/L), median (IQR)	35 (20–99)	59 (24–98)	0.5
Anemia (<12 g/dL in females, <13 g/dL in males), *n* (%)	38 (65.5)	17 (77.2)	0.3
Hemoglobin, mean (S.D.), g/dL	11.4 (1.6)	11.5 (1.4)	1.0
Cranial GCA	75 (77.3)	52 (82.5)	0.4
LV-GCA	22 (22.7)	11 (17.5)	0.4
Ischaemic GCA	28 (28.9)	8 (12.7)	0.02

time of referral was a predictor of positive CDS (43.8 vs. 10.0%; $P = 0.046$), and it was strongly correlated to a positive halo sign at the level of the temporal arteries (47.7 vs. 7.1%; $P = 0.006$), as well as to bilateral halo sign (51.7 vs. 24.1%; $P = 0.03$).

Forty-two patients who underwent CDS (66.7%) had previously received GC for a median time of 12 days (IQR 3–101). Twenty-two patients (34.9%) had been treated with high-dose GC therapy (≥30 mg/day) for a median time of 4 days (IQR 3–8). The median prednisone-equivalent dosage on the day of scan was 37.5 mg/day (IQR 10–50).

CDS sensitivity was lower in patients with high-dose GC doses protracted for >5 days ($N = 10$), reducing to 60.0% (95% C.I. 26.2–87.8%).

Follow-Up and Relapses

The median follow-up duration was 3.2 years (IQR 1.0–5.9 years), shorter in the FTA group compared with the conventional one [0.9 years (IQR 0.2–2.0) vs. 5.0 years (IQR 3.5–8.7); $P < 0.001$].

During the follow-up, 82 patients relapsed (51.3%). The median time to disease reoccurrence was 8 months (IQR 3–20 months). The calculated relapse rate per 10 person-years was 3.0 (95% C.I. 2.6–3.4 years). Fifty (31.3%) patients experienced more than one relapse. In the conventional group there were 64 (66%) relapses overall, over a longer follow-up duration; in the FTA 18 (28.6%) relapses were observed. The calculated relapse rate per 10 person-years did not differ between the two cohorts: [2.9 (95% C.I. 2.5–3.4) in the conventional group vs. 3.6 (95% C.I. 2.3–5.2) in the FTA (**Table 3**).

The cumulative incidence of relapse and time to first relapse did not change after FTA was implemented ($P = 0.23$) (**Figure 3**).

During follow-up there were no new cases of PVL related to disease relapses. Symptoms at the time of first relapse were different between the two groups. In the FTA cohort more patients were presenting with PMR-like symptoms (50.0 vs. 23.4%; $P = 0.03$), whereas cranial symptoms (22.2 vs. 64.1%; $P = 0.002$), especially headache (16.7 vs. 48.4%; $P = 0.02$), were more prominent in the historical cohort. Interestingly, none of the FTA patients with ischaemic GCA relapsed during follow-up (0.0% with ischaemic disease vs. 26.6% without ischaemic GCA; $P = 0.01$).

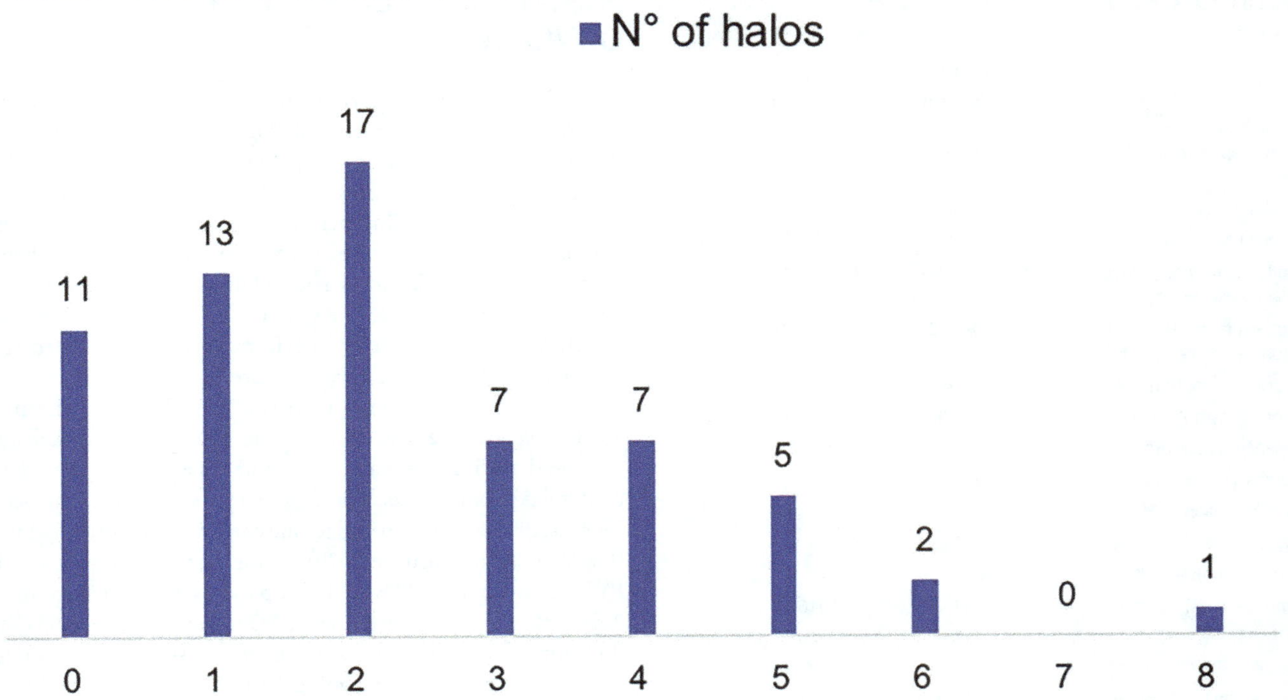

FIGURE 1 | CDS findings of patients evaluated with the FTA. Number of patients according to number of sites with halos (0–8 sites including the different branches of the temporal artery and the axillary arteries).

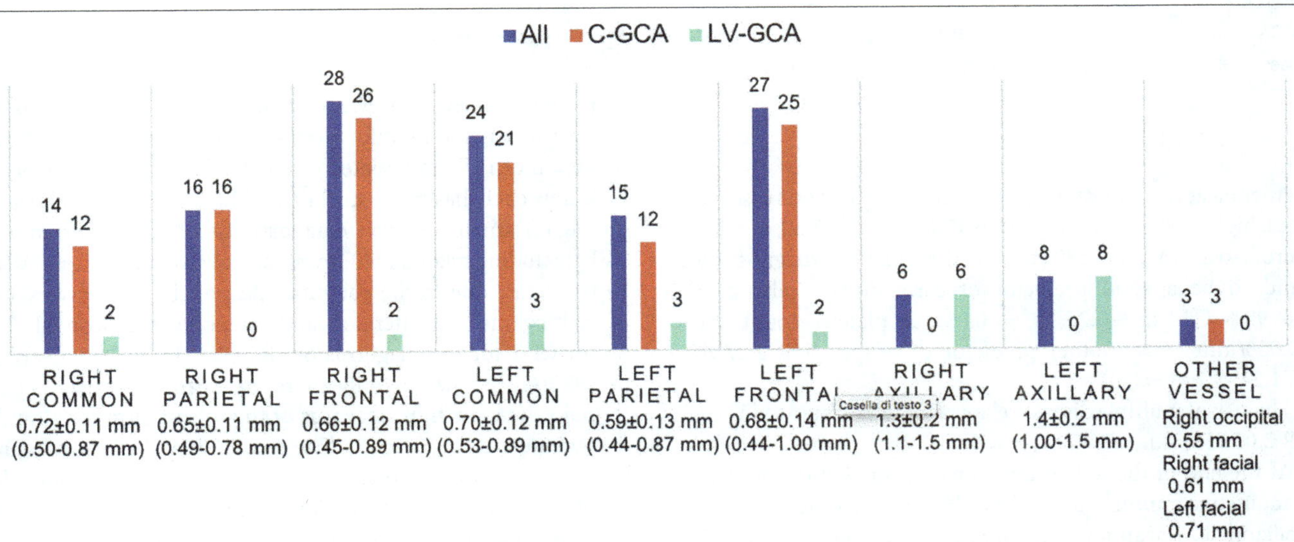

FIGURE 2 | CDS findings distribution and intima-media thickness of patients evaluated with the FTA. Number of patients with positive CDS in each vascular district, the average halo thickness (± S.D., range) is reported below. C-GCA, cranial giant cell arteritis; LV-GCA, large-vessel giant cell arteritis.

The ongoing therapy at the time of relapse was similar between the two groups. The median dose of prednisone was 12.5 vs. 13.75 mg/day between the two cohorts ($P = 0.4$).

Out of 18 patients of the FTA group with a confirmed GCA relapse, 14 CDS scans were performed (77.8%). Six scans had signs of active disease (42.9%) in patients with confirmed relapses. Bilateral halo was found in 2 patients with relapse (33.3%).

Regarding the non-FTA group, 13 patients were evaluated with CDS for relapse assessment. The total number of CDS was 22, with 10 of them showing a halo (45.5%) of which four were bilateral halos (40.0%).

TABLE 3 | Relapse characteristics between the conventional (No FTA) and the FTA cohorts.

	No FTA (*N* = 64)	FTA (*N* = 18)	*P*-value
Age at relapse, mean (S.D.), years	70.3 (8.1)	72.7 (7.7)	0.3
Females, *n* (%)	50 (80.0)	12 (66.7)	0.2
Previous PMR, *n* (%)	12 (18.8)	5 (27.7)	0.4
Time to 1st relapse (if any), median (IQR), months	8.5 (3.8–20.3)	7.5 (3.3–10.8)	0.4
Relapse rate per 10 person-years, median (95% C.I.)	2.9 (2.5–3.4)	3.6 (2.3–5.2)	0.3
Any cranial symptom, *n* (%)	41 (64.1)	4 (22.2)	0.002
Any ocular symptom, *n* (%)	4 (6.3)	0 (0.0)	0.3
Permanent visual loss, *n* (%)	0 (0.0)	0 (0.0)	nd
Amaurosis fugax, *n* (%)	4 (6.3)	0 (0.0)	0.3
Jaw claudication, *n* (%)	4 (6.3)	1 (5.6)	0.9
Tongue claudication, *n* (%)	0 (0.0)	0 (0.0)	nd
Scalp tenderness, *n* (%)	3 (4.7)	0 (0.0)	0.4
Headache, *n* (%)	31 (48.4)	3 (16.7)	0.02
PMR, *n* (%)	15 (23.4)	9 (50.0)	0.03
Increased ESR/CRP, *n* (%)	41 (67.2)	12 (66.6)	0.9
ESR, median (IQR), mm/h	36 (25–53)	32 (22–47)	0.2
CRP, median (IQR), mg/L	11.0 (5.4–18.6)	12.5 (5.2–26)	0.9
GC dose, median (IQR), mg/day	12.5 (7.5–25)	13.75 (10–25)	0.4
Immunosuppressive drug, *n* (%)	9 (14.1)	0 (0.0)	0.09
Cranial GCA	48 (75.0)	16 (88.9)	0.2
LV-GCA	16 (25.0)	2 (11.1)	0.2
Ischaemic GCA	17 (26.6)	0 (0.0)	0.01

Anemia at the time of diagnosis (Hb <11 g/dL) was associated with a higher relapse risk (HR 1.96 95% C.I. 1.04–3.69; $P = 0.04$). Microcytosis (MCV <80 fL) at the time of diagnosis was found to be a good predictor of early disease relapse (HR 2.80 95% C.I. 2.33–3.26; $P = 0.03$). A platelet count above 450,000/mm^3 was another predictor of relapse (HR 2.67 95% C.I. 1.24–5.7; $P = 0.01$).

The risk of multiple disease relapses was associated to LV-GCA (HR 2.02 95% C.I. 1.07–3.81; $P = 0.03$).

At the end of the follow-up, 38 patients (23.7%) were taking an adjunctive immunosuppressive (IS) agent (34 methotrexate, 3 Tocilizumab, 1 azathioprine) initiated after a median time of 10 months (IQR 5-29 months). There were no significant differences in the requirements for adjunctive IS between the two cohorts. LV-GCA patients were at higher risk of requiring IS (HR 2.42 95% C.I. 1.16–5.04; $P = 0.02$).

Chronic Complications

Large vessel complications (aneurysm, stenosis, vessel ectasia or dissection) were found to be more frequent in patients with LV-GCA (HR 4.58 95% C.I. 1.92–10.92; $P = 0.0006$) (**Figure 4**). There were no differences between the FTA and the conventional cohort.

FAST-TRACK CLINIC AT THE TIME OF COVID-19

During the lockdown period due the SARS-CoV-2 pandemic outbreak in Italy (March-April 2020) there was a significant decrease in the number of patients referred to the clinic compared to the preceding months (9 visits compared to 4) and to the corresponding period in the previous year (16 visits compared to 4) despite a regularly operating service (**Figure 5**). Since the end of the lockdown period the number of new referrals has increased again (15 new visits in the period May-June 2020), nevertheless, a delay in referral has been recorded since the pandemic outbreak. Overall there have been 10 confirmed diagnoses of GCA during this period, female (80%), mean age 76 ± 5 years. The rate of PVL due to GCA has significantly increased during the pandemic, and especially in the rate of bilateral AION which occurred in two patients during the period March-April 2020 compared to one case over the previous 4 years (October 2016-February 2020) of the fast-track clinic activity. PVL occurred in 4 (40%) of GCA patients assessed since March 2020 (vs. 12.7% in the previous FTA period; $P = 0.03$). The duration of symptoms prior to diagnosis since the COVID-19 outbreak in patients developing PVL has increased to 23 days (IQR 15–56) compared to 7 days (IQR 4–10) of the normal FTA activity; the two patients developing bilateral blindness were referred after a mean of 31 days since the symptoms onset.

DISCUSSION

Our data confirm that FTA including CDS assessment is an innovative disease-modifying strategy leading to a significant reduction of PVL and related disability. The effectiveness of the FTA approach has been further highlighted in our cohort by the significant increase in diagnostic delay and occurrence of PVL, including bilateral blindness, observed during the COVID-19 pandemic due to the patients', and possibly care givers' fear of seeking medical attention and attending the hospital. The use of CDS for the diagnosis of GCA has been first described in 1997 (12), however only in recent years there has been a formal validation and consensus of the role of ultrasound in the management of LVV (9, 13). The recognition of CDS as the first imaging modality in patients with cranial GCA was only included in International recommendations 2 years ago (9, 13). In Centers with the adequate expertise and machine equipment and settings, ultrasound has replaced TAB for the diagnosis of patients with suspected GCA and a highly suggestive clinical picture (7, 13, 14) As demonstrated by the change of practice in our two cohorts, the need for TAB reduced by 93% since the use of CDS as part of the FTA clinic. CDS has the advantage of being a quick, repeatable, low-cost procedure that allows to assess the whole length of the temporal artery (reducing false negatives related to the skipped nature of GCA inflammation) and to extent the examination to other cranial or extra-cranial arteries, optimizing the diagnostic yield (15, 16). CDS has been demonstrated to be more sensitive compared to TAB in the diagnosis of GCA (14), as confirmed by our study. The implementation of CDS into FTA clinics

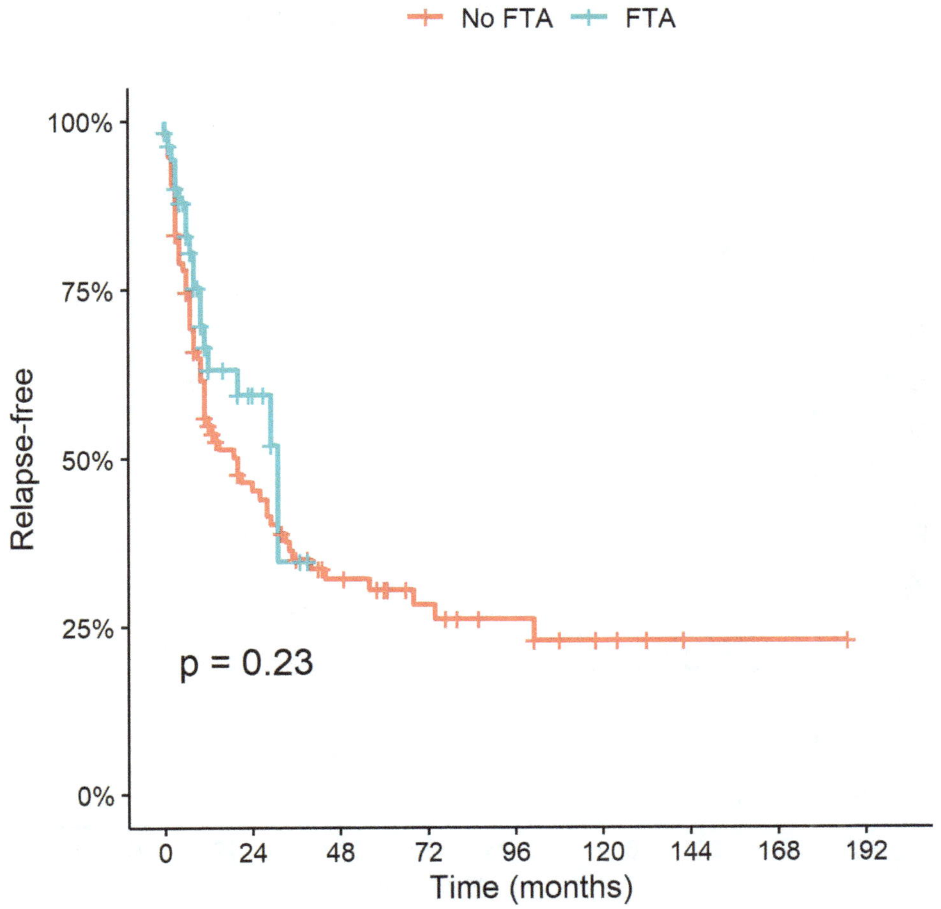

FIGURE 3 | Time to first relapse before and after FTA introduction.

allowing for a prompt and direct assessment and interpretation of imaging findings by the treating physician has led to the demonstration that very early diagnosis with the aid of CDS can significantly reduce the risk of PVL in patients with GCA (6, 17). Our data highlight the importance of early diagnostic assessment and treatment initiation through FTA, but also of early referral through the prompt recognition of prodrome symptoms possibly preceding the occurrence of ischaemic complications of GCA. In our cohort, patients assessed with FTA had less frequent comorbidities albeit being generally older. This characteristic might have contributed to reduce the confounding effect in case of presentation with unspecific symptoms and could have led to a more rapid referral compared to the conventional practice group. Blindness has been described in 15–30% of patients with GCA and is a complication that mostly occurs at the early stages of the disease, often being the presenting symptom leading to the diagnosis (18). Nevertheless, up to 28% of patients with PVL report premonitory reversible transient visual symptoms that can prompt the urgent referral if properly investigated and recognized (18). Other factors associated with PVL include jaw claudication, absence of constitutional symptoms or milder elevation of inflammatory markers (19, 20). Visual loss is usually irreversible in GCA, however, early initiation of GC, particularly if initiated within the 1st day of visual symptoms has been reported as the sole prognostic factor for a partial improvement of visual loss (9, 19). Diagnostic delay is known to be associated with the occurrence of bilateral PVL as confirmed by our data observed during COVID-19 outbreak (19). Clinical suspicion avoiding over-reliance on temporal headache alone is key to the early recognition of GCA. In our FTA cohort some symptoms were recorded as more frequent such as tongue claudication, scalp tenderness or weight loss. It is possible that patients with a clinical presentation more easily resembling GCA would be referred more rapidly, however, increased attention to rarer or less specific symptoms of GCA is pivotal to optimize the clinical suspicion. To further improve the outcome of LVV, the expedited process allowing for early access to specialist evaluation and confirmatory investigational tests obtained with FTA should be paralleled by educational programmes and clear recommendations for fast-track referral offered to primary care and other relevant specialists to further reduced the symptom latency period (21, 22). An improvement of the general public awareness of GCA could also be beneficial to reduce the diagnostic delay. During the COVID-19 pandemic several

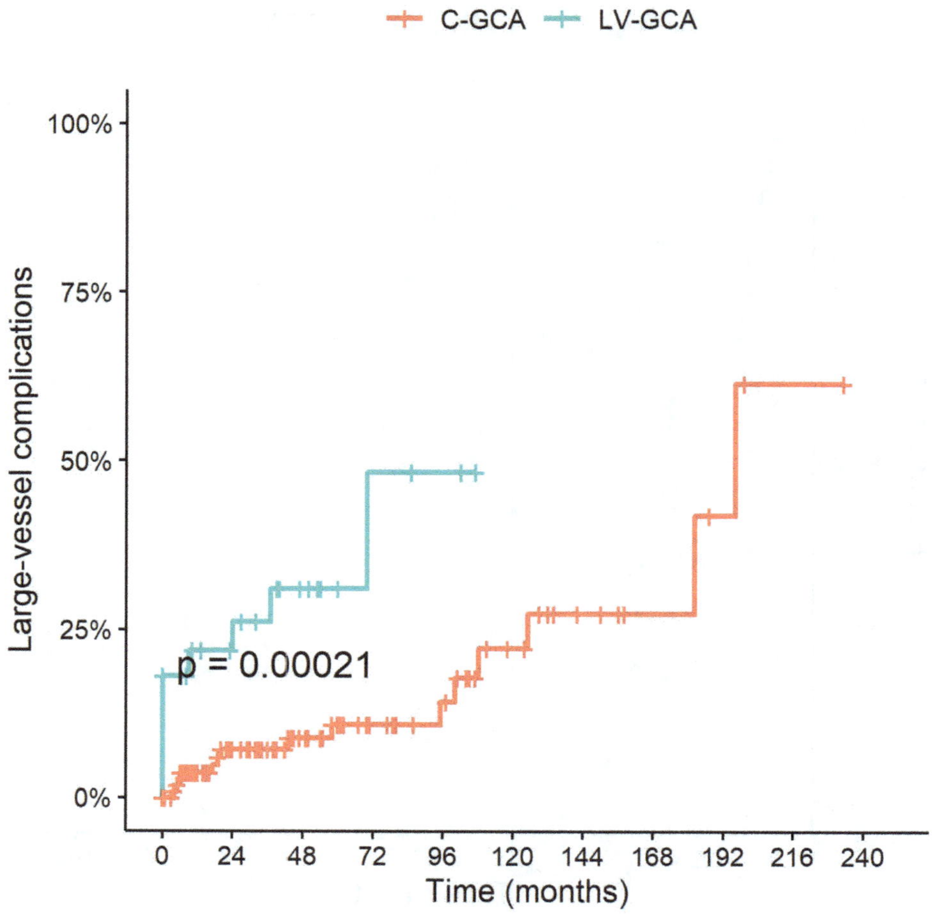

FIGURE 4 | Cumulative incidence of LV complications among LV-GCA compared to C-GCA. LV complications include thoracic/abdominal aortic aneurysm or dissection and stenosis, aneurysm or ectasia of other large arteries.

medical emergencies, including acute coronary syndromes, have recorded an unusual decrease in hospitalization and increased out-of-hospital mortality as a result of avoidance or delay in seeking medical attention (23, 24). Similarly, we have observed a significant increase in the rate of ischaemic complications (with 40% of PVL), including bilateral blindness with two new cases over a period of 2 months, compared to only one case over the 4-year activity of the FTA (25). The duration of symptom prior to the first evaluation for suspected GCA has increased during the COVID-19 outbreak despite a regularly operating fast-track clinic. The negative outcome of newly diagnosed patients with GCA observed during SARS-CoV-2 outbreak confirms once more that urgent referral and FTA are key in the management of LVV with a significant change in visual prognosis.

Nonetheless, our data suggest that FTA does not impact the long-term outcomes and relapse-risk. Our findings are in line with previous reports suggesting that early diagnosis of GCA does not seem to significantly improve the future risk of relapse (26). Predictors of relapse in LVV are poorly understood. Our data confirm that markers of inflammation, baseline anemia, and LV-GCA are associated with a higher risk of relapse (27–30). Increasing interest is emerging to find different predictors of relapse or future disease complications as part of the FTA approach, including quantitative analysis of CDS findings suggestive of more extensive or more severe vascular involvement at disease onset (31). A recently proposed ultrasonographic score combining information on the number of sites with halo and the halo thickness was suggested to be associated with ocular ischaemia (32). Nevertheless, to date, no reliable imaging biomarker has been identified to predict the risk of relapse or future ischaemic complications during follow-up (33, 34).

Our study has some limitations, including the retrospective collection of some of the data. Moreover, comparisons between the two cohorts regarding some of the rarer complications of GCA might have been limited by the small sample size.

The unmodified disease course despite the FTA and early diagnosis strategies in GCA suggest that a change in therapeutic strategy should be applied since the early stages of the disease to significantly modify the long-term outcome. Available evidence demonstrated a glucocorticoid-sparing effect and efficacy in reducing the risk of relapse in newly diagnosed or relapsing

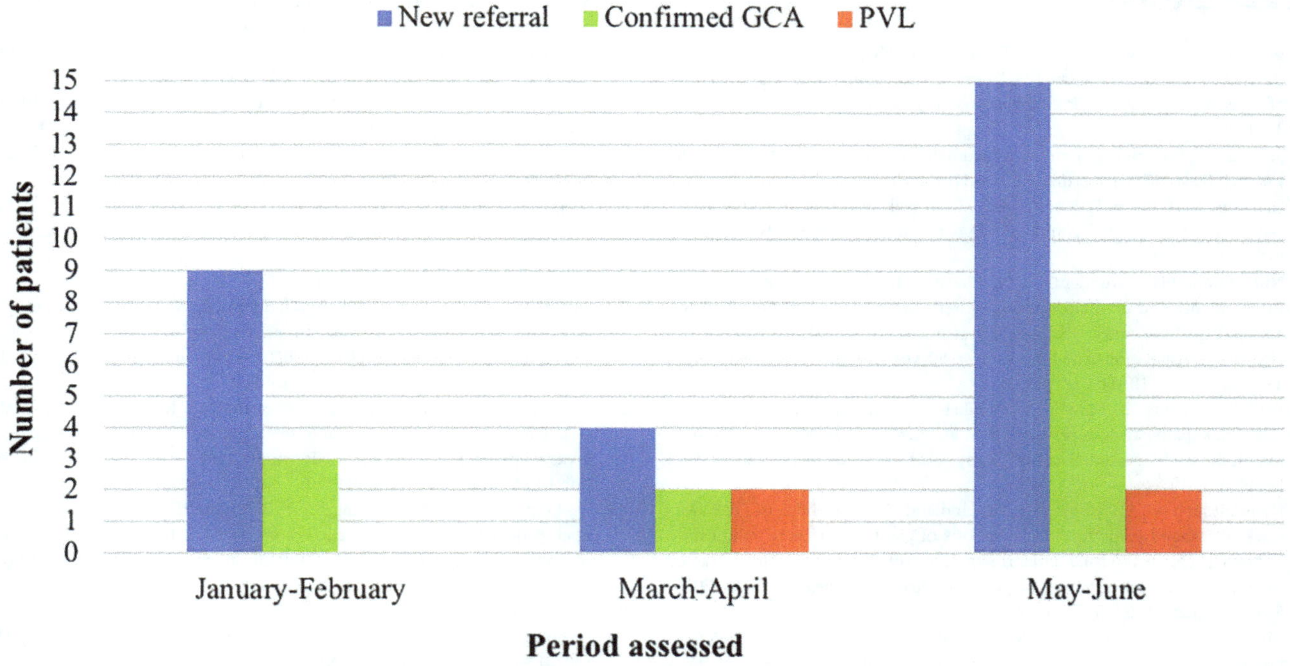

FIGURE 5 | Comparison of the fast-track clinic activity amongst different periods of 2020, including the lockdown months due to COVID-19 pandemic (March-April). GCA, giant cell arteritis; PVL, permanent visual loss.

patients with GCA treated with methotrexate or tocilizumab (35, 36). Nevertheless, in clinical practice patient-tailored evaluations of safety and cost-effectiveness issues are often taken into consideration in this elderly population group treated with concomitant high-dose glucocorticoids. Current recommendations suggest to reserve adjunctive therapy to selected patients with refractory or relapsing disease or with the presence or increased risk of glucocorticoid related adverse events and complications. A risk stratification process to select patients with poor prognosis to be treated more intensively upfront still requires further research. Data obtained from the FTA clinics suggest that the window of opportunity to obtain long-term modifications of the disease process in GCA is exceedingly short and should probably be associated with an optimization of the disease awareness to further accelerate referral and with a tailored therapeutic approach to potentiate treatment in patients at higher risk of relapse and complications.

CONCLUSION

FTA including CDS evaluation contributed to a substantial reduction of the PVL risk in GCA by shortening the time to diagnosis and treatment initiation. Relapse rate and LV-complications did not change upon FTA introduction, highlighting the need for better disease activity monitoring strategies and risk stratification at disease onset that would predict the occurrence of relapse during glucocorticoid de-escalation.

ETHICS STATEMENT

The studies involving human participants were reviewed and approved by University of Pavia Ethical Committee. The patients/participants provided their written informed consent to participate in this study.

AUTHOR CONTRIBUTIONS

SM, AB, EB, PD, and CM contributed equally to the ideation and realization of the research project and critically reviewed the manuscript. SM and AB wrote the manuscript. All authors contributed to the article and approved the submitted version.

SUPPLEMENTARY MATERIAL

The Supplementary Material for this article can be found online at: https://www.frontiersin.org/articles/10.3389/fmed.2020.589794/full#supplementary-material

Supplementary Figure 1 | Cumulative risk of blindness according to symptom latency in the whole cohort of patients (convenational approach, fast-track, and fast-track during COVID-19 pandemic).

Supplementary Figure 2 | Kaplan-Meyer curves of visual survival in the conventional group compared to the fast-track approach.

REFERENCES

1. Jennette JC, Falk RJ, Bacon PA, Basu N, Cid MC, Ferrario F, et al. 2012 Revised international chapel hill consensus conference nomenclature of vasculitides. *Arthritis Rheum.* (2013) 65:1–11. doi: 10.1002/art.37715
2. Salvarani C, Boiardi L. Polymyalgia rheumatica and giant-cell arteritis. *N Engl J Med.* (2002) 347:261–71. doi: 10.1056/NEJMra011913
3. Salvarani C, Cantini F, Hunder GG. Polymyalgia rheumatica and giant-cell arteritis. *Lancet.* (2008) 372:234–45. doi: 10.1016/S0140-6736(08)61077-6
4. Nuenninghoff DM, Hunder GG, Christianson TJH, McClelland RL, Matteson EL. Incidence and predictors of large-artery complication (aortic aneurysm, aortic dissection, and/or large-artery stenosis) in patients with giant cell arteritis: a population-based study over 50 years. *Arthritis Rheum.* (2003) 48:3522–31. doi: 10.1002/art.11353
5. Patil P, Williams M, Maw WW, Achilleos K, Elsideeg S, Dejaco C, et al. Fast track pathway reduces sight loss in giant cell arteritis: results of a longitudinal observational cohort study. *Clin Exp Rheumatol.* (2015) 33(2 Suppl. 89):S103–6.
6. Diamantopoulos AP, Haugeberg G, Lindland A, Myklebust G. The fast-track ultrasound clinic for early diagnosis of giant cell arteritis significantly reduces permanent visual impairment: towards a more effective strategy to improve clinical outcome in giant cell arteritis? *Rheumatology.* (2016) 55:66–70. doi: 10.1093/rheumatology/kev289
7. Monti S, Floris A, Ponte CB, Schmidt WA, Diamantopoulos AP, Pereira C, et al. The proposed role of ultrasound in the management of giant cell arteritis in routine clinical practice. *Rheumatology.* (2018) 57:112–9. doi: 10.1093/rheumatology/kex341
8. Mukhtyar C, Guillevin L, Cid MC, Dasgupta B, Groot K de, Gross W, et al. EULAR recommendations for the management of large vessel vasculitis. *Ann Rheum Dis.* (2009) 68:318–23. doi: 10.1136/ard.2008.088351
9. Hellmich B, Agueda A, Monti S, Buttgereit F, de Boysson H, Brouwer E, et al. 2018 Update of the EULAR recommendations for the management of large vessel vasculitis. *Ann Rheum Dis.* (2019) 79:19–30. doi: 10.1136/annrheumdis-2019-215672
10. Chrysidis S, Duftner C, Dejaco C, Schäfer VS, Ramiro S, Carrara G, et al. Definitions and reliability assessment of elementary ultrasound lesions in giant cell arteritis: a study from the OMERACT large vessel vasculitis ultrasound working Group. *RMD Open.* (2018) 4:e000598. doi: 10.1136/rmdopen-2017-000598
11. Aschwanden M, Daikeler T, Kesten F, Baldi T, Benz D, Tyndall A, et al. Temporal artery compression sign - a novel ultrasound finding for the diagnosis of giant cell arteritis. *Ultraschall Med.* (2013) 34:47–50. doi: 10.1055/s-0032-1312821
12. Schmidt WA, Kraft HE, Vorpahl K, Völker L, Gromnica-Ihle EJ. Color duplex ultrasonography in the diagnosis of temporal arteritis. *N Engl J Med.* (1997) 337:1336–42. doi: 10.1056/NEJM199711063371902
13. Dejaco C, Ramiro S, Duftner C, Besson FL, Bley TA, Blockmans D, et al. EULAR recommendations for the use of imaging in large vessel vasculitis in clinical practice. *Ann Rheum Dis.* (2018) 77:636–43. doi: 10.1136/annrheumdis-2017-212649
14. Luqmani R, Lee E, Singh S, Gillett M, Schmidt WA, Bradburn M, et al. The role of ultrasound compared to biopsy of temporal arteries in the diagnosis and Treatment of Giant Cell Arteritis (TABUL): a diagnostic accuracy and cost-effectiveness study. *Health Technol Assess.* (2016) 20:1–238. doi: 10.3310/hta20900
15. Germano G, Monti S, Ponte C, Possemato N, Caporali R, Salvarani C, et al. The role of ultrasound in the diagnosis and follow-up of large-vessel vasculitis: an update. *Clin Exp Rheumatol.* (2017) 35:S194–8.
16. Monti S, Agueda AF, Luqmani R. The use of ultrasound in the management of large-vessel vasculitis: an evolving concept. *Clin Exp Rheumatol.* (2018) 36:S96–102.
17. Patil P, Williams M, Maw WW, Achilleos K, Elsideeg S, Dejaco C, et al. Fast track pathway reduces sight loss in giant cell arteritis: results of a longitudinal observational cohort study. *Clin Exp Rheumatol.* (2015) 33(2 Suppl 89):S103–6.
18. Vodopivec I, Rizzo JF. Ophthalmic manifestations of giant cell arteritis. *Rheumatology.* (2018) 57:ii63–72. doi: 10.1093/rheumatology/kex428
19. González-Gay MA, Blanco R, Rodríguez-Valverde V, Martínez-Taboada VM, Delgado-Rodriguez M, Figueroa M, et al. Permanent visual loss and cerebrovascular accidents in giant cell arteritis: predictors and response to treatment. *Arthritis Rheum.* (1998) 41:1497–504. doi: 10.1002/1529-0131(199808)41:8<1497::AID-ART22>3.0.CO;2-Z
20. Singh AG, Kermani TA, Crowson CS, Weyand CM, Matteson EL, Warrington KJ. Visual manifestations in giant cell arteritis: trend over 5 decades in a population-based cohort. *J Rheumatol.* (2015) 42:309–15. doi: 10.3899/jrheum.140188
21. Mollan SP, Paemeleire K, Versijpt J, Luqmani R, Sinclair AJ. European headache federation recommendations for neurologists managing giant cell arteritis. *J Headache Pain.* (2020) 21:28. doi: 10.1186/s10194-020-01093-7
22. Helliwell T, Muller S, Hider SL, Prior JA, Richardson JC, Mallen CD. Challenges of diagnosis and management of giant cell arteritis in general practice: a multimethods study. *BMJ Open.* (2018) 8:e019320 doi: 10.1136/bmjopen-2017-019320
23. De Filippo O, D'Ascenzo F, Angelini F, Bocchino PP, Conrotto F, Saglietto A, et al. Reduced rate of hospital admissions for ACS during covid-19 outbreak in Northern Italy. *N Engl J Med.* (2020) 383:88–9. doi: 10.1056/NEJMc2009166
24. Baldi E, Sechi GM, Mare C, Canevari F, Brancaglione A, Primi R, et al. Out-of-hospital cardiac arrest during the Covid-19 outbreak in Italy. *N Engl J Med.* (2020) 383:496–8. doi: 10.1056/NEJMc2010418
25. Monti S, Delvino P, Bellis E, Milanesi A, Brandolino F, Montecucco C. Impact of delayed diagnoses at the time of COVID-19: increased rate of preventable bilateral blindness in giant cell arteritis. *Ann Rheum Dis.* (2020) 79:1658–9. doi: 10.1136/annrheumdis-2020-217915
26. Hocevar A, Rotar Z, Jese R, Semrl SS, Pizem J, Hawlina M, et al. Do early diagnosis and glucocorticoid treatment decrease the risk of permanent visual loss and early relapses in giant cell arteritis: a prospective longitudinal study. *Medicine.* (2016) 95:e3210. doi: 10.1097/MD.0000000000003210
27. Alba MA, García-Martínez A, Prieto-González S, Tavera-Bahillo I, Corbera-Bellalta M, Planas-Rigol E, et al. Relapses in patients with giant cell arteritis: prevalence, characteristics, and associated clinical findings in a longitudinally followed cohort of 106 patients. *Medicine.* (2014) 93:194–201. doi: 10.1097/MD.0000000000000033
28. Dumont A, Parienti J-J, Delmas C, Boutemy J, Maigné G, Martin Silva N, et al. Factors associated with relapse and dependence on glucocorticoids in giant cell arteritis. *J Rheumatol.* (2020) 47:108–16. doi: 10.3899/jrheum.181127
29. Kermani TA, Warrington KJ, Cuthbertson D, Carette S, Hoffman GS, Khalidi NA, et al. Disease relapses among patients with giant cell arteritis: a prospective, longitudinal cohort study. *J Rheumatol.* (2015) 42:1213–7. doi: 10.3899/jrheum.141347
30. Hernández-Rodríguez J, García-Martínez A, Casademont J, Filella X, Esteban M-J, López-Soto A, et al. A strong initial systemic inflammatory response is associated with higher corticosteroid requirements and longer duration of therapy in patients with giant-cell arteritis. *Arthritis Rheum.* (2002) 47:29–35. doi: 10.1002/art1.10161
31. Monti S, Ponte C, Pereira C, Manzoni F, Klersy C, Rumi F, et al. The impact of disease extent and severity detected by quantitative ultrasound analysis in the diagnosis and outcome of giant cell arteritis. *Rheumatology.* (2019) 59:2299–307. doi: 10.1093/rheumatology/kez554
32. van der Geest KSM, Borg F, Kayani A, Paap D, Gondo P, Schmidt W, et al. Novel ultrasonographic Halo Score for giant cell arteritis: assessment of diagnostic accuracy and association with ocular ischaemia. *Ann Rheum Dis.* (2020) 79:393–9. doi: 10.1136/annrheumdis-2019-216343
33. Ponte C, Serafim AS, Monti S, Fernandes E, Lee E, Singh S, et al. Early variation of ultrasound halo sign with treatment and relation with clinical features in patients with giant cell arteritis. *Rheumatology.* (2020) Keaa196. doi: 10.1093/rheumatology/keaa196

34. Schmidt WA, Krause A, Schicke B, Kuchenbecker J, Gromnica-Ihle E. Do temporal artery duplex ultrasound findings correlate with ophthalmic complications in giant cell arteritis? *Rheumatology.* (2009) 48:383–5. doi: 10.1093/rheumatology/ken515
35. Mahr AD, Jover JA, Spiera RF, Hernández-García C, Fernández-Gutiérrez B, Lavalley MP, et al. Adjunctive methotrexate for treatment of giant cell arteritis: an individual patient data meta-analysis. *Arthritis Rheum.* (2007) 56:2789–97. doi: 10.1002/art.22754
36. Stone JH, Tuckwell K, Dimonaco S, Klearman M, Aringer M, Blockmans D, et al. Trial of tocilizumab in giant-cell arteritis. *N Engl J Med.* (2017) 377:317–28. doi: 10.1056/NEJMoa1613849

9

Performance of Ultrasonography Compared to Conventional Radiography for the Diagnosis of Osteoarthritis in Patients With Knee Pain

Martin Brom [1], Ignacio J. Gandino [1], Johana B. Zacariaz Hereter [1], Marina Scolnik [1], Florencia B. Mollerach [1], Leandro G. Ferreyra Garrott [1], Josefina Marin [1], Santiago O. Ruta [1], Javier E. Rosa [1], Ricardo D. García-Mónaco [2] and Enrique R. Soriano [1]*

[1] *Rheumatology Department, Hospital Italiano de Buenos Aires, Buenos Aires, Argentina,* [2] *Radiology Department, Hospital Italiano de Buenos Aires, Buenos Aires, Argentina*

***Correspondence:**
Martin Brom
martin.brom@hospitalitaliano.org.ar

Purpose: To investigate the performance of ultrasonography (US) for the detection of knee osteoarthritis (OA) in patients suffering from knee pain, compared to conventional radiographs.

Methods: Cross-sectional study performed at a university teaching hospital. Consecutive patients complaining of unilateral or bilateral mechanical knee pain who signed an informed consent were included. All patients underwent simultaneously an ultrasonographic and a radiographic evaluation of the knee. Exclusion criteria were age under 18 years, prior diagnosis of knee OA, diagnosis of inflammatory arthritis, history of knee surgery or trauma, severe knee deformities, and corticosteroid injection within the last 2 months. The diagnostic properties of US for the detection of knee OA were evaluated using radiological data as the reference method. Evaluated test properties were sensitivity, specificity, positive predictive value (PPV), negative predictive value (NPV), and the positive and negative likelihood ratio (LR+ and LR–).

Results: Three-hundred twenty-two knees (281 patients) were included. Radiographic degenerative changes were present in 56.8% (183) of the evaluated knees. Regarding the diagnostic properties of the US, the presence of either osteophytes or the compromise of the femoral hyaline cartilage had the best sensitivity to detect OA (95%), with a NPV of 92% and a LR– of 0,07, while the combined identification of osteophytes and compromise of the femoral hyaline cartilage had the best specificity (94%), with 94% PPV and a LR+ of 13.

Conclusion: US demonstrated an excellent sensitivity with an adequate specificity for the detection of radiographic knee OA.

Keywords: radiography (D011859), ultrasonography (D014463), osteoarthritis (D010003), knee osteoarthritis (D020370), diagnostic imaging (D003952)

INTRODUCTION

Osteoarthritis (OA) is the most prevalent joint disorder, with a global age-standardized prevalence of knee OA of 3.8% (1), and it is one of the leading causes of global disability (2). It is characterized by mechanical joint pain and stiffness, and the most frequently affected joints are knees, hips, hands, and spine (3).

Although OA may be diagnosed merely by the presence of typical symptoms and signs in the at-risk group of patients (2, 4, 5), additional testing might be needed to rule out alternative diagnoses and especially, to stratify the degree of joint structural damage. The most frequently used imaging tool is conventional radiography since it is a widely available and cheap method that allows the detection of OA's classical features: marginal osteophytes, joint space narrowing, subchondral sclerosis, and cysts (5–7).

On the other hand, the use of X-Rays in OA has several limitations. Early diagnosis of OA cannot be achieved by this method since X-Rays can only identify late, non-reversible joint damage. Previous studies demonstrated that among patients with knee pain suspicious of OA, only 50% will have radiographic changes of OA (3), and moreover, there is only a moderate association between the degree of knee OA and the level of pain (4, 8) and only about 50% of the patients with knee OA experience pain (9). Pain in knee OA is multifactorial and it is influenced by mechanical, structural, inflammatory, bone-related, neurological and psychological factors (10, 11).

Considering the previously listed limitations of conventional radiography, it is important to have more sensitive tools for the diagnosis and assessment of knee OA. The most sensitive and specific diagnostic tool up to date is Magnetic Resonance Imaging (MRI), since it can evaluate all articular and periarticular structures—including bone marrow, and even biochemical composition of the articular tissues—but its use is limited to research due to the high cost and unavailability of MRI, and its contraindication on certain patients such as those with cardiac pacemakers (12).

Ultrasonography (US) is an attractive tool since, in contrast to conventional radiography, it can evaluate periarticular soft tissue structures and the presence of synovitis, and compared to MRI, it is a safe, inexpensive and less time-consuming method (13). Although US is an operator-dependent method, several studies demonstrated that the use of US in knee OA has good construct validity and moderate to good interobserver reliability (14–17).

In this context, we decided to investigate the properties and performance of US for the detection of knee OA in patients suffering from knee pain, compared to the conventional radiographic study of the knee.

PATIENTS AND METHODS

Cross-sectional study performed at a university teaching hospital in Buenos Aires, Argentina. Consecutive patients complaining of unilateral or bilateral mechanical knee pain who signed an informed consent were included. All patients underwent US and X-Ray evaluation of the knee. Exclusion criteria were age under 18 years, prior diagnosis of knee OA, diagnosis of inflammatory arthritis, history of knee surgery or trauma, severe knee deformities, and corticosteroid injection within the last 2 months. All procedures were in accordance with the ethical standards of the institutional research committee, and with the 1964 Helsinki declaration and its later amendments or comparable ethical standards.

US examinations were performed by 2 experienced rheumatologist ultrasonographists (SOR and JER), blinded to clinical and radiological data, using a MyLab 70 machine (Esaote) provided with a multi-frequency linear transducer (4–13 MHz). Patients were not allowed to speak to the ultrasonographist about their clinical condition. A standardized scanning method was adopted in order to evaluate the presence of osteophytes and degenerative femoral hyaline cartilage involvement. Patients were placed in supine position, and knees were evaluated in extension and in 30° flexion. Osteophytes were defined as protrusions at the joint margin seen in two planes. The degenerative femoral hyaline cartilage was defined by the presence of at least two of the following: loss of sharpness of the cartilage margins, loss of homogeneity of the cartilage layer or cartilage thinning (<2 mm) focal or extend to the entire cartilaginous layer.

Weight-bearing anteroposterior and lateral knee radiographs, acquired simultaneously to the US, were read by an experienced rheumatologist, blinded to the clinical and US data, who determined the presence or absence of radiological degenerative changes and classified the severity of knee OA using Kellgren-Lawrence (KL) grading scale (18).

Statistical analysis was performed using STATA V.14.1. Continuous variables were reported as mean and standard deviation (SD), according to the variable distribution. The Chi^2 Test was used for the comparison of the US features (osteophytes and hyaline cartilage involvement) with the radiographic KL grades, with a $p < 0.05$ considered significant. The diagnostic properties of US for the detection of osteophytes and degenerative cartilage involvement in the knee were evaluated using radiological data as the reference method. Evaluated test properties were sensitivity, specificity, positive predictive value (PPV), negative predictive value (NPV), and the positive and negative likelihood ratio (LR+ and LR–).

RESULTS

Two-hundred eighty-one patients were included, with a female-to-male ratio of 3:1 and a mean age of 64 years (*SD* 17). A total of 322 knees were evaluated since 41 patients complained of bilateral knee pain.

Table 1 shows the frequency of the US abnormal findings stratified by the radiographic extent of knee damage according to KL grading. Radiographic degenerative changes were present in 56.8% (183) of the evaluated knees, being KL 3 the most frequently observed grade. Regarding the US assessment, the presence of osteophytes or femoral hyaline cartilage involvement was more frequent in those knees with radiographic changes of OA, regardless of the severity according to the KL grading scale ($p < 0.001$ both for hyaline cartilage and osteophytes between

TABLE 1 | Frequency of the US abnormal findings according to radiographic features of knee OA.

	Presence of radiological degenerative changes, *n*: 183				Absence of radiological degenerative changes
	KL 1, *n*: 34	**KL 2, *n*: 20**	**KL 3, *n*: 115**	**KL 4, *n*: 14**	**KL 0, *n*: 139**
US femoral hyaline cartilage involvement, % (CI 95%)	77 (64–92)	70 (49–90)	97 (93–99)	100	24 (17–31)
US osteophytes, % (CI 95%)	62 (44–73)	90 (76–100)	85 (79–92)	100	14 (8–20)
US femoral hyaline cartilage involvement or US osteophytes, % (CI 95%)	92 (82–100)	100	95 (91–99)	100	24 (16–31)

US, ultrasound; OA, osteoarthritis; KL, Kellgren-Lawrence.

TABLE 2 | Diagnostic test properties of the US abnormal findings for the detection of knee OA using radiological data as the reference method.

	Sensitivity	**Specificity**	**PPV**	**NPV**	**LR+**	**LR-**
US femoral hyaline cartilage involvement, % (CI 95%)	90 (86–95)	75 (68–83)	84 (79–89)	85 (78–91)	3.6	0.13
US osteophytes, % (CI 95%)	82 (77–88)	86 (80–92)	89 (84–94)	78 (71–84)	5.85	0.21
US femoral hyaline cartilage involvement or US osteophytes, % (CI 95%)	95 (92–98)	76 (69–83)	85 (80–90)	92 (87–97)	3.96	0.07
US femoral hyaline cartilage and US osteophytes, % (CI 95%)	75 (68–81)	94 (89–97.5)	94 (89–97.6)	74 (67–80)	13	0.27

US, ultrasonography; PPV, positive predictive value; NPV, negative predictive value; CI, confidence interval; LR+, positive likelihood ratio; LR–, negative likelihood ratio.

all KL grades with radiographic damage and KL0, respectively). The damage of the femoral hyaline cartilage was significantly more frequently found in knees with radiographic knee OA KL 3 and 4 (97 and 100%, respectively; $p < 0.001$ between KL3 and KL4 compared with KL1), while the frequency of osteophytes detected by US was lowest in KL 1 (62%) compared to the other grades ($p = 0.0067$, and 0.0027 vs. KL3 and KL4, respectively). Noteworthy, 24% of the evaluated knees didn't show radiographic degenerative changes (KL 0) but did have ultrasonographic findings of knee OA. On the other hand, none of the patients with radiographic degenerative changes (KL $\geq$1) had a normal US.

Diagnostic test properties of the US abnormal findings for the detection of knee OA using radiological data as the reference method are shown in **Table 2**. The presence of osteophytes or the compromise of the femoral hyaline cartilage had the best sensitivity to detect OA (95%), with a NPV of 92% and a LR– of 0.07. The identification of osteophytes and compromise of the femoral hyaline cartilage the best specificity (94%), with 94% PPV and a LR+ of 13.

DISCUSSION

This cross-sectional study shows that US has very good diagnostic properties compared to the standard method, conventional radiography, for the diagnosis of knee OA. The definition and diagnosis of osteoarthritis has changed over time, driven by an increased understanding of the disease and the development of new technologies, which led to the appearance of concepts such as early OA (19). Ultrasonography has growing evidence as an alternative imaging method for the assessment of OA (14). Unlike conventional radiography, US has the ability to visualize articular and periarticular soft tissue structures such as cartilage thickness and soft tissues alterations such as joint effusion, synovitis, Baker's cyst, tendinopathy, bursitis, and meniscal lesions (8, 20–22). On the other hand, and in contrast to MRI, it is a widely available and inexpensive imaging method (13). Additionally, US features such as joint space narrowing and synovitis have been found to better correlate with pain than structural damage (23, 24), and US might be good tool to measure changes in clinical trials (13, 14, 25).

In this context we decided to perform a study to evaluate the diagnostic properties of US for the detection of knee OA in patients who sought medical attention due to knee pain. Although US allows the assessment of many soft tissue structures, the ultrasonographic evaluation of the knees in this cohort was limited to the presence of osteophytes and hyaline cartilage involvement since these are the only joint changes that can be observed both by US and conventional radiography, and therefore, these are the features that allow the comparison of the diagnostic properties of these 2 imaging methods.

Several studies have shown US to be reliable and valid for the evaluation of cartilage pathology in OA, and especially for large joints such as the knee (26–29), and US has demonstrated strong criterion validity with cartilage histology (25). The knee's hyaline cartilage has a normal thickness of 2 mm, and superficial regions can easily be evaluated by US (26, 27).

In this cohort, 56.8% of the patients with knee pain had radiological degenerative changes, and in concordance with previous studies (20, 30), KL 3 was the most frequently identified group. Interestingly, 24% of the patients without radiographic degenerative changes presented ultrasonographic findings of OA. Whether this represents a false positive result of US or the diagnosis of early OA can only be elucidated by following these knees in time, and cannot be answer by this study.

Previous studies demonstrated that US is as sensitive as MRI and more sensitive than conventional radiography for the detection of osteophytes (25, 26, 31–34), and showed a high intra and inter-reader agreement (26–28, 35). In this cohort, ultrasonography had a sensitivity of 95% (CI95% 92–98) for the detection of hyaline cartilage involvement or osteophytes, and a specificity of 86% (CI95% 80–92) for the identification of osteophytes, compared to conventional radiography. Using both features, as expected, increased specificity but decreased sensitivity (**Table 2**). On the other hand, if we had used US as gold standard, conventional radiography would have shown sensitivity of 83% and specificity of 93%.

There are some limitations that need mentioning. First, there are limitations that are inherent to the method: The visualization of the cartilage may be hindered by the acoustic window, which depends on the patient's joint anatomy, and US is an operator-dependent method (15). Second, inter and intraobserver agreement was not evaluated, which might affect reliability. Nevertheless, the participating ultrasonographists are part of the same group and share the same concepts on acquisition and reading of images. In addition, they have demonstrated a very good level of agreement (85%) in a previous studies (36). Third, although we are aware that looking for a correlation between the images and pain or clinical characteristics such as Body Mass Index (BMI), etc. would enrich the study, since the objective was the comparison of the diagnostic properties of US and radiographs and patients did not undergo an *ad hoc* physical examination, this was not possible. Finally, since this is a cross-sectional study, we cannot know if the changes found by US in knees with normal radiographs (KL 0) are false positive results or if it is an early diagnosis of OA.

On the other hand, this study has several strengths. This is a large cohort of patients, who were included consecutively and unselected. All patients were evaluated by 2 rheumatologists expert in ultrasonography, who were blinded to the KL grading. Likewise, the radiographic evaluators were expert rheumatologists, blinded to the US findings.

In conclusion, US demonstrated an excellent sensitivity with an adequate specificity for the detection of radiographic knee OA. The identification by US of femoral hyaline cartilage involvement or osteophytes showed the best sensitivity while the presence of both osteophytes and femoral hyaline cartilage showed the best specificity. We believe that ultrasonography is a valid method for the evaluation of patients with knee pain when OA is suspected. Its capability to identify early knee OA in patients with non-radiographic knee OA (KL 0) should be evaluated using as a more sensitive method, such as MRI, as the comparator group.

ETHICS STATEMENT

The studies involving human participants were reviewed and approved by Hospital Italiano de Buenos Aires. The patients/participants provided their written informed consent to participate in this study.

AUTHOR'S NOTE

This study was previously published as an abstract after being presented at an ACR meeting (37) (https://acrabstracts.org/abstract/radiographic-knee-osteoarthritis-in-patients-complaining-of-knee-pain-ultrasound-features/) and a PANLAR meeting (38) (https://journals.lww.com/jclinrheum/Fulltext/2018/04001/Abstracts_20th_PANLAR_Meeting__Buenos_Aires,0.1.aspx).

AUTHOR CONTRIBUTIONS

MB, IG, JZ, MS, FM, LF, JM, SR, JR, RG-M, and ES meet the ICMJE 4 criteria and the journal authorship criteria, and the final manuscript has been read and approved by all the authors.

REFERENCES

1. Cross M, Smith E, Hoy D, Nolte S, Ackerman I, Fransen M, et al. The global burden of hip and knee osteoarthritis: estimates from the Global Burden of Disease 2010 study. *Ann Rheum Dis.* (2014) 73:1323–30. doi: 10.1136/annrheumdis-2013-204763
2. Hunter DJ, Bierma-Zeinstra S. Osteoarthritis. *Lancet.* (2019) 393:1745–59. doi: 10.1016/S0140-6736(19)30417-9
3. Arden N, Nevitt MC. Osteoarthritis: epidemiology. *Best Pract Res Clin Rheumatol.* (2006) 20:3–25. doi: 10.1016/j.berh.2005.09.007
4. Bedson J, Croft PR. The discordance between clinical and radiographic knee osteoarthritis: a systematic search and summary of the literature. *BMC Musculoskelet Disord.* (2008) 9:116. doi: 10.1186/1471-2474-9-116
5. National Clinical Guideline Centre (UK). *Osteoarthritis: Care and Management in Adults.* National Institute for Health and Care Excellence (2014).
6. Hayashi D, Roemer FW, Guermazi A. Imaging for osteoarthritis. *Ann Phys Rehabil Med.* (2016) 59:161–9. doi: 10.1016/j.rehab.2015.12.003
7. Roemer FW, Eckstein F, Hayashi D, Guermazi A. The role of imaging in osteoarthritis. *Best Pract Res Clin Rheumatol.* (2014) 28:31–60. doi: 10.1016/j.berh.2014.02.002
8. Bevers K, Bijlsma JW, Vriezekolk JE, van den Ende CH, den Broeder AA. Ultrasonographic features in symptomatic osteoarthritis of the knee and relation with pain. *Rheumatology.* (2014) 53:1625–9. doi: 10.1093/rheumatology/keu030

9. Salaffi F, Ciapetti A, Carotti M. The sources of pain in osteoarthritis: a pathophysiological review. *Reumatismo.* (2014) 66:57–71. doi: 10.4081/reumatismo.2014.766
10. Claessens AAMC, Schouten JSAG, van den Ouweland FA, Valkenburg HA. Do clinical findings associate with radiographic osteoarthritis of the knee? *Ann Rheum Dis.* (1990) 49:771–4. doi: 10.1136/ard.49.10.771
11. Bijlsma JWJ, Berenbaum F, Lafeber FPJG. Osteoarthritis: an update with relevance for clinical practice. *Lancet.* (2011) 377:2115–26. doi: 10.1016/S0140-6736(11)60243-2
12. Hayashi D, Roemer FW, Guermazi A. Recent advances in research imaging of osteoarthritis with focus on MRI, ultrasound and hybrid imaging. *Clin Exp Rheumatol.* (2018) 36(Suppl. 1):43–52.
13. Bevers K, Bijlsma JWJ, Vriezekolk JE, van den Ende CHM, den Broeder AA. The course of ultrasonographic abnormalities in knee osteoarthritis: 1 year follow up. *Osteoarthr Cartil.* (2014) 22:1651–6. doi: 10.1016/j.joca.2014.06.012
14. Keen HI, Wakefield RJ, Conaghan PG. A systematic review of ultrasonography in osteoarthritis. *Ann Rheum Dis.* (2009) 68:611–9. doi: 10.1136/ard.2008.102434
15. Möller I, Bong D, Naredo E, Filippucci E, Carrasco I, Moragues C, et al. Ultrasound in the study and monitoring of osteoarthritis. *Osteoarthr Cartil.* (2008) 16(Suppl. 3):S4–7. doi: 10.1016/j.joca.2008.06.005
16. Bevers K, Zweers MC, van den Ende CHM, Martens HA, Mahler E, Bijlsma JWJ, et al. Ultrasonographic analysis in knee osteoarthritis: evaluation of inter-observer reliability. *Clin Exp Rheumatol.* (2012) 30:673–8.
17. Iagnocco A, Perricone C, Scirocco C, Ceccarelli F, Modesti M, Gattamelata A, et al. The interobserver reliability of ultrasound in knee osteoarthritis. *Rheumatology.* (2012) 51:2013–9. doi: 10.1093/rheumatology/kes161
18. Kellgren JH, Lawrence JS. Radiological assessment of osteo-arthrosis. *Ann Rheum Dis.* (1957) 16:494–502. doi: 10.1136/ard.16.4.494
19. Magnusson K, Kumm J, Turkiewicz A, Englund M. A naturally aging knee, or development of early knee osteoarthritis? *Osteoarthr Cartil.* (2018) 26:1447–52. doi: 10.1016/j.joca.2018.04.020
20. de Miguel Mendieta E, Cobo Ibáñez T, Usón Jaeger J, Bonilla Hernán G, Martín Mola E. Clinical and ultrasonographic findings related to knee pain in osteoarthritis. *Osteoarthr Cartil.* (2006) 14:540–4. doi: 10.1016/j.joca.2005.12.012
21. Mermerci BB, Garip Y, Uysal RS, Dogruel H, Karabulut E, Özoran K, et al. Clinic and ultrasound findings related to pain in patients with knee osteoarthritis. *Clin Rheumatol.* (2011) 30:1055–62. doi: 10.1007/s10067-011-1701-x
22. Meenagh G, Filippucci E, Delle Sedie A, Iagnocco A, Scirè CA, Riente L, et al. Ultrasound imaging for the rheumatologist XXX. Sonographic assessment of the painful knee. *Clin Exp Rheumatol.* (2010) 28:803–5.
23. Neogi T, Felson D, Niu J, Nevitt M, Lewis CE, Aliabadi P, et al. Association between radiographic features of knee osteoarthritis and pain: results from two cohort studies. *BMJ.* (2009) 339:b2844. doi: 10.1136/bmj.b2844
24. Torres L, Dunlop DD, Peterfy C, Guermazi A, Prasad P, Hayes KW, et al. The relationship between specific tissue lesions and pain severity in persons with knee osteoarthritis. *Osteoarthr Cartil.* (2006) 14:1033–40. doi: 10.1016/j.joca.2006.03.015
25. Oo WM, Linklater JM, Daniel M, Saarakkala S, Samuels J, Conaghan PG, et al. Clinimetrics of ultrasound pathologies in osteoarthritis: systematic literature review and meta-analysis. *Osteoarthr Cartil.* (2018) 26:601–11. doi: 10.1016/j.joca.2018.01.021
26. Mathiessen A, Cimmino MA, Hammer HB, Haugen IK, Iagnocco A, Conaghan PG. Imaging of osteoarthritis (OA): what is new? *Best Pract Res Clin Rheumatol.* (2016) 30:653–69. doi: 10.1016/j.berh.2016.09.007
27. Bruyn GAW, Naredo E, Damjanov N, Bachta A, Baudoin P, Hammer HB, et al. An OMERACT reliability exercise of inflammatory and structural abnormalities in patients with knee osteoarthritis using ultrasound assessment. *Ann Rheum Dis.* (2016) 75:842–6. doi: 10.1136/annrheumdis-2014-206774
28. Razek AAKA, El-Basyouni SR. Ultrasound of knee osteoarthritis: interobserver agreement and correlation with Western Ontario and McMaster Universities Osteoarthritis. *Clin Rheumatol.* (2016) 35:997–1001. doi: 10.1007/s10067-015-2990-2
29. Podlipská J, Guermazi A, Lehenkari P, Niinimäki J, Roemer FW, Arokoski JP, et al. Comparison of diagnostic performance of semi-quantitative knee ultrasound and knee radiography with MRI: Oulu Knee Osteoarthritis study. *Sci Rep.* (2016) 6:22365. doi: 10.1038/srep22365
30. Castaño Carou A, Pita Fernández S, Pértega Díaz S, de Toro Santos FJ. Clinical profile, level of affection and therapeutic management of patients with osteoarthritis in primary care: the spanish multicenter study EVALÚA. *Reumatol Clínica.* (2015) 11:353–60. doi: 10.1016/j.reumae.2015.03.007
31. Vlychou M, Koutroumpas A, Alexiou I, Fezoulidis I, Sakkas LI. High-resolution ultrasonography and 3.0 T magnetic resonance imaging in erosive and nodal hand osteoarthritis: high frequency of erosions in nodal osteoarthritis. *Clin Rheumatol.* (2013) 32:755–62. doi: 10.1007/s10067-013-2166-x
32. Roemer FW, Nevitt MC, Felson DT, Niu J, Lynch JA, Crema MD, et al. Predictive validity of within-grade scoring of longitudinal changes of MRI-based cartilage morphology and bone marrow lesion assessment in the tibio-femoral joint – the MOST study. *Osteoarthr Cartil.* (2012) 20:1391–8. doi: 10.1016/j.joca.2012.07.012
33. Wittoek R, Jans L, Lambrecht V, Carron P, Verstraete K, Verbruggen G. Reliability and construct validity of ultrasonography of soft tissue and destructive changes in erosive osteoarthritis of the interphalangeal finger joints: a comparison with MRI. *Ann Rheum Dis.* (2011) 70:278–83. doi: 10.1136/ard.2010.134932
34. Mathiessen A, Haugen IK, Slatkowsky-Christensen B, Bøyesen P, Kvien TK, Hammer HB. Ultrasonographic assessment of osteophytes in 127 patients with hand osteoarthritis: exploring reliability and associations with MRI, radiographs and clinical joint findings. *Ann Rheum Dis.* (2013) 72:51–6. doi: 10.1136/annrheumdis-2011-201195
35. Hammer HB, Iagnocco A, Mathiessen A, Filippucci E, Gandjbakhch F, Kortekaas MC, et al. Global ultrasound assessment of structural lesions in osteoarthritis: a reliability study by the OMERACT ultrasonography group on scoring cartilage and osteophytes in finger joints. *Ann Rheum Dis.* (2016) 75:402–7. doi: 10.1136/annrheumdis-2014-206289
36. Rosa JE, Ruta S, Bravo M, Pompermayer L, Marin J, Ferreyra-Garrot L, et al. Value of color Doppler ultrasound assessment of sacroiliac joints in patients with inflammatory low back pain. *J Rheumatol.* (2019) 46:694–700. doi: 10.3899/jrheum.180550
37. Gandino IJ, Ruta S, Scolnik M, Zacariaz J, Marin J, Rosa J, et al. Radiographic knee osteoarthritis in patients complaining of knee pain: ultrasound features [abstract]. *Arthritis Rheumatol.* (2016) 68(Suppl. 10). Available online at: https://acrabstracts.org/abstract/radiographic-knee-osteoarthritis-in-patients-complaining-of-knee-pain-ultrasound-features/ (accessed June 22, 2020).
38. Gandino IJ, Brom M, Ruta SO, Scolnik M, Zacariaz JB, Marin J, et al. Radiographic knee osteoarthritis in patients complaining of knee pain: ultrasound features. *JCR J Clin Rheumatol.* (2018) 24:S1–174. doi: 10.1097/RHU.0000000000000802

10

OrthoRehab: Development of a New Methodology for the Comparison Study Between Different Types of Ankle–Foot Orthoses in Foot Dysfunction

Cláudia Quaresma [1,2], Barbara Lopes [1,2], Jorge Jacinto [3], Tiago Robalo [3], Mariana Matos [3] and Carla Quintão [1,2]*

[1] *Instrumentation, Biomedical Engineering and Radiation Physics Laboratory (LIBPhys-UNL), Physics Department, NOVA School of Science and Technology, NOVA University of Lisbon, Caparica, Portugal,* [2] *Physics Department, NOVA School of Science and Technology, NOVA University of Lisbon, Caparica, Portugal,* [3] *Rehabilitation Medicine Center of Alcoitão, Alcabideche, Portugal*

***Correspondence:**
Cláudia Quaresma
q.claudia@.fct.unl.pt

Foot dysfunction is one of the most likely consequences of rheumatoid arthritis and stroke. It is characterized by severe changes in the gait pattern due to a significant increase in the plantar flexion. Some of these dysfunctions can be compensated by using an ankle–foot orthosis. However, the clinical decision about which orthosis best suits the patient creates a real problem for physicians/therapists.

Purpose: The main goal of this paper is to present a quantitative support tool that can assist the physicians/therapists in deciding which orthosis is most suitable for each subject.

Methodology: In order to achieve such goal, a platform named OrthoRehab was developed, and it was tested in three conditions: without any orthosis and with two different ankle–foot orthoses. The data were acquired in the Gait Laboratory of Rehabilitation Medicine Center of Alcoitão using a VICON NEXUS 1.8.5® motion capture system that allows the capturing of kinematic and kinetic data.

Results: The results reveal that OrthoRehab is a user-friendly, easy to apply tool that analyzes very relevant data for the clinical staff.

Conclusion: The developed decision support tool, OrthoRehab, offers a quantitative analysis and provides insight to which orthosis achieves the best performance in comparison with the patient's gait pattern with no orthosis.

Keywords: gait analysis, device, orthoses, rehabilitation, software, evaluation

INTRODUCTION

Major chronic diseases enumerated by the World Health Organization (WHO), for example, cancers, mental disorders, cardiovascular diseases, chronic respiratory diseases, and rheumatological diseases, have a huge impact on the quality of life of the individuals and represent the predominant health problems of the century (1, 2). Foot impairment is a major adverse condition in rheumatoid arthritis (RA) and stroke. Taking the total number of adult stroke patients into account, 10–20% have equinus foot as a severe consequence and >90% of patients with

RA have reported foot complaints during the course of the disease such as hallux valgus (65%), longitudinal arch (42%) flattening, and claw toe (39%) (3–7). This is one of the most dysfunctional deformities with a significant impact on gait and quality of life of individuals who have suffered from stroke or RA (5, 6, 8–12). The possible treatment for these dysfunctions/deformities is the use of ankle–foot orthoses (AFOs) or, in severe cases, surgical intervention. AFOs are external biomechanical devices capable of improving the gait and physical functioning of the affected lower limb.

Traditionally, the AFOs are chosen based on the therapist's knowledge and clinical experience, patient's needs, or the qualitative analysis of the patient's gait (13). Moreover, the guidelines for AFO prescription provide a general recommendation and are not specific for each type of orthosis. For that reason, current clinical criteria for choosing a particular AFO are limited and subjective (14). This has a huge impact on a patient's gait performance while using the device (13).

Currently, there is a considerable research gap regarding the complete analysis of gait pattern, including the quantitative assessment of spatiotemporal, kinematic, and kinetic parameters, at the same time, for each patient during the use of AFO. Moreover, research is also missing about which orthosis best fits the functional needs of each subject (9, 15). Efficacy studies of AFOs to promote walking ability should be developed, and they will support physicians/therapists to make more precise and reliable decisions on the rehabilitation process (13). Therefore, this paper presents the OrthoRehab—a clinical decision tool that supports physicians/therapists to define AFO for a patient with foot dysfunctions during the rehabilitation process. Thus, the main goals of this paper are (1) to describe the development process of the OrthoRehab and (2) to present the results of its application in the clinical environment.

MATERIALS AND METHODS

OrthoRehab was designed and developed for a multidisciplinary team, composed of physicians, therapists, and biomedical engineers from Rehabilitation Medicine Center of Alcoitão (CMRA) and NOVA University of Lisbon. This study was approved by the Portuguese Ethics Committees of this Center.

Regarding the methodology used for the development of the OrthoRehab, the following steps were performed with the contribution of all team members:

1. Choice of the requirements of the platform
2. A decision on what gait parameters should be analyzed
3. Division of these parameters by categories: spatiotemporal, kinematic, and kinetic
4. Structuring the platform according to the categories defined in the previous step
5. Defining the calculation of the parameters under analysis
6. Programming the graphical interface.

In order to define the requirements, we asked potential end users, including the physicians and therapists who participated in this project, what facilities they thought would be important for the platform to have (16). The results of this consultation allowed identifying the following specific needs:

- easy to use: the tool should be quick to learn, and physicians/therapists should be able to use it
- should be in digital format
- facilitate the analysis of the parameters
- provide reports
- be compatible with VICON NEXUS gait analysis files.

A platform (OrthoRehab) was developed to meet these requirements. The graphical user interface was developed using MATLAB 2014b® software. This allowed the introduction of VICON NEXUS 1.8.5® (software used for gait acquisitions in this study) files and performing the analysis of the spatiotemporal, kinematic, and kinetic parameters.

Thus, the platform OrthoRehab was organized in the following sections:

1. Import/export files (file compatibility)
2. Calculation of parameters
3. Visualization of results
4. Report creation.

Import/Export Files (File Compatibility)

The data acquisition is carried out using the software VICON NEXUS 1.8.5® adapted to a computer. Since this new platform was designed to be compatible with this system, it does not increase any workload on clinicians other than importing the generated files into the developed graphical interface. After the introduction of the files in the software, the data are studied and analyzed. Finally, the outputs were saved in a database.

Although the VICON NEXUS 1.8.5® software already analyzes all gait parameters, it considers only one gait cycle, in one condition (with or without orthoses), therefore being too general and unspecific.

Calculated Parameters

The analyzed parameters, divided into spatiotemporal, kinematic, and kinetic (**Table 1**), were chosen in partnership with the team (physicians and therapists) from of the CMRA and according to the methodology used by Boudarham (7), Kinsella (17), and Manca (18).

First of all, each condition (with and without orthosis) is verified whether the gait tests have adequate dynamic data of both lower limbs, that is, if there is at least a gait cycle without artifacts on the force platforms. Then, all the parameters listed below (**Table 1**) are calculated for each condition and for each gait cycle, and the average value of the parameters is determined for each condition. Finally, all values and curves are shown in the graphical interface corresponding to the average of all running cycles for the lower limb under analysis.

Spatiotemporal Analysis

The spatiotemporal parameters analyzed in each gait cycle are those related to time intervals, distances, velocity, cadence, and respective asymmetries. These asymmetries correspond to the differences in the values of each lower limb.

TABLE 1 | Analyzed spatiotemporal, kinematic, and kinetic parameters.

Spatiotemporal parameters	Step time and their asymmetry (s)	
	Step length and their asymmetry (m)	
	Step width and their asymmetry (m)	
	Velocity and global velocity (average velocity between both lower limbs) (m/s)	
	Cadence and their asymmetry (number of steps per minute)	
	Stance phase and their asymmetry (% gait cycle)	
	Swing phase (% gait cycle)	
	Single support phase and their asymmetry (% gait cycle)	
Kinematic parameters	Ankle joint's sagittal plane	Foot strike (")
		Dorsiflexion's maximum (")
		Plantar flexion's maximum (")
	Ankle joint's coronal plane	Foot strike (")
		Contralateral limb's foot off (")
	Vertical extension between maximum and minimum of pelvis's sagittal plane (")	
Kinetic parameters	Vertical ground reaction force	First maximum (N/kg)
		Second maximum (N/kg)
	Maximum of ankle joint's power (W/kg)	

For all conditions under analysis, each spatiotemporal parameter is calculated, and its values are firstly compared with normative ones. Afterward, the condition in which the patients show the best performance (i.e., higher velocities and lower asymmetries, is highlighted).

Kinematic Analysis

The kinematic analysis curves correspond to the average value over the gait cycles of the angles of movement by the percentage of each cycle.

The kinematic parameters analyzed by the OrthoRehab are:

- Sagittal plane of the tibiotarsal joint—defined by the points: initial contact, maximum dorsiflexion, and maximum plantar flexion
- Frontal plane of the tibiotarsal joint—defined by the points: initial contact and the release of the fingers of the contralateral lower limb
- Sagittal plane of the pelvis—defined by the vertical extension between the maximum and minimum points.

For ankle joint and ground reaction force, the developed interface shows charts with angle and force curves, respectively, for at most three conditions (without orthosis and with two different types of orthoses, generically denominated A and B). The kinematic analysis identifies which condition (without orthosis, with orthosis A or orthosis B) allows an increase in dorsiflexion amplitude, a decrease in the varus, and a lower energy expenditure of the gait of the individuals under analysis.

Kinetic Analysis

The kinetic parameters analyzed by the program are those related to force and energy, namely, vertical ground reaction force and a maximum of ankle joint's power.

The dynamic parameters analyzed by the program are:

- The vertical reaction force of the soil—the analyzed points are the first and second maxima
- Strength of the tibiotarsal joint—the point analyzed is the maximum of the curve that occurs just before the foot leaves the ground (of the lower limb under analysis). The purpose of studying the vertical force of the ground reaction is to assess the individual's ability to exert force on himself.

The dynamic analysis curves correspond to the mean value of the force per percentage of support phase and power and per cycle percentage. The vertical extension of the pelvis and the ankle joint force values are calculated for the three conditions and the lowest and highest values, respectively, are selected and highlighted. The values are presented in tables.

Graphical User Interface Visualization of Results

Since the visualization of the results is an essential issue for the usability of the interface, the graphical interface architecture and the functionalities were defined with physicians and therapists using a co-creation methodology.

Interface Design Requirements

The graphical interface was developed to fulfill the following requirements:

- Utility and functionality—should perform the calculations on the parameters of interest and functionally presents them
- Sequential and intuitional—all relevant information should be distributed in a simple, sequential, and intuitive way
- Innovative—an original tool that allows a comparative analysis between clinical results obtained for different types of orthoses
- Without additional work for physicians and therapists.

Graphical Interface Architecture

The graphical interface developed has an architecture that provides the following main sections: Main Menu, Import Files, and three tabs for data analysis: Space–Time Analysis; Kinematic Analysis; Dynamic Analysis.

The parameters under analysis are shown in tables and graphs. The program starts when the Main Menu window (**Figure 1**) opens. This window allows the user to introduce the data of each patient and import the files to be analyzed. After the files are imported, it is possible to access the three available types of analysis. Also, a support manual was also prepared to understand the design of the program, as well as all its functionalities.

Functionalities

The graphic interface developed has the following functionalities:

- Ability to read files in CSV format produced by VICON NEXUS 1.8.5® software

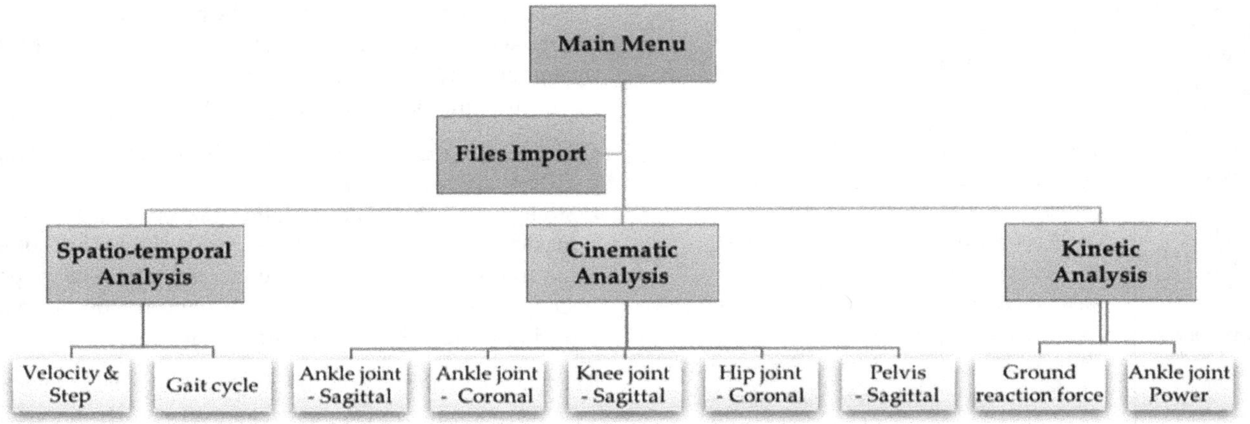

FIGURE 1 | Program structure.

- Perform spatiotemporal, kinematic, and kinetic analyses in three possible conditions: without orthosis, with orthosis A and with orthosis B—although the program is idealized to analyze three conditions, it is possible to perform the analyses with only two conditions under study
- Possibility to analyze one or both lower limbs
- Show the mean value of the parameters under analysis
- Present in the form of a table or graph the parameters analyzed for both lower limbs in the different conditions
- Highlight values that are closer to the normative standard (for example, higher speed) whenever possible
- Selection of the name of the dynamic orthoses under study, with no restriction for the type of the orthoses
- The option of activation of the non-pathological pattern in the graphs
- Graphical interactivity—zoom in and zoom out of the graphs, as well as display coordinates of points of the curves by placing the cursor
- Data recording capability
- Creation of a database (XLSX format) organized with all the parameters of interest
- Automatic addition of data from individuals to the database.

PILOT STUDY

The OrthoRehab tool was tested in three participants (two females and one male) with equinus foot dysfunction caused by a stroke (left hemiplegia). None of the subjects had previous experience with any of the orthoses under test (**Table 2**).

The inclusion criteria are the diagnosis of stroke with injury only in the right hemisphere (ability to understand and speech not compromised); equine foot, with dorsiflexion of the tibiotarsal joint up to 0° passively and modified Ashworth scale with scores: 0, 1, 1+, or 2; age between 55 and 65 years (excluding young strokes and degenerative motor disorders characteristic of older ages); ability to carry out independent walking by third parties in the minimum distance of 10 m, being allowed the use of a walking aid; ability to walk with shoes but without orthosis; the initial phase of training with orthosis: five training sessions or <1 week of use.

TABLE 2 | Participant's data.

Subject	1	2	3
Gender	Male	Female	Female
Age (years)	47	40	67
Height (±0.05 cm)	179.50	163.00	149.00
Body mass (±0.1 kg)	70.4	67.0	65.0
Time since stroke (days)	95	420	62
Ankle joint tone (1–4)	2	1	1
Passive joint range (Modified Ashword Scale)	Ankle joint dorsiflexion: +- 0"	No limitations	Ankle joint dorsiflexion: +- 0"
FAC - functional ambulatory category (1–6)	1	3	3
Dynamic balance in standing position (0–56) (Berg Balance Scale)	15	48	45

Procedure

Each subject was previously informed about the procedures and the objectives of the study and signed an informed consent.

The gait acquisitions were performed in the Biomechanics Laboratory of CMRA with controlled conditions of temperature and light and a regular floor. The acquisition procedure was performed in four steps:

1. Measurement of anthropometric parameters such as weight, height, distance between iliac crests, leg length, knee width, and ankle width
2. The software requires the placement of 16 reflective markers (eight on each lower limb) in specific anatomical places according to standard protocols for a lower body motion

analysis using the Vicon Plug-In Gait Model. In total, 16 reflective markers are placed, eight on each lower limb. These are placed in medial and lateral locations of the joints that are considered anatomical landmarks (19, 20).
3. The participants, wearing shoes, walked along the force platforms at a speed that they considered comfortable in the three conditions: (I) with no orthosis; (II) with orthosis A (posterior support); (III) with orthosis B (anterior support).
4. Point 3 was repeated two more times for each condition.

Kinetic data were collected with four force platforms from Advanced Mechanical Technology, Inc., AMTI OR6-7-2000 (50.8 × 46.4 cm) with four analogical amplifiers AMTI that were longitudinally oriented and embedded flush with the ground. Kinematic data were collected by six infrared cameras VICON T-Series T10 (1 megapixel). Additionally, there were two digital video cameras Basler piA1000-48gc GigE. All the equipment was connected to VICON NEXUS 1.8.5® software that allowed the simultaneous collection of kinematic and kinetic data of the gait of the subjects under analysis at a frequency of 100 Hz for infrared cameras and 1,000 Hz for force platforms.

RESULTS

In order to demonstrate the feasibility of OrthoRehab, as mentioned above, it was applied to three patients by a physician and a therapist. In this section, we present the end users' comments and the results from the pilot study.

End Users' Comments

The physician and the therapist who applied the OrthoRehab tool, during the proof-of-concept process, indicated that the tool is easy to be applied and it can support them to choose the most suitable type of orthosis according to the patient's needs. Additionally, the users mentioned that OrthoRehab can be used without workload and provide an evaluation that they cannot have in a conventional approach. Moreover, a high level of consensus was found with regard to whether there was a clinical need for the proposed new tool.

There was, also, a high level of agreement that the key to the success of the OrthoRehab was including physicians and therapists in the co-creation of this tool.

OrthoRehab Application

The analysis was performed only in the gait cycles of the left lower limb (affected limb) in the three conditions using OrthoRehab tool.

The average values, taking into account the three participants and the three trials performed for each one of them, were calculated.

Spatiotemporal Parameters

For velocity analysis, the highest value was selected. All participants presented values that were much lower than those referred to as non-pathological: 1.3 m/s (19). However, on average, the highest velocity was observed when the patients were using orthosis B.

Regarding the asymmetry of the cadence, the results show that A is the orthosis that causes the lowest values, while orthosis B reduced the asymmetry of time and step width. For step length, none of the orthoses proved to be efficient.

To reduce stance phase asymmetry, B is the orthosis that shows more benefits. To decrease the single support phase asymmetry, the best choice is A. In all participants, an increase of stance phase and a decrease of single support phase were also verified for both orthoses.

Kinematic Parameters

Maximum dorsiflexion and maximum plantar flexion of the sagittal plane of the ankle joint are taken into account to evaluate the increase of dorsiflexion. The gait performance was considered improved when the values of interest taken from the curves with orthosis are higher when compared with the values taken from the curves without orthosis.

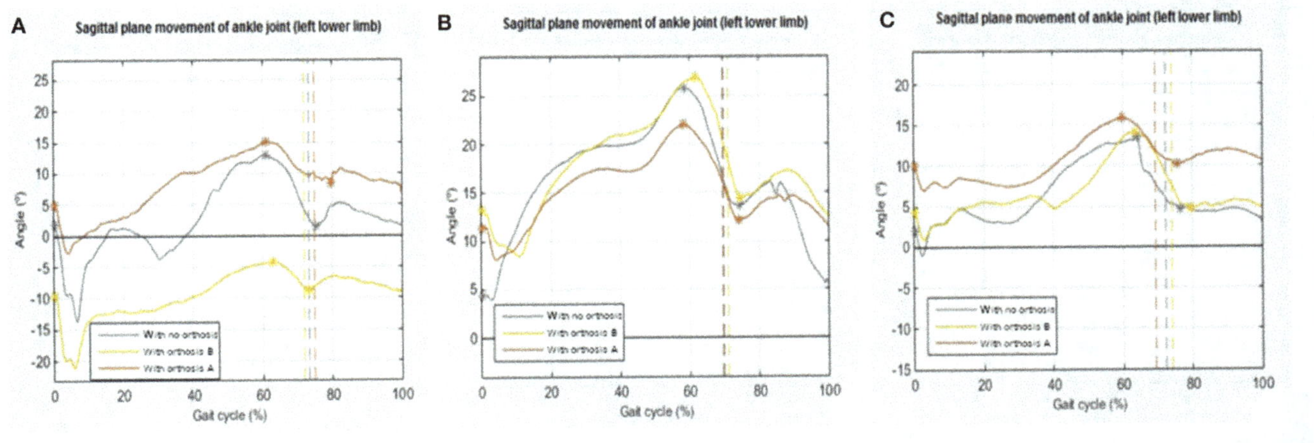

FIGURE 2 | Examples of plots representing the sagittal plane movement of the ankle joint of the pathological lower limb in the three conditions in the analysis. **(A)** Trial 1 of subject 1. **(B)** Trial 1 of subject 2. **(C)** Trial 1 of subject 3. The vertical line presents the contact phase, and the * is the higher value.

The angular results show that, on average, A is the orthosis that increases dorsiflexion [an increase of 6.133° (±0.001°) in foot impact, 0.614° (±0.001°) in maximum dorsiflexion, and 3.805° (±0.001°) in maximum plantar flexion]. Only subject 2 shows different results (**Figure 2**).

The increase in the stance phase was evaluated in order to analyze temporal behavior. The results obtained show that, on average, the use of orthoses does not improve temporal variation.

For angular analysis of foot impact and contralateral raised foot in the coronal plane of the ankle joint, we evaluated the increase in the *varus*.

The angular results show that, on average, both orthoses can decrease the characteristic *varus* of equinus foot dysfunction. However, the orthosis that shows quantitatively more significant improvement is B [an increase of 0.768° (±0.001°) in foot impact and 0.394° (±0.001°) on raised foot of contralateral limb]. Once again, subject 2 shows different results (**Figure 3**).

About the temporal variation, the methodology used is the same as the one used for the sagittal plane. Once again, the results show that, on average, the use of orthosis does not improve temporal variation.

The vertical extension of the angular pelvis in the sagittal plane is directly related to the gait's energy expenditure. We look for the lowest values of extension, since they mean lower energy expenditure and consequently more efficient gait. Although the data show that both orthoses impart a beneficial effect, on average, the A orthosis produces better results.

Kinetic Parameters

Concerning the ground reaction force, the higher force produced better performance. When the first and the last peaks were analyzed, on average, only A shows positive results in both peaks.

Regarding temporal variation, we can say that there is an improvement in the first peak of the curve if it is on the left of the corresponding peak without orthosis, and there is an improvement in the second peak if it is on the right. This criterion is adopted because it is verified, in the analyzed cases, that the first peak occurs later and the second peak occurs earlier relative to non-pathological behavior. The results show that, on average, no orthosis improves the first peak temporally and A shows benefits in the second peak (**Table 3**). It is also observed that the temporal relationship between the first and the second peak is much lower than the standard value of reference: 60% (21).

For the maximum force of the ankle joint, which occurs immediately before the raised foot, the results show that, on average, none of the orthoses can improve this parameter.

DISCUSSION/CONCLUSIONS

In this paper, we present the development of a decision support tool called OrthoRehab, as well as the steps involved in this process. Performance of the tool was evaluated in a clinical environment. Regarding the usability of the tool, the clinical team considered that OrthoRehab was easier to use without workload as well as user-friendly.

TABLE 3 | Mean values of the affected lower limb at the moment when the two peaks of reaction force of the soil occur.

		Average value (±0.01% support phase)		Normative reference value [17]
		Subject 1	**Subject 2**	
1st Peak	With no orthosis	48.01	42.37	20%
	Orthosis B	50.28	47.47	
	Orthosis A	49.79	50.25	
2nd Peak	With no orthosis	64.74	58.25	90%
	Orthosis B	67.59	56.00	
	Orthosis A	66.64	58.00	
Difference between the 1st and 2nd peak	With no orthosis	16.73	15.88	60%
	Orthosis B	17.31	8.52	
	Orthosis A	16.85	7.75	

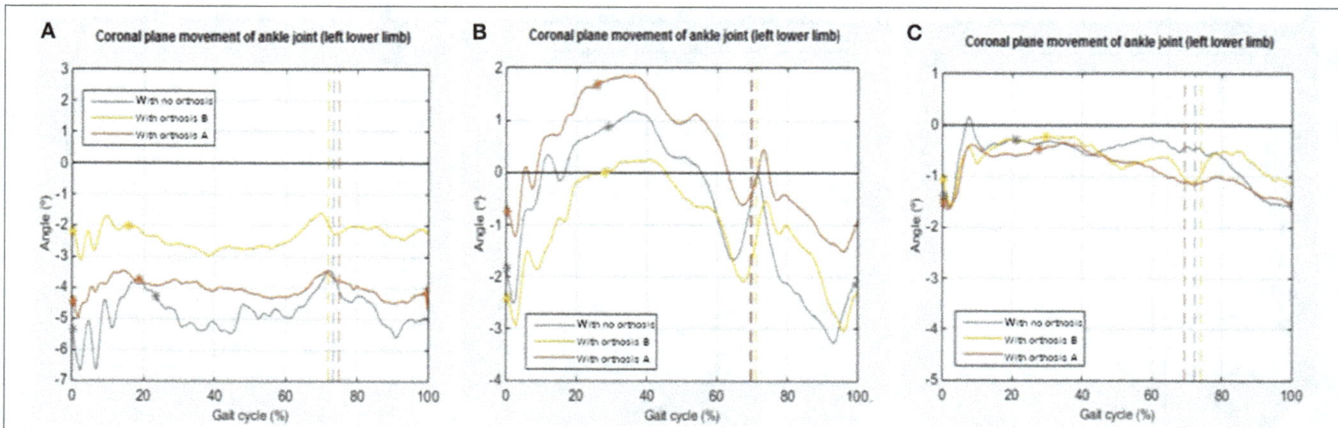

FIGURE 3 | Examples of plots representing the ankle joint's coronal plane of the pathological lower limb in the three conditions in the analysis. **(A)** Trial 1 of subject 1. **(B)** Trial 1 of subject 2. **(C)** Trial 1 of subject 3. The vertical line presents the contact phase, and the * is the higher value.

OrthoRehab provides simultaneous analysis for each subject in three conditions: with no orthosis and with two different AFOs. This tool gives a comparative and quantitative analysis of the most relevant gait parameters for foot dysfunction. Therefore, OrthoRehab contributes to the development of clinical plans for each subject with this dysfunction and, more specifically, it helps with the correct dynamic AFOs prescription.

The tool development methodology began with the decision about what were the most valuable kinematic and kinetic parameters for analysis of foot dysfunction and their distribution categories. This allowed developing a software that analyzes these parameters and plots them using an appropriate graphical interface. These two items (parameters and plots) provide physicians and therapists a global, integrated, and innovative evaluation of patient's gait in relation to the orthoses under study.

OrthoRehab was applied in a real clinical context, and it proved to be a reliable and suitable tool, fulfilling the objectives that were established.

OrthoRehab will help physicians and therapists in making a better, personalized, and reasoned decision about the AFO prescription. This tool can be useful in different clinical areas such as rheumatology, ortho-traumatologic, and also in populations of varying ages, since it can be applied to any person who has been prescribed a lower limb orthosis. Additionally, the OrthoRehab can be adapted to be applied to other dysfunctions/deformities and/or with different orthoses.

ETHICS STATEMENT

The studies involving human participants were reviewed and approved by Rehabilitation Medicine Center of Alcoitão. The patients/participants provided their written informed consent to participate in this study.

AUTHOR CONTRIBUTIONS

CQua, BL, JJ, and CQui contributed to the conception, design of the study, and participated in drafting the final manuscript. BL performed the tool and analyzed the data. All authors contributed to the conception, design of the review, contributed to manuscript revision, read, and approved the submitted.

ACKNOWLEDGMENTS

The authors would like to thank the teams from Rehabilitation Medicine Center of Alcoitão (CMRA) and from Nova School of Science and Technology of NOVA University of Lisbon that participated in the design and development of the OrthoRehab. This study was approved by the Portuguese Ethics Committees of the CMRA.

REFERENCES

1. World Health Organization. 2008–2013 action plan for the global strategy for the prevention and control of non-communicable diseases. Prevent and control cardiovascular diseases, cancers, chronic respiratory diseases diabetes. (2008). Available online at: https://apps.who.int/iris/bitstream/handle/10665/44009/9789241597418_eng.pdf?sequence=1 (accessed May 22, 2020).
2. Daïen D, Tubery A, Beurai-Weber M, Caila G, Picot M, Jaussent A, et al. Relevance and feasibility of a systematic screening of multimorbidities in patients with chronic inflammatory rheumatic diseases. *Joint Bone Spine.* (2019) 86:49–54. doi: 10.1016/j.jbspin.2018.03.016
3. Trieb K. Management of the foot in rheumatoid arthritis. *J Bone Joint Surg Br.* (2005) 87:1171e1177. doi: 10.1302/0301-620X.87B9.16288
4. Yano K, Ikari K, Inoue E, Sakuma Y, Mochizuki T, Koenuma N, et al. Features of patients with rheumatoid arthritis whose debut joint is a foot or ankle joint: a 5,479-case study from the IORRA cohort. *PLoS ONE.* (2018) 13:e0202427. doi: 10.1371/journal.pone.0202427
5. Mochizuki T, Yano K, Ikari K, Okazaki K. Effect of an orthosis on foot center of pressure translation for treatment of hallux valgus in patients with rheumatoid arthritis: a report of 17 cases. *Asia-Pacific J Sports Med Arthroscopy Rehabil Technol.* (2020) 19:7e10. doi: 10.1016/j.asmart.2019.10.003
6. Son SM, Park IS, Yoo JSJ. Short-term effect of botulinum toxin an injection on spastic equinovarus foot in cerebral palsy patients: a study using the foot pressure measurement system. *Ann Rehabil Med.* (2015) 39:1. doi: 10.5535/arm.2015.39.1.1
7. Boudarham J, Pradon D, Roche N, Bensmail D, Zory R, et al. Effects of a dynamic-ankle-foot orthosis (Liberte®) on kinematics and electromyographic activity during gait in hemiplegic patients with spastic foot equinus. *NeuroRehabilitation.* (2014) 35:369–79. doi: 10.3233/NRE-141128
8. de Quervain IAK, Simon SR, Leurgans S, Pease WS, McAllister D, et al. Gait pattern in the early recovery period after stroke. *J Bone Joint Surg Am.* (1996) 78:1506–14. doi: 10.2106/00004623-199610000-00008
9. Bollens B, Gustin T, Stoquart G, Detrembleur C, Lejeune T, Deltombe T, et al. A randomized controlled trial of selective neurotomy vs. botulinum toxin for spastic equinovarus foot after stroke. *Neurorehabil Neural Repair.* (2013) 27:695–703. doi: 10.1177/1545968313491002
10. Cinone N, Letizia S, Santoro L, Facciorusso S, Armiento R, Picelli A, et al. Combined effects of isokinetic training and botulinum toxin type A on spastic equinus foot in patients with chronic stroke: a pilot, single-blind, randomized controlled trial. *Toxins.* (2019) 11:210. doi: 10.3390/toxins11040210
11. Sung, K, Chung C, Lee K, Kwon K, Lee JH, Park MS, et al. Discrepancy between true ankle dorsiflexion and gait kinematics and its association with severity of planovalgus foot deformity. *BMC Musculoskeletal Disord.* (2020) 21:250. doi: 10.1186/s12891-020-03285-3
12. Jafarian F, Payehdar S, Forghany S. Effects of ankle foot orthoses on restricted ankle joint dorsiflexion due to plantarflexors stiffness in people with stroke: a scoping review. *J Rehabil Sci Res.* (2019) 6:59–62. doi: 10.30476/jrsr.2019.75366
13. Totah D, Menon M, Jones-Hershinow C, Barton K, Gates DH. The impact of ankle-foot orthosis stiffness on gait: a systematic literature review. *Gait Posture.* (2019) 69:101–11. doi: 10.1016/j.gaitpost.2019.01.020
14. Chisholm A, Perry S. Ankle-foot orthotic management in neuromuscular disorders: recommendations for future research. *Disabil Rehabil.* (2012) 7:437–49. doi: 10.3109/17483107.2012.680940
15. Kobayashi T, Leung AK, Akazawa Y, Hutchins SW. Correlations between Berg balance scale and gait speed in individuals with stroke wearing

ankle-foot orthoses-a pilot study. *Disabil Rehabil Assist Technol.* (2016) 11:219–22. doi: 10.3109/17483107.2014.932019
16. Barrett LF, Barrett DJJSSCR. An introduction to computerized experience sampling in psychology. *Soc Sci Comput Rev.* (2001) 19:175–85. doi: 10.1177/089443930101900204
17. Kinsella S, Moran KJG. Gait pattern categorization of stroke participants with equinus deformity of the foot. *Gait Posture.* (2008) 27:144–51. doi: 10.1016/j.gaitpost.2007.03.008
18. Manca M, Ferraresi G, Cosma M, Cavazzuti L, Morelli M, Benedetti MG. Gait patterns in hemiplegic patients with equinus foot deformity. *Adv Neuromotor Stroke Rehabil.* (2014) 2014:939316. doi: 10.1155/2014/939316
19. Richards J. *Biomechanics in Clinic and Research.* London: Churchill Livingstone (2008).
20. Vicon Motion Systems Limited. *Plug-inGait: ProductGuide—Foundation Notes.* (2010). Available online at: https://www.vicon.com/downloads/documen-tation/vicon-documentation/plug-in-gait-product-guide (accessed June 30, 2016).
21. Ferreira LAB, Neto HP, Christovão TCL, Duarte NAC, Lazzari RD, Galli M, et al. Effect of ankle-foot orthosis on gait velocity and cadence of stroke patients: a systematic review. *J Phys Therapy Sci.* (2013) 25:1503–8. doi: 10.1589/jpts.25.1503

11

Peripheral Enthesitis Detected by Ultrasonography in Patients with Axial Spondyloarthritis—Anatomical Distribution, Morphology and Response to Tumor Necrosis Factor-Inhibitor Therapy

Sengul Seven [1,2], Susanne Juhl Pedersen [1,2], Mikkel Østergaard [1,2], Sara Kamp Felbo [1,2], Inge Juul Sørensen [1], Uffe Møller Døhn [1] and Lene Terslev [1,2]*

[1] Copenhagen Center for Arthritis Research and Center for Rheumatology and Spine Diseases, Centre of Head and Orthopaedics, Rigshospitalet, Glostrup, Denmark, [2] Department of Clinical Medicine, University of Copenhagen, Copenhagen, Denmark

***Correspondence:**
Sengul Seven
sengul.seven@dadlnet.dk

Objectives: To investigate the anatomical distribution, morphological abnormalities and response to adalimumab therapy of ultrasound(US)-detected peripheral enthesitis in patients with axial spondyloarthritis (SpA).

Methods: In a randomized, placebo-controlled, double-blinded, investigator-initiated trial (NCT01029847), patients with axial SpA according to the Assessment of Spondyloarthritis International Society criteria were randomized to subcutaneous adalimumab 40 mg every other week or placebo from baseline to week 6. From week 6 to 24, all patients received adalimumab 40 mg every other week. Of 49 patients enrolled, 21 patients participated in our observational US sub-study. US assessment applying the OMERACT US definitions for enthesitis of 10 peripheral entheseal regions of the upper and lower extremities and clinical examination were performed at baseline, weeks 6 and 24. US was performed by one experienced investigator. Hypo-echogenicity, increased thickness and Doppler activity of the enthesis were considered signs of active inflammation, whereas insertional bone erosions, intratendinous calcifications, and enthesophytes were regarded as signs of structural lesions.

Results: Enthesitis on US was mostly present in the lower limbs, especially in the Achilles tendon (81%), the quadriceps tendon (62%), and the greater femoral trochanter (52%). Structural lesions were predominant (38 vs. 12% of examined entheses with inflammatory changes), particularly in the entheses of the lower limbs, and exhibited no change during treatment.

Conclusion: US-detected structural lesions were common while inflammatory lesions were relatively rare in patients initiating adalimumab due to axial SpA. Structural lesions did not appear to change during 24 weeks follow-up, suggesting that these lesions may not be helpful outcome measures in short-term clinical trials.

Keywords: imaging, ultrasound, enthesitis, spondyloarthritis, inflammation

INTRODUCTION

Enthesitis is typically defined as inflammation of the insertion of tendons, ligaments, aponeurosis, and capsules into the bone, and it is considered a pathological, clinical, and imaging hallmark of the spondyloarthritis (SpA) group, including psoriatic arthritis (PsA) (1–3). The Assessments in the SpondyloArthritis International Working Group (ASAS) and the Group for Research and Assessment of Psoriasis and Psoriatic Arthritis (GRAPPA) have recommended enthesitis as one of the key domains for assessing disease activity and response in SpA (axial and peripheral) and PsA (4, 5). The Outcome Measures in Rheumatology (OMERACT) Ultrasound (US) Working Group (WG), has developed and validated consensus-based US definitions for enthesitis lesions in SpA including PsA (1, 2) of which some are related to inflammation and some to inactive structural lesions.

Enthesitis lesions may be detected by US at clinically asymptomatic entheses and with a greater sensitivity than clinical examination (3–5). Since 1994, US has been used for evaluating peripheral enthesitis in SpA patients in both lower and upper limb entheses (6–9). B-mode and Doppler US (color and power) both depict the morphological features and vascularity of the enthesis and may aid in the diagnosis and evaluation of treatment effect (10–12), however, in most studies the inclusion criterion was symptomatic entheses in addition to US verified Doppler activity in the entheses. Different clinical enthesitis scores (13–15) and US enthesitis scores (5, 16, 17) exist in literature, but currently there is no consensus on which clinical scores and US scores to apply. Additionally, little is known about the presence and response to treatment of US-detected enthesitis (inflammatory lesions and/or structural lesions) in axial SpA patients initiating TNF-I therapy due to axial inflammatory activity.

The aim of the study was to investigate the anatomical distribution, morphological abnormalities and response to Tumor Necrosis Factor-inhibitor (TNF-I) therapy of US-detected peripheral enthesitis lesions in a cohort of patients with axial SpA, with or without symptomatic peripheral enthesitis, initiating adalimumab therapy, applying the OMERACT US definitions for enthesitis lesions.

PATIENTS AND METHODS

Study Design

The main study (the ASIM study) was a randomized, double-blinded, placebo-controlled investigator-initiated, 52 weeks longitudinal trial (ClinicalTrials.gov, NCT01029847) conducted in Denmark at five rheumatology outpatient clinics from 2010 to 2014. Fifty patients were included and randomized to receive subcutaneous adalimumab 40 mg every other week or placebo from baseline to week 6. From week 6 to 24, all patients received adalimumab 40 mg every other week. Participants in our observational US sub-study were recruited among patients in the main study. The US sub-study was conducted at Rigshospitalet, Glostrup. The study was approved by the local ethical committee, approval number H1-2013-118, and conducted according to the Declaration of Helsinki V and the Danish legislation. All participants gave written informed consent before study inclusion.

Inclusion and Exclusion Criteria

All patients had axial SpA according to the Assessment of Spondyloarthritis International Society (ASAS) classification criteria, sacroiliitis on X-ray or MRI, disease activity assessed by BASDAI >4 (0–10) despite NSAID treatment and a clinical indication for TNF-I treatment. Treatment with glucocorticoids and/or initiation or changes in csDMARD were not allowed 4 weeks prior to inclusion. Entheseal involvement was not an inclusion criterion.

Patient Evaluation

Patient demographics, clinical and biochemical data were obtained for all participants at every visit. The clinical examination included 66/68 joint count, the Bath Ankylosing Spondylitis Metrology Index (BASMI) and assessment of entheses according to the Leeds enthesitis index (LEI) (13), Maastricht Ankylosing Spondylitis Enthesitis Score (MASES) (15) and the Spondyloarthritis Research Consortium of Canada (SPARCC) enthesitis index (14). A standardized approach to clinical examination of entheses based on a predefined illustrated set of instructions was developed (18). Blood samples were analyzed for serum C-reactive protein (CRP) and Human Leukocyte Antigen B27 (HLA-B27). US assessments were performed at baseline, and weeks 6 and 24.

Ultrasound

All US scans were performed with General Electric Logiq 9 US machine. A ML 12 high-frequency linear probe was used with a center frequency of 14 megahertz (MHz). Doppler setting was adjusted for slow flow according to published recommendations (19). US was performed blinded to clinical and biochemical data according to a standardized protocol by an experienced investigator (LT), who has previously participated in reliability exercises on patients with enthesitis showing high inter- and intrareader reliability (2). Twenty entheseal sites were examined by greyscale and color Doppler; the common extensor, and flexor tendons of the elbow, insertions of supraspinatus tendon, triceps, greater femoral trochanter, quadriceps, proximal, and distal patellar and Achilles tendon, and plantar fascia. Enthesitis was defined according to the OMERACT definitions (2). Hypo-echogenicity, increased thickness (morphologic abnormalities) and Doppler activity of the enthesis were considered signs of active inflammation, whereas insertional bone erosions, intra-tendinous calcifications, and enthesophytes were regarded as signs of structural lesions (2). All lesions were scored dichotomously. US enthesitis was scored according to the Glasgow Ultrasound Enthesitis Scoring System (GUESS) (5), Spanish Enthesitis Index (SEI) (16) and the Madrid Sonography Enthesitis Index (MASEI) (17).

TABLE 1 | Demographic, clinical, and laboratory characteristics of the study population.

	All patients	Placebo	Adalimumab	P-value*
Number of participants	21	10	11	
Demographics				
Age, years	39.4 (9.4)	34.3 (5.5)	44.1 (10.0)	**0.02**
Female sex, *N* (%)	9 (42.9)	5 (50.0)	4 (36.4)	0.5
Symptom duration, years	14.1 (12.8)	11.1 (6.8)	16.8 (16.4)	0.9
Biochemical characteristics				
HLA-B27 positive, *N* (%)	15 (71.4)	8 (80.0)	7 (63.6)	0.4
C-reactive protein (mg/L)	8.5 (15.9)	3.8 (3.5)	12.8 (21.3)	0.3
Clinical characteristics				
Physician VAS global (0–10)[a]	6.8 (2.0)	7.7 (1.4)	5.9 (2.2)	0.2
SJC66	0.2 (0.6)	0.2 (0.6)	0.3 (0.7)	0.6
TJC68	3.6 (7.0)	3.6 (4.3)	3.6 (9.0)	0.4
MASES (0–13)	3.9 (3.8)	4.6 (4.0)	2.9 (3.7)	0.3
LEI (0–6)	0.9 (1.0)	0.7 (1.0)	1.1 (1.1)	0.5
SPARCC enthesitis index (0–16)	3.0 (3.2)	3.2 (3.8)	2.6 (2.9)	1.0
Patient reported outcomes				
HAQ	1.0 (0.5)	1.1 (0.7)	1.0 (0.4)	0.6
VAS pain (0–10)[a]	7.3 (2.0)	7.7 (1.8)	6.9 (2.1)	0.4
VAS patient global (0–10)[a]	7.2 (2.1)	7.6 (2.2)	6.8 (2.1)	0.3
BASDAI (0–10)	6.6 (1.6)	7.0 (1.9)	6.3 (1.3)	0.4
BASFI (0–10)	5.9 (2.1)	5.9 (2.5)	5.8 (1.9)	0.9
BASMI (0–10)	3.2 (2.1)	2.7 (2.0)	3.7 (2.2)	0.2

*N (%) for female sex and HLA-B27 status, mean (SD) for all others. Chi²-test for female gender and HLA-B27, Mann-Whitney U-tests for all others. *P < 0.05 is considered significant and indicated in bold.*

[a]According to Bath Ankylosing Spondylitis Questionnaire.

BASDAI, Bath Ankylosing Spondylitis Disease Activity Index; BASFI, Bath Ankylosing Spondylitis Functional Index; BASMI, Bath Ankylosing Spondylitis Metrology Index; HAQ, Health Assessment Questionnaire; HLA-B27, Human Leukocyte Antigen B27; LEI, Leeds Enthesitis Index; MASES, Maastricht Ankylosing Spondylitis Enthesitis Score; SJC, Swollen Joint Count; SPARCC, Spondyloarthritis Research Consortium of Canada; TJC, Tender Joint Count; VAS, Visual Analog Scale.

STATISTICS

Descriptive statistics were applied for analysis of demographics, clinical, biochemical, and US data. Statistical analyses were performed using non-parametric tests. Differences in the two study populations were analyzed by applying Chi^2-test and Mann-Whitney *U*-test, and the Wilcoxon Rank test was used to analyze differences in treatment effect over time. To determine the agreement between clinical enthesitis vs. US enthesitis and US inflammation, respectively, Cohen's Kappa was calculated, and Spearman's Rho was performed to calculate correlations between clinical scores vs. US enthesitis scores at baseline. We considered Kappa values of <0 as indicating no agreement, 0–0.20 as slight, 0.21–0.40 fair, 0.41–0.60 moderate, 0.61–0.80 good, and 0.81–1 as excellent agreement. A $p < 0.05$ was considered statistically significant. All statistical analyses were performed in IBM SPSS version 22.0.

RESULTS

Demographics, Clinical, and Biochemical Characteristics

Of the 49 patients enrolled in the main study, 21 participated in the US sub-study. The number of patients randomized to receive adalimumab and placebo were 11 and 10, respectively. The patients were 57% males with a mean age of 39.4 years, and 71% were HLA-B27 positive. Baseline demographics, clinical and biochemical characteristics are shown in **Table 1**. The two randomization groups were comparable in baseline characteristics apart from age where patients in the adalimumab group were statistically significantly older than in the placebo group.

The Distribution of US Enthesitis at Baseline

The distribution of clinical and US signs of enthesitis in all 21 patients at baseline is provided in **Table 2**, including the Kappa agreement between clinical enthesitis vs. US enthesitis (i.e., inflammatory lesions and/or structural lesions) and clinical enthesitis vs. US inflammatory lesions alone. Overall, enthesitis (inflammatory lesions and/or structural lesions) was found in 95% of patients. Inflammatory lesions were found in 52% of patients (12% of examined entheses—2% with Doppler activity), while 95% of patients (38% of examined entheses) had structural lesions perceived to be inactive. In comparison 67% of patients had clinical signs of enthesitis. The US-inflammatory lesions in the lower extremities were most frequently found in the insertions of the Achilles tendon (19%) and plantar fascia (19%), while in the upper extremities in the insertion of triceps tendon (5%) and the common extensor tendon of the elbow (5%). Inflammatory lesions were not seen at the greater femoral trochanter and at the insertion of the common flexor tendon.

US enthesitis (inflammation and/or structural US changes) was predominantly found in the lower extremities, especially in the Achilles tendon (81%), the quadriceps tendon (62%) and at the insertion onto the greater femoral trochanter (52%), and these were mostly structural lesions (76, 62, 52%, respectively). In the upper extremities US enthesitis was mostly recorded in the supraspinatus tendon insertion (29%) and at the insertion of the common extensor tendon of the elbow (24%).

When evaluating the different types of inflammatory and structural lesions (**Table 3**), at the upper extremities we observed the presence of erosion only at the insertion of the supraspinatus tendon (18%) and the common extensor tendon of the elbow (5%), while erosions were recorded at nearly all entheses of the lower extremities, especially at the greater femoral trochanter (33%), although never in the distal insertion of the patellar tendon. Calcifications and/or enthesophytes were present across all entheseal regions, except for the common flexor tendon of the elbow and the plantar fascia. Increased thickness and/or

TABLE 2 | Distribution of clinical and US entheseal findings and enthesitis scores at baseline ($n = 21$).

Entheseal region	US			Clinical enthesitis[c]
	Inflammatory lesions[a]	Structural lesions[b]	Enthesitis (inflammatory and/or structural lesions)	
Supraspinatus tendon	0	6 (28.6)	6 (28.6)[##]	8 (38.1)
Triceps tendon	1 (4.8)	1 (4.8)	2 (9.5)	NA
Common extensor tendon, elbow	1 (4.8)[$]	5 (23.8)	5 (23.8)[#]	3 (14.3)
Common flexor tendon, elbow	0	0	0	6 (28.6)
Greater femoral trochanter	0	11 (52.4)	11 (52.4)[##]	12 (57.1)
Quadriceps tendon	3 (14.3)[$]	13 (61.9)	13 (61.9)[#]	3 (14.3)
Proximal insertion of the patellar tendon	1 (4.8)[$]	2 (9.5)	3 (14.3)[#]	4 (19.0)
Distal insertion of the patellar tendon	2 (9.5)[$]	2 (9.5)	3 (14.3)[#]	2 (9.5)
Achilles tendon	4 (19.0)[$$$]	16 (76.2)	17 (81.0)[#]	4 (19.0)
Plantar fascia	4 (19.0)[$]	0	4 (19.0)[#]	6 (28.6)
US enthesitis score				
GUESS (0–36)			3.1 (1.9)	
SEI (0–76)			1.8 (2.1)	
MASEI (0–136)			6.7 (4.6)	

N (%) participants with lesions.
[a]Inflammation: Doppler activity, hypo-echogenicity or increased thickness.
[b]Chronic lesions: Erosions, calcifications or enthesophytes.
[c]Entheses with tenderness.
Kappa agreement was calculated for US enthesitis vs. clinical enthesitis. Kappa value<0 no[#], 0–0.20 slight[##], 0.21–0.40 fair, 0.41–0.60 moderate, 0.61–0.80 good, 0.81–1 excellent agreement, respectively.
Kappa agreement was calculated for US inflammatory lesion vs. clinical enthesitis. Kappa value<0 no[$], 0–0.20 slight[$$], 0.21–0.40 fair[$$$], 0.41–0.60 moderate, 0.61–0.80 good, 0.81–1 excellent agreement, respectively.
GUESS, The Glascow Ultrasound Enthesitis Scoring System; LEI, Leeds Enthesitis Index; MASEI, Madrid Sonography Enthesitis Index; MASES, Maastricht Ankylosing Spondylitis Enthesitis Score; NA, not applicable; SEI, Spanish Enthesitis Index; SPARCC, Spondyloarthritis Research Consortium of Canada; US, ultrasound.

hypoechoic features were mostly seen at the Achilles tendon insertion and the plantar fascia (14 and 15%, respectively), while completely absent at the supraspinatus tendon, common flexor tendon of the elbow, and the greater femoral trochanter. Doppler was only recorded at the quadriceps tendon (7%) and the distal insertion of the patellar tendon (2%).

Agreement Between US Enthesitis and Clinical Assessment

A fair agreement for US inflammatory lesions vs. clinical enthesitis was seen at the Achilles tendon insertion, while none to poor agreement was found between US structural lesions and inflammatory lesions vs. clinical enthesitis for all other entheses (**Table 2**). Overall, 10% of non-tender entheses showed US signs of inflammation and on the contrary 18% of tender entheses did not show US signs of inflammation. The different clinical scores of enthesitis and the different US enthesitis scores at baseline are also seen in **Table 2**. When performing the Spearmann's rho, we only found a statistically significant correlation between the LEI clinical enthesitis score vs. SEI US enthesitis score.

TABLE 3 | US findings at baseline ($n = 21$).

Entheseal region	Erosion	Calcifications / enthesophytes	Increased thickness / hypoechoic	Doppler
Supraspinatus tendon	7 (18)	2 (5)	0	0
Triceps tendon	0	1 (3)	1 (2)	0
Common extensor tendon, elbow	2 (5)	6 (14)	2 (5)	0
Common flexor tendon, elbow	0	0	0	0
Greater femoral trochanter	14 (33)	6 (14)	0	0
Quadriceps tendon	3 (7)	20 (48)	2 (5)	3 (7)
Proximal insertion of the patellar tendon	3 (7)	2 (5)	1 (2)	0
Distal insertion of the patellar tendon	0	3 (7)	1 (2)	1 (2)
Achilles tendon	3 (7)	28 (67)	6 (14)	0
Plantar fascia ($n = 20$)	1 (3)	0	6 (15)	0

N (%) of entheses with lesions.

US and Clinical Enthesitis Changes During Treatment

The clinical findings and US enthesitis (inflammatory and/or structural lesions) scores in the two randomization groups at weeks 0, 6, and 24 are provided in **Table 4**. A statistically significant decrease in BASDAI was seen at both weeks 6 and 24 in the adalimumab group, while only at week 24 in in the placebo group. The SPARCC enthesitis index had decreased significantly from baseline at weeks 6 and 24. No other changes in clinical indices was observed in either of the groups. Regarding the US findings, the only statistically significant changes were for the common extensor tendon of the elbow from baseline to weeks 6 and 24 in the adalimumab group, and for the SEI US score from baseline to week 24 in the placebo group.

DISCUSSION

In this observational US sub-study of axial SpA patients who initiated TNF-I treatment based on axial inflammation, a high prevalence of structural lesions was observed in peripheral entheses (95% of patients, 38% of examined entheses), whereas the prevalence of inflammatory entheseal changes was fairly low (52% of patients, 12% of examined entheses, and 2% with Doppler activity). US signs of enthesitis were mainly identified in the lower extremities, mostly as structural lesions. No change in structural lesions were found during treatment, indicating a low ability to change and supporting the perception of being inactive lesions.

TABLE 4 | Clinical and US findings during study period.

	Placebo			Adalimumab		
	Week 0	**Week 6**	**Week 24**	**Week 0**	**Week 6**	**Week 24**
Number of patients	10	9	10	11	11	10
Clinical enthesitis scores						
MASES (0–13)	4.6 (4.0)	4.0 (3.3)	2.2 (3.7)	3.0 (3.7)	2.1 (2.5)	2.0 (3.0)
LEI (0–6)	0.7 (0.9)	0.9 (1.0)	0.6 (0.9)	1.1 (1.1)	0.7 (0.9)	0.3 (0.7)
SPARCC enthesitis index (0–16)	3.2 (3.8)	3.6 (2.6)	2.2 (2.8)	2.6 (2.9)	1.6 (1.9)**	0.8 (1.1)***
BASDAI	7.0 (1.9)	6.4 (2.5)	4.3 (2.7)***	6.3 (1.3)*	4.2 (2.3)**	2.9 (2.5)***
US findings[a]						
Supraspinatus tendon	3 (30)	2 (22)	1 (10)	3 (27)	2 (18)	1 (10)
Common extensor tendon, elbow	0	0	0	5 (46)*	0	1 (10)***
Common flexor tendon, elbow	0	0	0	0	0	0
Triceps tendon, elbow	1 (10)	0	1 (10)	1 (9)	0	2 (20)
Greater femoral trochanter	6 (60)	6 (67)	6 (60)	5 (46)	6 (55)	6 (60)
Quadriceps tendon	4 (40)	1 (11)	4 (40)	9 (82)	8 (73)	6 (60)
Proximal insertion of the patellar tendon	1 (10)	0	0	2 (18)	1 (9)	1 (10)
Distal insertion of the patellar tendon	2 (20)	1 (11)	1 (10)	1 (9)	1 (9)	0
Achilles tendon	7 (70)	7 (78)	8 (80)	10 (91)	7 (64)	7 (70)
Plantar fascia	1 (10)	0	0	3 (27)	3 (27)	2 (20)
US enthesitis scores						
GUESS (0–36)	2.90 (2.33)	2.56 (1.59)	2.22 (1.39)	3.18 (1.60)	3.09 (1.92)	2.56 (1.81)
SEI (0–76)	2.10 (2.13)	1.22 (1.30)	0.89 (1.54)***	1.55 (2.16)	1.18 (0.98)	0.89 (1.05)
MASEI (0–136)	6.00 (4.92)	4.89 (3.06)	5.00 (3.87)	7.36 (4.46)	7.36 (4.59)	6.89 (5.13)

Mean (SD) for clinical and US enthesitis scores, n (%) participants with US findings.
[a]Inflammatory and/or structural lesions.
*Wilcoxon Rank test was applied. $P < 0.05$ is considered significant. *$p < 0.05$ week 0–6; **$P < 0.05$ week 6–24; ***$P < 0.05$ week 0–24.*
BASDAI, Bath Ankylosing Spondylitis Disease Activity Index; GUESS, The Glascow Ultrasound Enthesitis Scoring System; LEI, Leeds Enthesitis Index; MASEI, Madrid Sonography Enthesitis Index; MASES, Maastricht Ankylosing Spondylitis Enthesitis Score; SEI, Spanish Enthesitis Index; SPARCC, Spondyloarthritis Research Consortium of Canada; US, Ultrasound.

The high frequency of US structural lesions in our population with long-standing disease is in line with previous US studies of enthesitis in SpA patients by Naredo et al. (3) and D'Agostino et al. (20) and in AS patients by Wink et al. (6) and Spadaro et al. (7) Calcifications/enthesophytes can also be seen in healthy subjects (8–11), with the highest frequency in the lower limbs, possibly increasing with increasing age, but with a lower prevalence than in SpA patients.

Regarding US signs of entheseal inflammation, the study by Wink et al. (6), which included AS patients, found Doppler activity in 55% of examined entheses, (i.e., more frequently compared with our study). Wink et al. did not include the insertions of triceps or supraspinatus but included the pes anserine. The latter may explain the high frequency of Doppler findings, as this was the most frequent site for Doppler activity. The proximity of the pes anserine to the inferior geniculate artery might increase the risk of overestimation of the inflammation. Since this study also looked at combinations of inflammatory lesions and included adjacent bursitis and effusion in this definition, results are therefore not comparable. Spadaro et al. (7) found a frequency of entheseal Doppler activity (6%) more similar to ours. However, Naredo et al. (20) also found a high prevalence of inflammatory changes with morphologic abnormalities in 61% of the SpA patients and intra-entheseal Doppler activity in 47% of the patients, both most commonly at the Achilles tendon insertion (29 and 16%, respectively). Our population, however, was selected based on axial manifestations, while peripheral findings were not required. This explains the low frequency of inflammatory US findings. The frequently registered high frequency of structural changes in peripheral entheses documents that most patients with axial SpA at some stage in their disease course get entheseal affection which is severe enough to leave recognizable structural damage.

Entheseal Doppler activity has been found in healthy subjects (8, 12, 21), also at the quadriceps insertion, where most Doppler activity was also found in our population. Other studies did not find any entheseal Doppler activity in healthy subjects (9, 22).

Although not an inclusion criterion, the patients in our study had clinically peripheral enthesis involvement with a MASES index of 3.9 (3.8), however, there were none to poor agreement between clinical entheses assessment and US findings of enthesitis. Further, no agreement was seen when evaluating different clinical enthesis scores and different US enthesitis scores. This is in line with several previous studies that have found US to be more sensitive than clinical evaluation for detection of inflammation (4). The tenderness at the clinically tender entheses that did not show US signs of inflammation may originate from other tender structures close to the entheses.

An outcome measure needs to possess ability to change during effective therapies (23). Wink et al. found no statistically significant decrease in inflammatory lesions (6). In the present study US enthesitis was not sensitive to change during adalimumab therapy, which is probably at least partially explained by the low number of inflammatory lesions. The lack of documented responsiveness supports that future studies should both test the current US measures in more actively inflamed cohorts and investigate new and potentially more sensitive measures.

The strength of this study is the placebo-controlled study design applying a standardized clinical and US protocol performed by an experienced sonographer. However, the study was observational and included axial SpA patients regardless of the presence of US enthesitis findings. Additionally, the low number of patients and low number of inflammatory lesions are the primary limitation, since the statistical power to show significant changes over time and differences between the groups was low.

In conclusion, we found by US a high prevalence of structural lesions and a very low prevalence of inflammatory lesions in a population of axial SpA patients with or without clinical peripheral enthesitis. In our study US structural lesions did not appear to have ability to change during 24 weeks of TNF-I treatment, suggesting that US-structural enthesitis lesions may not be helpful outcome measures in short-term clinical trials.

ETHICS STATEMENT

The studies involving human participants were reviewed and approved by the Videnskabsetiske Komiteer in the Capital Region of Denmark. The patients/participants provided their written informed consent to participate in this study.

AUTHOR CONTRIBUTIONS

LT, SP, and MØ contributed to the conception and design of the study. SS, SF, and LT wrote sections of the manuscript. SS and LT wrote the first draft of the manuscript. SS, LT, SF, and SP performed the statistical analysis and interpretation. SS organized the database. LT, IS, SP, and UD contributed to the acquisition of data. All authors contributed to manuscript revision, read, and approved the submitted version.

ACKNOWLEDGMENTS

The abstract has previously been presented at the EULAR conference [abstract no. OP0287 (24)].

REFERENCES

1. Terslev L, Naredo E, Iagnocco A, Balint PV, Wakefield RJ, Aegerter A. et al. Defining enthesitis in spondyloarthritis by ultrasound: results of a Delphi process and of a reliability reading exercise. *Arthritis Care Res.* (2014) 66:741–8. doi: 10.1002/acr.22191
2. Balint PV, Terslev L, Aegerter P, Bruyn GW, Valckenaere IC, Gandjbakhch F, et al. Reliability of a consensus-based ultrasound definition and scoring for enthesitis in spondyloarthritis and psoriatic arthritis: an OMERACT US initiative. *Ann Rheum Dis.* (2018) 77:1730–35. doi: 10.1136/annrheumdis-2018-213609
3. D'Agostino M-A, Said-Nahal R, Hacquard-Bouder C, Brasseur JL, Dougados M, Bredan M. Assessment of peripheral enthesitis in the spondylarthropathies by ultrasonography combined with power aoppler: a cross-sectional study. *Arthritis Rheum.* (2003) 48:523–33. doi: 10.1002/art.10812
4. Lehtinen A, Taavitsainen M, Leirisalo-Repo M. Sonographic analysis of enthesopathy in the lower extremities of patients with spondylarthropathy. *Clin Exp Rheumatol.* (1994) 12:143–8.
5. Balint PV, Kane D, Wilson H, McInnes IB, Sturrock RD. Ultrasonography of entheseal insertions in the lower limb in spondyloarthropathy. *Ann Rheum Dis.* (2002) 61:905–10. doi: 10.1136/ard.61.10.905
6. Wink F, Bruyn GA, Maas F, Griep EN, van der Veer E, Bootsma H, et al. Ultrasound evaluation of the entheses in daily clinical practice during tumor necrosis factor-alpha blocking therapy in patients with ankylosing spondylitis. *J Rheumatol.* (2017) 44:587–93. doi: 10.3899/jrheum.160584
7. Spadaro A, Iagnocco A, Perrotta FM, Modesti M, Scarno A, Valesini G. Clinical and ultrasonography assessment of peripheral enthesitis in ankylosing spondylitis. *Rheumatology.* (2011) 50:2080–6. doi: 10.1093/rheumatology/ker284
8. Guldberg-Moller J, Terslev L, Nielsen SM, Kønig MJ, Torp-Pedersen ST, Torp-Pedersen A, et al. Ultrasound pathology of the entheses in an age and gender stratified sample of healthy adult subjects: a prospective cross-sectional frequency study. *Clin Exp Rheumatol.* (2019) 37:408–13.
9. Queiro R, Alonso S, Alperi M, Fernández M, Tejón P, Riestra JL, et al. Entheseal ultrasound abnormalities in patients with SAPHO syndrome. *Clin Rheumatol.* (2012) 31:913–9. doi: 10.1007/s10067-012-1959-7
10. Gutierrez M, Luccioli F, Salaffi F, Bartoloni E, Bertolazzi C, Bini V, et al. Ultrasound revealing subclinical enthesopathy at the greater trochanter level in patients with spondyloarthritis. *Clini Rheumatol.* (2012) 31:463–8. doi: 10.1007/s10067-011-1875-2
11. Jaen-Diaz JI, Cerezo-Lopez E, Lopez-de Castro F, Mata-Castrillo M, Barceló-Galíndez, JP, de la Fuente J, et al. Sonographic findings for the common extensor tendon of the elbow in the general population. *J Ultrasound Med.* (2010) 29:1717–24. doi: 10.7863/jum.2010.29.12.1717
12. Lin C, Diab M, Milojevic D. Grey-scale ultrasound findings of lower extremity entheses in healthy children. *Pediatr Rheumatol Online J.* (2015) 13:14. doi: 10.1186/s12969-015-0012-1
13. Healy PJ, Helliwell PS. Measuring clinical enthesitis in psoriatic arthritis: assessment of existing measures and development of an instrument specific to psoriatic arthritis. *Arthritis Rheum.* (2008) 59:686–91. doi: 10.1002/art.23568
14. Maksymowych WP, Mallon C, Morrow S, Shojania K, Olszynski WP, Wong RL, et al. Development and validation of the spondyloarthritis research consortium of Canada (SPARCC) enthesitis index. *Ann Rheum Dis.* (2009) 68:948–53. doi: 10.1136/ard.2007.084244

15. Heuft-Dorenbosch L, Spoorenberg A, van Tubergen A, Landewé R, van ver Tempel H, Mielants H, et al. Assessment of enthesitis in ankylosing spondylitis. *Ann Rheum Dis.* (2003) 62:127–32. doi: 10.1136/ard.62.2.127
16. Alcalde M, Acebes JC, Cruz M, González-Hombrado L, Herrero-Beaumont G, Sánchez-Pernaute O. A sonographic enthesitic index of lower limbs is a valuable tool in the assessment of ankylosing spondylitis. *Ann Rheum Dis.* (2007) 66:1015–9. doi: 10.1136/ard.2006.062174
17. de Miguel E, Cobo T, Munoz-Fernandez S, Naredo E, Usón J, Acebes JC, et al. Validity of enthesis ultrasound assessment in spondyloarthropathy. *Ann Rheum Dis.* (2009) 68:169–74. doi: 10.1136/ard.2007.084251
18. Poggenborg RP, Eshed I, Ostergaard M, Sørensen IJ, Møller JM, Madsen OK, et al. Enthesitis in patients with psoriatic arthritis, axial spondyloarthritis and healthy subjects assessed by 'head-to-toe' whole-body MRI and clinical examination. *Ann Rheum Dis.* (2015) 74:823–9. doi: 10.1136/annrheumdis-2013-204239
19. Torp-Pedersen ST, Terslev L. Settings and artefacts relevant in colour/power Doppler ultrasound in rheumatology. *Ann Rheum Dis.* (2008) 67:143–49. doi: 10.1136/ard.2007.078451
20. Naredo E, Batlle-Gualda E, Garcia-Vivar ML, García-Aparicio AM, Fernández-Sueiro JL, Fernández-Prada M, et al. Power doppler ultrasonography assessment of entheses in spondyloarthropathies: response to therapy of entheseal abnormalities. *J Rheumatol.* (2010) 37:2110–7. doi: 10.3899/jrheum.100136
21. Krogh TP, Fredberg U, Ammitzbol C, Ellingsen T. Ultrasonographic characteristics of the common extensor tendon of the elbow in asymptomatic individuals: thickness, color doppler activity, and bony spurs. *Orthop J Sports Med.* (2017) 5:2325967117704186. doi: 10.1177/2325967117704186
22. Jousse-Joulin S, Morvan J, Devauchelle-Pensec V, Saraux A. Ultrasound assessment of the entheses in primary Sjogren syndrome. *Ultrasound Med Biol.* (2013) 39:2485–7. doi: 10.1016/j.ultrasmedbio.2013.05.013
23. Terslev L, Naredo E, Keen HI, Bruyn GAW, Iagnocco A, Wakefield RJ, et al. The OMERACT stepwise approach to select and develop imaging outcome measurement instruments: the musculoskeletal ultrasound example. *J Rheumatol.* (2019) 46:1394–400. doi: 10.3899/jrheum.181158
24. Seven S, Pedersen SJ, Østergaard M, Sørensen IJ. OP0287 ultrasonography-detected peripheral enthesitis in patients with axial spondyloarthritis – anatomical distribution, morphology and response to anti-tnf therapy. *Ann Rheum Dis.* (2017) 76:175.1–75. doi: 10.1136/annrheumdis-2017-eular.2781

12

Establishing Classification Tree Models in Rheumatoid Arthritis Using Combination of Matrix-Assisted Laser Desorption/Ionization Time-of-Flight Mass Spectrometry and Magnetic Beads

Dan Ma [1†], ***Nana Liang*** [2†] ***and Liyun Zhang*** [1*]

[1] *Department of Rheumatology, Shanxi Bethune Hospital, Shanxi Academy of Medical Sciences, Shanxi Bethune Hospital Affiliated to Shanxi Medical University, Taiyuan, China,* [2] *First Hospital/First Clinical Medical College of Shanxi Medical University, Taiyuan, China*

***Correspondence:**
Liyun Zhang
1315710223@qq.com

† These authors have contributed equally to this work and share first authorship

Background: There is no simple method for early diagnosis and evaluation of rheumatoid arthritis (RA). This study aimed to determine potential biomarkers and establish diagnostic patterns for RA using proteomic fingerprint technology combined with magnetic beads.

Methods: The serum protein profiles of 97 RA patients and 76 healthy controls (HCs) were analyzed by matrix-assisted laser desorption/ionization time-of-flight mass spectrometry (MALDI-TOF-MS) with weak cationic exchange (WCX) magnetic beads. Samples were randomly divided into training (83 RA patients and 56 HCs) and test sets (14 RA patients and 20 HCs). Patients were classified according to their Disease Activity Score: in remission, $n = 28$; with low disease activity, $n = 17$; with moderate disease activity, $n = 21$; with high disease activity, $n = 31$. There are 44 RA patients alone, 22 RA patients with interstitial lung disease (RA-ILD), 18 RA patients with secondary Sjögren's syndrome (RA-sSS), 6 RA patients with osteonecrosis of the femoral head (RA-ONFH), and 7 RA patients with other complications. Eleven patients were treated with etanercept only for half a year, after which their serum protein profiles were detected. The proteomic pattern was identified by Biomarker Patterns Software, and the potential biomarkers for RA diagnosis were further identified and quantified by enzyme-linked immunosorbent assay.

Results: The diagnostic pattern with four potential protein biomarkers, mass-to-charge (m/z) 3,448.85, 4,716.71, 8,214.29, and 10,645.10, could accurately recognize RA patients from HCs (specificity, 91.57%; sensitivity, 92.86%). The test set were correctly classified by this model (sensitivity, 95%; specificity, 100%). The components containing the four biomarkers were preliminarily retrieved through the ExPasy database, including the C-C motif chemokine 24 (CCL24), putative metallothionein (MT1DP), sarcolipin (SLN), and C-X-C motif chemokine 11 (CCXL11). Only the CCL24 level was detected to have a significant decrease in the serum of RA patients as compared with HCs ($p < 0.05$). No significant difference was found in others, but a decreasing trend consistent with the down-regulation of the four biomarkers detected by MALDI-TOF-MS was observed. The diagnostic models could effectively discriminate between RA alone and RA with complications (RA-ILD: m/z 10,645.10 and 12,595.86; RA-sSS: m/z 6,635.62 and 33,897.72; RA-ONFH: m/z 2,071.689). The classification model, including m/z 1,130.776, 1,501.065, 2,091.198, and 11,381.87, could distinguish between RA patients with disease activity and those in remission. RA with low disease activity could be efficiently discriminated from other disease activity patients by specific protein biomarkers (m/z 2,032.31, 2,506.214, and Z9286.495). Two biomarkers (m/z 2,032.31 and 4,716.71) were applied to build the classification model for RA patients with moderate and high disease activities. Biological markers for etanercept (m/z 2,671.604064, 5,801.840579, 8,130.195641, and 9,286.49499) were observed between the responder ($n = 7$) and non-responder groups ($n = 4$) ($p < 0.05$).

Conclusion: We successfully established a series of diagnostic models involving RA and RA with complications as well as assessed disease activity. Furthermore, we found that CCL24 may be a valuable auxiliary diagnostic indicator for RA. These results provide reference values for clinical practice in the future.

Keywords: rheumatoid arthritis, MALDI-TOF-MS, weak cationic exchange magnetic beads, biomarkers, classification tree model

INTRODUCTION

Rheumatoid arthritis (RA) is a chronic systemic autoimmune and inflammatory disease characterized by synovitis and vasculitis, which lead to the destruction of cartilage, joint deformation, loss of joints function, and systemic organ damages, and it affects approximately 0.5–1% of population (1). Pulmonary involvement is a common extraarticular manifestation of RA (2), particularly interstitial lung disease (ILD), which occurs in 1–58% of RA patients and has significant effect on morbidity and mortality (3, 4). In addition, both secondary Sjögren's syndrome (sSS) (5, 6) and osteonecrosis of the femoral head (ONFH) in RA have a pooled prevalence of 19.5 and 5.75–53.8%, respectively (7, 8).

Diagnosis of RA according to the American College of Rheumatology (ACR) criteria in 1987 is based on clinical symptoms, presence of rheumatoid factor (RF), and imaging tests; however, such criteria are not suitable for early-stage RA patients. Compared with the 1987 ACR diagnosis guideline, the sensitivity of the ACR/2010 European League Against Rheumatism (EULAR) classification standard is higher mainly due to the addition of anti-citrullinated protein antibodies. However, the specificity of anti-citrullinated protein antibodies in RA is only 60–75%, which suggests low diagnostic efficacy (9). A population-based incidence study revealed that the incidence of RF-negative RA has significantly increased and RF-positive RA has significant decreases (10). These can lead to difficulty in early diagnosis. Furthermore, disease activity is evaluated by the Disease Activity Score (DAS) tool and others, which are complex, inconvenient, or maybe not suitable for general clinical practice. High-resolution computer tomography, which is used for diagnosing early possible complications such as ILD (11), is expensive and has radiation risk (12). Although magnetic resonance has been demonstrated to be a useful imaging test in diagnosing ONFH, it is also expensive (13, 14). Meanwhile, due to low sensitivity and specificity of anti-Ro and anti-La antibodies and considering the invasiveness of lip biopsy, diagnosis of early RA-sSS is difficult (15, 16). Therefore, there has been increasing interest in identifying specific and powerful biomarkers for both the diagnosis of RA, RA-ILD, RA-sSS, and RA-ONFH and the evaluation of disease activity in order to increase the diagnostic efficiency and early treatment.

Early intervention (≤3 months) using biologic agents was the strongest predictor of successful remission, as confirmed in clinical practice. However, clinical applications of biological agents have been limited by their expensive cost (17). Therefore, it is important to explore promising biomarkers to evaluate the potential clinical effects of etanercept and determine which patient would benefit the most, with the possibility of modulating treatment for RA patients who are not responding to the drug in order to reduce their economic burden.

Matrix-assisted laser desorption/ionization time-of-flight mass spectrometry (MALDI-TOF-MS) (18) is currently one of the most important and key proteomic technologies (19). It can be used to make high-throughput protein analysis of large samples, and it has high sensitivity, resolving capability, and reproducibility (20). Weak cation exchange (WCX) magnetic beads (21) use their large surface to capture proteins and small molecular peptides of interest (22). The use of MALDI-TOF-MS and WCX magnetic beads, especially combined with bioinformatics tools, is appropriate for setting up the classification tree model to assist in preliminary biomarker discovery (23).

Many researchers have already applied MALDI-TOF-MS to generate protein fingerprints and build serological classification tree models in certain diseases, including rheumatic diseases [early RA (24), RA (25), systemic lupus erythematosus (26), and SS (27)] and other diseases (28, 29), and these were highly effective in discriminating patients and controls (30). However, these studies only built the diagnostic model for RA patients, but they did not have database retrieval, and some studies lacked further validation for the classification tree models. This study aimed to detect a series of specific proteomic diagnostic model for RA, RA-ILD, RA-sSS, and RA-ONFH as well as the potential biomarkers to distinguish the RA disease activity and to identify etanercept's clinical effect using proteomic fingerprint technology (MALDI-TOF-MS) combined with WCX magnetic beads. For the potential protein for diagnosis of RA, we made a further preliminary retrieval through the ExPasy database and verified these biomarkers by enzyme-linked immunosorbent assay (ELISA).

METHODS

Patients and Healthy Controls

A total of 173 serum samples were collected in our study from May 2015 to July 2017 at Shanxi Bethune Hospital. The study population included 97 RA patients (RA alone, $n = 44$; RA-ILD, $n = 22$; RA-sSS, $n = 18$; RA-ONFH, $n = 6$; RA with other complications, $n = 7$) and 76 healthy controls (HCs). All patients were diagnosed using the 1987 ACR or the 2010 ACR/EULAR criteria. All patients were classified according to their DAS, as calculated from the online Disease Activity Score-28 (DAS28) for Rheumatoid Arthritis with ESR tool based on 28 joints: in remission (DAS28 < 2.6, $n = 28$), with low disease activity ($2.6 <$ DAS28 ≤ 3.2, $n = 17$), with moderate disease activity ($3.2 <$ DAS28 ≤ 5.1, $n = 21$), and with high disease activity (DAS28 > 5.1, $n = 31$). All ILD cases were diagnosed by high-resolution computer tomography of the chest. Meanwhile, all sSS patients were diagnosed based on the American-European Consensus Group classification criteria (2002) and the 2012 ACR classification criteria. ONFH diagnosis was based on the detection of marrow foci with decreased signals on T1-weighted images and the characteristic "double-line sign" on T2-weighted images. None of the patients had any active or latent bacterial, fungal, or viral infection at the time of enrolment. Eleven patients only received the same etanercept treatment after inclusion, and their clinical outcome was assessed at week 24. They never received anti-tumor necrosis factor therapy before then. Their ACR 20/70% improvement criteria (ACR20/70), which were used to determine the therapeutic effects of etanercept, C-reactive protein level, erythrocyte sedimentation rate, and presence of RF were evaluated. Finally, four non-responders (as defined by ACR20 negative) and seven responders (ACR70 positive) to etanercept at week 24 were evaluated in our research.

We use two cohorts to build and test the RA diagnostic model. Cohort 1 (training set) included 83 RA patients and 56 HCs to establish a serological classification tree mode to distinguish them. Cohort 2 (blinded testing set) included 14 RA patients and 20 healthy individuals to test the classification efficiency of this RA diagnosis model. The detailed clinical and demographic features of the study subjects are provided in **Table 1**. Furthermore, we used serum samples from RA patients ($n = 22$) and HCs ($n = 22$) for ELISA to verify the results of MALDI-TOF-MS.

TABLE 1 | Clinical and demographic characteristics of patients and healthy controls.

Characteristic	RA	HCs
Age (years, $\bar{x} \pm s$)	56 ± 13	53 ± 12
Sex (male/female)	68\29	57\19
Disease duration (M (Q1, Q3), months)	84 (7,120)	–
Tender joint counts (M (Q1, Q3), numbers)	4 (0,24)	–
Swollen joint counts (M (Q1, Q3), numbers)	2 (0,24)	–
Erythrocyte sedimentation rate (M (Q1, Q3), mm/h)	42 (5,108)	–
C-reactive protein (M (Q1, Q3), mg/dL)	42 (5,108)	–
Rheumatoid factor, positive (%)	59 (71.1%)	–
Anti-CCP antibody, positive (%)	51 (61.4%)	–
DAS28ESR ($\bar{x} \pm s$)	4.93 ± 1.30	–
Only Treatment of Recombinant Human Tumor Necrosis Factor-α ReceptorII:IgG Fc Fusion Protein for Injection(%)	11 (11%)	–

TABLE 2 | Biomarker statistics for RA vs. HCs spectra in the decision tree classification.

M/Z	RA (Mean ± SD)	HCs (Mean ± SD)	P
10,645.10	10.39 ± 5.81	7.44 ± 5.06	0.002
4,716.71	2.27 ± 1.49	5.92 ± 4.25	0.000
3,448.85	2.37 ± 2.02	3.76 ± 2.10	0.000
8,214.28	1.39 ± 0.83	2.76 ± 1.66	0.000

Sera Collection and Preparation

Blood samples (4 mL) were collected and centrifuged at 3,000 rpm for 5 min at 4°C. All serum samples was divided and immediately stored at 80°C. The collection and analysis interval was within 3 months.

Magnetic Bead–Based Sample Preparation for MALDI-TOF-MS

Serum samples were pretreated with magnetic beads. In brief, 10 μL of each serum sample was mixed with 20 μL of U9 (9 mol urea, 2% CHAPS) in a 0.5-mL EP tube. After incubating for 30 min at 4°C, the sample was diluted 1:40 by adding 370 μL of buffer (containing 50 mmol NaAC, pH 4.0). Then, 50 μL of WCX magnetic beads (50 mg/mL) was added to a polymerase chain reaction tube, which was placed in a magnet separator for 1 min, and the supernatant was carefully removed using a pipette. The magnetic beads were then washed twice with 100 μL buffer. A 100-μL diluted serum sample was carefully added and mixed with the activated magnetic beads by pipetting up and down several times; this was, incubated for 1 h at 4°C and washed twice with 100 μL buffer. After binding and washing,

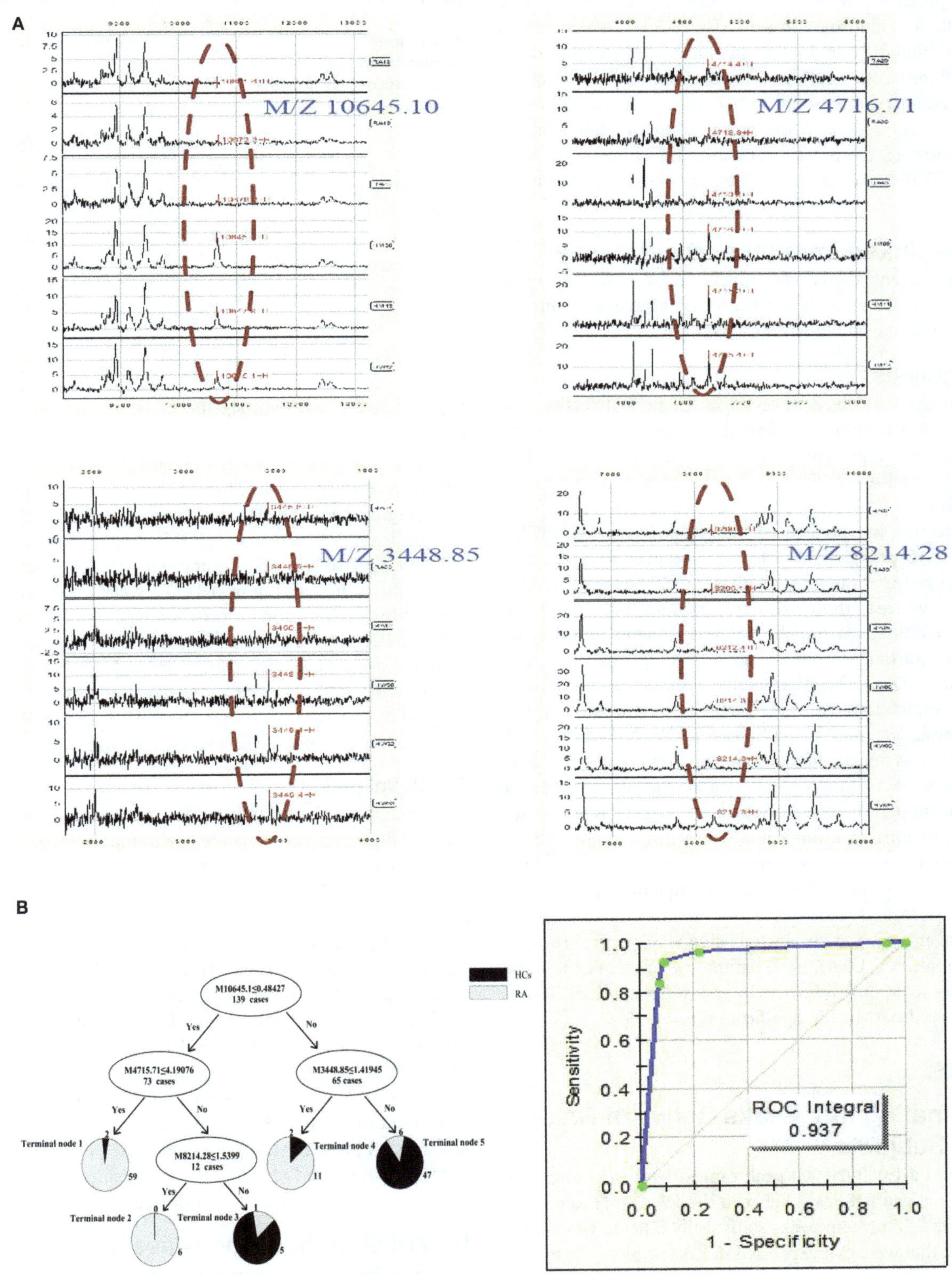

FIGURE 1 | (A) Serum protein/peptide spectrum of RA patients and HCs. **(B)** Dot plots and ROC curve of selected biomarker candidates in patients with RA and healthy controls. The mass-to-charge value in the nodes was followed by lower or equal to intensity value. If the answer to the question in a node of the tree was yes, it proceeded down to the left node, otherwise it proceeded down to the right node. When samples allocated to terminal node 1, 2, and 4 were assigned as RA, whereas those classified into terminal node 3 and 5 were assigned as HCs.

the bound proteins were eluted from the magnetic beads using 10 μL of 0.5% trifluoroacetic acid. Then, 5 μL of the eluted sample was diluted 1:2 in 5 μL of sinapic acid (50% acetonitrile + 0.5% trifluoroacetic acid), and 1 μL of the resulting mixture was aspirated and spotted onto 8 spots of prestructured sample support (Au-chip). After air-drying for approximately 5 min at room temperature, the protein crystal on the chip was detected by MALDI-TOF-MS (PBS IIc; Ciphergen Biosystems, Fremont, CA, USA).

Enzyme-Linked Immunosorbent Assay

The serum concentrations were measured by ELISA using an ELISA kit provided by Xinqaun Company (Taiyuan, China) in accordance with the manufacturer's instructions.

Data Analysis

The data analysis involved three stages: (i) peak detection and alignment; (ii) selection of differently expressed peaks among groups that may represent potential biomarkers of RA, RA-ILD, RA-SS, and RA-ONPH; (iii) data analysis using a decision tree algorithm.

Peak detection was performed using Ciphergen ProteinChip version 3.0.2 (Ciphergen Biosystems). The protein peaks with mass-to-charge (m/z) ranging from 2,000 to 50,000 were selected for analysis, whereas those with m/z ranging between 0 and 2,000 were eliminated from the analysis to avoid interference from adducts, artifacts from energy-absorbing molecules, and other possible chemical contaminants. Peak detection involved (i) baseline subtraction, (ii) mass accuracy calibration, and (iii) automatic peak detection. Using Biomarker Wizard version 3.1.0 (Ciphergen Biosystems), biomarkers that represent consistent protein peak sets across multiple spectra were generated. Baseline subtraction was performed on all spectra. The peak m/z of 4,901 was selected to normalize dimension. The settings for auto-detect peaks to cluster were as follows: first pass: signal-to-noise ratio, 5; minimum peak threshold, 10%; cluster completion: cluster mass window, 0.3%; second pass: signal-to-noise ratio, 2.

Statistical analysis was conducted using SPSS version 18 (IBM Corp., Armonk, NY, USA). Both parametric Student's t test and non-parametric Mann–Whitney U test were applied. Results were considered statistically significant if $p < 0.05$.

RESULTS

Discriminating m/z Peaks Between RA and Control Subjects

Among the m/z 1,000–20,000 peak range, there were a total of 115 differential protein peaks between the RA and HCs groups. Of these peaks, 58 protein peaks statistically differed ($p < 0.05$), including 22 that were overexpressed in RA samples ($p < 0.05$).

Establishment of the Serological Classification Tree Model for RA

RA Patients and HCs

A total of 22 protein peaks were used by the Biomarker Patterns Software (BPS) version 5.0 (Ciphergen Biosystems) to establish the most optimal classification tree based on the lowest error cost of misclassification (represented as relative cost of 0.462). The most optimal tree model consisted of m/z peaks 3,448.85, 4,716.71, 8,214.28, and 10,645.10 (**Table 2**), all of which were down-regulated in patients with RA compared with HCs (**Figure 1A**). The classical protein/peptide spectra of serum sample from RA patients and HCs are shown in **Figure 1A**. All 139 spectra of the training set were differentiated into five terminal nodes (**Figure 1B**). This classification tree had a specificity of 91.57% and a sensitivity of 92.86% for distinguishing between RA patients and HCs (**Table 3**). All 14 RA spectra and 20 HCs in the test set were correctly classified by this model, yielding a sensitivity of 95.00% and a specificity of 100% (**Table 3**). The integral of receiver operating characteristic curve (ROC) of this decision tree supplied by BPS version 5.0 was 0.937 (**Figure 1B**).

TABLE 3 | Prediction success of classification tree model for RA.

Actual class (according decision tree classification class to clinical diagnosis)	Decision tree classification class	
	RA, *n* (%)	**HCs, *n* (%)**
In the training set		
RA ($n = 83$)	76 (91.57)	7 (8.43)
HCs ($n = 56$)	4 (7.143)	52 (92.86)
In the blinded testing set		
RA ($n = 14$)	14 (100)	0 (0)
HCs ($n = 20$)	1 (5)	19 (95)

ELISA Validation

The components containing four targeted protein peaks of the RA diagnostic model were preliminarily retrieved through the ExPasy database. The proteins of m/z 10,645.10, 4,716.71, 3,448.85, and 8,214.28 might correspond to C-C motif chemokine 24 (CCL24; code: O00175), putative metallothionein (MT1DP; code: A1L3X4), sarcolipin (SLN; code: O00631), and C-X-C motif chemokine 11 (CCXL-11; code: O14625), respectively.

Therefore, the above targeted biomarkers were further identified and quantified through ELISA. A significant decrease was observed in the CCL24 level in the serum of RA patients (75.12 ± 69.59 ng/mL) as compared with HCs (125.3 ± 41.9 ng/mL) ($p < 0.05$) (**Figure 2A**). No significant difference was found in MT1DP, SLN, and CXCL-11 between RA patients and HCs (**Figures 2B–D**). Remarkably, the ELISA results, i.e., the four biomarkers had lower levels in RA patients than HCs, were consistent with the MALDI-TOF-MS results.

Establishment of the Classification Tree Model for Assessing Disease Activity in RA Patients

RA Patients With Remission and Disease Activity

This classification tree model was established from 28 RA patients with remission and 69 disease activity patients and had m/z 1,130.776, 1,501.065, 2,091.198, and 11,381.87 (**Table 4**) and six terminal nodes (**Figure 3A**). It had a sensitivity of 94.12% and a

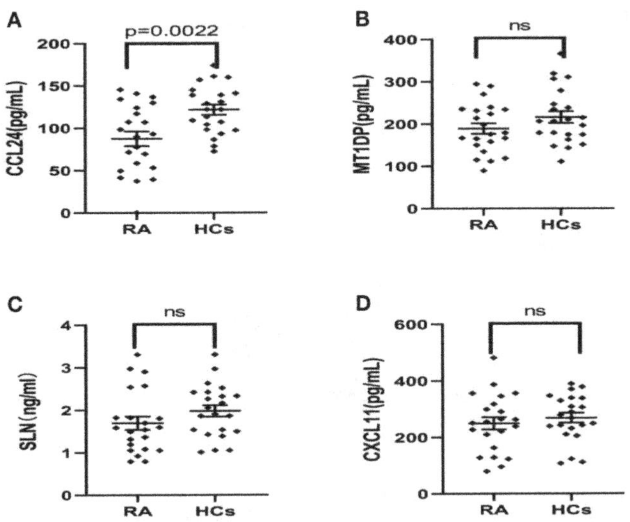

FIGURE 2 | (A–D) ELISA results of CCL24, MT1DP, SLN, and CXCL11 in the serum of RA patients ($n = 22$) and health controls ($n = 22$), indicated the CCL24 level has a significantly decreased expression in the RA serum and other biomarkers had not a difference. Plots indicate individual protein level of each group. Data are presented as mean±SEM. ns, no significant.

TABLE 4 | Biomarker statistics for assessing the activity of disease in RA patients.

M/Z	Remission (Mean ± SD)	Disease activity (Mean ± SD)	P
1,130.78	1.01 ± 1.75	1.18 ± 1.54	0.013
1,501.70	1.56 ± 1.79	−0.19 ± 1.26	0.003
2,091.20	3.08 ± 1.34	4.52 ± 2.01	0.025
11,381.87	0.02 ± 0.16	0.16 ± 0.13	0.014
M/Z	**Low disease activity (Mean ± SD)**	**Other disease activity (Mean ± SD)**	***p***
2,013.49	3.71 ± 1.80	5.52 ± 2.59	0.019
8,765.23	4.25 ± 4.48	2.09 ± 1.91	0.026
M/Z	**Moderate disease activity (Mean ± SD)**	**High disease activity (Mean ± SD)**	***P***
2,032.31	1.57 ± 1.44	2.59 ± 1.95	0.047
8,214.28	2.65 ± 1.43	1.83 ± 1.35	0.042

specificity of 93.33% (**Table 5**). The integral of ROC was 0.990 (**Figure 4**).

RA Patients With Low Disease Activity and Other Disease Activity

This classification tree model was built from the serum samples of 17 RA patients with low disease activity and 52 patients with other disease activity and had m/z 2,032.31, 2,506.21, and 9,286.50 (**Table 4**) and five terminal nodes (**Figure 3B**). It had a sensitivity of 86.67% and a specificity of 80.65% (**Table 5**). The integral of ROC was 0.898 (**Figure 4**).

RA Patients With Moderate Disease Activity and High Disease Activity

This classification tree model was established to detect a distinction between RA patients with moderate disease activity and those with high disease activity and had m/z 2,032.31 and 4,716.71 (**Table 4**) and three terminal nodes (**Figure 3C**) It had a sensitivity of 74.19% and a specificity of 76.19% (**Table 5**). The integral of ROC was 0.786 (**Figure 4**).

Discriminating m/z Peaks Between RA and RA With Complications (RA-ILD, RA-sSS, and RA-ONFH)

RA and RA-ILD

A total of 13 protein peaks from serum samples including 22 RA-ILD and 44 RA patients without complications were detected ($p < 0.05$) by MALDI-TOF-MS combined with WCX magnetic beads, which were down-regulated in patients with RA-ILD. We also used BPM5.0 to establish the most optimal tree model to distinguish between RA-ILD and RA without complications, which had m/z 10,645.10 and 12,595.86 (**Table 6**) and included three terminal nodes (**Figure 3D**). It has a sensitivity of 86.36% and a specificity of 84.09%, respectively (**Table 7**). The integral of ROC was 0.856 (**Figure 5**).

RA and RA-sSS

Thirteen proteins from serum samples of 18 RA-sSS and 44 RA patients without complications were detected ($p < 0.05$). All were down-regulated in patients with RA-sSS. We also established the classification tree model by BPM5.0, which comprised m/z 6,635.62 and 33,897.72 (**Table 6**). The RA-sSS classification tree model included 3 terminal nodes (**Figure 3E**). After identification using the model, the patients were classified as having RA and RA-sSS with a specificity of 77.78% and a sensitivity of 79.55% (**Table 7**). The integral of ROC of this RA-sSS decision tree was 0.794 (**Figure 5**).

RA and RA-ONFH

There were two differential protein peaks/spot detected between 6 RA-ONFH and 44 RA patients without complications ($p < 0.05$). They were down-regulated in patients with RA-ONPH and were added into BPM5.0 to generate the classification tree model, which had m/z 2,071.69 (**Table 6**). The classification tree model included two terminal nodes (**Figure 3F**), which had a sensitivity of 66.67% and a specificity of 95.45% (**Table 7**). The integral of ROC was 0.811 (**Figure 5**).

Developing Biological Markers for Etanercept Used in RA Patients

A total of four protein peaks were detected in RA patients between the responder ($n = 7$) and non-responder groups ($n = 4$) ($p < 0.05$), which included m/z 2,671.60, 5,801.84, 8,130.19, and

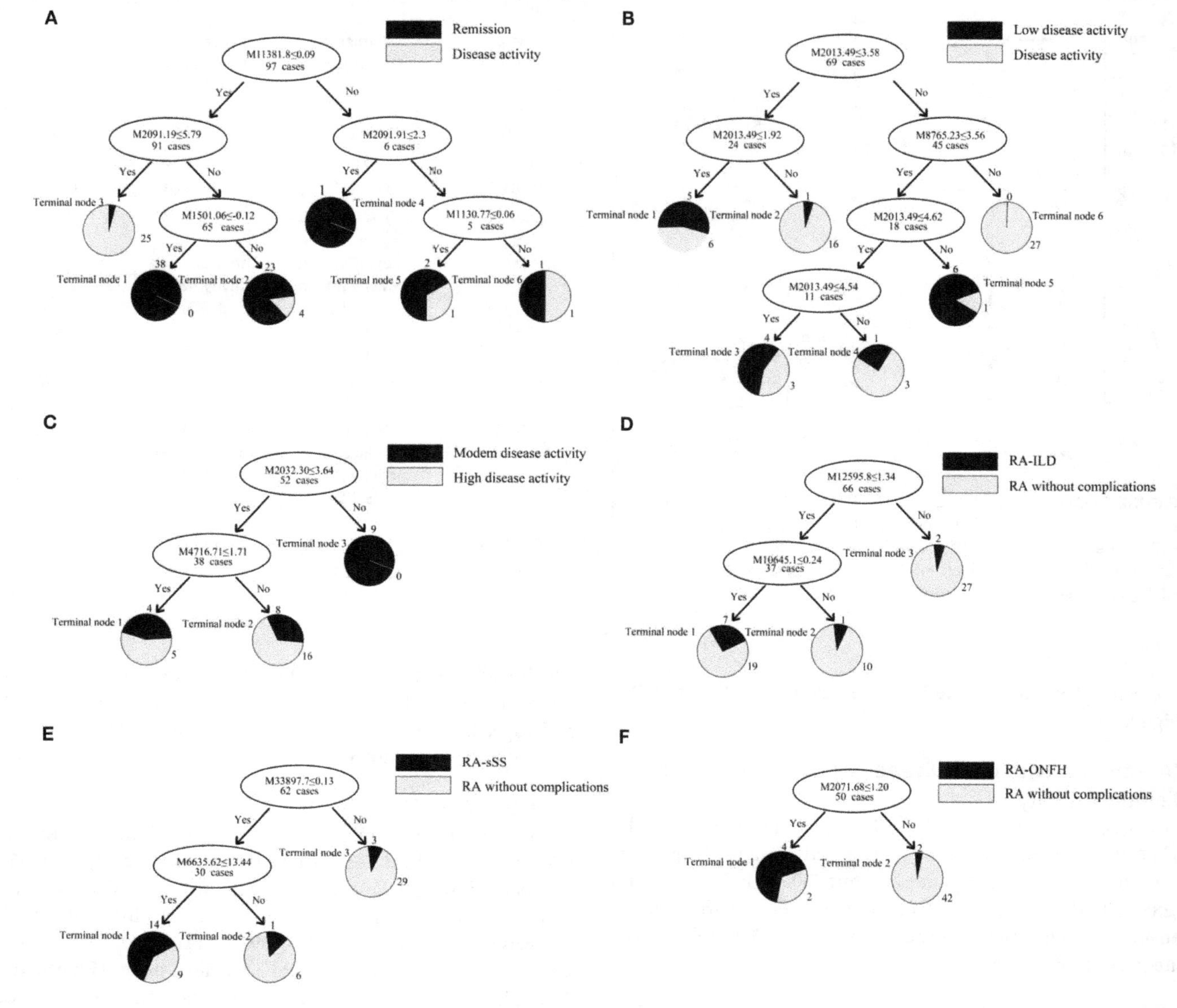

FIGURE 3 | (A–F) Classification tree model for assessing disease activity in RA patients and distinguishing RA patients with complications. The mass-to-charge value in the nodes was followed by lower or equal to intensity value. If the answer to the question in a node of the tree was yes, it proceeded down to the left node, otherwise it proceeded down to the right node. When proceeding to the terminal nodes, the decision tree assigned to samples to different groups. **(A)**: patients with remission (terminal node 2, 4, and 5) and disease activity (terminal node 1, 3, and 6); **(B)**: RA patients with low disease activity (terminal node 1, 3, and 5) and other disease activity (terminal node 2, 4, and 6); **(C)**: RA patients with moderate disease activity (terminal node 2) and high disease activity (terminal node 1 and 3); **(D)**: RA-ILD (terminal node 1); **(E)**: RA-sSS (terminal node 1); **(F)**: RA-ONFH (terminal node 1).

9,286.49. Three proteins at m/z 5,801.84, 8,130.19, and 9,286.49 were decreased in the responder group, whereas one at m/z 2,671.60 was overexpressed in the responder population.

DISCUSSION

We developed a classification tree model for early RA diagnosis by MALDI-TOF-MS with WCX magnetic beads, which included m/z 3,448.85, 4,716.71, 8,214.28, and 10,645.10. This diagnostic model was applied for RA and had a much higher specificity (91.566%) and sensitivity (92.857%). In addition, the classification tree model was tested among 14 RA patients and 20 HCs in blinded test set and had a sensitivity of 95.0% and a specificity of 100%. The four peaks might be critical peptides or proteins involved in the pathogenesis. Similar to the study by Zhang et al. (31), clinically useful biomarkers for RA were identified with this approach to discriminate patients with RA from HCs. Zhang et al. (32) reported that m/z 15,715.5, 7,771.4, 8,959.4, 8,469.8, and 8,710.8 in serum are of certain value for differential diagnosis of RA from osteoarthritis (OA) and HCs. Compared with these prior studies, we not only completed the building of the RA diagnostic model but also determined the origin and full identity of the biomarkers for RA diagnosis.

We preliminarily retrieved components comprising these four protein peaks of diagnostic model from the ExPasy database, which was used to discriminate RA patients from the HCs. The four biomarkers may probably be CCL24, MT1DP, SLN, and CXCL-11, which were further identified and quantified through ELISA. Only the CCL24 level was detected to have a significant decrease in the serum of RA patients as compared with HCs ($p < 0.05$). No significant difference was found in others, but a decreasing trend consistent with the down-regulation of the four biomarkers detected by MALDI-TOF-MS was observed. The results agreed with previous reports. In Aloush et al. study, a significant decrease was observed in the level of CCR3 receptor in the serum of RA patients compared with HCs (33). CCL24/eotaxin-2 acts via highly specific activation of the CCR3 receptor. Another study observed that anti-eotaxin-2 antibody has a significant protective effect in adjuvant-induced arthritis in rats (34). Noticeably, a specific pattern was observed for mRNA expression in CCL24/eotaxin-2, which was higher among RA patients with lower X-ray scores than those with severe X-ray scores. The same results were also found in the comparison between the two groups with RA with low and medium disease activity and the subgroup with high activity (35). Combined with the above results, CCL24 may play a vital role in the pathogenesis of RA. The lower level of CCL24 in our result may be due to the reaction of eotaxin-2 to therapeutic manipulation in RA. However, in study by Uchida et al. (36), who detected discriminatory biomarkers to differentiate RA from OA using synovial fluid, they purified the protein based the detected specific peaks and the result revealed that m/z 10,850 was the clearest signal found specifically in RA and that it is myeloid-related protein 8, which might be related to the disease activity in RA. Despite the different results among research, these results highlighted that the CCL24, as a biomarker of this model, may be vital proteins or peptides that participate in the pathogenesis of RA and may be a promising potential therapeutic target for arthritis (37).

Although other biomarkers for the RA diagnostic model did not significantly differ in our result, the ELISA results, i.e.,

TABLE 5 | Establishment of the classification tree models for assessing the activity of disease in RA patients.

	Classification tree model	Accuracy (%)	Sensitivity (%)	Specificity (%)
Remission/ Disease activity(28/69)	M/Z1130.78, 1,501.07, 2,091.20, 11,381.87	92.78	94.12	93.33
Low disease activity/Other disease activity (17/52)	M2013.49, 8,765.23	82.61	86.67	80.65
Moderate disease activity/High disease activity (21/31)	M/Z2032.31, 4,716.71	75.00	74.19	76.19

TABLE 6 | Biomarker statistics for RA vs. RA with complications spectra in the decision tree classification.

M/Z	RA + ILD (Mean ± SD)	RA (Mean ± SD)	P
10,645.10	0.12 ± 0.36	0.47 ± 0.70	0.003
12,595.86	0.84 ± 0.44	1.55 ± 0.84	0
M/Z	**RA+sSS (Mean ± SD)**	**RA (Mean ± SD)**	***p***
6,635.62	11.38 ± 6.10	14.79 ± 5.89	0.045
33,897.72	0.11 ± 0.06	0.15 ± 0.05	0.037
M/Z	**RA+ONFH (Mean ± SD)**	**RA (Mean ± SD)**	***P***
2,071.69	1.73 ± 2.11	3.43 ± 1.63	0.025

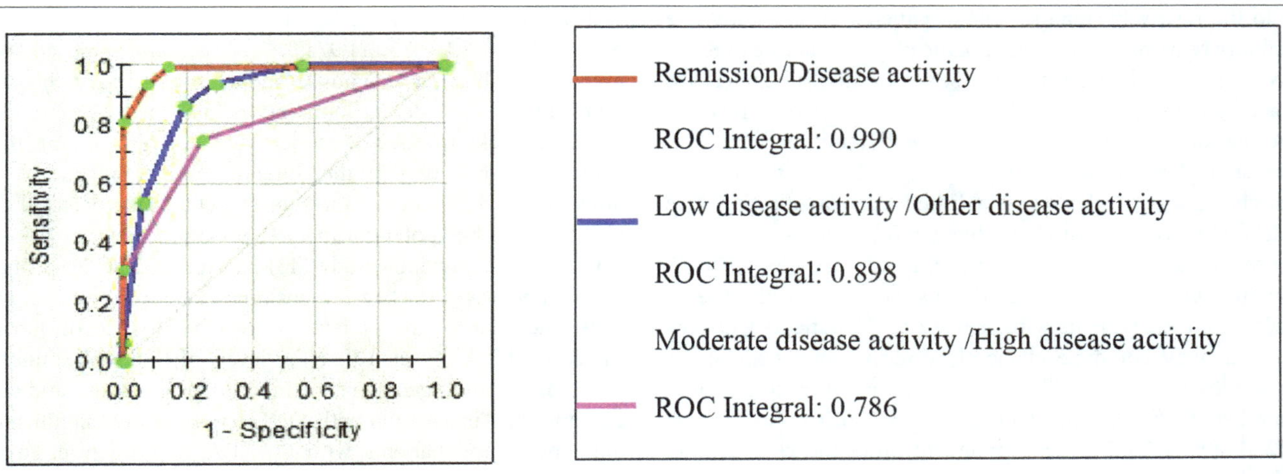

FIGURE 4 | The ROC of the diagnostic models for assessing the activity of disease in RA patients.

TABLE 7 | The classification tree models for RA and RA with complications.

	Classification tree model	Accuracy	Sensitivity	Specificity
RA/RA- ILD(44/22)	M/Z10645.10, 12,595.86	84.85%	86.36%	84.09%
RA/RA-sSS(44/18)	M/Z6635.62, 33,897.72	79.03%	77.78%	79.55%
RA/RA-ONFH(44/6)	M/Z2071.69	92.00%	66.67%	95.45%

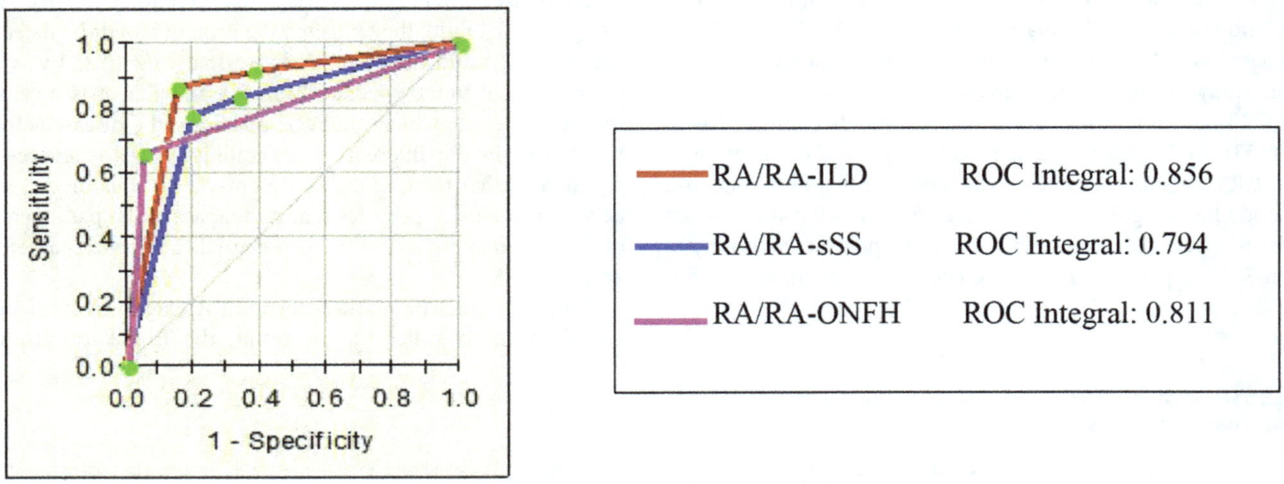

FIGURE 5 | The ROC of the diagnostic models of RA with complications.

the four biomarkers had lower levels in RA patients than in HCs, were consistent with the MALDI-TOF-MS results. Thus far, MT1DP and SLN as the possible components, are not reported in studies about autoimmune disease. According to previous studies, the fourth protein, CXCL11, is believed to be the dominant CXCR3 agonist because it is more potent (38), and it has been believed to play a vital role in directing Th1 cells to sites of inflammation (39). Recent studies strongly concluded that the CXCR3 receptor is a potential therapeutic target for treating autoimmune diseases, such as RA and multiple sclerosis (40). Although we were not able to identify other biomarkers, possibly due to the relatively small sample of patients in this study, the possibility remains that this chemokine plays a vital role in RA.

We also aimed to construct a series of clinical models for an accurate assessment model of disease activity. Thus far, there are no studies about it, and we did not find relevant conclusions for the assessment model of RA in the present research. Consequently, we established the classification tree model for assessing the disease activity in RA patients. At first, we can use the classification model including m/z 1,130.78, 1,501.07, 2,091.20, and 11,381.87 to distinguish patients with disease activity from RA patients with remission. RA patients with low disease activity could be efficiently discriminated from other disease activity patients with the combined use of specific protein biomarkers (m/z 2,032.31, 2,506.21, and 9,286.50). Finally, m/z 2,032.31 and 4,716.71 were applied to build the classification model for RA patients with moderate disease activity and high disease activity. These models are possibly the most convenient and efficient clinical methods for RA patients.

After assessing and diagnosing RA patients using the established model, they should be comprehensively assessed to determine other complications, which can prompt early treatment. Therefore, we built the classification tree model for to accurately recognize RA-ILD, RA-sSS, and RA-ONFH from RA. The most optimal tree model to distinguish between RA-ILD and RA without complication had m/z 10,645.10, and 12,595.86. In the present research, the diagnostic model was applicable for RA-sSS and/or SS-ILD (41), but no biomarkers discriminating for RA-ILD were found. The RA-sSS model had m/z 6,635.62 and 33,897.72 and had a specificity of 77.78% and a sensitivity of 79.55%. In the study of Li et al. (42), m/z peaks at 8,133.85, 11,972.8, 2,220.81, and 4,837.66 were used to establish a diagnostic model for Primary Sjögren's syndrome from systemic lupus erythematosus, RA, and HCs. The m/z peaks of RA-sSS model were different among these studies. We believe that the difference might be due to the different characteristics of the subjects. Our study detected that m/z 2,071.68 has potential in discriminating between RA and RA-ONFH. A previous study (43) showed that seven proteins were found based on two-dimensional electrophoresis patterns from the sera of 10 patients with ONFH and 10 normal subjects. ELISA revealed that the levels of tissue plasminogen activator, plasminogen activator inhibitor 1, crosslaps, and anti-p53 antibody in patients with ONFH were always significantly different among patients with OA, RA, and fracture. In the diagnostic models of RA with complications, all had different protein peaks; thus, further research is needed to clarify its specific components.

The biological markers for etanercept used in RA patients were also generated in our study. A total of 4 protein peaks, including m/z 2,671.60, 5,801.84, 8,130.20, and 9,286.49, were detected in RA patients between the responder ($n = 7$) and non-responder groups ($n = 4$). The study of Trocme et al. (44) revealed factors predictive of infliximab therapeutic response. Five proteins at 3.86, 7.77, 7.97, 8.14, and 74.07 kDa were overexpressed in the non-responder group ($n = 28$), whereas one at 28 kDa was increased in the responder group ($n = 32$). Biomarker characterization showed that apolipoprotein A-1 was predictive of a good response to infliximab, whereas platelet factor four was associated with non-response, thereby providing some thoughts to the scientific research in our future study.

These data suggested that MALDI-TOF-MS combined with WCX magnetic beads could be helpful in clinical applications for efficient diagnosis and accurate assessment of disease activity, and it is useful for differentiating RA patients with complications, which plays an important role in providing early treatment to RA patients, thereby preventing worse symptoms in the future. Nevertheless, the identification of these biomarkers is essential in understanding the pathogenesis of RA, on which they may play a vital role. Therefore, our future study will complete the identification of other potential diagnostic biomarkers for RA, and their identification will further improve the usefulness of the model, shed further light on the pathogenesis of RA, and promote the study on the diagnostic biomarkers for RA.

In many health-care systems, the medical treatment of patients comprises three phases (clinical diagnosis, assessment, and treatment), to which the proposed models we established above are applied. Unlike findings about biomarkers discovered in previous studies, this study not only explored the diagnostic criteria established by proteomic technology to accurately recognize RA patients from HCs but also assessed the disease activity and developed classification tree models for comprehensive assessment of patient's condition and to determine whether they have other complications. Our study detected the potential biomarkers for etanercept used in RA patients, which can help solve future clinical problems. We further identified and quantified the biomarkers for RA and found that the CCL24 level was lower in the RA group than in HCs. In future study, we will complete the identification of other potential diagnostic biomarkers to explore their role in the pathogenesis and to detect the precise therapeutic target.

However, this study has some limitations. The tested sample size is small and should be increased. To identify the discovered protein peak, the sample size should be increased. Furthermore, no pathological controls with undifferentiated arthritis, OA, or inflammatory joint diseases were assayed in this study. Thus, these should be considered in future research. More effort in future studies should be done, including increasing the sample size and completing other molecular identification of the potential specific biomarkers reported in this study for a better understanding of RA.

CONCLUSION

Our study successfully established a series of specific proteomic diagnostic models for RA, RA-ILD, RA-sSS, and RA-ONFH and detected the potential biomarkers to distinguish RA disease activity and to identify etanercept's clinical effect using proteomic fingerprint technology (MALDI-TOF-MS) combined with WCX magnetic beads. Furthermore, we have also demonstrated the differential expression of CCL24 in RA serum and HCs, which appears to have a pathogenetic role in RA and may serve as therapeutic targets in the future. Further exploration of these findings requires a larger sample size.

ETHICS STATEMENT

The studies involving human participants were reviewed and approved by Ethics Committee of the Shanxi Bethune Hospital. The patients/participants provided their written informed consent to participate in this study.

AUTHOR CONTRIBUTIONS

LZ: study concept and design. DM, NL, and LZ: acquisition, analysis and interpretation of data, statistical analysis, drafting of the manuscript, and critical revision of the manuscript. All authors read and approved the final manuscript.

REFERENCES

1. McInnes I, Schett G. The pathogenesis of rheumatoid arthritis. *N Engl J Med.* (2011) 365:2205–19. doi: 10.1056/NEJMra1004965
2. Turesson C, O'Fallon W, Crowson C, Gabriel S, Matteson E. Extra-articular disease manifestations in rheumatoid arthritis: incidence trends and risk factors over 46 years. *Ann Rheum Dis.* (2003) 62:722–7. doi: 10.1136/ard.62.8.722
3. Spagnolo P, Lee J, Sverzellati N, Rossi G, Cottin V. The Lung in rheumatoid arthritis: focus on interstitial lung disease. *Arthritis Rheumatol.* (2018) 70:1544–54. doi: 10.1002/art.40574
4. Gochuico B, Avila N, Chow C, Novero L, Wu H, Ren P, et al. Progressive preclinical interstitial lung disease in rheumatoid arthritis. *Arch Intern Med.* (2008) 168:159–66. doi: 10.1001/archinternmed.2007.59
5. Hajiabbasi A, Shenavar Masooleh I, Alizadeh Y, Banikarimi A, Ghavidel Parsa P. Secondary Sjogren's syndrome in 83 patients with rheumatoid arthritis. *Acta Med Iran.* (2016) 54:448–53.

6. Gilboe I, Kvien T, Uhlig T, Husby G. Sicca symptoms and secondary Sjögren's syndrome in systemic lupus erythematosus: comparison with rheumatoid arthritis and correlation with disease variables. *Ann Rheum Dis.* (2001) 60:1103–9. doi: 10.1136/ard.60.12.1103
7. Weinstein R. Clinical practice. Glucocorticoid-induced bone disease. *N Engl J Med.* (2011) 365:62–70. doi: 10.1056/NEJMcp1012926
8. Watanabe Y, Kawai K, Hirohata K. Histopathology of femoral head osteonecrosis in rheumatoid arthritis: the relationship between steroid therapy and lipid degeneration in the osteocyte. *Rheumatol Int.* (1989) 9:25–31.doi: 10.1007/bf00270286
9. Mun S, Lee J, Park A, Kim H, Lee Y, Son H, et al. Proteomics approach for the discovery of rheumatoid arthritis biomarkers using mass spectrometry. *Int J Mol Sci.* (2019) 20:4368. doi: 10.3390/ijms20184368
10. Myasoedova E, Davis J, Matteson E, Crowson C. Is the epidemiology of rheumatoid arthritis changing? Results from a population-based incidence study, 1985-2014. *Ann Rheum Dis.* (2020) 79:440–4. doi: 10.1136/annrheumdis-2019-216694
11. Travis W, Costabel U, Hansell D, King T, Lynch D, Nicholson A, et al. An official American Thoracic Society/European Respiratory Society statement: update of the international multidisciplinary classification of the idiopathic interstitial pneumonias. *Am J Respir Crit Care Med.* (2013) 188:733–48. doi: 10.1164/rccm.201308-1483ST
12. Assayag D, Elicker B, Urbania T, Colby T, Kang B, Ryu J, et al. Rheumatoid arthritis-associated interstitial lung disease: radiologic identification of usual interstitial pneumonia pattern. *Radiology.* (2014) 270:583–8. doi: 10.1148/radiol.13130187
13. Saini A, Saifuddin A. MRI of osteonecrosis. *Clin Radiol.* (2004) 59:1079–93. doi: 10.1016/j.crad.2004.04.014
14. Jones L, Hungerford D. Osteonecrosis: etiology, diagnosis, and treatment. *Curr Opin Rheumatol.* (2004) 16:443–9.doi: 10.1097/01.moo.0000127829.34643.fd
15. Baldini C, Talarico R, Tzioufas A, Bombardieri S. Classification criteria for Sjogren's syndrome: a critical review. *J Autoimmun.* (2012) 39:9–14.doi: 10.1016/j.jaut.2011.12.006
16. Kyriakidis N, Kapsogeorgou E, Tzioufas A. A comprehensive review of autoantibodies in primary Sjögren's syndrome: clinical phenotypes and regulatory mechanisms. *J Autoimmun.* (2014) 51:67–74. doi: 10.1016/j.jaut.2013.11.001
17. Gremese E, Salaffi F, Bosello S, Ciapetti A, Bobbio-Pallavicini F, Caporali R, et al. Very early rheumatoid arthritis as a predictor of remission: a multicentre real life prospective study. *Ann Rheum Dis.* (2013) 72:858–62.doi: 10.1136/annrheumdis-2012-201456
18. Tsuchida S, Umemura H, Nakayama T. Current status of Matrix-Assisted Laser Desorption/Ionization-Time-of-Flight Mass Spectrometry (MALDI-TOF MS) in clinical diagnostic microbiology. *Molecules.* (2020) 25:4775. doi: 10.3390/molecules25204775
19. Angeletti S, Ciccozzi M. Matrix-assisted laser desorption ionization time-of-flight mass spectrometry in clinical microbiology: an updating review. *Infect Genet Evol.* (2019) 76:104063.doi: 10.1016/j.meegid.2019.104063
20. Baumann S, Ceglarek U, Fiedler G, Lembcke J, Leichtle A, Thiery J. Standardized approach to proteome profiling of human serum based on magnetic bead separation and matrix-assisted laser desorption/ionization time-of-flight mass spectrometry. *Clin Chem.* (2005) 51:973–80. doi: 10.1373/clinchem.2004.047308
21. Whiteaker J, Zhao L, Zhang H, Feng L, Piening B, Anderson L, et al. Antibody-based enrichment of peptides on magnetic beads for mass-spectrometry-based quantification of serum biomarkers. *Anal Biochem.* (2007) 362:44–54.doi: 10.1016/j.ab.2006.12.023
22. Peter J, Otto A. Magnetic particles as powerful purification tool for high sensitive mass spectrometric screening procedures. *Proteomics.* (2010) 10:628–33.doi: 10.1002/pmic.200900535
23. Li Y, Hu C, Leng X, Zhao G, Li N, Xu Y. Promising diagnostic biomarkers for primary biliary cirrhosis identified with magnetic beads and MALDI-TOF-MS. *Anat Rec.* (2009) 292:455–60. doi: 10.1002/ar.20870
24. Goëb V, Thomas-L'Otellier M, Daveau R, Charlionet R, Fardellone P, Le Loët X, et al. Candidate autoantigens identified by mass spectrometry in early rheumatoid arthritis are chaperones and citrullinated glycolytic enzymes. *Arthritis Res Ther.* (2009) 11:R38.doi: 10.1186/ar2644
25. de Seny D, Fillet M, Meuwis M, Geurts P, Lutteri L, Ribbens C, et al. Discovery of new rheumatoid arthritis biomarkers using the surface-enhanced laser desorption/ionization time-of-flight mass spectrometry ProteinChip approach. *Arthritis Rheum.* (2005) 52:3801–12. doi: 10.1002/art.21607
26. Huang Z, Shi Y, Cai B, Wang L, Wu Y, Ying B, et al. MALDI-TOF MS combined with magnetic beads for detecting serum protein biomarkers and establishment of boosting decision tree model for diagnosis of systemic lupus erythematosus. *Rheumatology (Oxford).* (2009) 48:626–31. doi: 10.1093/rheumatology/kep058
27. Giusti L, Baldini C, Bazzichi L, Bombardieri S, Lucacchini A. Proteomic diagnosis of Sjögren's syndrome. *Expert Rev Proteomics.* (2007) 4:757–67. doi: 10.1586/14789450.4.6.757
28. Lin X, Yang S, Du J, Tian Y, Bu L, Huo S, et al. Detection of lung adenocarcinoma using magnetic beads based matrix-assisted laser desorption/ionization time-of-flight mass spectrometry serum protein profiling. *Chin Med J.* (2010) 123:34–9. doi: 10.3760/cma.j.issn.0366-6999.2010.01.006
29. Li J, Zhang Z, Rosenzweig J, Wang Y, Chan D. Proteomics and bioinformatics approaches for identification of serum biomarkers to detect breast cancer. *Clin Chem.* (2002) 48:1296–304. doi: 10.1016/S0009-8981(02)00170-5
30. Cheng A, Chen L, Chien K, Chen Y, Chang J, Wang H, et al. Oral cancer plasma tumor marker identified with bead-based affinity-fractionated proteomic technology. *Clin Chem.* (2005) 51:2236–44. doi: 10.1373/clinchem.2005.052324
31. Yan Z, Chaojun H, Chuiwen D, Xiaomei L, Xin Z, Yongzhe L, et al. Establishing serological classification tree model in rheumatoid arthritis using combination of MALDI-TOF-MS and magnetic beads. *Clin Exp Med.* (2015) 15:19–23.doi: 10.1007/s10238-013-0265-2
32. Zhang X, Yuan Z, Shen B, Zhu M, Liu C, Xu W. Discovery of serum protein biomarkers in rheumatoid arthritis using MALDI-TOF-MS combined with magnetic beads. *Clin Exp Med.* (2012) 12:145–51. doi: 10.1007/s10238-011-0154-5
33. Aloush V, George J, Elkayam O, Wigler I, Oren S, Entin-Meer M, et al. Decreased levels of CCR3 in CD4+ lymphocytes of rheumatoid arthritis patients. *Clin Exp Rheumatol.* (2010) 28:462–7. doi: 10.1186/1471-2474-11-143
34. Ablin J, Entin-Meer M, Aloush V, Oren S, Elkayam O, George J, et al. Protective effect of eotaxin-2inhibition in adjuvant-induced arthritis. *Clin Exp Immunol.* (2010) 161:276–83. doi: 10.1111/j.1365-2249.2010.04172.x
35. Zhebrun D, Totolyan A, Maslyanskii A, Titov A, Patrukhin A, Kostareva A, et al. Synthesis of some CC chemokines and their receptors in the synovium in rheumatoid arthritis. *Bull Exp Biol Med.* (2014) 158:192–6.doi: 10.1007/s10517-014-2720-9
36. Uchida T, Fukawa A, Uchida M, Fujita K, Saito K. Application of a novel protein biochip technology for detection and identification of rheumatoid arthritis biomarkers in synovial fluid. *J Proteome Res.* (2002) 1:495–9. doi: 10.1021/pr025531w
37. Cole K, Strick C, Paradis T, Ogborne K, Loetscher M, Gladue R, et al. Interferon-inducible T cell alpha chemoattractant (I-TAC): a novel non-ELR CXC chemokine with potent activity on activated T cells through selective high affinity binding to CXCR3. *J Exp Med.* (1998) 187:2009–21. doi: 10.1084/jem.187.12.2009
38. Karin N, Razon H. Chemokines beyond chemo-attraction: CXCL10 and its significant role in cancer and autoimmunity. *Cytokine.* (2018) 109: 24–8. doi: 10.1016/j.cyto.2018.02.012
39. C. Jenh, M. Cox, L. Cui, E. Reich, L. Sullivan, S. Chen, et al. A selective and potent CXCR3 antagonist SCH 546738 attenuates the development of autoimmune diseases and delays graft rejection. *BMC immunology.* (2012) 13:2.doi: 10.1186/1471-2172-13-2
40. Korniejewska A, McKnight A, Johnson Z, Watson M, Ward S. Expression and agonist responsiveness of CXCR3 variants in human T lymphocytes. *Immunology.* (2011) 132:503–15.doi: 10.1111/j.1365-2567.2010.03384.x
41. Li Y, Sun X, He J, Jia R, Yang D, Zhang X, et al. Screening for serum specific biomarkers in patients with primary Sjögren's syndrome and interstitial lung disease using proteomic fingerprint techniques. *Beijing Da Xue Xue Bao.* (2012) 44:240–3. doi: 10.3969/j.issn.1671-167X.2012.02.017

diagnostic model for Sjögren's syndrome by proteomic fingerprinting. *Clin Rheumatol.* (2014) 33:1745–50. doi: 10.1007/s10067-014-2762-4

43. Tan X, Cai D, Wu Y, Liu B, Rong L, Chen Z, et al. Comparative analysis of serum proteomes: discovery of proteins associated with osteonecrosis of the femoral head. *Transl Res.* (2006) 148:114–9. doi: 10.1016/j.trsl.2006.05.001
44. Trocmé C, Marotte H, Baillet A, Pallot-Prades B, Garin J, Grange L, et al. Apolipoprotein A-I and platelet factor 4 are biomarkers for infliximab response in rheumatoid arthritis. *Ann Rheum Dis.* (2009) 68:1328–33. doi: 10.1136/ard.2008.093153

13

High-Resolution Peripheral Quantitative Computed Tomography for Bone Evaluation in Inflammatory Rheumatic Disease

Rasmus Klose-Jensen[1,2], *Justin J. Tse*[3,4], *Kresten Krarup Keller*[5], *Cheryl Barnabe*[3,6], *Andrew J. Burghardt*[7], *Stephanie Finzel*[8,9], *Lai-Shan Tam*[10], *Ellen-Margrethe Hauge*[1,2], *Kathryn S. Stok*[11] and *Sarah L. Manske*[3,4*]

[1] Department of Rheumatology, Aarhus University Hospital, Aarhus, Denmark, [2] Department of Clinical Medicine, Faculty of Health, Aarhus University, Aarhus, Denmark, [3] Cumming School of Medicine, McCaig Institute for Bone and Joint Health, University of Calgary, Calgary, AB, Canada, [4] Department of Radiology, Cumming School of Medicine, University of Calgary, Calgary, AB, Canada, [5] Diagnostic Centre, Silkeborg Regional Hospital, Silkeborg, Denmark, [6] Department of Medicine, Cumming School of Medicine, University of Calgary, Calgary, AB, Canada, [7] Department of Radiology and Biomedical Imaging, University of California, San Francisco, San Francisco, CA, United States, [8] Department of Rheumatology and Clinical Immunology, Medical Centre - University of Freiburg, Freiburg, Germany, [9] Faculty of Medicine, University of Freiburg, Freiburg, Germany, [10] Department of Medicine and Therapeutics, The Chinese University of Hong Kong, Hong Kong, China, [11] Department of Biomedical Engineering, The University of Melbourne, Parkville, VIC, Australia

***Correspondence:**
Sarah L. Manske
smanske@ucalgary.ca

High resolution peripheral quantitative computed tomography (HR-pQCT) is a 3-dimensional imaging modality with superior sensitivity for bone changes and abnormalities. Recent advances have led to increased use of HR-pQCT in inflammatory arthritis to report quantitative volumetric measures of bone density, microstructure, local anabolic (e.g., osteophytes, enthesiophytes) and catabolic (e.g., erosions) bone changes and joint space width. These features may be useful for monitoring disease progression, response to therapy, and are responsive to differentiating between those with inflammatory arthritis conditions and healthy controls. We reviewed 69 publications utilizing HR-pQCT imaging of the metacarpophalangeal (MCP) and/or wrist joints to investigate arthritis conditions. Erosions are a marker of early inflammatory arthritis progression, and recent work has focused on improvement and application of techniques to sensitively identify erosions, as well as quantifying erosion volume changes longitudinally using manual, semi-automated and automated methods. As a research tool, HR-pQCT may be used to detect treatment effects through changes in erosion volume in as little as 3 months. Studies with 1-year follow-up have demonstrated progression or repair of erosions depending on the treatment strategy applied. HR-pQCT presents several advantages. Combined with advances in image processing and image registration, individual changes can be monitored with high sensitivity and reliability. Thus, a major strength of HR-pQCT is its applicability in instances where subtle changes are anticipated, such as early erosive progression in the presence of subclinical inflammation. HR-pQCT imaging results could ultimately impact decision making to uptake aggressive treatment strategies and prevent progression of joint damage. There are several potential areas where HR-pQCT evaluation of inflammatory arthritis still requires development. As a highly sensitive imaging technique, one of the major challenges has been motion artifacts;

motion compensation algorithms should be implemented for HR-pQCT. New research developments will improve the current disadvantages including, wider availability of scanners, the field of view, as well as the versatility for measuring tissues other than only bone. The challenge remains to disseminate these analysis approaches for broader clinical use and in research.

Keywords: HR-pQCT (high-resolution peripheral quantitative computed tomography), arthritis, joint space, erosions, osteophytes, bone mineral density, bone microstructure

INTRODUCTION

Imaging is playing an increasing role in the diagnosis and monitoring of inflammatory disease. For many years the only imaging modality for joint assessment was conventional radiographs (CR); however, newer technologies have revolutionized the diversity of medical imaging capabilities in rheumatic diseases. Magnetic resonance imaging (MRI) and ultrasound (US) are now used regularly in both research and clinical practice for investigating joint diseases, particularly for the identification of soft tissue pathology and inflammation. In contrast, computed tomography (CT) capitalizes on the ability of bone to attenuate x-rays, thus providing excellent bone contrast in three dimensions with high spatial resolution but is limited by poor soft-tissue contrast. High-resolution peripheral quantitative computed tomography (HR-pQCT) imaging was designed to examine volumetric bone mineral density and microstructure of the radius and tibia and has been used extensively in osteoporosis research. HR-pQCT uses the same principles as traditional CT but can achieve a much higher spatial resolution and still has a very low radiation dose. The total effective dose for the metacarpophalangeal (MCP) joint and wrist scans is ~0.025 mSv (1). For comparison, the radiation dose for a conventional chest X-ray is 0.1 mSv. Still, HR-pQCT has a smaller field of view. Isotropic voxel sizes of 61 or 82 μm lead to spatial resolutions of 100 or 142 μm, respectively, approximately the thickness of an individual human trabecula. The high resolution allows segmentation of the bone at the microstructural level, permitting quantification of architecture and micro-scale pathological features, such as erosions. Initially limited by a gantry size that limited imaging to distal joints in the hands (**Figure 1**), wrist, foot, and ankles only, the newest generation HR-pQCT permits more proximal imaging of the elbows and knee, expanding capabilities to important anatomic sites in the context of inflammatory arthritis.

In 2011 the Study grouP for x-trEme Computed Tomography in Rheumatoid Arthritis (SPECTRA) was formed to facilitate the worldwide collaboration of periarticular image acquisition standards, image interpretation and analysis guides, and applications in clinical research. A systematic review was published in 2016, detailing the published research of HR-pQCT imaging and arthritis (2). Since then, the number of published papers has more than doubled, suggesting the importance of this review to update the current knowledge and expanded uses of this technology. We have structured this review to summarize pathological findings observed at the metacarpophalangeal (MCP) and wrist joints in different types of peripheral inflammatory arthritis using HR-pQCT, compare HR-pQCT imaging outcomes with other modalities in terms of erosions, joint space width, bony proliferations, bone density and microstructure, summarize the reproducibility of the quantitative outcome measures assessed with HR-pQCT imaging, investigate early detection of arthritis, the longitudinal changes over time for the quantitative outcome measures, and finally discuss the implications of the use of HR-pQCT in inflammatory arthritis and future directions.

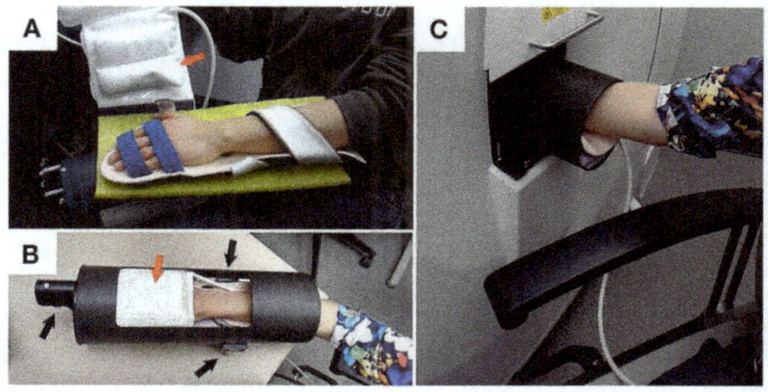

FIGURE 1 | Example demonstrating how a participant is positioned for XtremeCTII scanning. **(A)** Participant's hand is positioned on a rigid-formed mold, with straps securing the distal and proximal ends of the forearm. An additional x-ray compatible, inflatable, pad-based positioning system (red arrows) is positioned above the hand to further reduce accidental motion during scan acquisitions. **(B)** The secured appendage is then placed within a cylindrical, annular, carbon-fiber molded sample holder. Using three spherical landmarks (black arrows), and with the participant resting comfortably, the supported participants' hand and sample holder is then securely and accurately placed within the scanner **(C)**.

MATERIALS AND METHODS

Search Strategy

US National Library of Medicine Medical Subject Heading (MeSH) terms, keywords, and acronyms for HR-pQCT were selected. We combined this search with MeSH terms, keywords, and acronyms for the metacarpophalangeal joints (MCP) and/or radius and/or wrist, to specify the periarticular regions of interest, and MeSH terms and keywords for arthritis (search terms available in **Appendix 1** in Supplementary Material). PubMed (1966–January 2020) and Embase (1980–January 2020) searches were conducted to identify potentially relevant studies. Filters were applied to eliminate animal studies and identify English language studies and full-length articles. Web of Science was used to identify articles which referenced the articles found through PubMed and Embase. References from identified articles were checked manually. Authors from the SPECTRA Collaboration aided in identifying any potential studies we did not find through the other searches.

Inclusion Criteria

Any studies reporting original results of HR-pQCT imaging of the MCP and/or wrist joints were selected through the title/abstract search. These studies could report on the normal state or any arthritis conditions [including RA, osteoarthritis (OA), PsA], as well as "pre-arthritis" states [e.g., persons positive for anticitrullinated protein antibodies (ACPA) with arthralgia]. At the full-text review stage, we selected articles for data extraction if they reported on any of the following outcomes: (1) pathology findings, determined a priori to include bone mineral architecture, bone mineral density (BMD), erosions, vascular channels, cortical breaks, joint space, bony proliferations, or surface changes; (2) comparison to other imaging modalities; and (3) reproducibility. Article selection and data extraction were performed by one author (RKJ).

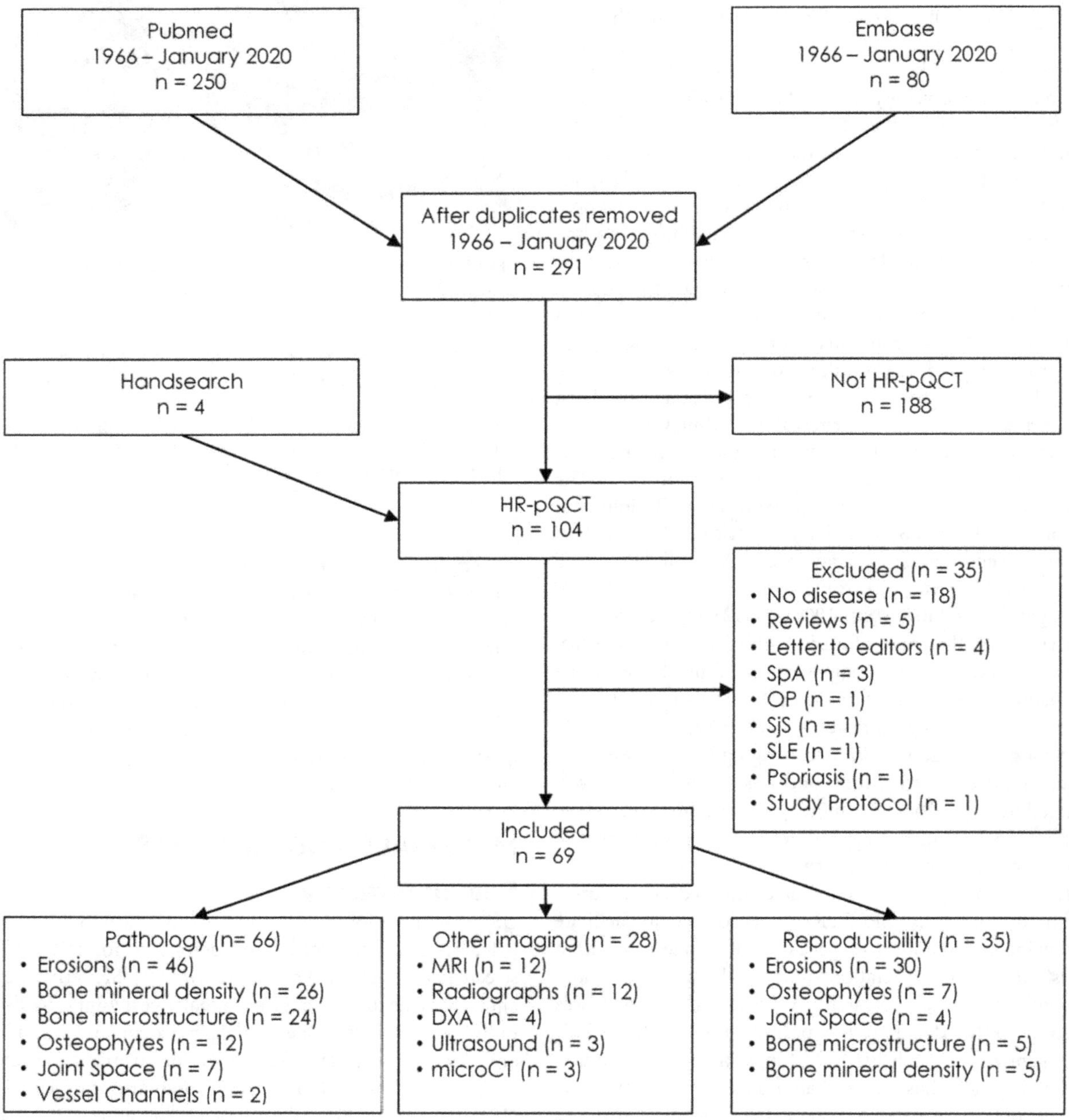

FIGURE 2 | Flow diagram for study inclusion. DXA, Dual x-ray absorptiometry; HR-pQCT, High-resolution peripheral quantitative computed tomography; OP, Osteoporosis; SjS, Sjogren's syndrome; SpA, Spondyloarthritis; SLE, Systemic lupus erythematosus; microCT, Micro-computed tomography.

Analysis

Owing to the heterogeneity of case definitions for different pathologies, variations in analysis techniques, and the identification of studies in a variety of normal and disease states, it was not possible to perform a meta-analysis. Therefore, a narrative summary of the work was performed following pathology descriptions and comparisons to other imaging modalities and reproducibility.

PATHOLOGY

A total of 291 unique publications were identified, each subject to selection based on the title and abstract. One hundred and three met eligibility for full-text review, with 69 selected for data extraction (**Figure 2**). Of these 69 articles, 66 described pathology findings, 28 related comparisons of HR-pQCT findings to another imaging modality, and 35 described precision or reproducibility. All the studies meeting inclusion criteria are detailed in **Table 1**.

Erosion Detection by HR-pQCT

Bone erosions were originally defined radiographically as breaks in the cortical bone surface, typically accompanied by loss of underlying trabecular bone (71–73).

Erosions on HR-pQCT have been defined in a diverse manner; the early studies simply defined erosion as a clear juxta-articular break of the cortical shell (4, 5) while others stated that the break had to be seen in a minimum number of consecutive slices (3). Not until 2016 was a clear definition proposed by the SPECTRA Collaboration following a consensus exercise (63). Erosions were defined as (1) a definite break in the cortical bone; (2) the cortical break must extend over at least two consecutive slices; (3) the cortical break must be detectable in two perpendicular planes; (4) the cortical interruption must have a loss of underlying trabecular bone, and (5) the cortical interruption must be non-linear in shape to differentiate from vascular channels penetrating the cortices (**Figure 3**). In contrast, cortical breaks or interruptions have been defined as a clear interruption of the cortex, seen on two consecutive slices on two orthogonal planes but without the need to demonstrate loss of trabecular bone or shape (34). Such, cortical breaks or interruptions have not been incorporated in the SPECTRA definition of erosions.

The high spatial resolution of HR-pQCT images has allowed deeper investigation into the role of these erosions in the inflammatory arthritis disease course. Forty-six publications characterizing erosions or cortical breaks/interruptions were found. Erosions have been assessed in a variety of arthritic conditions including early inflammatory arthritis (3, 33, 37, 53, 58, 59, 67), RA (1, 3–7, 9, 10, 12, 15, 23, 26, 28–30, 34, 39, 40, 44, 46–48, 52, 54, 55, 61, 64, 65, 67), PsA (5, 7, 14, 49, 61, 66, 69), and erosive hand OA (21), as well as healthy controls (3, 5, 7, 16, 33, 39, 40, 44, 45, 52, 54, 55, 60, 61, 64, 67) and subjects with ACPA antibodies but no features of arthritis (32, 50, 62).

Erosions are most abundant in patients with RA (3, 4, 16, 33, 52, 54, 55, 57, 64, 65, 69), especially ACPA and rheumatoid factor (RF) positive RA patients (26). The erosions exhibit a clear predilection for the radial and ulnar quadrant of the 2nd and 3rd MCP joints. Erosions are most common in the metacarpal head but are also prevalent in the proximal interphalangeal (PIP) bases (4, 15). Although patients with PsA also exhibited a high degree of erosive damage (69), erosions are not as prevalent in PsA patients when compared with RA patients (5, 7, 61). For patients with PsA, erosions are most common in the radial quadrant. However, PsA erosions were also found to a high degree in the dorsal and palmar quadrant of the MCP joint (5, 69). Differences in erosion morphology have also been described in RA compared with PsA patients. In one study, erosions in RA patients were typically U-shaped in appearance, while erosions in PsA patients are more often tubule and Ω-shaped (5); these findings have not been confirmed in other studies. The possible differences in shape may reflect different pathophysiological mechanisms, leading to greater erosion repair in PsA than RA, or alternatively, these morphological phenotypes may reflect differences in disease severity. Further investigation is needed to explore differences between morphologies observed in RA and PsA.

Typically, erosion presence has been assessed manually by an experienced reader. However, manual scoring is laborious and requires substantial training and standardization. An automated detection algorithm has been developed, named the Cortical Interruption Detection Algorithm (39, 40, 52, 53, 64). The Cortical Interruption Detection Algorithm detects the presence of cortical interruptions, directing the reader to lesion locations to verify that they meet the erosion definition as opposed to those that merely represent physiological breaks in the cortical bone, i.e., vascular channels (**Figure 4A**) or stack misalignment (**Figure 4B**) and osteophyte formation (**Figure 4C**). This algorithm also captures very small cortical breaks (>0.246 mm in diameter) that can be challenging to detect through visual inspection (39, 40).

Comparison of Erosion Detection With Other Imaging Modalities

Erosion detection by HR-pQCT has been compared with other pre-clinical and clinical imaging modalities. An image review showing erosions on HR-pQCT, MRI, and CR have also been published for patients with RA (33).

Micro-computed tomography (microCT) applies the same technology as HR-pQCT for pre-clinical investigations but uses a smaller field of view to acquire even higher spatial resolution images (<10 μm, depending on the size of the sample and scanner characteristics) that can be performed on *ex vivo* samples only. Two studies compared cortical interruption detection using HR-pQCT with microCT as a gold standard. The sensitivity of HR-pQCT in detecting cortical interruptions was 82% (34). MicroCT has also been used as a gold standard in order to investigate the ability of the Cortical Interruption Detection Algorithm to find the minimum diameter to detect and quantify cortical interruptions on HR-pQCT. This algorithm performed best for the detection of cortical interruptions with a minimum diameter of 0.16 mm (40).

Additional research has been performed comparing clinical CR and MRI with HR-pQCT, as a gold standard, for the detection of erosions (**Figure 5**). In a clinical setting, CR is still the gold standard. The sensitivity of erosion detection by CR was 61 to 68% when HR-pQCT was considered as a reference (1, 12). Face validity of HR-pQCT identification of erosions

TABLE 1 | Studies included in the systematic review.

Author, year (ref)	Participants	Type of study	Joints included	Outcomes	Other modalities
Fouque-Aubert, 2010 (3)	RA (*n* = 57); eRA (*n* = 36); control (*n* = 43)	Cross-sectional	MCP	Erosions, BMD, microstructure	
Stach, 2010 (4)	RA (*n* = 58); control (*n* = 30)	Cross-sectional	MCP; Radius	Erosions, Osteophyte	
Finzel, 2011 (5)	RA (*n* = 58); PsA (*n* = 30)	Cross-sectional	MCP	Erosions, Osteophyte	
Finzel, 2011 (6)	RA (*n* = 30)	Cohort	MCP	Erosions	
Finzel, 2011 (7)	RA (*n* = 14); PsA (*n* = 6); control (*n* = 6)	Cross-sectional	MCP	Erosions	US
Zhu, 2012 (8)	RA (*n* = 100)	Cross-sectional	MCP; Radius	BMD, microstructure	DXA
Albrech, 2013 (9)	RA (*n* = 50)	Cross-sectional	MCP	Erosions	MRI
Aschenberg, 2013 (10)	RA (*n* = 40)	Cohort	MCP	Erosions, Osteophyte	
Barnabe, 2013 (11)	eRA (*n* = 10)	Cross-sectional	MCP	JSW	
Barnabe, 2013 (12)	RA (*n* = 15); control (*n* = 15)	Cross-sectional	MCP; PIP	Erosions, JSW, BMD, microstructure	CR
Burghardt, 2013 (13)	RA (*n* = 16); control (*n* = 7)	Cross-sectional	MCP; Radius	JSW	CR
Finzel, 2013 (14)	PsA [(*n* = 41) TNFi/MTX *n* = 28/13]	Cohort	MCP	Erosions, Osteophyte	
Finzel, 2013 (15)	RA (*n* = 20)	Cohort	MCP	Erosions	
Srikhum, 2013 (16)	RA (*n* = 16); control (*n* = 7)	Cross-sectional	MCP; Radius	Erosions	MRI
Zhu, 2013 (17)	RA (*n* = 66); control (*n* = 66)	Cross-sectional	Radius	BMD, microstructure	DXA
Kleyer, 2014 (18)	ACPA+ (*n* = 15); ACPA– (*n* = 15)	Cross-sectional	MCP	BMD, microstructure	
Kocijan, 2014 (19)	RA (*n* = 90); control (*n* = 70)	Cross-sectional	Radius	BMD, microstructure	
Kocijan, 2014 (20)	RA (*n* = 60); PsA (*n* = 50)	Cross-sectional	Radius	BMD, microstructure	
Finzel, 2014 (21)	PsA (*n* = 25); HOA (*n* = 25); control (*n* = 20)	Cross-sectional	MCP	Osteophyte	
Teruel, 2014 (22)	RA (*n* = 16)	Cross-sectional	Radius	BMD, microstructure	MRI
Töpfer, 2014 (23)	RA (*n* = 18)	Cross-sectional	MCP	Erosions	
Zhu, 2014 (24)	RA (*n* = 50); control (*n* = 50)	Cross-sectional	Radius	BMD, microstructure	
Zhu, 2015 (25)	PsA (*n* = 53); control (*n* = 53)	Cross-sectional	Radius	BMD, microstructure	DXA
Hecht, 2015 (26)	RA (*n* = 242)	Cross-sectional	MCP	Erosions	
Kocijan, 2015 (27)	PsA (*n* = 50); PsO (*n* = 30); control (*n* = 70)	Cross-sectional	Radius	BMD, microstructure	
Lee, 2015 (1)	RA (*n* = 16)	Cross-sectional	MCP; Radius	Erosions	MRI; CR
Regensburger, 2015 (28)	RA (*n* = 103)	Cross-sectional	MCP; Radius	Erosions	MRI
Töpfer, 2015 (29)	RA (*n* = 22)	Cohort	MCP	Erosions, BMD	
Barnabe, 2016 (30)		Cross-sectional	MCP	Erosions	
Figueriredo, 2016 (31)	ACPA+ RA (*n* = 202)	Cohort	MCP	Erosions, Osteophytes	
Kleyer, 2016 (32)	ACPA+ (*n* = 20); ACPA– (*n* = 13)	Cross-sectional	MCP	Erosions	MRI
Scharmga, 2016 (33)	RA (*n* = 34); eRA (*n* = 10); control (*n* = 38)	Cross-sectional	MCP	Erosions	MRI; CR
Scharmga, 2016 (34)	Cadaver (*n* = 10)	Cross-sectional	MCP; PIP	Erosions	μCT
Shen, 2016 (35)	PsA (*n* = 80)	Cross-sectional	Radius	BMD, BMS	DXA
Tom, 2016 (36)	Cadaver (*n* = 7)	Cross-sectional	MCP	JSW	
Feehan, 2017 (37)	eRA (*n* = 30); control (*n* = 30)	Cohort	MCP; Radius	BMD, BMS	
Kleyer, 2017 (38)	RA (*n* = 15); PsA (*n* = 15); control (*n* = 15)	Cross-sectional	MCP	3D printing	
Peters, 2017 (39)	RA (*n* = 7); control (*n* = 3)	Cross-sectional	MCP	Erosions	
Peters, 2017 (40)	RA (*n* = 32); control (*n* = 32)	Cohort	MCP	Erosions	μCT
Scharmga, 2017 (41)	Cadaver (*n* = 7)	Cross-sectional	MCP	Erosions, VC	
Shimizu, 2017 (42)	RA [(*n* = 27) TNFi/MTX *n* = 17/10]	Cohort	MCP; Radius	Erosions, JSW, BMD	MRI; CR
Simon, 2017 (43)	RA (*n* = 106); control (*n* = 103); Cadaver (*n* = 6)	Cross-sectional	MCP; Radius	BMD, BMS	
Werner, 2017 (44)	RA (*n* = 107); control (*n* = 105); Cadaver (*n* = 6)	Cross-sectional	MCP; Radius	Erosions, VC	μCT

(Continued)

TABLE 1 | Continued

Author, year (ref)	Participants	Type of study	Joints included	Outcomes	Other modalities
Yang, 2017 (45)	RA (*n* = 12); control (*n* = 20)	Cross-sectional	MCP; Radius	BMD, microstructure	
Yue, 2017 (46)	RA (*n* = 20); RA (*n* = 20)	Cohort	MCP	Erosions	
Figueriredo, 2018 (47)	RA (*n* = 65)	Cross-sectional	MCP	Erosions	
Ibrahim-Nasser, 2018 (48)	RA (*n* = 29)	Cross-sectional	MCP	Erosions, BMD, microstructure	CR
Kampylafka, 2018 (49)	PsA [(*n* = 20) IL17 = 20)	Cohort	MCP; PIP; Radius	Erosions, Osteophytes, BMD, microstructure	MRI; US
Keller, 2017 (50)	Control [ACPA+ (*n* = 29); ACPA– (*n* = 29)]	Cross-sectional	MCP	Erosions, BMD, microstructure	
Kong, 2018 (51)	RA [(*n* = 32) US+/– *n* = 20/12]	Cross-sectional	MCP	BMD, microstructure	US
Peters, 2018 (52)	RA (*n* = 41); control (*n* = 38)	Cross-sectional	MCP; PIP	Erosions	MRI; CR
Peters, 2018 (53)	eRA (*n* = 17); undifferentiated arthritis (*n* = 4)	Cross-sectional	MCP	Erosions	
Scharmga, 2018 (54)	RA (*n* = 39); control (*n* = 38)	Cross-sectional	MCP; PIP	Erosions	MRI; CR
Scharmga, 2018 (55)	RA (*n* = 20); control (*n* = 10)	Cross-sectional	MCP; PIP	Erosions	CR
Simon, 2018 (56)	RA ACPA + (*n* = 106); RA ACPA – (*n* = 30); CD (*n* = 43); UC (*n* = 27); PsO (*n* = 74); PsA (*n* = 88); control (*n* = 108)	Cross-sectional	MCP	BMD, microstructure	
Simon, 2018 (57)	PsA (*n* = 55); PsO (*n* = 55); control (*n* = 47)	Cross-sectional	MCP	Erosions, Osteophytes	
Yue, 2018 (58)	eRA (*n* = 63); Remission/not remission	Cohort	MCP	Erosions, BMD, microstructure	
Finzel, 2019 (59)	eRA (*n* = 66 TOC/TNFi *n* = 33/33)	Cohort	MCP; Radius	Erosions	
Berlin, 2019 (60)	Control (*n* = 120)	Cross-sectional	MCP; PIP	Erosions, Osteophytes	
Henchie, 2019 (61)	RA (*n* = 17); PsA (*n* = 17); control (*n* = 12)	Cross-sectional	MCP	Erosions, Osteophytes	
Keller, 2019 (62)	Control [ACPA+ (*n* = 22); ACPA– (*n* = 23)]	Cohort	MCP; Radius	Erosions	
Manske, 2019 (63)	RA (*n* = 43)	Cross-sectional	MCP	JSW	CR
Peters, 2019 (64)	RA (*n* = 32); control (*n* = 32)	Cohort	MCP; PIP	Erosions, BMD, microstructure	CR
Shimizu, 2019 (65)	RA [(*n* = 28) TNFi+/– *n* = 18/10]	Cohort	Radius	Erosions	MRI
Wu, 2019 (66)	PsA (*n* = 60)	Cohort	MCP	Erosions, Osteophytes.	
Yue, 2019 (67)	eRA (*n* = 117)	Cohort	MCP	Erosions	
Simon, 2019 (68)	PsA [(*n* = 165) None/MTX/bDMARD *n* = 79;52;34]	Cross-sectional	Radius	BMD, microstructure	
Wu, 2020 (69)	PsA (*n* = 62); control (*n* = 62)	Cross-sectional	MCP	Erosions, Osteophytes, BMD, microstructure	
Stok, 2020 (70)	RA (*n* = 30)	Cross-Sectional	MCP	JSW	

RA, Rheumatoid arthritis; PsA, Psoriasis arthritis; PSO, Psoriasis; ACPA, Anticitrullinated protein antibodies; US, Ultrasound; IL, interleukin; TNFi, Tumor necrosis factor inhibitors; TOC, tocilizumab; UC, Ulcerative colitis; CD, Crohn's disease; MTX, Methotrexate; bDMARD, biological Disease-modifying antirheumatic drug; BMD, Bone mineral density; MCP, Metacarpophalangeal; PIP, proximal interphalangeal.

was supported by one study that reported that the Sharp/van der Heijde (SvH) score based on MCP and PIP joints using CR were significantly associated with the number and size of erosions by HR-pQCT (52). However, the HR-pQCT scanner has a much smaller field of view, and it remains unknown if the added benefit of the greater sensitivity can make up for the fewer joints examined.

Twelve studies have compared erosion detection by HR-pQCT and MRI, with HR-pQCT as the gold standard, in patients with RA, PsA as well as ACPA positive arthralgia patients without arthritis. The sensitivity for MRI erosion detection ranged from 60 to 86% (1, 9, 16, 28), while the specificity was 97 to 100% (1, 9, 28, 32). HR-pQCT was superior at detecting erosions of less than 10 mm^3 (9).

HR-pQCT has also been used as a reference for erosion detection in order to compare it with US (7). US and HR-pQCT were consistent in the measurement of the width of erosions. However, there was a 10% false-negative rate, and 29% false-positive rate for erosion detection by US. False-negative

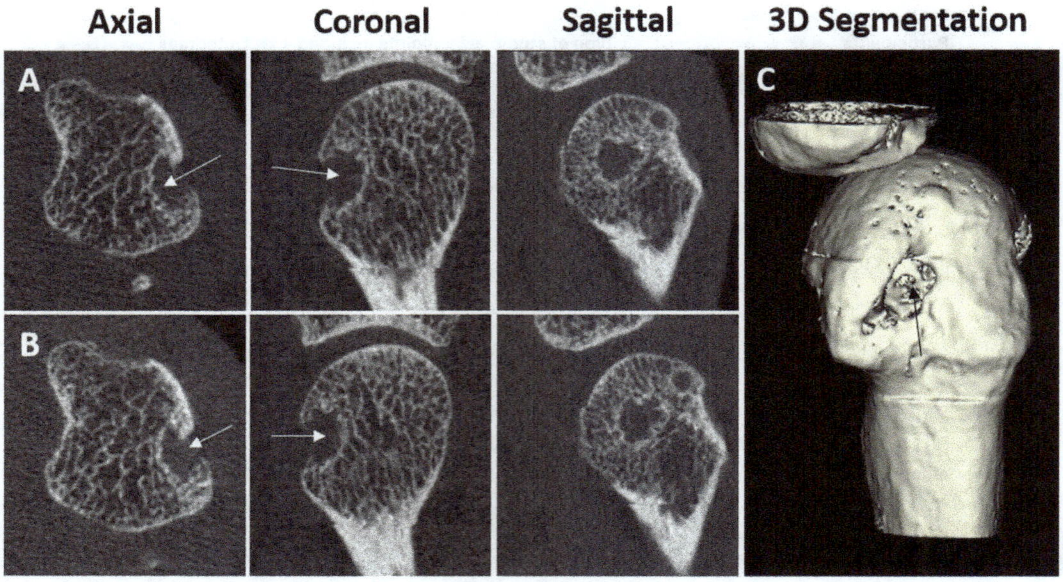

FIGURE 3 | Example of a cortical break meeting the SPECTRA definition of erosion by high-resolution peripheral quantitative computed tomography imaging in the radial quadrant of the second metacarpophalangeal joint from a 54-year-old female patient with rheumatoid arthritis. Arrows indicate the cortical break. **(A,B)** Are the grayscale, consecutive slices. **(C)** Is the 3D segmentation, performed using thresholding (3D Slicer, http://www.slicer.org). Images provided courtesy of Aarhus University (RKJ, KKK, EMH).

results recorded with US were due to its limited resolution to detect cortical lesions <2 mm in width. It was interpreted that the false-positive results occurred because of surface irregularities suggestive of bone erosions on US (7). US has a crucial drawback, as some quadrants of the joints are hard to visualize due to the acoustic window, e.g., radial or ulnar quadrant of the 3rd MCP.

Overall, these findings indicate that HR-pQCT detects more erosions and cortical interruptions than any other clinical imaging modality. However, with increased spatial resolution, more cortical interruptions are observed; this likely includes more physiological cortical interruptions, i.e., vascular channels. However, the higher resolution could also help distinguish pathological from physiological cortical interruptions.

Quantitative Evaluation of Erosions From HR-pQCT Imaging

As a result of the high spatial resolution and 3D imaging, accurate quantification of erosion size is possible. Several published methods exist, including semiquantitative scores (1, 4, 16), manual measures of the maximal dimension of width and depth (5, 7, 15, 30, 46, 48, 58), sphericity (23, 29), and surface area (23, 52, 64). Erosion volume is the most commonly used method due to the ability to detect changes (progression or repair) in three dimensions. However, there is presently no consensus on how to quantify erosion volume. Erosion width and depth have been manually assessed using OsiriX medical imaging software (Pixmeo, Bernex, Switzerland) (48, 50, 62, 65). The erosion volume can then be estimated from a half-ellipsoid formula (9, 23, 26, 28, 47, 57) or ellipsoid formula (**Figure 6A**) (42). More recently, semi-automated and automated algorithms have been introduced. These include Medical Image Analysis Framework (MIAF) (custom software developed at the University of Erlangen; **Figure 6B**) (23, 29), modified Evaluation Script for Erosions (mESE; using Image Processing Language, Scanco Medical) (47), Cortical Interruption Detection Algorithm (custom analysis developed at Maastricht University and Eindhoven University of Technology using Image Processing Language, Scanco Medical; **Figure 7**) (39, 40, 52, 53, 64) and a surface transformation algorithm (custom software developed at Worcester Polytechnic Institute; **Figure 8**) (61). MIAF, mESE, and the Cortical Interruption Detection Algorithm perform a segmentation of the bone and an estimation of the location of the cortical break. Based on this segmentation, the number of voxels in the erosion are counted, producing a true volumetric measure of erosion size. In contrast, the surface transformation algorithm uses statistical shape modeling to compare surface deformities of inflammatory arthritis joints with healthy joints, producing measurements of erosion depth (**Figure 8**) (61).

A single study compared erosion volumes measured manually (estimated from width and depth and calculated assuming the erosion approximated a half-ellipsoid) and using MIAF and mESE. While erosion volumes were similar when measured with the semi-automated methods, manual measurements yield significantly lower absolute volume measures compared with semi-automated methods, particularly for irregularly shaped erosions, illustrating that the erosions should not be assumed to be shaped like a half-ellipsoid (47). To date, no other studies have compared other erosion measurement algorithms.

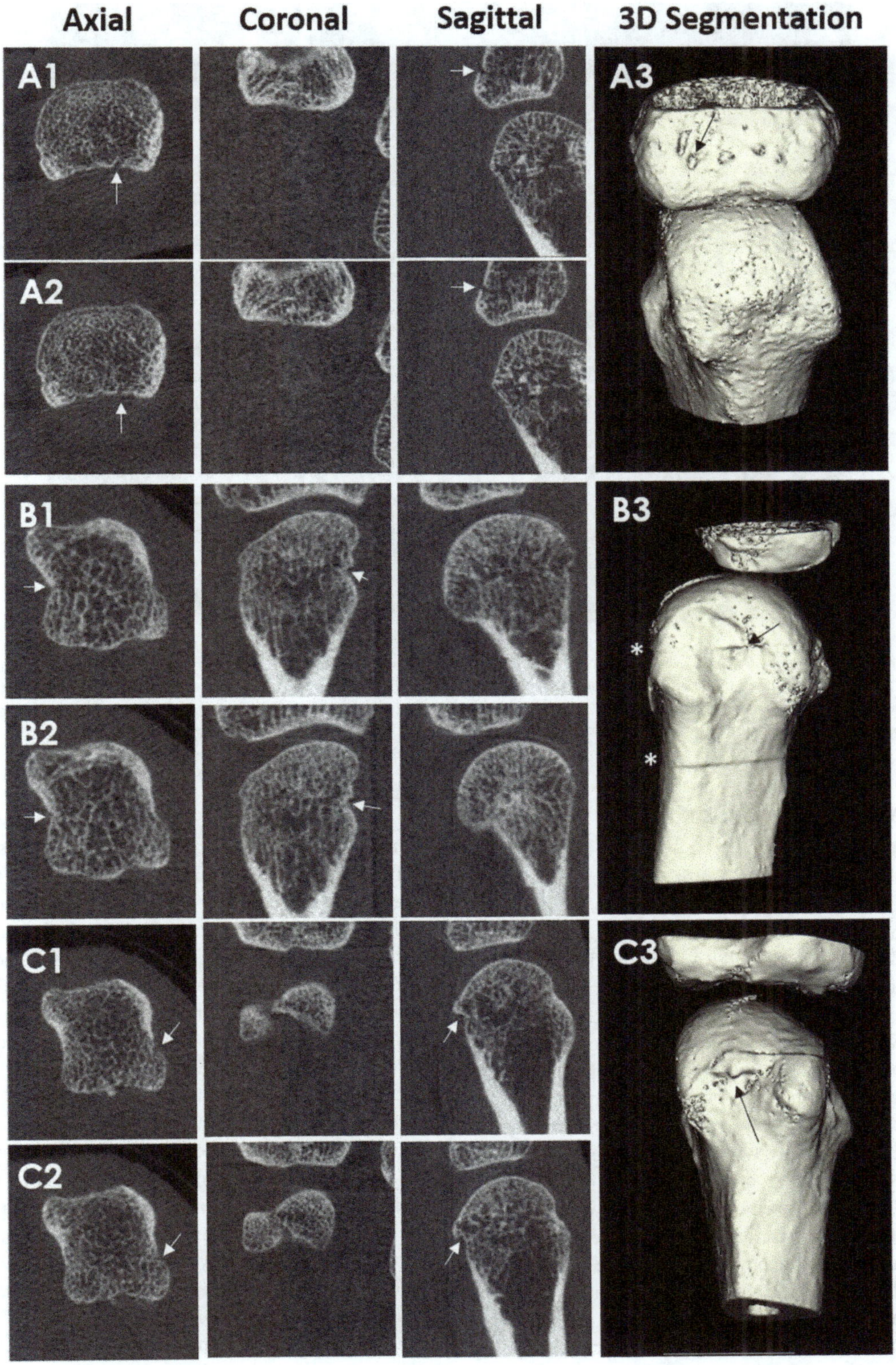

FIGURE 4 | HR-pQCT images of cortical breaks, which do not meet the SPECTRA definition for erosions. Arrows indicate the cortical break. Patient A, where **(A1,A2)** are consecutive slices and **(A3)** is the 3D segmentation. Third MCP Joint from a 67-year-old male patient with rheumatoid arthritis. The cortical break is linear in shape. Therefore, the cortical break is defined as a vascular channel Patient B, where **(B1,B2)** are consecutive slices, and **(B3)** is the 3D segmentation. Second MCP Joint from a 51-year-old female patient with rheumatoid arthritis. Cortical break in relation to stack misalignment represented by *. Patient C, where **(C1,C2)** are consecutive slices and **(C3)** are 3D segmentation. Second MCP Joint from a 51-year-old female patient with rheumatoid arthritis. Cortical break in relation to a bony proliferation. Images provided courtesy of Aarhus University (RK-J, KK, and E-MH).

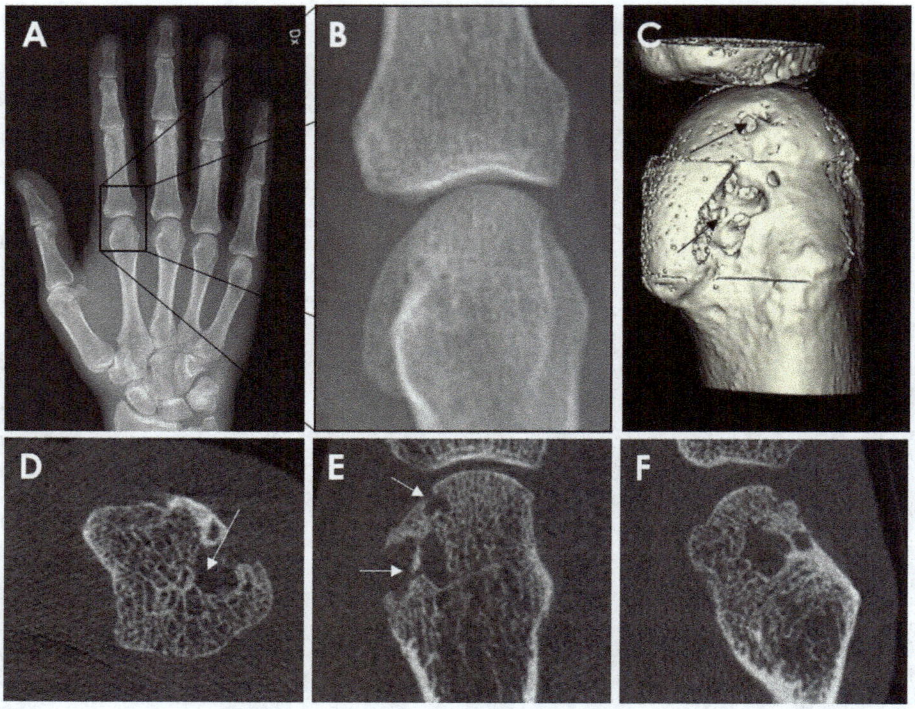

FIGURE 5 | Conventional Radiography **(A,B)** and HR-pQCT imaging **(C–E)** from a 62-year-old male patient with rheumatoid arthritis. Anterior-posterior view of the right hand **(A)**. Enlargement of the second metacarpophalangeal joint **(B)**. High-resolution peripheral quantitative computed tomography images of the second MCP joint as 3D segmentations performed using thresholding **(C)** (3D Slicer, http://www.slicer.org) and the axial **(D)**, coronal **(E)**, and sagittal **(F)** plane, congruent with the corresponding radiograph. The arrow demonstrates the erosion location. Images provided courtesy of Aarhus University (RKJ, KKK, EMH).

Vascular Channels and Cortical Micro-Channels

The high resolution of HR-pQCT not only reveals cortical interruptions meet the definition of erosions but also interruptions which have been hypothesized to be vascular channels. According to the SPECTRA erosion definition, the cortical interruption was suspected to be vascular channels if the interruption was characterized by a parallel cortical lining seen on two consecutive slices and two orthogonal planes (41).

Efforts have been made to test this hypothesis. One study investigated 10 cadaveric fingers, not necessarily affected by inflammatory arthritis, imaged by HR-pQCT with subsequent histological evaluation. Fifty-two vascular channels were identified by histology, and 11 of these fulfilled the definition of erosions on HR-pQCT. Seven cortical breaks which fulfilled the SPECTRA definition of vascular channels were located. Five could be evaluated with histology, and only one of these was a true vascular channel. While they are not vascular channels, these microchannels may provide a link between the synovium and the bone marrow (41). Another approach for investigating vascular channels was to inject the contrast agent Imeron into the ulnar and radial artery of six cadaveric hands prior to HR-pQCT scanning (44). This technique detected very small intraarticular vascular channels. The vascular channels, however, were located proximal to the cortical micro-channels. With both studies, it is possible that very small vascular channels escaped detection due to the challenges of visualizing by perfusion and casting, microCT contrast or standard histological stains (44).

These findings do support the suggestion that bone has a large number of channels passing from the inside to the outside of the bone that is not necessarily linked to erosions, nor do all channels contain vessels. The shape of cortical interruptions cannot be used to accurately decide if cortical breaks contain vessels, as many cortical interruptions, that do not have a classic linear shape, contain vessels (41). Understanding the role of these various channels may be important to understand RA pathology. Traditionally, it has been postulated that synovitis is an initial process that is succeeded by bone involvement known as the "outside-in hypothesis." Conversely, it has been suggested that RA is primarily a bone marrow disease which subsequently affects the synovial membrane; this is known as the "inside-out hypothesis" (74). The cortical micro-channels connect the synovial compartment with the bone marrow and might be important in investigating whether bone damage begins from the inside-out or outside-in (75, 76). HR-pQCT will be useful in combination with other imaging techniques to understand some of these pathological mechanisms.

Bony Proliferations

Bony proliferation is another common pathologic feature of many arthritic diseases, including PsA, primary hand OA and secondary OA due to inflammatory arthritis. There is currently

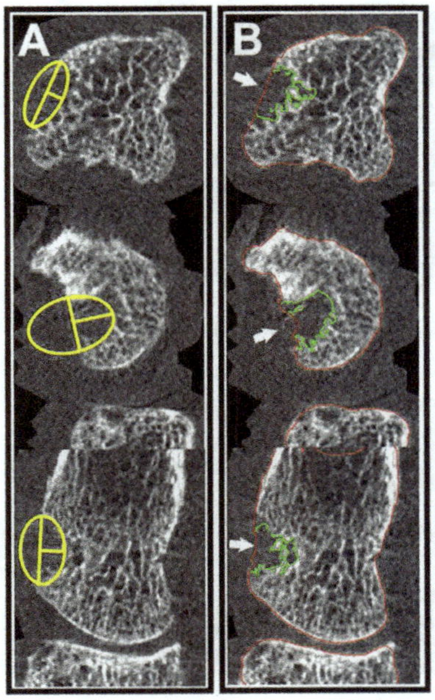

FIGURE 6 | (A) Manual measurement of erosion width and depth. **(B)** Semi-automated erosion volume assessment using MIAF (University of Erlangen). Images provided courtesy of the University of Calgary (JJT, CB, SLM).

no consensus on how to define or quantify the assessment of bony proliferations. However, most studies have defined osteophytes and enthesophytes in a similar fashion; these include bony protrusions from the juxta-articular cortical shell (4, 5, 10, 14, 21, 57) (**Figure 9**), bony proliferation at specific anatomical sites (57), or bone formation arising from the periosteal bone cortex at the insertion sites of the capsule, ligament, or tendons (66, 69). Thirteen publications characterizing osteophytes or enthesophytes with HR-pQCT were found; 8 of which were cross-sectional studies. In three of the studies, the osteophytes or enthesophytes were graded on a semi-quantitative scale (0–3) according to the height measured as the maximum distance between the original and the new cortical lining (4, 5, 21). Two of these three studies also presented direct measurements of the height. The remaining five studies measured osteophyte or enthesophyte height directly (5, 14, 21, 57), and one of these also segmented the osteophyte volume (69). Two studies found that chronic RA patients had a greater number and larger osteophytes than healthy subjects (4, 61); these osteophytes were found mostly in the palmar and dorsal quadrant of the joints. PsA patients had a greater number and size of osteophytes relative to RA patients (5, 61). The highest number of osteophytes in PsA patients was observed in the radial quadrant, closely followed by the dorsal and palmar quadrants. Enthesophytes in patients with PsA is more abundant and greater in size compared to healthy subjects. The majority of enthesophytes in patients with PsA were found at the palmar and dorsal quadrants of the metacarpal heads (57). The volume of enthesophytes is also significantly greater in patients with PsA compared to healthy controls (69). Patients with PsA had a similar number and size of osteophytes compared to those with hand OA. The osteophytes of patients with hand OA were seen predominantly in the palmar and dorsal quadrant, while the distribution of osteophytes in patients with PsA was more widespread (21). In addition, patients with PsA have significantly taller and more abundant bony proliferations (5). There have also been attempts to study bony proliferations according to age. In healthy subjects, the number of osteophytes in the 2nd and 3rd MCP and PIP joints were found to increase with age (60). The number and height of enthesophytes also increase with age; these have been observed not only in patients with PsA but also in healthy subjects. Therefore, the progression of osteophytes may not solely signify disease severity but may also indicate normal age-related change (57). Like erosions, the sensitivity for enthesophyte detection by HR-pQCT is far higher than MRI as 89% of PsA patients had enthesophytes by HR-pQCT, while they were observed in only 30% of the PsA patients on MRI (49). Presently, it is unknown whether there is a benefit of HR-pQCT imaging for tracking the progression of bony proliferation compared to conventional radiographs since no studies have compared the sensitivity and osteophytes seem to progress despite therapy.

Joint Space Width

HR-pQCT images can also be used to quantify joint space width and volume based on the 3D volume between the bones rather than the 2D analysis that is typically applied to conventional radiographs. Seven publications with joint space analysis were found; all but one has investigated the validity of proposed semi-automatic scripts. Three different algorithms were developed using a similar methodology (11, 13). A consensus method has recently been published by the SPECTRA Collaboration (**Figure 10**), this method is proposed for universal use in ongoing and future clinical trials of arthritic conditions (70). The established joint space width (JSW) metrics include mean, minimum and maximum JSW as well as standard deviation, asymmetry (maximum/minimum) and joint space volume. A single study has investigated the validity of a JSW script on cadaveric MCP joints at different flexion angles. The study found in order to have reliable joint space measures, the acquisition of the joints had to be < 10 degrees flexion for longitudinal studies (36). Whether the joint space analysis is affected by other factors such as joint swelling, is currently under investigation.

Lastly, two studies evaluated relationships between joint space narrowing assessed from CR and 3D joint space analysis on HR-pQCT. Minimum JSW, JSW standard deviation, and JSW asymmetry assessed by HR-pQCT were associated with SvH joint space score (13, 63).

The minimum joint space width has been shown to be significantly smaller in patients with RA compared to healthy subjects, which is suggestive of a loss of cartilage thickness in the affected patients (13). However, larger studies are needed to reliably investigate group differences.

Bone Mineral Density and Microstructure

HR-pQCT provides 3D images, so volumetric bone mineral density (vBMD, g/cm^3) is assessed rather than areal BMD (aBMD) that is reported by dual-energy x-ray absorptiometry (DXA). Microstructural features of trabecular bone, including

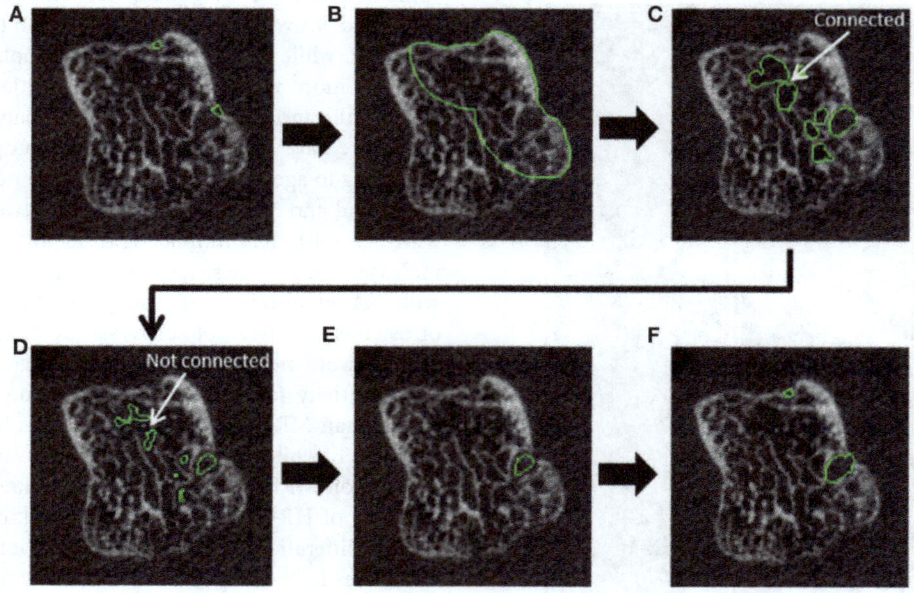

FIGURE 7 | Steps incorporated in the automated cortical interruption detection algorithm and measurement of underlying loss of trabecular bone, as visualized on a 2D grayscale image. **(A)** Detection of two cortical interruptions ≥0.41 mm. **(B)** Region of interest (ROI) identified by dilating the cortical interruptions by 48 voxels (corresponding to 3.936 mm), and masking with the periosteal contour. **(C)** Only voids that are ≥0.738 in diameter are selected by performing a distance transformation within the ROI. **(D)** Voids are eroded by 2 voxels to detach connections of ≤0.328 mm and prevent leakage into the trabecular bone. **(E)** Inclusion of voids that remain connected to a cortical interruption after erosion. **(F)** Dilation of voids to the original size, and inclusion of cortical interruptions that were originally detected. Reproduced with permission from (53).

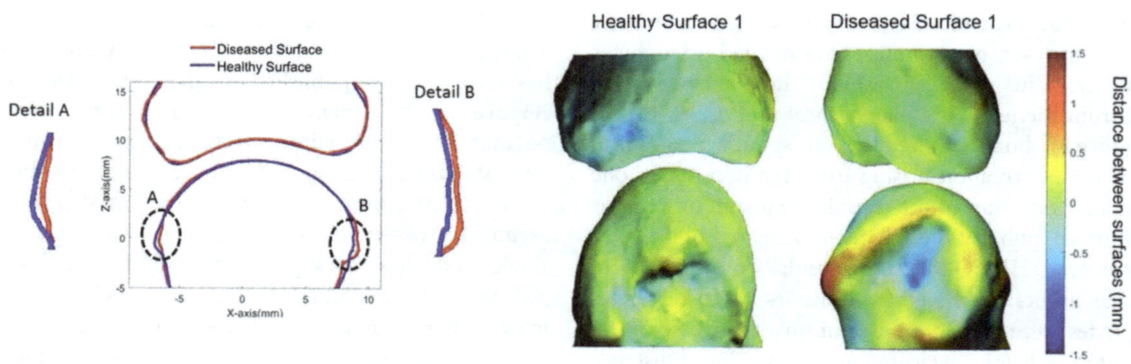

FIGURE 8 | Surface deformation model (61) showing: **(Left)** cross-section of MCP joint with the diseased surface (red) overlaid on the average healthy surface (blue). **(Right)** 3D heat map representing distances between diseased (top) and healthy (bottom) surfaces. Positive distances reflect bony proliferations, while negative distances represent erosive damage. Image provided courtesy of Worcester Polytechnic Institute (Kyle Murdock and Karen Troy).

trabecular thickness, number and separation, have been measured directly and with greater accuracy using the second-generation scanners compared to the first-generation scanner (77). BMD and microstructure imaged by HR-pQCT have been investigated in several different groups of patients and with focus on different joints of interest as well as the typical measurements of the distal radius and distal tibia applied in osteoporosis studies. Most of these studies were cross-sectional, and the majority of studies were done with either RA or PsA patients. One study assessed the relationship of periarticular osteoporosis in the wrist and MCP joint by HR-pQCT imaging with BMD in axial skeletal sites by DXA. Areal BMD in the axial skeleton was moderately correlated with vBMD assessed by HR-pQCT in both the radius and 2nd metacarpal head while microarchitecture only had a weak to moderate correlation in patients with RA (8). Finally, one study investigated the correlation between bone density and bone microstructure parameters measured at the MCP joint and SvH score in patients with RA, but only found a significant correlation between trabecular separation and SvH score (3).

Six cross-sectional studies compared RA patients with healthy subjects. Cortical and trabecular vBMD was significantly lower in female and male patients with RA when compared to healthy subjects at the distal radius, even though no difference in axial

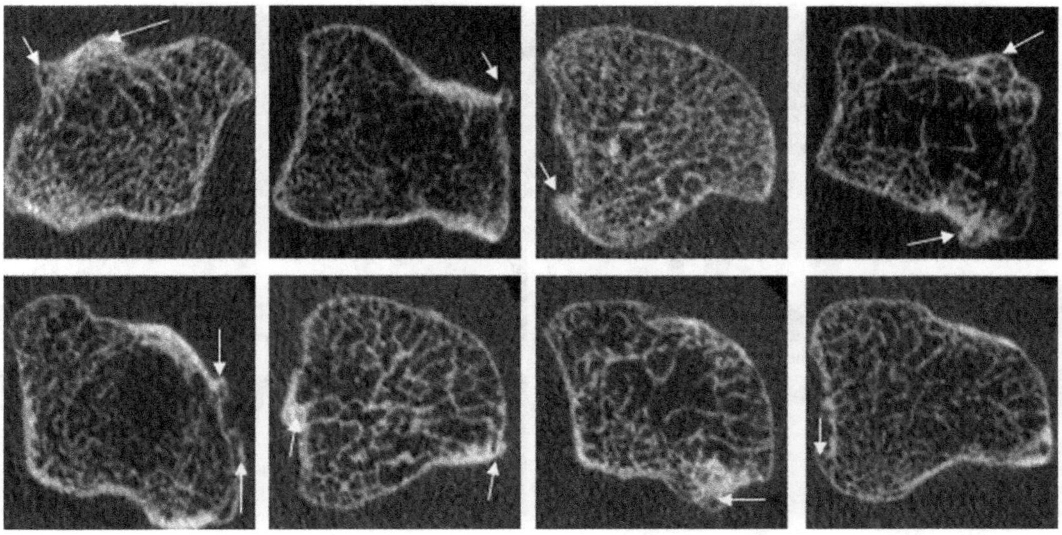

FIGURE 9 | Examples of osteophytes in the metacarpal head of PsA patients, which commonly show widespread involvement of the cortical bone. Images provided courtesy of The Chinese University of Hong Kong (L-ST).

aBMD measured by DXA could be observed (17, 24). In the same population, the cortical porosity and trabecular separation were significantly greater, and bone volume fraction significantly lower, in the RA patients (17, 19, 24). Volumetric BMD and microarchitecture were similarly different at the MCP joints in three of four studies. The trabecular vBMD, bone volume fraction and thickness was significantly lower, while trabecular separation was significantly higher in patients with RA compared to healthy subjects (3, 12, 43, 45).

Five cross-sectional studies have investigated bone density and microarchitecture in patients with PsA. At the radius, cortical vBMD was significantly lower, while cortical porosity was significantly higher in PsA patients compared to healthy subjects. By DXA, the PsA patients had significantly higher aBMD at the lumbar spine compared to healthy subjects; this difference, however, became insignificant after adjusting for Body Mass Index (BMI), suggesting BMI may have confounded the relationship (4). Other studies have found a significant loss of periarticular trabecular bone in PsA patients compared to healthy subjects with regards to both vBMD (69) and bone structure (27). Compared to treatment naïve PsA patients, patients with a history of biological disease-modifying anti-rheumatic drugs (DMARD) treatment had significantly higher vBMD, BV/TV as well as greater trabecular number and thickness. No significant differences in bone density or microarchitecture outcomes were observed in patients previously treated with MTX compared to treatment naïve PsA patients (68).

The trabecular number and vBMD were significantly lower, while trabecular separation was significantly higher for PsA patients when compared with RA patients. However, this difference was only seen between ACPA positive RA patients and PsA patients. The ACPA positive RA patients had a significantly longer disease duration. Therefore, this difference is more likely attributed to disease duration rather than the underlying condition (20). In contrast, when comparing patients with various chronic inflammatory diseases (ACPA-positive RA, ACPA-negative RA, Crohn's Disease, ulcerative colitis, psoriasis and PsA) and healthy participants, vBMD differed only between ACPA-positive RA and healthy subjects (56). Together these findings suggest that to date, the bone density and microstructure seems to be affected in different kinds of inflammatory diseases, but the nature of these findings are unclear as the periarticular bone density and microstructure are influenced by other factors independent of the inflammatory nature of the disease, such as genetic factors, sex, physical activity, height, weight, BMI, smoking and alcohol consumption, and daily calcium intake.

Reproducibility of the Pathological Measures

Reproducibility has been reported for erosion measurements, osteophytes, joint space width, bone mineral density and microstructure (**Table 2**). Reproducibility is most often presented as Intraclass correlation coefficients (ICC), root mean square coefficient of variance (CV_{RMS}%), but also as the coefficient of variation. The reproducibility for bone mineral density, microstructure, and most joint space width metrics are excellent (**Table 2**). Reproducibility for erosion measures is generally good but does show some variation. Due to the distinct methods used for erosion quantification, these values are hard to compare. Osteophyte assessment has the lowest values for reproducibility (69).

When compared with reproducibility for semi-quantitative scoring systems on MRI (RAMRIS) (78) and CR (SvH) (79), HR-pQCT offers many advantages by using quantitative tools for outcome measurement that require fewer operator inputs. The reliability for erosion count was higher for HR-pQCT than MRI. However, the ICC was excellent for both modalities (9, 28), while only moderate for CR (55). The semi-automated or fully-automated assessments of bone mineral density, microstructure, joints space width and cortical interruptions result in intra-reader and inter-reader differences that are non-existent, or

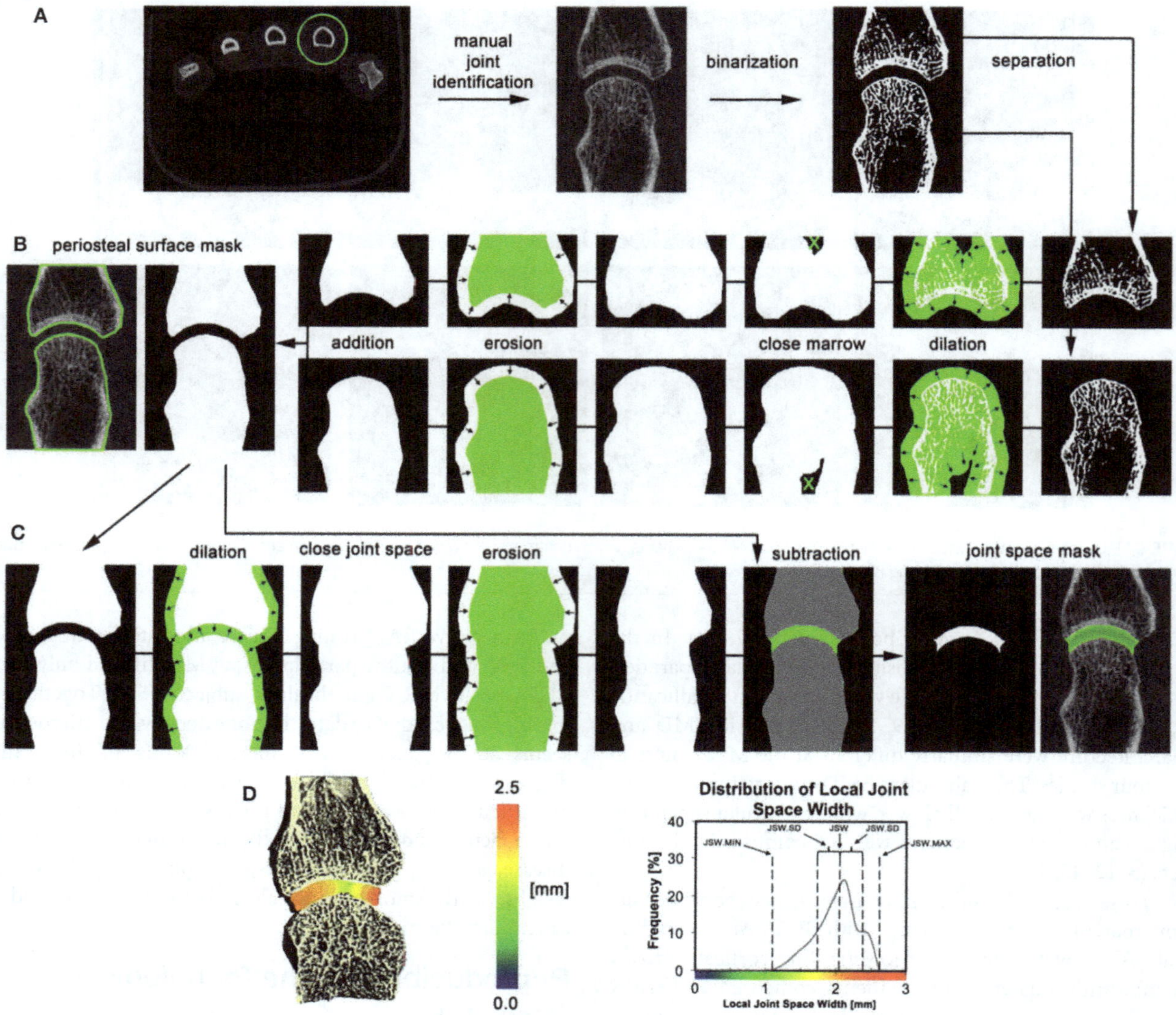

FIGURE 10 | 3D volumetric joint space width analysis by HR-pQCT. **(A)** The relevant joint is identified; bone is segmented by thresholding, and bones are separated based on their relevant position (distal and proximal). **(B)** Periosteal surfaces for each bone in the joint are identified using an automated process. **(C)** Joint space volume is identified through a series of morphological operations and subtraction of the original bone volumes. **(D)** Joint space metrics are derived from the 3D map of local joint space widths. The 3D map is shown in pseudo color (left), and as a distribution (right) for the 2nd metacarpal of an RA patient. Reproduced with permission from (13).

nearly negligible because the analyses are automated, with the exception of an allowance for corrections of bone segmentation. Scan-rescan reproducibility for JSW minimum is similar to that obtained with inter-reader ratings on 2D radiographs (RMSSD 0.18 mm) but far superior for mean JSW (RMSSD 0.05 mm) (80). Intra- and inter-reader reproducibility and reliability for erosion detection and volume are comparable to reproducibility and reliability reported for the erosion domain of the RAMRIS scoring system (9, 28, 81, 82).

Longitudinal Changes of the Pathological Measures

While the diagnostic uses of HR-pQCT might be limited at present, the research applications are vast. Several clinical trials have been conducted using erosion volume by HR-pQCT as an outcome measure. One of the major advantages is the potential for shorter monitoring times to evaluate erosion progression or repair. Fifteen studies have reported longitudinal changes in the number and/or size of erosions. Of these, three investigated PsA (14, 49, 66), 10 investigated patients with RA (6, 10, 15, 29, 42, 46, 58, 59, 64, 65), and one study examined ACPA+ individuals without arthritis (62). Seven studies investigated intervention with different therapies either as an open-label study or secondary analysis in a randomized controlled trial. Five of the seven studies were done on patients with RA (12, 19, 43, 55, 69), and two in PsA (21, 60). In patients with established RA, two studies of patients with mean disease duration more than 5 years did not detect any change in erosions at 1-year follow-up (10, 64). However, longitudinal changes are diverse.

Studies which traced changes of individual erosions in patients receiving care according to treat-to-target strategy over a 1-year period have shown that 15–31% of erosions progress in size, 48–65% were stable in size and 20–21% show partial repair after 1 year (29, 58, 67).

The shortest time interval over which significant changes have been evaluated is 3 months. This study was conducted enrolling patients with RA and a mean disease duration of more than 5 years who were receiving either a TNF inhibitor (TNFi) in combination with methotrexate or methotrexate alone. While no significant changes in MRI outcome measures were observed, a significant increase in erosion volume assessed by HR-pQCT was observed for the methotrexate-treated patients, and those on combination therapy with treatment response had a demonstrated decrease in erosion volume (42). In this same study, joint space did decrease significantly in patients in combination therapy only. Paradoxically, this was not seen in methotrexate-treated patients. However, methotrexate-treated patients had smaller joint space at baseline, which may explained why no change was seen after the 3-month follow-up (42). Change in erosion volume after 3 and 6 months has also been investigated for patients with RA and a mean disease duration of roughly 10 years receiving either alendronate or denosumab together with their regular DMARD treatment (46). No significant change was observed after 3 months. Conversely, erosion volume increased significantly in patients receiving alendronate, while decreasing significantly in patients receiving denosumab after 6 months. While these represent the shortest time interval over which changes in erosion volume and JSW have been observed, two studies have shown decreases in erosion volume in response to tocilizumab in combination with methotrexate for both patients with newly diagnosed RA (59) and established RA (15); this has also been observed for patients with established RA treated with TNFi in combination with methotrexate (6) over a 1-year follow-up. Stabilization in erosion size with therapy has also been demonstrated, in newly diagnosed patients with RA on treatment with a TNFi in combination with methotrexate (59). PsA studies have shown slower erosion changes than RA; no significant progression in erosions was seen in patients with established PsA after 24 weeks (49) or 1-year (14). However, one study found progression of erosion number and size after 5-years in patients with established PsA and a mean disease duration of 14 years (66).

While the measurement of erosion size has been the most commonly used outcome metric, osteophytes and bone quality have also been assessed. Five longitudinal studies investigated changes in osteophytes over time. In RA patients, no significant change in osteophyte number or score was seen after a year (10). However, an 18-month follow-up study did find an increase in both osteophytes number and volume in RA patients in open-label treatment (31). No change in osteophyte size was observed in PsA patients treated with secukinumab for 24 weeks (49). However, in patients treated with MTX and TNFi osteophyte height increased over 1 year (14), and volume increased over 5 years in patients in open-label treatment (66).

Only six longitudinal studies of bone density and microarchitecture in the MCP joint or the radius have been reported. In longitudinal studies of RA or PsA patients without a healthy control group, conducted with 3-month or 1-year follow-up, no significant changes in vBMD or microstructure were observed (42, 49, 58). In one study, greater decreases in vBMD and microstructure over 1 year were observed in RA patients compared to healthy controls (64), while two other studies found comparable decreases in both early RA patients and healthy controls (37, 62). Differences in disease duration, treatment status, and the anatomic site measured may explain the variable findings across studies. More extensive longitudinal studies are needed to reveal the critical anatomic locations, time course, and mechanisms of bone loss that should be strategically targeted for observation.

Combined with advances in image processing and image registration, individual spatially localized changes can be monitored with high sensitivity and reliability (**Table 2**) (64). To date, the published studies report data for the joint region captured in the field of view, and not for the local changes such as the peri-articular region. Furthermore, these techniques can be applied where only subtle changes are anticipated, such as understanding bony damage progression in the presence of subclinical inflammation.

Early Detection of Articular Damage in Inflammatory Arthritis by HR-pQCT Imaging

The sensitive detection of erosive damage and bony proliferation suggests that HR-pQCT may have utility in the early detection of articular damage in inflammatory arthritis. For conventional radiographs, erosions have been observed to be prevalent in ~50% of RA patients at clinical diagnosis, and up to 60% of patients have erosions after 1 year (83). Therefore, the higher sensitivity of HR-pQCT compared to conventional radiographs is promising not only in assessing longitudinal changes but may also be useful for early detection in patients where the diagnosis is suspected but cannot be made clinically. However, the ability to image multiple joints is limited by the acquisition speed. Although many erosions occur in the standard scan sites of the 2nd and 3rd metacarpals of the dominant hand, other joints will be missed. Further, the contrast is insufficient to detect inflammation (synovitis and osteitis, also referred to as bone marrow oedema in RA patients) believed to be key precursors to clinical disease. Nonetheless, two cross-sectional studies found a significantly thinner trabecular bone in the MCP joints of ACPA positive individuals with arthralgia compared with ACPA negative healthy individuals (18, 50). Kleyer et al. also observed significantly lower trabecular number, bone volume fraction and vBMD in ACPA positive individuals with arthralgia compared with ACPA negative healthy individuals (18), suggesting that periarticular bone loss may be an early sign of clinical disease. Changes to bone mineral density and microstructure, however, is very non-specific to arthritis, as possible changes can be attributed to many other factors. Therefore, the use of bone mineral density and microstructure for early detection of articular damage in inflammatory arthritis

TABLE 2 | Reproducibility measures.

Author, year (ref)	Participants	Reproducibility feature	Method	Findings
Erosion count				
Albrecht, 2013 (9)	RA (*n* = 50)	Inter-reader reliability	Erosion count	ICC range: metacarpal head: 0.936–1.00. ICC range: phalangeal Base: 0.948–1.00.
Aschenberg, 2013 (10)	RA (*n* = 40)	Inter-reader reliability	Erosion score	ICC (range): 0.79 (0.57–0.95)
Hecht, 2015 (26)	RA (*n* = 242)	Inter-reader agreement	Erosion count	ICC: [0.87–1.00]
Regensburger, 2015 (28)	RA (*n* = 103)	Inter-reader reliability	Erosion count	ICC [95% CI]: 0.98 [0.98–0.98]
Scharmga, 2016 (34)	RA (*n* = 44); control (*n* = 38)	Intra- and inter-reader reliability	Cortical break count	ICC [95% CI]: 0.61 [0.49–0.70] ICC [95% CI]: 0.55 [0.43–0.65]
Peters, 2017 (40)	RA (*n* = 32); control (*n* = 32)	Inter-reader reliability	Cortical break count 1>0.16 mm, 2>0.33 mm 3>0.53 mm	ICC [95% CI]: 0.91 [0.65–0.97] ICC [95% CI]: 0.81 [0.52–0.92] ICC [95% CI]: 0.52 [0.11–0.78]
Scharmga, 2017 (41)	Cadaver (*n* = 7)	Intra- and inter-reader reliability	Cortical break count	ICC range: 0.52–0.75 ICC range: 0.37–0.55
Peters, 2017 (39)	RA (*n* = 7); control (*n* = 3)	Inter-reader reliability	Cortical break count	ICC [95%CI]: 0.97 [0.90–0.99]
Peters, 2018 (53)	eRA (*n* = 17); undifferentiated arthritis (*n* =4)	Inter-reader reliability and reproducibility	Cortical interruptions count	ICC [95%CI]: 0.96[0.89–0.97] ICC [95%CI]: 0.94[0.89–0.97] ICC [95%CI]: 0.96[0.92–0.98] ICC [95%CI]: 0.94[0.89–0.97]
Scharmga, 2018 (54)	RA (*n* = 39); control (*n* = 38)	Intra- and inter-reader reliability	Cortical interruptions	ICC [95%CI]: 0.69[0.65–0.73] ICC [95%CI]: 0.56[0.49–0.62]
Scharmga, 2018 (55)	RA (*n* = 20); control (*n* = 10)	Intra- and inter-reader reliability	Cortical interruptions	ICC [95%CI]: 0.88 [0.83–0.92] ICC [95%CI]: 0.48 [0.20–0.67]
Simon, 2018 (57)	PsA (*n* = 55); PsO (*n* = 55); control (*n* = 47)	Inter-reader agreement	Erosions number	ICC: 0.96
Berlin, 2019 (60)	Control (*n* = 120)	Inter-reader agreement	Erosion count	ICC [95%CI]: 0.76 [0.62–0.86]
Erosion score				
Aschenberg, 2013 (10)	RA (*n* = 40)	Inter-reader reliability	Erosion and osteophyte count and score	ICC (range): 0.79 (0.57–0.95)
Erosions width and depth				
Finzel, 2013 (15)	RA (*n* = 20)	Intra- and inter-reader reproducibility	Width and depth	ICC: 0.99 ICC: 0.99 ICC: 0.93 ICC: 0.94
Lee, 2015 (1)	RA (*n* = 16)	Intra- and inter-reader reproducibility	Sum maximum dimension.	ICC: 0.89 ICC: 0.99
Barnabe, 2016 (30)		Inter-reader reliability	Width and depth	CV_{RMS}%: 12.3–20.6 CV_{RMS}%: 22.2–24.0
Yue, 2017 (46)	RA (*n* = 20); RA (*n* = 20)	Intra- and inter-reader reliability	Width and depth	ICC [95%CI]: 0.99 [0.94–1.00] ICC [95%CI]: 0.99 [0.96–1.00] ICC [95%CI]: 0.98 [0.96–0.99] ICC [95%CI]: 0.98 [0.97–0.99
Keller, 2017 (50)	Control [ACPA+ (*n* = 29); ACPA– (*n* = 29)]	Intrareader reproducibility	Width and depth	CV%: 14.9 CV%:10.8%
Ibrahim-Nasser, 2018 (48)	RA (*n* = 29)	Inter-reader precision	Width and depth	CV_{RMS}%: 16.0–20 CV_{RMS}%: 17.5–23.4
Yue, 2018 (58)	eRA (*n* = 63); Remission/not remission	Intra- and inter-reader reliability	Width and depth	ICC [95%CI]: 0.97 [0.93–0.99] ICC [95%CI]: 1.00 [0.99–1.00] ICC [95%CI]: 0.98 [0.93–0.99] ICC [95%CI]: 0.92 [0.70– 0.98]
Henchie, 2019 (61)	RA (*n* = 17); PsA (*n* = 17); control (*n* = 12)	Inter-reader precision	Depth.	RMSE: 4+/−3% Precision error: 50 μm
Erosion volume				
Töpfer, 2014 (23)	RA (*n* = 18)	Inter-reader precision	Volume (Half-ellipsoid). Volume. (MIAF).	CV_{RMS}%: 15.4 CV_{RMS}%: 7.78
Regensburger, 2015 (28)	RA (*n* = 103)	Inter-reader reliability	Volume (Half-ellipsoid).	ICC [95% CI]: 0.95 [0.94–0.96]

(Continued)

TABLE 2 | Continued

Author, year (ref)	Participants	Reproducibility feature	Method	Findings
Töpfer, 2015 (29)	RA (*n* = 22)	Inter-reader precision	Volume. (MIAF).	CV_{RMS}%: 6 – 8.3
Figueriredo, 2016 (31)	ACPA+ RA (*n* = 202)	Inter-reader reliability	Volume (Half-ellipsoid).	ICC [95%CI]: 0.96 [0.94–0.97]
Shimizu, 2017 (42)	RA [(*n* = 27) TNFi/MTX *n* = 17/10)	Intra- and inter reader agreement	Volume	CV_{RMS}%: 3.43 CV_{RMS}%: 3.92
Yue, 2017 (46)	RA (*n* = 20); RA (*n* = 20)	Intra- and inter-reader reliability	Volume	ICC [95%CI]: 0.98 [0.87–1.00] ICC [95%CI]: 0.96 [0.73–1.00]
Keller, 2017 (50)	Control [ACPA+ (*n* = 29); ACPA– (*n* = 29)]	Intrareader reproducibility	Volume (Osirix)	CV%20.6%,
Figueriredo, 2018 (47)	RA (*n* = 65)	Inter-reader reliability	Volume (Half-ellipsoid) Volume (MIAF) Volume (mESE)	ICC [95%CI]: 0.95 [0.92–0.97] ICC [95%CI]: 0.92 [0.79–0.97] ICC [95%CI]: 0.99 [0.99–0.99]
Ibrahim-Nasser, 2018 (48)	RA (*n* = 29)	Inter-reader precision error	Volume (Osirix)	CV_{RMS}%: 16.0–20 CV_{RMS}%: 17.5–23.4 CV_{RMS}%: 14.0–21.2
Peters, 2018 (53)	eRA (*n* = 17); undifferentiated arthritis (*n* =4)	Intra- Inter-reader reliability and Intra- Inter-reader reproducibility	Cortical interruptions (CIDA)	ICC [95%CI]: 0.99[0.99–1.00] ICC [95%CI]: 0.91[0.81–0.96] ICC [95%CI]: 1.00[0.99–1.00] ICC [95%CI]: 0.91[0.81–0.96]
Simon, 2018 (57)	PsA (*n* = 55); PsO (*n* = 55); control (*n* = 47)	Inter-reader agreement	Volume	ICC: 0.90
Yue, 2018 (58)	eRA (*n* = 63); Remission/not remission	Intra- and inter-reader reliability	Volume	ICC [95%CI]: 0.95 [0.79–0.99] ICC [95%CI]: 0.98 [0.83–1.00]
Shimizu, 2019 (65)	RA [(*n* = 28) TNFi+/– *n* = 18/10]	Intra- and Inter-reader reproducibility	Volume (Osirix)	ICC: 0.93 ICC: 0.80
Wu, 2020 (69)	PsA (*n* = 62); control (*n* = 62)	Inter-reader reliability	Volume	ICC [95%CI]: 1.00 [0.99–1.00]
Erosion surface area				
Töpfer, 2014 (23)	RA (*n* = 18)	Inter-reader precision	Surface Area (MIAF)	CV_{RMS}%: 9.89
Peters, 2017 (40)	RA (*n* = 32); control (*n* = 32)	Inter-reader reliability	Cortical interruptions 1>0.16 mm, 2>0.33 mm 3>0.53 mm	1.ICC [95% CI]:0.93 [0.82–0.97 2.ICC [95% CI]:0.86 [0.67–0.94] 3.ICC [95% CI]:0.21 [–0.15–0.56]
Peters, 2017 (39)	RA (*n* = 7); control (*n* = 3)	Inter-reader reliability	Cortical break Surface area	ICC [95%CI]: 0.98 [0.92–1.00]
Peters, 2018 (53)	eRA (*n* = 17); undifferentiated arthritis (*n* =4)	Intra- Inter-reader reliability and Intra- Inter-reader reproducibility	Cortical interruptions surface area (CIDA)	ICC [95%CI]: 0.95[0.92–0.98] ICC [95%CI]: 0.70[0.41–0.84] ICC [95%CI]: 0.95[0.92–0.98] ICC [95%CI]: 0.70[0.41–0.86]
Erosion sphericity				
Töpfer, 2014 (23)	RA (*n* = 18)	Inter-reader precision	Sphericity. (MIAF).	CV_{RMS}%: 5.46
Erosion marginal osteosclerosis				
Yue, 2017 (46)	RA (*n* = 20); RA (*n* = 20)	Intra- and inter-reader reliability	Marginal osteosclerosis	ICC [95%CI]: 0.98 [0.96–0.99] ICC [95%CI]: 0.97 [0.90–0.99]
Yue, 2018 (58)	eRA (*n* = 63); Remission/not remission	Intra- and inter-reader reliability	Marginal osteosclerosis	ICC [95%CI]: 0.99 [0.91–1.00] ICC [95%CI]: 0.94 [0.73–0.99]
Osteophyte count				
Aschenberg, 2013 (10)	RA (*n* = 40)	Inter-reader reliability	Count	ICC (range): 0.79 (0.57–0.95)
Finzel, 2013 (21)	PsA (*n* = 25); HOA (*n* = 25); control (*n* = 20)	Intra- Inter-reader reproducibility	Count	Spearman's rho (0.95–1.00) ICC 0.91
Simon, 2018 (57)	PsA (*n* = 55); PsO (*n* = 55); control (*n* = 47)	Inter-reader agreement	Count	ICC: 0.95
Berlin, 2019 (60)	Control (*n* = 120)	Inter-reader agreement	Count	ICC [95%CI]: 0.96 [0.92–0.98]
Osteophyte score				
Aschenberg, 2013 (10)	RA (*n* = 40)	Inter-reader agreement	Score	ICC (range): 0.79 (0.57–0.95)
Finzel, 2013 (21)	PsA (*n* = 25); HOA (*n* = 25); control (*n* = 20)	Intra- and Inter-reader reproducibility	Score	Spearman's rho (0.95–1.00) ICC 0.92

(Continued)

TABLE 2 | Continued

Author, year(ref)	Participants	Reproducibility feature	Method	Findings
Osteophyte height				
Finzel, 2013 (14)	PsA [(*n* = 41) TNFi/MTX *n* = 28/13]; RA (*n* = 43)	Inter-reader reproducibility Intra-reader reliability	Height	*r* = 0.9692 *r* = 0.9722
Finzel, 2013 (21)	PsA (*n* = 25); HOA (*n* = 25); control (*n* = 20)	Inter-reader reproducibility	Height	ICC 0.96
Simon, 2018 (57)	PsA (*n* = 55); PsO (*n* = 55); control (*n* = 47)	Inter-reader agreement	Height	ICC: 0.94
Henchie, 2019 (61)	RA (n = 17); PsA (n = 17); control (n = 12)	Inter-reader precision	Periosteal bone growth height	RMSE: 20+/−13% Precision error:210 μm
Wu, 2020 (69)	PsA (*n* = 62); control (*n* = 62)	Inter-reader reliability	Entesophyte height	ICC [95%CI]: 0.74 [0.42–0.89]
Osteophyte volume				
Wu, 2020 (69)	PsA (*n* = 62); control (*n* = 62)	Inter-reader reliability	Entesophyte volume	ICC [95%CI]: 0.99 [0.97–0.99]
Bone mineral density				
Fouque-Aubert, 2010 (3)	RA (*n* = 14); control (*n* = 14)	Repositioning and scan/rescan	BMD	CV%: ≤ 1.8
Barnabe, 2013 (12)	RA (*n* = 15); control (*n* = 15)	Intrareader reproducibility	BMD	CV_{RMS}%: < 0.83
Keller, 2017 (50)	Control [ACPA+ (*n* = 29); ACPA– (*n* = 29)]	Intrareader reproducibility	BMD	CV%: 0.6–3.53
Peters, 2018 (53)	eRA (*n* = 17); undifferentiated arthritis (*n* = 4)	Inter-reader reliability and Intra- Inter-reader reproducibility	BMD	ICC [95%CI]: 0.99[0.99–1.00] ICC [95%CI]: 0.99[0.99–1.00] ICC [95%CI]: 0.99[0.99–1.00] ICC [95%CI]: 1.00[1.00–1.00]
Wu, 2020 (69)	PsA (*n* = 62); control (*n* = 62)	Inter-reader reliability	BMD	CV%: 0.38–1.03
Bone microstructure				
Fouque-Aubert, 2010 (3)	RA (*n* = 14); control (*n* = 14)	Repositioning and scan/rescan	Microstructure	CV%: ≤ 12.5
Barnabe, 2013 (12)	RA (*n* = 15); control (*n* = 15)	Intrareader reproducibility	Microstructure	CV_{RMS}%: < 0.83
Keller, 2017 (50)	Control [ACPA+ (*n* = 29); ACPA– (*n* = 29)]	Intrareader reproducibility	Microstructure	CV%: 0.6–3.53
Peters, 2018 (53)	eRA (*n* = 17); undifferentiated arthritis (*n* =4)	Inter-reader reliability and Intra- and inter-reader reproducibility	Microstructure	ICC [95%CI]: 0.99[0.99–1.00] ICC [95%CI]: 0.99[0.99–1.00] ICC [95%CI]: 1.00[1.00–1.00] ICC [95%CI]: 1.00[1.00–1.00]
Wu, 2020 (69)	PsA (*n* = 62); control (*n* = 62)	Inter-reader reliability	Microstructure	CV%: 0.38–1.03
Joint space				
Barnabe, 2013 (12)	RA (*n* = 15); control (*n* = 15)	Intrareader	JSW	CV_{RMS}%: 17.1
Burghardt, 2013 (13)	RA (*n* = 16); control (*n* = 7)	Repositioning and scan/rescan	JSV JSW JSW.SD JSW.Min JSW.MAX JSW.AS	CV_{RMS}%: 3.5 CV_{RMS}%: 2.1 CV_{RMS}%: 10.4 CV_{RMS}%: 12.5 CV_{RMS}%: 2.2 CV_{RMS}%: 13.9
Tom, 2016 (36)	Cadaver (*n* = 7)	Repositioning and scan/rescan	JSV JSW JSW.Min JSW.Max	CV_{RMS}%: 2.2 CV_{RMS}%: 3.8 CV_{RMS}%: 8.0 CV_{RMS}%: 4.4
Stok, 2020 (70)	RA (*n* = 30)	Repositioning and scan/rescan	JSV JSW JSW.Minimum JSW.Maximum JSW.Asymmetry	ICC [95%CI]: 0.99 [0.98–0.99] ICC [95%CI]: 0.95 [0.91–0.97] ICC [95%CI]: 0.66 [0.36–0.82] ICC [95%CI]: 0.73 [0.50–0.86] ICC [95%CI]: 0.75 [0.54–0.87]

ACPA, Anti-citrullinated protein antibodies; BMD, Bone mineral density; CV, coefficient of variance; CIDA, Cortical interruption detection algorithm; eRA, Early Rheumatoid arthritis; ICC, Intra-class correlation coefficient; JSW, Joint space width; JSV, Joint space volume; MTX, Methotrexate; MIAF-finger, Medical Image Analysis Framework – Finger; mESE, modified Evaluation Script for Erosions; PsO, Psoriasis; PsA, Psoriatic arthritis; RA, Rheumatoid arthritis; RMSE, root-mean-square error; $CV_{RMS\%}$*, root mean square coefficient of variance; TNFi, Tumor necrosis factor inhibitors.*

is still limited. The number and volume of erosions have been shown to increase over a 1-year period in ACPA positive individuals with arthralgia but with no sign of arthritis and when compared with an ACPA negative control group (62). Therefore, erosion number and size may be a sensitive measure for early RA progression.

CURRENT LIMITATIONS AND FUTURE DIRECTIONS FOR IMPROVEMENT

Availability of an Accessible Tool for Erosion Quantification

Clinical studies have been successfully performed using HR-pQCT and a variety of custom software packages for analysis. The detection of clinical erosive features is demonstrated, as well as the reproducibility and sensitivity to measure change. However, while erosion volume quantification shows clear promise as an outcome measure, one of the challenges has been the heterogeneity of approaches to identify erosions and measure their size. This also includes distinguishing erosions from other physiological features. An ideal tool would require minimal operator input but allow corrections when necessary. Furthermore, current approaches have been built with a variety of proprietary and/or custom software packages which are typically only accessible to individual research groups. To improve reproducibility and consistency of definitions, as well as the widespread adoption of semi-automated techniques, a new approach must be developed in an open-source, user-friendly software platform. Machine learning approaches may also better automate erosion detection (84).

Segmentation to Assess the Cortical and Trabecular Bone Density and Microstructure

The current standard approach for segmentation to assess bone mineral density and microstructure is a semi-automated slice-by-slice hand contouring approach or semi-automated edge detection algorithm (85). The algorithms were developed for the distal radius and tibia with the assumption that cortical bone is thicker and denser than trabecular bone, which is not necessarily appropriate for the MCP and PIP joints (86). As well, joints with low bone mineral density and high cortical porosity, such as seen in advanced RA, have proven problematic for the algorithms. The presence of cortical breaks and erosions is also problematic for the existing segmentation approaches, i.e., there exists no consensus as to whether the site of an erosion should be included or excluded. Another important consideration for the examined joint is how much of the bone should be segmented, some have used a volume of interest that spans the majority of the metaphysis, and is standardized to be 10% of the metacarpal length (45). However, presently, there is no consensus on this matter.

To date, significant differences in bone mineral density and microstructure between patients with inflammatory arthritis and healthy controls were primarily reported for the trabecular bone compartment. It is possible that further development of the segmentation algorithms and the imaging resolution could improve segmentation accuracy and might reveal greater differences in the cortical bone of inflammatory arthritis patients.

Motion Compensation

One disadvantage of HR-pQCT imaging is that the lengthy, but highly sensitive acquisition process renders it susceptible to motion artifacts, which can impair the ability to accurately and precisely quantify bone and joint outcomes (87, 88). To date, the number of scans excluded for patient motion is rarely reported with sufficient detail, and as such, it is challenging to know the impact of motion on outcomes.

Motion artifact is particularly problematic for longitudinal studies or when implementing more advanced analyses, such as quantifying bone structure, formation, and resorption (89, 90). While this technique holds promise to identify erosions undergoing repair or progression (64), the technique is currently limited to cross-sectional studies because motion artifact typically occurs in the multi-acquisition scan (multi-stack) for joints, and might falsely detect repair or progression. A partial solution to this problem has been implemented by overlapping the acquisitions. However, this simply serves to smooth the effects of motion on scan quality rather than eliminate it (90). Ideally, existing motion compensation algorithms could be implemented in HR-pQCT image reconstruction software to reduce data loss and maximize the utility of acquired data (91, 92).

Joints of Interest

Conventional radiographs assess erosions in 16 joints in each hand and six joints in each foot. Presently, the image acquisition protocol recommended by the SPECTRA Collaboration for the MCP joints specifies that at a minimum, both the 2nd and 3rd MCP should be imaged (93). There is currently no standard image acquisition protocol for the PIP joints. In spite of this, a limited number of published studies have investigated the PIP joint in a similar fashion as the MCP joints (12, 34, 49, 52, 54, 55, 60, 64). The wrist is also examined in multiple studies with the intention of evaluation of bone mineral density and microstructure of the radius, and JSW in the wrist (13). Still, no protocol for assessing erosions in the radius have been published. Whether there is any benefit to include other joints such as the knee, elbow, ankle or foot remains unclear, but are accessible for HR-pQCT imaging. For the HR-pQCT to be a viable modality for assessing progression in clinical practice, further research to explicitly investigate the number and which specific joints needed for the HR-pQCT scanner to have an added benefit compared to CR are needed.

Disadvantages of HR-pQCT Scanning and the Limited Field of View

The HR-pQCT scanner is not widely available to most researchers or clinicians. Presently, HR-pQCT scanners are only developed by Scanco Medical (Bruttisellen, Switzerland). Worldwide only 93 HR-pQCT scanners are installed (46 of the first-generation and 47 of the second-generation), and about 20 research groups use the technology in rheumatological research, this limits the feasibility of implementing the method in clinical practice at this time. However, the existing HR-pQCT models use cone-beam configurations (conical x-ray beam which projects onto a flat panel detector), the term "cone-beam CT" has been adopted in reference to scanners with a very large detector that commonly uses this hardware configuration. Cone-beam CT provides higher spatial resolution at lower costs than conventional multi-detector CT systems (94). Acquisition times can be much faster (<1 min vs. 6 to 9 min) than HR-pQCT due to the larger detector sizes. Improvements to image reconstruction can advance the accuracy of bone microarchitectural measurement to be comparable with HR-pQCT (95, 96). Therefore, cone-beam CT could be a viable modality to complement HR-pQCT imaging, thereby increasing access. The outcome measures described throughout this review could be widely implemented for cone-beam CT. Another limitation of exclusively using HR-pQCT for inflammatory arthritis is the inability to visualize soft tissue and inflammation. Dual-energy CT scans acquire projections at two different energy levels to take advantage of differing attenuation coefficients for different tissues at each energy (97–99). Approaches have been implemented in commercial multi-detector CT scanners (100) and have been used to identify tophi and other crystal arthropathies (101–103), as well as more recently to identify bone marrow edema (104, 105). While not currently available in HR-pQCT scanners, there is the potential that future extremity CT scanners will additionally be able to quantify soft tissue and inflammatory abnormalities.

Using Multi-Modal Imaging to Link Erosive Damage to Inflammatory Markers

Investigators have proceeded with evaluating if HR-pQCT images and findings can be used in conjunction with those obtained using US or MRI to provide a comprehensive overview of soft tissue and bone in the same joint. A complimentary paper on this topic is included in this issue (Tse et al., submitted). In particular, the presence of hyperintense signals on MRI linked to inflammation in RA patients, such as osteitis (106) and synovitis is associated with more pronounced erosive damage in patients with RA (52, 54). In the radius of patients with RA, bone mineral density, trabecular thickness and number were significantly higher, while trabecular separation was lower in regions with MRI-defined osteitis than without (22). Similarly, US Doppler-positive RA patients identified with ultrasound had a lower trabecular number and vBMD alongside higher trabecular separation and distribution of trabecular separation in the MCP joints compared to Doppler negative patients (51).

Education for Patients and Students

Lastly, the use of HR-pQCT imaging as possible pedagogical tool should not be overlooked. The spatial and high-resolution imaging are useful for developing 3D models of the periarticular changes of the joint. 3D printed prototypes of arthritic and healthy joints from HR-pQCT data have been investigated as a tool to demonstrate joint disease to address an eventual gap in patient education and disease understanding (38). The HR-pQCT data have also been used with Virtual Reality application for student training (107).

CONCLUSIONS

In conclusion, owing to the ability to detect change over time periods as short as 3 months, there is a great capacity to utilize HR-pQCT measurements as outcomes in future clinical trials. In addition, HR-pQCT provides uniquely high *in-vivo* sensitivity for erosion detection compared to other modalities. The erosion measures, joint space narrowing, bone density and microstructure have high to excellent reproducibility, whereas osteophytes measure only showed moderate to high reproducibility. The highly sensitive assessment of bone microstructure and damage has the potential to better understand bone changes, particularly in the early stages of inflammatory diseases. Finally, new research developments will improve the accessibility of scanners, the field of view of the imaging, analysis tools such as automatic methods for longitudinally evaluating distinct erosions, as well as the versatility for measuring tissues other than only bone.

AUTHOR CONTRIBUTIONS

RK-J performed the systematic literature review. RK-J and SM drafted the manuscript. All authors contributed conception and design of the review and contributed to manuscript revision, and read and approved the submitted version.

FUNDING

Funding to support the review was provided by a grant from the University of Calgary and Canadian Institutes for Health Research (Planning and Dissemination). JT received salary support from the T. Chen Fong Postdoctoral Fellowship; SM received support from the Arthritis Society Stars Early Career Investigator Award. RK-J received support from Aarhus University, The Danish Rheumatism Association and A.P. Møller Fonden. E-MH received support from the Danish Rheumatism Association and the Novo Nordic Foundation.

REFERENCES

1. Lee CH, Srikhum W, Burghardt AJ, Virayavanich W, Imboden JB, Link TM, et al. Correlation of structural abnormalities of the wrist and metacarpophalangeal joints evaluated by high-resolution peripheral quantitative computed tomography, 3 Tesla magnetic resonance imaging and conventional radiographs in rheumatoid arthritis. *Int J Rheum Dis.* (2015) 18:628–39. doi: 10.1111/1756-185X.12495
2. Nagaraj S, Finzel S, Stok KS, Barnabe C. High-resolution peripheral quantitative computed tomography imaging in the assessment of periarticular bone of metacarpophalangeal and wrist joints. *J Rheumatol.* (2016) 43:1921–34. doi: 10.3899/jrheum.160647
3. Fouque-Aubert A, Boutroy S, Marotte H, Vilayphiou N, Bacchetta J, Miossec P, et al. Assessment of hand bone loss in rheumatoid arthritis by high-resolution peripheral quantitative CT. *Ann Rheum Dis.* (2010) 69:1671–76. doi: 10.1136/ard.2009.114512
4. Stach CM, Bäuerle M, Englbrecht M, Kronke G, Engelke K, Manger B, et al. Periarticular bone structure in rheumatoid arthritis patients and healthy individuals assessed by high resolution computed tomography. *Arthritis Rheum.* (2010) 62:330–9. doi: 10.1002/art.27252
5. Finzel S, Englbrecht M, Engelke K, Stach C, Schett G. A comparative study of periarticular bone lesions in rheumatoid arthritis and psoriatic arthritis. *Ann Rheum Dis.* (2011) 70:122–27. doi: 10.1136/ard.2010.132423
6. Finzel S, Rech J, Schmidt S, Engelke K, Englbrecht M, Stach C, et al. Repair of bone erosions in rheumatoid arthritis treated with tumour necrosis factor inhibitors is based on bone apposition at the base of the erosion. *Ann Rheum Dis.* (2011) 70:1587–93. doi: 10.1136/ard.2010.148395
7. Finzel S, Ohrndorf S, Englbrecht M, Stach C, Messerschmidt J, Schett G, et al. A detailed comparative study of high-resolution ultrasound and micro-computed tomography for detection of arthritic bone erosions. *Arthritis Rheum.* (2011) 63:1231–6. doi: 10.1002/art.30285
8. Zhu TY, Griffith JF, Qin L, Hung VWY, Fong TN, Kwok AW, et al. Bone density and microarchitecture: relationship between hand, peripheral, and axial skeletal sites assessed by HR-pQCT and DXA in rheumatoid arthritis. *Calcif Tissue Int.* (2012) 91:343–55. doi: 10.1007/s00223-012-9644-z
9. Albrecht A, Finzel S, Englbrecht M, Rech J, Hueber A, Schlechtweg P, et al. The structural basis of MRI bone erosions: An assessment by microCT. *Ann Rheum Dis.* (2013) 72:1351–7. doi: 10.1136/annrheumdis-2012-201982
10. Aschenberg S, Finzel S, Schmidt S, Kraus S, Engelke K, Englbrechtl M, et al. Catabolic and anabolic periarticular bone changes in patients with rheumatoid arthritis: a computed tomography study on the role of age, disease duration and bone markers. *Arthritis Res Ther.* (2013) 15:R62. doi: 10.1186/ar4235
11. Barnabe C, Buie H, Kan M, Szabo E, Barr SG, Martin L, et al. Reproducible metacarpal joint space width measurements using 3D analysis of images acquired with high-resolution peripheral quantitative computed tomography. *Med Eng Phys.* (2013) 35:1540–44. doi: 10.1016/j.medengphy.2013.04.003
12. Barnabe C, Szabo E, Martin L, Boyd SK, Barr SG. Quantification of small joint space width, periarticular bone microstructure and erosions using high-resolution peripheral quantitative computed tomography in rheumatoid arthritis. *Clin Exp Rheumatol.* (2013) 31:243–50. doi: 10.1016/j.bone.2010.05.034
13. Burghardt AJ, Lee CH, Kuo D, Majumdar S, Imboden JB, Link TM, et al. Quantitative *in vivo* HR-pQCT imaging of 3D wrist and metacarpophalangeal joint space width in rheumatoid arthritis. *Ann Biomed Eng.* (2013) 41:2553–64. doi: 10.1007/s10439-013-0871-x
14. Finzel S, Kraus S, Schmidt S, Hueber A, Rech J, Engelke K, et al. Bone anabolic changes progress in psoriatic arthritis patients despite treatment with methotrexate or tumour necrosis factor inhibitors. *Ann Rheum Dis.* (2013) 72:1176–81. doi: 10.1136/annrheumdis-2012-201580
15. Finzel S, Rech J, Schmidt S, Engelke K, Englbrecht M, Schett G. Interleukin-6 receptor blockade induces limited repair of bone erosions in rheumatoid arthritis: a micro CT study. *Ann Rheum Dis.* (2013) 72:396–400. doi: 10.1136/annrheumdis-2011-201075
16. Srikhum W, Virayavanich W, Burghardt AJ, Yu A, Link TM, Imboden JB, et al. Quantitative and semiquantitative bone erosion assessment on high-resolution peripheral quantitative computed tomography in rheumatoid arthritis. *J Rheumatol.* (2013) 40:408–16. doi: 10.3899/jrheum.120780
17. Zhu TY, Griffith JF, Qin L, Hung VWY, Fong TN, Au SK, et al. Structure and strength of the distal radius in female patients with rheumatoid arthritis: a case-control study. *J Bone Miner Res.* (2013) 28:794–806. doi: 10.1002/jbmr.1793
18. Kleyer A, Finzel S, Rech J, Manger B, Krieter M, Faustini F, et al. Bone loss before the clinical onset of rheumatoid arthritis in subjects with anticitrullinated protein antibodies. *Ann Rheum Dis.* (2014) 73:854–60. doi: 10.1136/annrheumdis-2012-202958
19. Kocijan R, Finzel S, Englbrecht M, Engelke K, Rech J, Schett G, et al. Decreased quantity and quality of the periarticular and nonperiarticular bone in patients with rheumatoid arthritis: a cross-sectional HR-pQCT study. *J Bone Miner Res.* (2014) 29:1005–14. doi: 10.1002/jbmr.2109
20. Kocijan R, Finzel S, Englbrecht M, Engelke K, Rech J, Schett G. Differences in bone structure between rheumatoid arthritis and psoriatic arthritis patients relative to autoantibody positivity. *Ann Rheum Dis.* (2014) 73:2022–28. doi: 10.1136/annrheumdis-2013-203791
21. Finzel S, Sahinbegovic E, Kocijan R, Engelke K, Englbrecht M, Schett G. Inflammatory bone spur formation in psoriatic arthritis is different from bone spur formation in hand osteoarthritis. *Arthritis Rheumatol.* (2014) 66:2968–75. doi: 10.1002/art.38794
22. Teruel JR, Burghardt AJ, Rivoire J, Srikhum W, Noworolski SM, Link TM, et al. Bone structure and perfusion quantification of bone marrow edema pattern in the wrist of patients with rheumatoid arthritis: a multimodality study. *J Rheumatol.* (2014) 41:1766–73. doi: 10.3899/jrheum.131564
23. Töpfer D, Finzel S, Museyko O, Schett G, Engelke K. Segmentation and quantification of bone erosions in high-resolution peripheral quantitative computed tomography datasets of the metacarpophalangeal joints of patients with rheumatoid arthritis. *Rheumatology.* (2014) 53:65–71. doi: 10.1093/rheumatology/ket259
24. Zhu TY, Griffith JF, Qin L, Hung VW, Fong TN, Au SK, et al. Alterations of bone density, microstructure, and strength of the distal radius in male patients with rheumatoid arthritis: a case-control study with HR-pQCT. *J Bone Miner Res.* (2014) 29:2118–29. doi: 10.1002/jbmr.2221
25. Zhu TY, Griffith JF, Qin L, Hung VWY, Fong TN, Au SK, et al. Density, structure, and strength of the distal radius in patients with psoriatic arthritis: the role of inflammation and cardiovascular risk factors. *Osteoporos Int.* (2014) 26:261–72. doi: 10.1007/s00198-014-2858-3
26. Hecht C, Englbrecht M, Rech J, Schmidt S, Araujo E, Engelke K, et al. Additive effect of anti-citrullinated protein antibodies and rheumatoid factor on bone erosions in patients with RA. *Ann Rheum Dis.* (2015) 74:2151–6. doi: 10.1136/annrheumdis-2014-205428
27. Kocijan R, Englbrecht M, Haschka J, Simon D, Kleyer A, Finzel S, et al. Quantitative and qualitative changes of bone in psoriasis and psoriatic arthritis patients. *J Bone Miner Res.* (2015) 30:1775–83. doi: 10.1002/jbmr.2521
28. Regensburger A, Rech J, Englbrecht M, Finzel S, Kraus S, Hecht K, et al. A comparative analysis of magnetic resonance imaging and high-resolution peripheral quantitative computed tomography of the hand for the detection of erosion repair in rheumatoid arthritis. *Rheumatology.* (2015) 54:1573–81. doi: 10.1093/rheumatology/kev031
29. Töpfer D, Gerner B, Finzel S, Kraus S, Museyko O, Schett G, et al. Automated three-dimensional registration of high-resolution peripheral quantitative computed tomography data to quantify size and shape changes of arthritic bone erosions. *Rheumatology.* (2015) 54:2171–80. doi: 10.1093/rheumatology/kev256
30. Barnabe C, Toepfer D, Marotte H, Hauge EM, Scharmga A, Kocijan R, et al. Definition for rheumatoid arthritis erosions imaged with high resolution peripheral quantitative computed tomography and interreader reliability for detection and measurement. *J Rheumatol.* (2016) 43:1935–40. doi: 10.3899/jrheum.160648
31. Figueiredo CP, Simon D, Englbrecht M, Haschka J, Kleyer A, Bayat S, et al. Quantification and impact of secondary osteoarthritis in patients with anti-citrullinated protein antibody-positive rheumatoid arthritis. *Arthritis Rheumatol.* (2016) 68:2114–21. doi: 10.1002/art.39698
32. Kleyer A, Krieter M, Oliveira I, Faustini F, Simon D, Kaemmerer N, et al. High prevalence of tenosynovial inflammation before

onset of rheumatoid arthritis and its link to progression to RA—A combined MRI/CT study. *Semin Arthritis Rheum.* (2016) 46:143–50. doi: 10.1016/j.semarthrit.2016.05.002

33. Scharmga A, Peters M, van Tubergen A, van den Bergh J, Barnabe C, Finzel S, et al. Heterogeneity of cortical breaks in hand joints of patients with rheumatoid arthritis and healthy controls imaged by high-resolution peripheral quantitative computed tomography. *J Rheumatol.* (2016) 43:1914–20. doi: 10.3899/jrheum.160646
34. Scharmga A, Peters M, van Tubergen A, Van Den Bergh J, De Jong J, Loeffen D, et al. Visual detection of cortical breaks in hand joints: reliability and validity of high-resolution peripheral quantitative CT compared to microCT. *BMC Musculoskelet Disord.* (2016) 17:271. doi: 10.1186/s12891-016-1148-y
35. Shen J, Shang Q, Wong C-K, Li EK, Kun EW, Cheng IT, et al. Carotid plaque and bone density and microarchitecture in psoriatic arthritis: the correlation with soluble ST2. *Sci Rep.* (2016) 6:32116. doi: 10.1038/srep32116
36. Tom S, Frayne M, Manske SL, Burghardt AJ, Stok KS, Boyd SK, et al. Determining metacarpophalangeal flexion angle tolerance for reliable volumetric joint space measurements by high-resolution peripheral quantitative computed tomography. *J Rheumatol.* (2016) 43:1941–4. doi: 10.3899/jrheum.160649
37. Feehan LM, Li LL, McKay HA. Micro-structural bone changes in early rheumatoid arthritis persist over 1-year despite use of disease modifying anti-rheumatic drug therapy. *BMC Musculoskelet Disord.* (2017) 18:521. doi: 10.1186/s12891-017-1888-3
38. Kleyer A, Beyer L, Simon C, Stemmler F, Englbrecht M, Beyer C, et al. Development of three-dimensional prints of arthritic joints for supporting patients' awareness to structural damage. *Arthritis Res Ther.* (2017) 19:34. doi: 10.1186/s13075-017-1234-z
39. Peters M, Scharmga A, De Jong J, van Tubergen A, Geusens P, Arts JJ, et al. An automated algorithm for the detection of cortical interruptions on high resolution peripheral quantitative computed tomography images of finger joints. *PLoS ONE.* (2017) 12:e0175829. doi: 10.1371/journal.pone.0175829
40. Peters M, Scharmga A, van Tubergen A, Arts J, Loeffen D, Weijers R, et al. The reliability of a semi-automated algorithm for detection of cortical interruptions in finger joints on high resolution CT compared to microct. *Calcif Tissue Int.* (2017) 101:132–40. doi: 10.1007/s00223-017-0264-5
41. Scharmga A, Keller KK, Peters M, Van Tubergen A, Van Den Bergh JP, Van Rietbergen B, et al. Vascular channels in metacarpophalangeal joints: a comparative histologic and high-resolution imaging study. *Sci Rep.* (2017) 7:8966. doi: 10.1038/s41598-017-09363-2
42. Shimizu T, Choi HJ, Heilmeier U, Tanaka M, Burghardt AJ, Gong J, et al. Assessment of 3-month changes in bone microstructure under anti-TNFα therapy in patients with rheumatoid arthritis using high-resolution peripheral quantitative computed tomography (HR-pQCT). *Arthritis Res Ther.* (2017) 19:222. doi: 10.1186/s13075-017-1430-x
43. Simon D, Kleyer A, Stemmler F, Simon C, Berlin A, Hueber AJ, et al. Age- and sex-dependent changes of intra-articular cortical and trabecular bone structure and the effects of rheumatoid arthritis. *J Bone Miner Res.* (2017) 32:722–30. doi: 10.1002/jbmr.3025
44. Werner D, Simon D, Englbrecht M, Stemmler F, Simon C, Berlin A, et al. Early changes of the cortical micro-channel system in the bare area of the joints of patients with rheumatoid arthritis. *Arthritis Rheumatol.* (2017) 69:1580–87. doi: 10.1002/art.40148
45. Yang H, Yu A, Burghardt AJ, Virayavanich W, Link TM, Imboden JB, et al. Quantitative characterization of metacarpal and radial bone in rheumatoid arthritis using high resolution- peripheral quantitative computed tomography. *Int J Rheum Dis.* (2017) 20:353–62. doi: 10.1111/1756-185X.12558
46. Yue J, Griffith JF, Xiao F, Shi L, Wang D, Shen J, et al. Repair of bone erosion in rheumatoid arthritis by denosumab: a high-resolution peripheral quantitative computed tomography study. *Arthritis Care Res.* (2017) 69:1156–63. doi: 10.1002/acr.23133
47. Figueiredo CP, Kleyer A, Simon D, Stemmler F, D'Oliveira I, Weissenfels A, et al. Methods for segmentation of rheumatoid arthritis bone erosions in high-resolution peripheral quantitative computed tomography (HR-pQCT). *Semin Arthritis Rheum.* (2018) 47:611–18. doi: 10.1016/j.semarthrit.2017.09.011
48. Ibrahim-Nasser N, Marotte H, Valery A, Salliot C, Toumi H, Lespessailles E. Precision and sources of variability in the assessment of rheumatoid arthritis erosions by HRpQCT. *Jt Bone Spine.* (2018) 85:211–17. doi: 10.1016/j.jbspin.2017.02.011
49. Kampylafka E, D'Oliveira I, Linz C, Lerchen V, Stemmler F, Simon D, et al. Resolution of synovitis and arrest of catabolic and anabolic bone changes in patients with psoriatic arthritis by IL-17A blockade with secukinumab: results from the prospective PSARTROS study. *Arthritis Res Ther.* (2018) 20:153. doi: 10.1186/s13075-018-1653-5
50. Keller KK, Thomsen J, Stengaard-Pedersen K, Nielsen A, Schiøttz-Christensen B, Svendsen L, et al. Local bone loss in patients with anti-citrullinated peptide antibody and arthralgia, evaluated with high-resolution peripheral quantitative computed tomography. *Scand J Rheumatol.* (2018) 47:110–16. doi: 10.1080/03009742.2017.1333629
51. Kong S, Locrelle H, Amouzougan A, Denarie D, Collet P, Pallot-Prades B, et al. Remaining local subclinical joint inflammation is associated with deteriorated metacarpeal head bone microarchitecture in rheumatoid arthritis patients low disease activity. *Joint Bone Spine.* (2018) 85:569–72. doi: 10.1016/j.jbspin.2017.11.010
52. Peters M, van Tubergen A, Scharmga A, Driessen A, van Rietbergen B, Loeffen D, et al. Assessment of cortical interruptions in the finger joints of patients with rheumatoid arthritis using HR-pQCT, radiography, and MRI. *J Bone Miner Res.* (2018) 33:1676–85. doi: 10.1002/jbmr.3466
53. Peters M, de Jong J, Scharmga A, van Tubergen A, Geusens P, Loeffen D, et al. An automated algorithm for the detection of cortical interruptions and its underlying loss of trabecular bone; a reproducibility study. *BMC Med Imaging.* (2018) 18:13. doi: 10.1186/s12880-018-0255-7
54. Scharmga A, Geusens P, Peters M, van den Bergh JP, Loeffen D, Schoonbrood T, et al. Structural damage and inflammation on radiographs or magnetic resonance imaging are associated with cortical interruptions on high-resolution peripheral quantitative computed tomography: a study in finger joints of patients with rheumatoid arthritis and h. *Scand J Rheumatol.* (2018) 47:431–9. doi: 10.1080/03009742.2018.1424234
55. Scharmga A, Peters M, van den Bergh JP, Geusens P, Loeffen D, van Rietbergen B, et al. Development of a scoring method to visually score cortical interruptions on high-resolution peripheral quantitative computed tomography in rheumatoid arthritis and healthy controls. *PLoS ONE.* (2018) 13:e0200331. doi: 10.1371/journal.pone.0200331
56. Simon D, Kleyer A, Englbrecht M, Stemmler F, Simon C, Berlin A, et al. A comparative analysis of articular bone in large cohort of patients with chronic inflammatory diseases of the joints, the gut and the skin. *Bone.* (2018) 116:87–93. doi: 10.1016/j.bone.2018.07.017
57. Simon D, Kleyer A, Faustini F, Englbrecht M, Haschka J, Berlin A, et al. Simultaneous quantification of bone erosions and enthesiophytes in the joints of patients with psoriasis or psoriatic arthritis - effects of age and disease duration. *Arthritis Res Ther.* (2018) 20:203. doi: 10.1186/s13075-018-1691-z
58. Yue J, Griffith JF, Xu J, Xiao F, Shi L, Wang D, et al. Effect of treat-to-target strategies on bone erosion progression in early rheumatoid arthritis: An HR-pQCT study. *Semin Arthritis Rheum.* (2018) 48:374–83. doi: 10.1016/j.semarthrit.2018.05.001
59. Finzel S, Kraus S, Figueiredo CP, Regensburger A, Kocijan R, Rech J, et al. Comparison of the effects of tocilizumab monotherapy and adalimumab in combination with methotrexate on bone erosion repair in rheumatoid arthritis. *Ann Rheum Dis.* (2019) 78:1186–91. doi: 10.1136/annrheumdis-2018-214894
60. Berlin A, Simon D, Tascilar K, Figueiredo C, Bayat S, Finzel S, et al. The ageing joint-standard age- and sex-related values of bone erosions and osteophytes in the hand joints of healthy individuals. *Osteoarthr Cartil.* (2019) 27:1043–47. doi: 10.1016/j.joca.2019.01.019
61. Henchie TF, Gravallese EM, Bredbenner TL, Troy KL. An image-based method to measure joint deformity in inflammatory arthritis: development and pilot study. *Comput Methods Biomech Biomed Eng.* (2019) 22:942–52. doi: 10.1080/10255842.2019.1607315
62. Keller KK, Thomsen JS, Stengaard-Pedersen K, Therkildsen J, Nielsen AW, Schiøtz-Christensen B, et al. One-year progression of erosive disease in patients with anti-citrullinated peptide antibodies and arthralgia. *Joint Bone Spine.* (2019) 87:181–3. doi: 10.1016/j.jbspin.2019.09.006

63. Manske SL, Brunet SC, Finzel S, Stok KS, Conaghan PG, Boyd SK, et al. The SPECTRA collaboration OMERACT working group: construct validity of joint space outcomes with high-resolution peripheral quantitative computed tomography. *J Rheumatol.* (2019) 46:1369–73. doi: 10.3899/jrheum.180870
64. Peters M, van den Bergh JP, Geusens P, Scharmga A, Loeffen D, Weijers R, et al. Prospective follow-up of cortical interruptions, bone density, and micro-structure detected on HR-pQCT: a study in patients with rheumatoid arthritis and healthy subjects. *Calcif Tissue Int.* (2019) 104:571–81. doi: 10.1007/s00223-019-00523-2
65. Shimizu T, Cruz A, Tanaka M, Mamoto K, Pedoia V, Burghardt AJ, et al. Structural changes over a short period are associated with functional assessments in rheumatoid arthritis. *J Rheumatol.* (2019) 46:676–84. doi: 10.3899/jrheum.180496
66. Wu D, Griffith JF, Lam SHM, Wong PCH, Shi L, Li EK, et al. Progressive structural bone changes and their relationship with treatment in patients with psoriatic arthritis: a longitudinal HR-pQCT study. *Arthritis Res Ther.* (2019) 21:265. doi: 10.1186/s13075-019-2043-3
67. Yue J, Lau TCK, Griffith JF, Xu J, Xiao F, Shi L, et al. Circulating miR-99b-5p as a novel predictor of erosion progression on high-resolution peripheral quantitative computed tomography in early rheumatoid arthritis: a prospective cohort study. *Int J Rheum Dis.* (2019) 22:1724–33. doi: 10.1111/1756-185X.13644
68. Simon D, Kleyer A, Bayat S, Tascilar K, Kampylafka E, Meinderink T, et al. Effect of disease-modifying anti-rheumatic drugs on bone structure and strength in psoriatic arthritis patients. *Arthritis Res Ther.* (2019) 21:162. doi: 10.1136/annrheumdis-2019-eular.7249
69. Wu D, Griffith JF, Lam SHM, Wong P, Yue J, Shi L, et al. Comparison of bone structure and microstructure in the metacarpal heads between patients with psoriatic arthritis and healthy controls: an HR-pQCT study. *Osteoporos Int.* (2020) 31:941–50. doi: 10.1007/s00198-020-05298-z
70. Stok KS, Burghardt AJ, Boutroy S, Peters MPH, Manske SL, Stadelmann VA, et al. Consensus approach for 3D joint space width of metacarpophalangeal joints of rheumatoid arthritis patients using high-resolution peripheral quantitative computed tomography. *Quant Imaging Med Surg.* (2020) 10:314–325. doi: 10.21037/qims.2019.12.11
71. Sharp JT, Lidsky MD, Collins LC, Moreland J. Methods of scoring the progression of radiologic changes in rheumatoid arthritis. Correlation of radiologic, clinical and laboratory abnormalities. *Arthritis Rheum.* (1971) 14:706–20. doi: 10.1002/art.1780140605
72. Schett G, Gravallese E. Bone erosion in rheumatoid arthritis: mechanisms, diagnosis and treatment. *Nat Rev Rheumatol.* (2012) 8:656–64. doi: 10.1038/nrrheum.2012.153
73. Geusens P, Van den Bergh J. Bone erosions in rheumatoid arthritis. *Rheumatology.* (2014) 53:4–5. doi: 10.1093/rheumatology/ket358
74. Ten Brinck RM, Van Steenbergen HW, Van Der Helm-Van Mil AHM. Sequence of joint tissue inflammation during rheumatoid arthritis development. *Arthritis Res Ther.* (2018) 20:1–8. doi: 10.1186/s13075-018-1756-z
75. Hetland ML, Ejbjerg B, Hørslev-Petersen K, Jacobsen S, Vestergaard A, Jurik AG, et al. MRI bone oedema is the strongest predictor of subsequent radiographic progression in early rheumatoid arthritis. Results from a 2-year randomised controlled trial (CIMESTRA). *Ann Rheum Dis.* (2009) 68:384–90. doi: 10.1136/ard.2008.088245
76. McInnes IB, Schett G. The pathogenesis of rheumatoid arthritis. *N Engl J Med.* (2011) 365:2205–19. doi: 10.1056/NEJMra1004965
77. Manske SL, Zhu Y, Sandino C, Boyd SK. Human trabecular bone microarchitecture can be assessed independently of density with second generation HR-pQCT. *Bone.* (2015) 79:213–21. doi: 10.1016/j.bone.2015.06.006
78. Conaghan P, Bird P, Ejbjerg B, O'Connor P, Peterfy C, McQueen F, et al. The EULAR-OMERACT rheumatoid arthritis MRI reference image atlas: the metacarpophalangeal joints. *Ann Rheum Dis.* (2005) 64:i11–21. doi: 10.1136/ard.2004.031815
79. Van Der Heijde D. How to read radiographs according to the sharp/van der heijde method. *J Rheumatol.* (2000) 27:261–3. doi: 10.1097/00002281-200007000-00005
80. Neumann G, DePablo P, Finckh A, Chibnik LB, Wolfe F, Duryea J. Patient repositioning reproducibility of joint space width measurements on hand radiographs. *Arthritis Care Res.* (2011) 63:203–7. doi: 10.1002/acr.20374
81. Døhn UM, Conaghan PG, Eshed I, Boonen A, Boyesen P, Peterfy CG, et al. The OMERACT-RAMRIS rheumatoid arthritis magnetic resonance imaging joint space narrowing score: Intrareader and interreader reliability and agreement with computed tomography and conventional radiography. *J Rheumatol.* (2014) 41:392–7. doi: 10.3899/jrheum.131087
82. Crowley AR, Dong J, McHaffie A, Clarke AW, Reeves Q, Williams M, et al. Measuring bone erosion and edema in rheumatoid arthritis: a comparison of manual segmentation and RAMRIS methods. *J Magn Reson Imaging.* (2011) 33:364–71. doi: 10.1002/jmri.22425
83. Hørslev-Petersen K, Hetland ML, Ørnbjerg LM, Junker P, Pødenphant J, Ahlquist P, et al. Clinical and radiographic outcome of a treat-to-target strategy using methotrexate and intra-articular glucocorticoids with or without adalimumab induction: A 2-year investigator-initiated, double-blinded, randomised, controlled trial (OPERA). *Ann Rheum Dis.* (2016) 75:1645–53. doi: 10.1136/annrheumdis-2015-208166
84. Lauze FB, Ren J, Moaddel HA, Hauge EM, Keller KK, Jensen RK. Automatic detection and localization of bone erosion in hand HR-pQCT. In: Hahn HK, Mori K, editors. *Medical Imaging 2019: Computer-Aided Diagnosis (SPIE),* (San Diego, CA), 74. doi: 10.1117/12.2512876
85. Burghardt AJ, Buie HR, Laib A, Majumdar S, Boyd SK. Reproducibility of direct quantitative measures of cortical bone microarchitecture of the distal radius and tibia by HR-pQCT. *Bone.* (2010) 47:519–28.
86. Buie HR, Campbell GM, Klinck RJ, MacNeil JA, Boyd SK. Automatic segmentation of cortical and trabecular compartments based on a dual threshold technique for *in vivo* micro-CT bone analysis. *Bone.* (2007) 41:505–15. doi: 10.1016/j.bone.2007.07.007
87. Pauchard Y, Liphardt AM, Macdonald HM, Hanley DA, Boyd SK. Quality control for bone quality parameters affected by subject motion in high-resolution peripheral quantitative computed tomography. *Bone.* (2012) 50:1304–10. doi: 10.1016/j.bone.2012.03.003
88. Sode M, Burghardt AJ, Pialat J-B, Link TM, Majumdar S. Quantitative characterization of subject motion in HR-pQCT images of the distal radius and tibia. *Bone.* (2011) 48:1291–7. doi: 10.1016/j.bone.2011.03.755
89. Christen P, Boutroy S, Ellouz R, Chapurlat R, Van Rietbergen B. Least-detectable and age-related local *in vivo* bone remodelling assessed by time-lapse HR-pQCT. *PLoS ONE.* (2018) 13:e0191369. doi: 10.1371/journal.pone.0191369
90. Brunet SC, Kuczynski MT, Bhatla JL, Sophie L, Pauchard Y, Salat P, et al. The utility of multi-stack alignment and 3D longitudinal image registration to assess bone remodeling in rheumatoid arthritis patients from second generation HR-pQCT scans. *BMC Med Imaging.* (2020) 20:36. doi: 10.1186/s12880-020-00437-8
91. Sisniega A, Stayman JW, Yorkston J, Siewerdsen JH, Zbijewski W. Motion compensation in extremity cone-beam CT using a penalized image sharpness criterion. *Phys Med Biol.* (2017) 62:3712–34. doi: 10.1088/1361-6560/aa6869
92. Sisniega A, Thawait GK, Shakoor D, Siewerdsen JH, Demehri S, Zbijewski W. Motion compensation in extremity cone-beam computed tomography. *Skeletal Radiol.* (2019) 48:1999–2007. doi: 10.1007/s00256-019-03241-w
93. Barnabe C, Feehan L. High-resolution peripheral quantitative computed tomography imaging protocol for metacarpophalangeal joints in inflammatory arthritis: the SPECTRA collaboration. *J Rheumatol.* (2012) 39:1494–5. doi: 10.3899/jrheum.120218
94. Posadzy M, Desimpel J, Vanhoenacker F. Cone beam CT of the musculoskeletal system: clinical applications. *Insights Imaging.* (2018) 9:35–45. doi: 10.1007/s13244-017-0582-1
95. Mys K, Varga P, Gueorguiev B, Hemmatian H, Stockmans F, van Lenthe GH. Correlation between cone-beam computed tomography and high-resolution peripheral computed tomography for assessment of wrist bone microstructure. *J Bone Miner Res.* (2019) 34:867–74. doi: 10.1002/jbmr.3673
96. Mys K, Stockmans F, Vereecke E, van Lenthe GH. Quantification of bone microstructure in the wrist using cone-beam computed tomography. *Bone.* (2018) 114:206–14. doi: 10.1016/j.bone.2018.06.006
97. Granton PV, Pollmann SI, Ford NL, Drangova M, Holdsworth DW. Implementation of dual- and triple-energy cone-beam micro-CT for postreconstruction material decomposition. *Med Phys.* (2008) 35:5030–42. doi: 10.1118/1.2987668

98. Patino M, Prochowski A, Agrawal MD, Simeone FJ, Gupta R, Hahn PF, et al. Material separation using dual-energy CT: current and emerging applications. *Radiographics*. (2016) 36:1087–105. doi: 10.1148/rg.2016150220
99. Johnson TRC. Dual-energy CT: general principles. *AJR Am J Roentgenol.* (2012) 199:3–8. doi: 10.2214/AJR.12.9116
100. Graser A, Johnson TRC, Bader M, Staehler M, Haseke N, Nikolaou K, et al. Dual energy CT characterization of urinary calculi: initial *in vitro* and clinical experience. *Invest Radiol.* (2008) 43:112–9. doi: 10.1097/RLI.0b013e318157a144
101. Diekhoff T, Kiefer T, Stroux A, Pilhofer I, Juran R, Mews J, et al. Detection and characterization of crystal suspensions using single-source dual-energy computed tomography: a phantom model of crystal arthropathies. *Invest Radiol.* (2015) 50:255–60. doi: 10.1097/RLI.00000000000 00099
102. Davies J, Riede P, van Langevelde K, Teh J. Recent developments in advanced imaging in gout. *Ther Adv Musculoskelet Dis.* (2019) 11:1759720X19844429. doi: 10.1177/1759720X19844429
103. McQueen FM, Doyle A, Dalbeth N. Imaging in gout - what can we learn from MRI, CT, DECT and US? *Arthritis Res Ther.* (2011) 13:246. doi: 10.1186/ar3489
104. Diekhoff T, Scheel M, Hermann S, Mews J, Hamm B, Hermann KGA. Osteitis: a retrospective feasibility study comparing single-source dual-energy CT to MRI in selected patients with suspected acute gout. *Skeletal Radiol.* (2017) 46:185–90. doi: 10.1007/s00256-016-2533-1
105. Jans L, De Kock I, Herregods N, Verstraete K, Van den Bosch F, Carron P, et al. Dual-energy CT: a new imaging modality for bone marrow oedema in rheumatoid arthritis. *Ann Rheum Dis.* (2018) 77:958–60. doi: 10.1136/annrheumdis-2018-213152
106. McQueen FM. Bone marrow edema and osteitis in rheumatoid arthritis: the imaging perspective. *Arthritis Res Ther.* (2012) 14:224. doi: 10.1186/ar4035
107. Kleyer A, Simon D, Hartmann F, Schuster L, Hueber AJ. "Virtual rheumatology": a new teaching concept for rheumatology of the future? *Z Rheumatol.* (2019) 78:112–15. doi: 10.1007/s00393-019-0594-y

14

Artificial Intelligence for Ultrasound Informative Image Selection of Metacarpal Head Cartilage

Edoardo Cipolletta[1*†], *Maria Chiara Fiorentino*[2†], *Sara Moccia*[2,3†], *Irene Guidotti*[2], *Walter Grassi*[1], *Emilio Filippucci*[1†] *and Emanuele Frontoni*[2†]

[1] Rheumatology Unit, Department of Clinical and Molecular Sciences, Polytechnic University of Marche, Ancona, Italy, [2] Department of Information Engineering, Polytechnic University of Marche, Ancona, Italy, [3] Department of Advanced Robotics, Italian Institute of Technology, Genoa, Italy

Correspondence:
Edoardo Cipolletta
edoardocipolletta@gmail.com

†ORCID:
Edoardo Cipolletta
orcid.org/0000-0002-6881-8197
Maria Chiara Fiorentino
orcid.org/0000-0002-7397-803X
Sara Moccia
orcid.org/0000-0002-4494-8907
Emilio Filippucci
orcid.org/0000-0002-7251-7784
Emanuele Frontoni
orcid.org/0000-0002-8893-9244

Objectives: This study aims to develop an automatic deep-learning algorithm, which is based on Convolutional Neural Networks (CNNs), for ultrasound informative-image selection of hyaline cartilage at metacarpal head level. The algorithm performance and that of three beginner sonographers were compared with an expert assessment, which was considered the gold standard.

Methods: The study was divided into two steps. In the first one, an automatic deep-learning algorithm for image selection was developed using 1,600 ultrasound (US) images of the metacarpal head cartilage (MHC) acquired in 40 healthy subjects using a very high-frequency probe (up to 22 MHz). The algorithm task was to identify US images defined informative as they show enough information to fulfill the Outcome Measure in Rheumatology US definition of healthy hyaline cartilage. The algorithm relied on VGG16 CNN, which was fine-tuned to classify US images in informative and non-informative ones. A repeated leave-four-subject out cross-validation was performed using the expert sonographer assessment as gold-standard. In the second step, the expert assessed the algorithm and the beginner sonographers' ability to obtain US informative images of the MHC.

Results: The VGG16 CNN showed excellent performance in the first step, with a mean area (AUC) under the receiver operating characteristic curve, computed among the 10 models obtained from cross-validation, of 0.99 ± 0.01. The model that reached the best AUC on the testing set, which we named "MHC identifier 1," was then evaluated by the expert sonographer. The agreement between the algorithm, and the expert sonographer was almost perfect [Cohen's kappa: 0.84 (95% confidence interval: 0.71–0.98)], whereas the agreement between the expert and the beginner sonographers using conventional assessment was moderate [Cohen's kappa: 0.63 (95% confidence interval: 0.49–0.76)]. The conventional obtainment of US images by beginner sonographers required 6.0 ± 1.0 min, whereas US videoclip acquisition by a beginner sonographer lasted only 2.0 ± 0.8 min.

Conclusion: This study paves the way for the automatic identification of informative US images for assessing MHC. This may redefine the US reliability in the evaluation of MHC integrity, especially in terms of intrareader reliability and may support beginner sonographers during US training.

Keywords: hyaline cartilage, ultrasonography, metacarpal head, artificial intelligence, deep learning, convolutional neural network, rheumatoid arthritis, osteoarthritis

INTRODUCTION

Hyaline cartilage is a highly specialized connective tissue characteristic of synovial joints. Its principal function is to provide low-friction articular surfaces and to act as a shock absorber during the joint movement (1). Hyaline cartilage lacks blood vessels, thus it has a limited capacity for intrinsic healing and repair. In this regard, the integrity of this noble tissue is essential to joint health. The chondrocyte, the unique cell type in adult hyaline cartilage, maintains a stable equilibrium between the synthesis and the degradation of extracellular matrix components. With age and/or in the presence of various rheumatic diseases, such as rheumatoid arthritis and osteoarthritis, this balance is undermined, and the catabolic activity exceeds the anabolic one, thus leading to dehydration, degeneration, and thinning of the cartilage layer (2).

Although conventional radiography is the most adopted imaging method for the assessment of joint damage in daily clinical practice, it provides only an indirect visualization of the hyaline cartilage through the evaluation of the joint space narrowing. The accuracy of conventional radiography has been questioned in non-weight-bearing joints such as the ones of hands and wrists, which are commonly involved in different rheumatic diseases (3, 4). Moreover, in several studies, conventional radiography was found to be less sensitive than ultrasonography (US) in the detection of joint damage (5–11).

Recently, US has been suggested as a reliable and reproducible tool for the assessment of the hyaline cartilage of the small joints of the hand (4, 11–17). One of the main drawbacks of US is its subjectivity in the interpretation of US findings and the consequent variable inter- and intraobserver reliability (18–20). This issue is particularly relevant for the beginner musculoskeletal sonographer (18–20). Thus, the development of a tool that can enhance the US learning process is noteworthy (21).

In the last few years, artificial intelligence has been gaining importance in US, and a number of advantages have been claimed for this alternative method over the conventional acquisition and interpretation of US images, including faster performance, higher reliability and better standardization of image acquisition (22–27). Only a few studies have applied artificial intelligence in the field of musculoskeletal diseases (28–32), and no studies explored the artificial intelligence (AI) in the US assessment of hyaline cartilage, except our previous preliminary work (33).

To date, deep learning (DL) has shown its value in the healthcare domain for computer-assisted medical image analysis (24). DL is a branch of AI, and its algorithms are inspired by human brain, being able to learn from a large amount of data by itself. In fact, DL has the advantage of directly learning image features from raw data, avoiding the need to design hand-crafted features as for traditional machine learning approaches (23). In particular, Convolutional Neural Networks (CNNs), one of the most popular DL algorithms, are widely used for medical image analysis tasks such as classification, segmentation, detection, and biometric measurements, with applications in diagnosis and image-guided interventions and therapy (23). CNNs are able to recognize complex structures in an image by applying convolutional filters (each defined by a kernel matrix) whose weights are iteratively learned during CNN training. Training a CNN relies on labeled data, which are used to learn the mapping from the input to the desired output. Training a CNN from scratch requires a large amount of labeled data, which may not always be available, especially in the medical image analysis domain where image labeling by expert clinicians is a resource-expensive procedure. Moreover, training a CNN from scratch may often lead to overfitting issues (i.e., CNN inability to generalize on new sets of data). A feasible alternative is to exploit transfer learning. Transfer learning consists of extracting knowledge from one task (where large annotated datasets are available) and using the extracted knowledge for a second one. It has been demonstrated that using transfer learning is particularly useful for medical image analysis since limited training data are usually available (34, 35).

Driven by this last consideration, we decided to use transfer learning for training a CNN for US informative-frame selection. We investigated CNNs pretrained on ImageNet, a large image database that includes more than 1 million of annotated natural images (e.g., cats, dogs, cars).

The main aim of this study was to develop an automatic DL algorithm for US informative-image selection of hyaline cartilage at metacarpal head level. An image was defined informative when it shows enough information to fulfill the Outcome Measure in Rheumatology US definition of healthy hyaline cartilage (36). The algorithm performance and that of three beginner sonographers were compared with an expert assessment, which was considered the gold standard.

MATERIALS AND METHODS

Study Design

The study was conducted from January 2019 to March 2020. The study was divided in two steps. In the first one, a CNN algorithm for informative image selection was developed and trained using 1,600 static US images. The US images were acquired by an expert

(E.F.) in musculoskeletal US who evaluated the metacarpal head cartilage (MHC) from the 2nd to the 5th digit bilaterally in 40 healthy subjects.

In the second step of the study, the CNN output was compared with the conventional assessment of the MHC carried out independently by three beginner (E.M., F.F., and J.D.B.) and the expert (E.F.) sonographers. A beginner sonographer was defined as a sonographer with limited experience (<1 year) in the US assessment of hyaline cartilage. MHC from the 2nd to the 5th digit of both hands of eight healthy subjects was independently evaluated on the same day by the beginner and the expert sonographers. The beginner sonographers were asked to provide a set of eight US images per subject (one US image per each metacarpal head) for a total of 192 static images and a set of eight 10-s videoclips on the same healthy subjects for a total of 192 videoclips. A random sample of 128 static images and 64 videoclips were used in the reliability analysis. The US images evaluated by the beginners (each beginner judged a third of the US images) and the videoclips assessed by the algorithm were tested against the expert opinion who had to state whether the US images were informative or not. Expert was blinded to the US images authorship (i.e., beginner sonographer or artificial intelligence algorithm). The time required for each US examination was registered.

Subjects

Healthy subjects were selected from relatives visiting or accompanying in- and out-patients, friends of the authors, and medical students attending the "Carlo Urbani" Hospital (Jesi, Ancona, Italy). Healthy subjects were enrolled because they had the lowest probability to present US abnormalities indicative of cartilage damage. In fact, pathologic findings may generate a bias in the interpretation of US images by both the beginner sonographers and the algorithm.

Exclusion criteria were as follows: (i) previous diagnosis of inflammatory/degenerative arthropathies; (ii) joint pain [visual analog scale (VAS) ≥10/100] and/or analgesic or non-steroidal anti-inflammatory drugs' intake in the 4 weeks preceding the visit; (iii) age <18 years old; and (iv) hard tissue enlargement or deformity of the metacarpophalangeal, proximal, or distal interphalangeal joints suggestive of hand osteoarthritis and/or joint inflammation at physical examination. The following demographic data were recorded: sex, age, handedness, height, weight, and body mass index.

US Image Acquisition and Interpretation

US examinations were carried out using a MyLab Class C (Esaote SpA, Genoa, Italy), equipped with a very high-frequency broadband linear probe (10–22 MHz). A grayscale standard setting was adopted (B-mode frequency: 22 MHz, master gain: 70%, mechanical index: 0.3, dynamic range: 12, depth 15 mm, focus position at the area of interest).

The hands were placed on the table, with the metacarpophalangeal joints in maximal flexion (>60°) (14, 36, 37). The metacarpal head from the 2nd to the 5th digit of both hands was scanned on the dorsal aspect from radial to ulnar and from proximal to distal sides to ensure the maximal exploration of the hyaline cartilage using the EULAR standard scans (38). Particular attention was paid to ensure a perpendicular insonation of the cartilage surface (14, 36, 37).

The normal appearance of the hyaline cartilage is characterized by a homogenous hypo-anechoic layer delimited by two regular, sharp, and bright margins where insonated orthogonally (36, 37). An US image displaying such characteristics was defined informative. The detection in the videoclip by the algorithm or by the expert of at least a frame showing US features of healthy hyaline cartilage was a sufficient criterion to classify it as informative. **Figure 1** provides a pictorial evidence of a healthy MHC.

CNN Algorithm for Informative Frame Selection

A VGG16 CNN, pre-trained on the ImageNet dataset, was used for transfer learning. The VGG16 architecture was chosen for two main reasons: (1) its sequential architecture results to be particularly suitable for small-size training set and low image variability (2, 39) its shallow architecture (only 3 × 3 convolutional layers stacked on top of each other in increasing depth) is associated with low computation cost.

In the original VGG16 architecture implementation, the ImageNet images are processed through 13 convolutional (conv) layers to perform feature extraction. The filters used in each conv layer have very small receptive field (3 × 3) (the smallest size to capture notion about left/right, up/down and center),

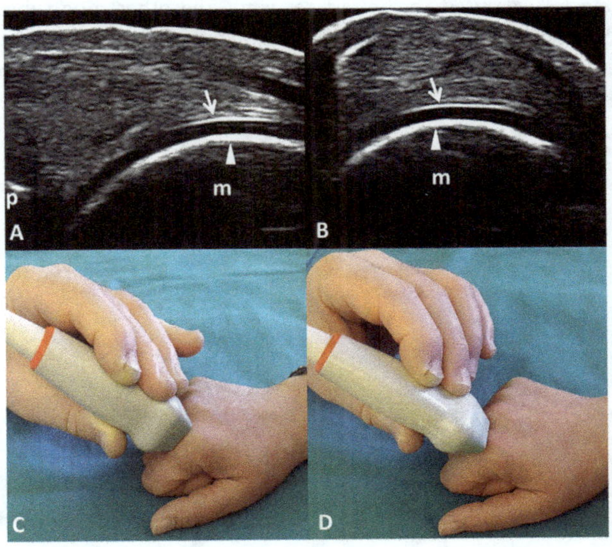

FIGURE 1 | Healthy hyaline cartilage. Dorsal longitudinal **(A)** and transverse **(B)** scans of the hyaline cartilage of the 2nd metacarpal head in a healthy subject. Hyaline cartilage appears as a homogeneously hypo-anechoic layer delimited by two regular, sharp, continuous, and hyperechoic interfaces where insonated orthogonally. Arrows indicate the outer margin (i.e., the chondrosynovial interface); arrowheads indicate the inner margin (i.e., the osteochondral interface). **(C,D)** The position of the probe in the dorsal longitudinal **(C)** and transverse **(D)** scans. m, metacarpal head; p, base of the proximal phalanx.

followed by a rectified linear unit (ReLU) activation function. After the convolutional layers, three fully connected (FC) layers (4,096 neurons in the first two layers and 1,000 neurons in the last one) followed by a softmax layer are used to predict class probability.

In this work, the ImageNet pretrained weights were used as a starting point for the CNN training process. We modified the three FC layers using 1,024, 512, and 2 neurons in the first, second, and third FC layers, respectively, to adapt the architecture to our binary classification problem (informative—non-informative image classification) (**Figure 2**). The architecture was trained freezing the first 10 conv layers and tuning the remaining ones. In this way, we managed to exploit the knowledge encoded in the VGG16 trained on the large ImageNet dataset.

Training Strategy

Prior training the VGG16, US images were resized to 224 × 224 pixels and converted to RGB images, repeating the grayscale channel for three times, to match the image input dimension required by the pre-trained VGG16. Intensity mean was removed from each image.

The mini-batch gradient descent, with a momentum of 0.9, was used as optimizer using the categorical cross-entropy as loss function. The batch size was set to 64 as a balance between training speed and gradient convergence. Training was performed for 100 epochs with a learning rate of 0.0001.

A leave-four-subject out cross-validation was performed for testing the classification. The dataset was divided into 10 subsets of subjects. In turn, one of the 10 subsets (containing four subjects) was used as the test set while the other nine subsets were used as training set. The validation was performed selecting randomly four subjects from the training set, obtaining in such a way 10 models.

The analyses were performed using Keras with TensorFlow library as backend on Google Colaboratory (https://colab.research.google.com/).

Performance Metrics

To measure the performance of our approach, we computed the mean area under the curve (AUC) of the operating characteristic curve (ROC) and the mean classification Precision (*Prec*), Recall (*Rec*), and f1-score (*f1*) for the *i*th class, with $i \in C$ (informative, non-informative), where TP_i, FP_i, FN_i were the true positives, false positives, and the false negatives, respectively.

$$Prec_i = \frac{TP_i}{TP_i + FP_i} \quad (1)$$

$$Rec_i = \frac{TP_i}{TP_i + FN_i} \quad (2)$$

$$f1_i = \frac{2\ x\ Prec_i\ x\ Rec_i}{Prec_i + Rec_i} \quad (3)$$

Statistical Analysis

Results are expressed as number and/or corresponding percentage for qualitative variables and as mean and standard deviation (SD) for quantitative variables. The Chi-square test and the Mann-Whitney test were used to compare the qualitative and quantitative variables, respectively. The agreement in the informative image selection between the expert (i.e., the gold standard) and the algorithm, and between the expert and the conventional assessment of the beginners was calculated using an unweighted Cohen's kappa and interpreted according to Landis and Koch (40).

Two-tailed *p*-values <0.05 were considered significant. Statistical analysis was performed using Statistical Package for the Social Sciences (SPSS) software (version 26.0 for Windows, Chicago, Illinois, USA).

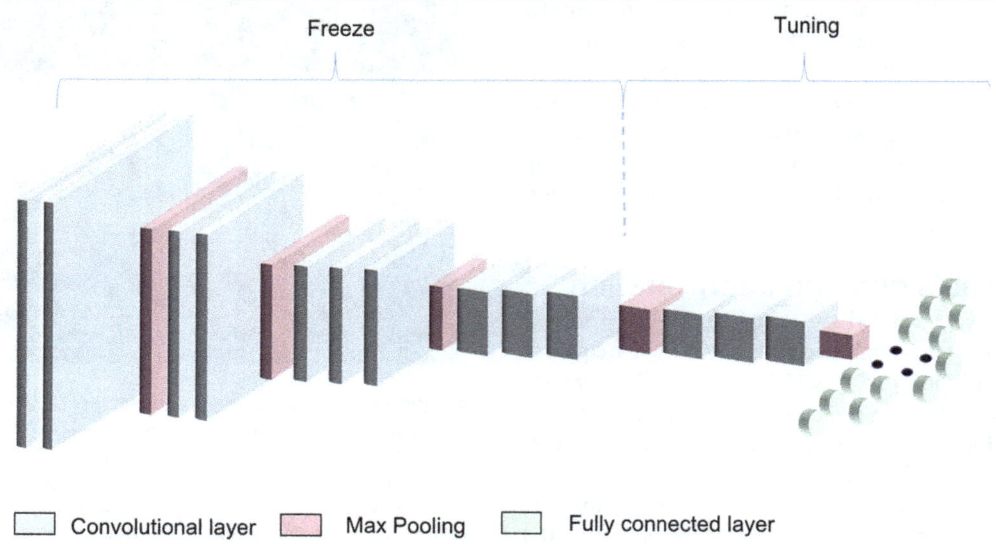

FIGURE 2 | VGG16 transfer-learning strategy. The algorithm was obtained by freezing the first four blocks of the VGG16 pretrained on the ImageNet dataset and training the remaining blocks along with the dense layers.

RESULTS

Subjects

A total of 48 healthy subjects were included in this monocentric and cross-sectional study: 40 in the training and testing of the algorithm (first step) and 8 in the reliability analysis (second step). **Table 1** shows the main demographic characteristics of the participants.

Artificial-Intelligence Algorithm: Training and Testing

In the first step of the study, the VGG16 CNN showed excellent performance in the informative image selection task, with an AUC of 0.99 ± 0.01 (**Figure 3**) computed among the 10 models.

Table 2 shows the classification results for both informative and non-informative frame obtained from the cross-validation procedure.

Figure 4 shows an example of informative and non-informative frames selected by the model that reached the best AUC, which we named "MHC identifier 1."

TABLE 1 | Demographic characteristics of the healthy participants.

Sex (female/male)	33/15
Age (years, mean ± SD)	54.6 ± 5.6
Handedness (right/left)	40/8
Height (cm, mean ± SD)	170.7 ± 9.5
Weight (kg, mean ± SD)	72.4 ± 6.4
Body mass index (kg/m^2, mean ± SD)	24.8

SD, standard deviation.

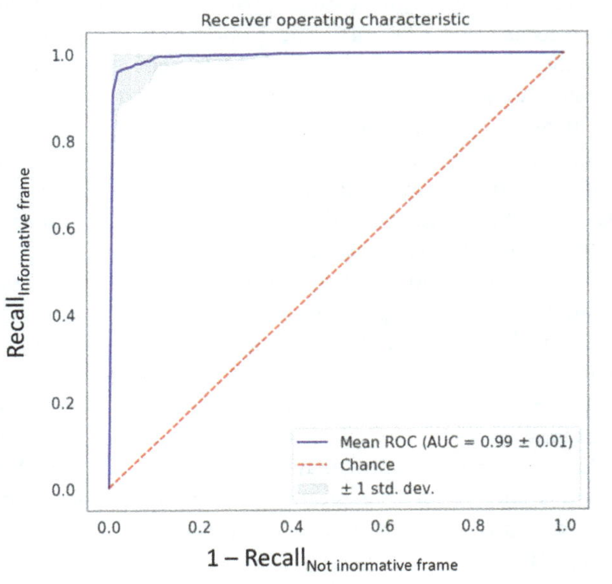

FIGURE 3 | Receiving operating characteristic curve obtained with the fine-tuned VGG16 CNN algorithm "MHC identifier 1." AUC, area under the curve; ROC, receiving operating characteristics; std dev, standard deviation.

Feasibility

The average time required to complete the conventional US assessment was 6.0 ± 1.0 and 4.0 ± 0.5 min for beginners and expert sonographer, respectively ($p < 0.01$). On the other hand, the time spent to acquire the videoclips was 2.0 ± 0.8.

Reliability Analysis

The agreement between the automatic algorithm and the expert sonographer was almost perfect (Cohen's kappa: 0.84, 95% confidence interval: 0.71–0.98); whereas, the agreement between the expert and the beginners using conventional assessment was moderate (Cohen's kappa: 0.63, 95% confidence interval: 0.49–0.76) ($p < 0.01$) (**Table 3**) without significant difference in the interobserver agreement between the expert and each beginner sonographer ($p = 0.14$).

TABLE 2 | Classification metrics for precision, recall, and f1-score, with i ∈ C (informative, non-informative).

	i	Precision	Recall	f1-score
VGG16 CNN algorithm "MHC identifier 1"	Informative	0.94 (0.07)	0.98 (0.02)	0.97 (0.05)
	Non-informative	0.98 (0.02)	0.96 (0.06)	0.97 (0.04)

Values in brackets are the standard deviation.
MHC, metacarpal head cartilage.

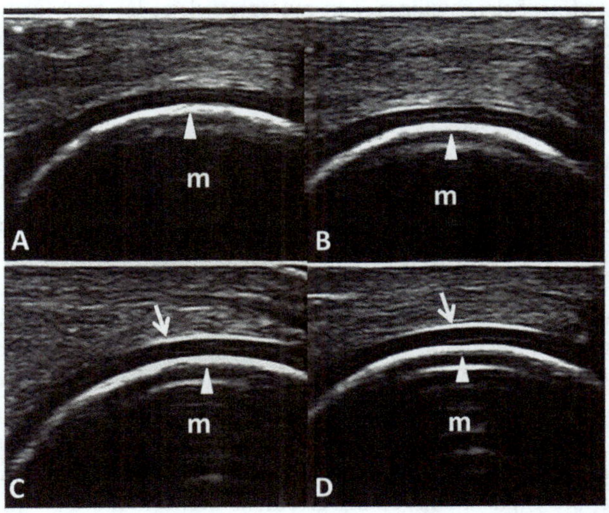

FIGURE 4 | Informative and non-informative US frame selected by the VGG16 CNN algorithm "MHC identifier 1." Dorsal longitudinal scans acquired at the metacarpal head level in healthy subjects. **(A,B)** Examples of non-informative frames; **(C,D)** Examples of informative frames. In fact, while the inner margin (arrowheads) is evident in all the panels, the chondrosynovial (arrows) interface is clearly visible only in the lower images **(C,D)**. m, metacarpal head; arrows, chondrosynovial interface; arrowheads, osteochondral interface.

TABLE 3 | Interobserver agreement.

		Beginners	
US static images (*n* = 128)		**Informative**	**Non-informative**
Expert	Informative	56 (43.8)	8 (6.3)
	Non-informative	16 (12.5)	48 (37.5)
	Total agreement: 81.3%		
		MHC Identifier 1	
10-s videoclips (*n* = 64)		**Informative**	**Non-informative**
Expert	Informative	31 (48.4)	2 (3.1)
	Non-informative	3 (4.7)	28 (43.8)
	Total agreement: 92.2%		

Values in brackets are percentages.
MHC, metacarpal head cartilage; US, ultrasound.
The beginner sonographers and the VGG16 CNN algorithm "MHC identifier 1" agreement with the expert sonographer considered the gold standard.

DISCUSSION

Last-generation US systems allow the real-time identification of otherwise undetectable musculoskeletal abnormalities, which have a growing impact in the management of many rheumatic diseases (41, 42). However, US is a highly operator-dependent technique, and sonographer skills and experience may affect both acquisition and interpretation processes (19, 20). Several international initiatives were undertaken to ensure the standardization of US assessment and to increase its reproducibility in rheumatological setting (36, 38, 43, 44). The use of artificial intelligence in musculoskeletal US may further increase its reproducibility and may save sonographers time as shown in cardiological setting (45).

The correct acquisition of an US image is the essential step to ensure an accurate and reliable assessment of the image itself (31, 39, 46). Thus, we believe that the availability of an algorithm facilitating the identification of the region of interest during the acquisition process of US images represents a further step toward the standardization of US examination.

This study describes the first steps taken to develop an algorithm that can identify informative US images for the assessment of the MHC. The application of such an algorithm, that we called "MHC identifier 1," may redefine the US reliability in the evaluation of the MHC integrity, especially in terms of intrareader reproducibility. MHC identifier 1 showed an almost perfect agreement with the expert sonographer. Here are some possible explanations of disagreement between the algorithm and the expert: while processing an US videoclip, the algorithm may detect even just one frame to define it as informative, which may be missed or considered not relevant by the expert assessment. Conversely, the expert may consider sufficiently assessable US images even if rejected by the algorithm for not strictly fulfilling all the morphostructural criteria. The choice to use both videoclips and static images could be considered a limit of the present study. However, we decided to test the performance of the algorithm using videoclips instead of pictures, since its task will be to support the sonographer during a real-time US examination and not only in the interpretation of static images. Conversely, the sonographer selects a representative US image which conveys the message of a part of the US examination. Finally, according to the data we recorded, the use of this algorithm may shorten the time required to obtain informative US images up to one-third. However, it should be borne in mind that, to date, MHC identifier 1 cannot be routinely applied to clinical practice. In fact, the images must be manually exported from the US system and transferred in a computer where the algorithm can analyze them. A future development may include the incorporation of MHC identifier1 into an US machine to test the clinical value and the feasibility of this method in real-life setting. Thus, the feasibility of this method, including easiness of its use, costs, and availability are yet to be determined.

Our study presents some limitations. First, the same expert sonographer, who served as the imaging "gold standard," was also the teacher and tutor of the beginner sonographers. This fact may imply a possible risk of systematic bias. Second, only a relatively low number of US images were used in the reliability exercise. However, this limit should be read in light of the fact that it is a pilot study. Third, its monocentric design may limit the generalizability of our results. Fourth, the impact of machine-assisted acquisition of US images was not evaluated. Furthermore, the intrareader reliability of both the sonographers and the algorithm was not tested. Finally, the impact of using different US systems needs to be tested, as images in this study were all obtained with the same US system.

The assessment of MHC status is progressively gaining a relevant role in the management of patients with different chronic arthropathies. In fact, in 2019, the Outcome Measure in Rheumatology US Working Group proposed the US definitions of cartilage damage in patients with rheumatoid arthritis and osteoarthritis (36, 44). The same group of experts is currently carrying out a Delphi exercise to define and quantify the structural joint damage (including cartilage lesion) in rheumatoid arthritis by US.

Although preliminary, our results open up new horizons in the use of artificial intelligence in the US evaluation of hyaline cartilage. In fact, the algorithm MHC identifier 1 could enhance the learning process improving the awareness of the beginner sonographer regarding the probe positioning required to obtain images conveying essential information to assess the MHC. In addition, the ability of this algorithm to identify informative frame on videoclips may suggest its use as a tool that could assist the sonographer during the real time US examination.

Further implementation may allow to measure the MHC thickness and to evaluate the hyaline cartilage of other sites commonly involved by rheumatic diseases such as the knee and the hip (16, 17, 47).

The possibility of identifying, evaluating, and measuring the hyaline cartilage in a reliable and faster way may reduce the US examination time, shorten the learning curve of beginner sonographers by taking advantage of AI feedbacks, and promote new studies in this field (e.g., aimed to compare the semiquantitative scoring system of cartilage damage and the quantitative assessment, and to follow-up the progression of cartilage damage).

In conclusion, this study describes the first steps in the development of an algorithm identifying informative US images for assessing the MHC. The automatic selection of US images acquired by beginner sonographers resulted reliable and feasible, as shown by the comparison with an expert sonographer. The application of such an algorithm may redefine the US reliability in the evaluation of the MHC integrity, especially in terms of intrareader reliability and may support beginner sonographers during US training. However, this algorithm needs further validation before its use in clinical practice.

ETHICS STATEMENT

Ethical review and approval was not required for the study on human participants in accordance with the local legislation and institutional requirements. The patients/participants provided their written informed consent to participate in this study.

AUTHOR CONTRIBUTIONS

EC, EFi, MF, and SM substantially contributed to study conception and design, acquisition, analysis, and interpretation of data. IG substantially contributed to acquisition, analysis, and interpretation of data. EFr and WG substantially contributed to analysis and interpretation of data. All the authors revised the paper and approved the final version of the article to be published.

ACKNOWLEDGMENTS

We would like to thank Dr. Jacopo Di Battista, Dr. Francesca Francioso, and Dr. Erica Moscioni for acting as beginner sonographers in the agreement exercise.

REFERENCES

1. Fox SAJ, Bedi A, Rodeo SA. The basic science of articular cartilage: structure, composition, and function. *Sports Health.* (2009) 1:461–8. doi: 10.1177/1941738109350438
2. Pap T, Korb-Pap A. Cartilage damage in osteoarthritis and rheumatoid arthritis-two unequal siblings. *Nat Rev Rheumatol.* (2015) 11:606–15. doi: 10.1038/nrrheum.201595
3. Navarro-compán V, Landewé R, Provan SA, Ødegård S, Uhlig T, Kvien TK, et al. Relationship between types of radiographic damage and disability in patients with rheumatoid arthritis in the EURIDISS cohort: a longitudinal study. *Rheumatology.* (2014) 54:83–90. doi: 10.1093/rheumatology/keu284
4. Mandl P, Supp G, Baksa G, Radner H, Studenic P, Gyebnar J, et al. Relationship between radiographic joint space narrowing, sonographic cartilage thickness and anatomy in rheumatoid arthritis and control joints. *Ann Rheum Dis.* (2015) 74:2022–7. doi: 10.1136/annrheumdis-2014-205585
5. Døhn UM, Ejbjerg BJ, Court-Payen M, Hasselquist M, Narvestad E, Szkudlarek M, et al. Are bone erosions detected by magnetic resonance imaging and ultrasonography true erosions? A comparison with computed tomography in rheumatoid arthritis metacarpophalangeal joints. *Arthritis Res Ther.* (2006) 8:R110. doi: 10.1186/ar1995
6. Wakefield RJ, Gibbon WW, Conaghan PG., O'Connor P, McGonagle D, Pease C, et al. The value of sonography in the detection of bone erosions in patients with rheumatoid arthritis: a comparison with conventional radiography. *Arthritis Rheum.* (2000) 43:2762–70. doi: 10.1002/1529-0131(200012)43:12<2762::AID-ANR16>3.0.CO;2
7. Szkudlarek M, Klarlund M, Narvestad E., Court-Payen M, Strandberg C, Jensen KE, et al. Ultrasonography of the metacarpophalangeal and proximal interphalangeal joints in rheumatoid arthritis: a comparison with magnetic resonance imaging, conventional radiography and clinical examination. *Arthritis Res Ther.* (2006) 8:R52. doi: 10.1186/ar1904
8. Scheel AK, Hermann KGA, Ohrndorf S, Werner C, Schirmer C, Detert J, et al. Prospective 7 year follow up imaging study comparing radiography, ultrasonography, and magnetic resonance imaging in rheumatoid arthritis finger joints. *Ann Rheum Dis.* (2006) 65:595–600. doi: 10.1136/ard.2005041814
9. Funck-Brentano T, Etchepare F, Joulin SJ, Gandjbakch F, Pensec VD, Cyteval C, et al. Benefits of ultrasonography in the management of early arthritis: a cross-sectional study of baseline data from the ESPOIR cohort. *Rheumatology.* (2009) 48:1515–9. doi: 10.1093/rheumatology/kep279
10. Wiell C, Szkudlarek M, Hasselquist M., Møller JM, Vestergaard A, Nørregaard J, et al. Ultrasonography, magnetic resonance imaging, radiography, and clinical assessment of inflammatory and destructive changes in fingers and toes of patients with psoriatic arthritis. *Arthritis Res Ther.* (2007) 9:R119. doi: 10.1186/ar2327
11. Hurnakova J, Filippucci E, Cipolletta E, Matteo Di. A, Salaffi F, Carotti M, et al. Prevalence and distribution of cartilage damage at the metacarpal head level in rheumatoid arthritis and osteoarthritis: an ultrasound study. *Rheumatology.* (2019) 58:1206–13. doi: 10.1093/rheumatology/key443
12. Möller B, Bonel H, Rotzetter M, Villiger PM, Ziswiler H. Measuring finger joint cartilage by ultrasound as a promising alternative to conventional radiograph imaging. *Arthritis Rheum.* (2009) 61:435–41. doi: 10.1002/art24424
13. Filippucci E, da Luz KR, Di Geso L, Salaffi F, Tardella M, Carotti M, et al. Interobserver reliability of ultrasonography in the assessment of cartilage damage in rheumatoid arthritis. *Ann Rheum Dis.* (2010) 69:1845–8. doi: 10.1136/ard.2009125179
14. Cipolletta E, Filippucci E, Matteo Di. A, Tesei G, Cosatti M, Di Carlo M, et al. The reliability of ultrasound in the assessment of hyaline cartilage in rheumatoid and healthy metacarpal heads. *Ultraschall Med.* (2020). doi: 10.1055/a-1285-4602. [Epub ahead of print].
15. Iagnocco A, Conaghan PG, Aegerter P, Moller I, Bruyn GAW, Chary-Valckenaere I, et al. The reliability of musculoskeletal ultrasound in the detection of cartilage abnormalities at the metacarpo-phalangeal joints. *Osteoarthritis Cartilage.* (2012) 20:1142–6. doi: 10.1016/j.joca.2012.07003
16. Cipolletta E, Filippucci E, Matteo Di A, Hurnakova J, Di Carlo M, Pavelka K, et al. FRI0634 standard reference values of metacarpal head cartilage thickness measurement by ultrasound in healthy subjects. *Ann Rheum Dis.* (2019) 78:1014–5. doi: 10.1136/annrheumdis-2019-eular5807
17. Cipolletta E, Hurnakova J, Matteo Di A, Di Carlo M, Pavelka K, Grassi W, et al. Prevalence and distribution of cartilage and bone damage at metacarpal head in healthy subjects. *Clin Exp Rheumatol* (2020). [Epub ahead of print].
18. Hammer HB, Iagnocco A, Mathiessen A, Filippucci E, Gandjbakhch F, Kortekaas MC, et al. Global ultrasound assessment of structural lesions in osteoarthritis: a reliability study by the OMERACT ultrasonography group

on scoring cartilage and osteophytes in finger joints. *Ann Rheum Dis.* (2016) 75:402–7. doi: 10.1136/annrheumdis-2014-206289
19. Gutiérrez M, Di Geso L, Rovisco J, Di Carlo M, Ariani A, Filippucci E, et al. Ultrasound learning curve in gout: a disease-oriented training program. *Arthritis Care Res.* (2013) 65:1265–74. doi: 10.1002/acr22009
20. Gutierrez M, Filippucci E, Ruta S, Salaffi F, Blasetti P, di Geso L, et al. Inter-observer reliability of high-resolution ultrasonography in the assessment of bone erosions in patients with rheumatoid arthritis: experience of an intensive dedicated training programme. *Rheumatology.* (2011) 50:373–80. doi: 10.1093/rheumatology/keq320
21. Filippucci E, Meenagh G, Ciapetti A, Iagnocco A, Taggart A, Grassi W. E-learning in ultrasonography: a web-based approach. *Ann Rheum Dis.* (2007) 66:962–5. doi: 10.1136/ard.2006064568
22. Akkus Z, Cai J, Boonrod A, Zeinoddini A, Weston AD, Philbrick KA., et al. A survey of deep-learning applications in ultrasound: artificial intelligence-powered ultrasound for improving clinical workflow. *J Am Coll Radiol.* (2019) 16:1318–28. doi: 10.1016/j.jacr.2019.06004
23. Liu S, Wang Y, Yang X, Lei B, Liu L, SX Li, et al. Deep learning in medical ultrasound analysis: a review. *Engineering.* (2019) 5:261–75. doi: 10.1016/j.eng.2018.11020
24. Litjens G, Kooi T, Bejnordi BE, Setio AAA, Ciompi F, Ghafoorian M, et al. A survey on deep learning in medical image analysis. *Med Image Anal.* (2017) 42:60–88. doi: 10.1016/j.media.2017.07005
25. Stoel B. Use of artificial intelligence in imaging in rheumatology – current status and future perspectives. *RMD Open.* (2020) 6:e001063. doi: 10.1136/rmdopen-2019-001063
26. Zaffino P, Moccia S, De Momi E, Spadea MF. A review on advances in intra-operative imaging for surgery and therapy: imagining the operating room of the future. *Ann Biomed Eng.* (2020) 48:2171–91. doi: 10.1007/s10439-020-02553-6
27. Moccia S, De Momi E, El Hadji S, Mattos LS. Blood vessel segmentation algorithms - review of methods, datasets and evaluation metrics. *Comput Methods Programs Biomed.* (2018) 158:71–91. doi: 10.1016/j.cmpb.2018.02001
28. Chang RF, Lee CC, Lo CM. Computer-aided diagnosis of different rotator cuff lesions using shoulder musculoskeletal ultrasound. *Ultrasound Med Biol.* (2016) 42:2315–22. doi: 10.1016/j.ultrasmedbio.2016.05016
29. Klauser AS, Franz M, Bellmann WR, Gruber J, Hartig F, Mur E, et al. Contrast-enhanced ultrasonography for the detection of joint vascularity in arthritis - subjective grading versus computer-aided objective quantification. *Ultraschall der Medizin.* (2011). 32:E31–7. doi: 10.1055/s-0031-1281671
30. Chang RF, Lee CC, Lo CM. Quantitative diagnosis of rotator cuff tears based on sonographic pattern recognition. *PLoS ONE.* (2019) 14:e0212741. doi: 10.1371/journal.pone0212741
31. Andersen JKH, Pedersen JS, Laursen MS, Holtz K, Grauslund J, Savarimuthu TR, et al. Neural networks for automatic scoring of arthritis disease activity on ultrasound images. *RMD Open.* (2019) 5:e000891. doi: 10.1136/rmdopen-2018-000891
32. Christensen ABH, Just SA, Andersen JKH, Savarimuthu TR. Applying cascaded convolutional neural network design further enhances automatic scoring of arthritis disease activity on ultrasound images from rheumatoid arthritis patients. *Ann Rheum Dis.* (2020) 79:1189–93. doi: 10.1136/annrheumdis-2019-216636
33. Fiorentino MC, Moccia S, Cipolletta E, Filippucci E, Frontoni E. A learning approach for informative-frame selection in US rheumatology images. In: Autexier S, Campbell J, Rubio J, Sorge V, Suzuki M, Wiedijk F, editors. *Lecture Notes in Computer Science (including subseries Lecture Notes in Artificial Intelligence and Lecture Notes in Bioinformatics).* New York, NY: Springer Verlag (2019). p. 228–36. doi: 10.1007/978-3-030-30754-7_23
34. Esteva A, Kuprel B, Novoa RA, Ko J, Swetter SM, Blau HM, et al. Dermatologist-level classification of skin cancer with deep neural networks. *Nature.* (2017) 542:115–8. doi: 10.1038/nature21056
35. Tajbakhsh N, Shin JY, Gurudu SR, Hurst RT, Kendall CB, Gotway MB, et al. Convolutional neural networks for medical image analysis: full training or fine tuning? *IEEE Trans Med Imaging.* (2016) 35:1299–312. doi: 10.1109/TMI.2016253 5302
36. Mandl P, Studenic P, Filippucci E, Bachta A, Backhaus M, Bong D, et al. Development of semiquantitative ultrasound scoring system to assess cartilage in rheumatoid arthritis. *Rheumatology.* (2019) 58:1802–11. doi: 10.1093/rheumatology/ke z153
37. Torp-Pedersen S, Bartels E, Wilhjelm J, Bliddal H. Articular Cartilage thickness measured with US is not as easy as it appears: a systematic review of measurement techniques and image interpretation. *Ultraschall der Medizin - Eur J Ultrasound.* (2010) 32:54–61. doi: 10.1055/s-0029-1245386
38. Möller I, Jan I, Backhaus M, Ohrndorf S, Bong DA, Martinoli C, et al. The 2017 EULAR standardised procedures for ultrasound imaging in rheumatology. *Ann Rheum Dis.* (2017) 76:1974–9. doi: 10.1136/annrheumdis-2017-211585
39. Patrini I, Ruperti M, Moccia S, Mattos LS, Frontoni E, De Momi E. Transfer learning for informative-frame selection in laryngoscopic videos through learned features. *Med Biol Eng Comput.* (2020) 58:1225–38. doi: 10.1007/s11517-020-02127-7
40. Landis JR, Koch GG. The measurement of observer agreement for categorical data. *Biometrics.* (1977) 33:159–74. doi: 10.2307/2529310
41. Filippucci E, Cipolletta E, Mashadi Mirza R, Carotti M, Giovagnoni A, Salaffi F, et al. Ultrasound imaging in rheumatoid arthritis. *Radiol Med.* (2019) 124:1087–100. doi: 10.1007/s11547-019-01002-2
42. Ruta S, Reginato AM, Pineda C, Gutierrez M. Pan-American League Against Rheumatisms (PANLAR) Ultrasound Study Group. General applications of ultrasound in rheumatology: why we need it in our daily practice. *J Clin Rheumatol.* (2015) 21:133–43. doi: 10.1097/RHU0000000000000230
43. Naredo E, D'Agostino MA, Conaghan PG, Backhaus M, Balint P, Bruyn GAW, et al. Current state of musculoskeletal ultrasound training and implementation in Europe: results of a survey of experts and scientific societies. *Rheumatology.* (2010) 49:2438–43. doi: 10.1093/rheumatology/keq243
44. Bruyn GA, Iagnocco A, Naredo E, Balint PV, Gutierrez M, Hammer HB, et al. OMERACT definitions for ultrasonographic pathologies and elementary lesions of rheumatic disorders 15 years on. *J Rheumatol.* (2019) 46:1388–93. doi: 10.3899/jrheum181095
45. Davis A, Billick K, Horton K, Jankowski M, Knoll P, Marshall JE, et al. Artificial intelligence and echocardiography: a primer for cardiac sonographers. *J Am Soc Echocardiogr.* (2020) 33:1061–6. doi: 10.1016/j.echo.2020. 04025
46. Moccia S, Vanone GO, Momi E, Laborai A, Guastini L, Peretti G, et al. Learning-based classification of informative laryngoscopic frames. *Comput Methods Programs Biomed.* (2018) 158:21–30. doi: 10.1016/j.cmpb.2018.01030
47. Martel-Pelletier J, Barr AJ, Cicuttini FM, Conaghan PG, Cooper C, Goldring MB, et al. Osteoarthritis. *Nat Rev Dis Primers.* (2016) 2:16072. doi: 10.1038/nrdp.201672

15

Novel Muscle Imaging in Infammatory Rheumatic Diseases—A Focus on Ultrasound Shear Wave Elastography and Quantitative MRI

Matthew Farrow[1,2,3], *John Biglands*[2,4], *Abdulrahman M. Alfuraih*[5], *Richard J. Wakefield*[1,2] *and Ai Lyn Tan*[1,2*]

[1] Leeds Institute of Rheumatic and Musculoskeletal Medicine, Chapel Allerton Hospital, University of Leeds, Leeds, United Kingdom, [2] NIHR Leeds Biomedical Research Centre, Leeds Teaching Hospitals NHS Trust, Leeds, United Kingdom, [3] School of Pharmacy and Medical Sciences, University of Bradford, Bradford, United Kingdom, [4] Medical Physics and Engineering, Leeds Teaching Hospitals NHS Trust, Leeds, United Kingdom, [5] Radiology and Medical Imaging Department, Prince Sattam Bin Abdulaziz University, Al-Kharj, Saudi Arabia

***Correspondence:**
Ai Lyn Tan
a.l.tan@leeds.ac.uk

In recent years, imaging has played an increasing role in the clinical management of patients with rheumatic diseases with respect to aiding diagnosis, guiding therapy and monitoring disease progression. These roles have been underpinned by research which has enhanced our understanding of disease pathogenesis and pathophysiology of rheumatology conditions, in addition to their key role in outcome measurement in clinical trials. However, compared to joints, imaging research of muscles is less established, despite the fact that muscle symptoms are very common and debilitating in many rheumatic diseases. Recently, it has been shown that even though patients with rheumatoid arthritis may achieve clinical remission, defined by asymptomatic joints, many remain affected by lingering constitutional systemic symptoms like fatigue, tiredness, weakness and myalgia, which may be attributed to changes in the muscles. Recent improvements in imaging technology, coupled with an increasing clinical interest, has started to ignite new interest in the area. This perspective discusses the rationale for using imaging, particularly ultrasound and MRI, for investigating muscle pathology involved in common inflammatory rheumatic diseases. The muscles associated with rheumatic diseases can be affected in many ways, including myositis—an inflammatory muscle condition, and myopathy secondary to medications, such as glucocorticoids. In addition to non-invasive visual assessment of muscles in these conditions, novel imaging techniques like shear wave elastography and quantitative MRI can provide further useful information regarding the physiological and biomechanical status of the muscle.

Keywords: muscle, myositis, myopathy, MRI, ultrasound, shear wave elastography, imaging, rheumatic

INTRODUCTION

Advances in diagnostic imaging in rheumatology, particularly in the area of arthritis, have contributed to significant clinical benefits to patients and improved knowledge in disease pathogenesis. Despite the usefulness of ultrasound and magnetic resonance imaging (MRI) in diagnosing arthritis and monitoring disease progression in joints and related joint structures, the role of muscle imaging has conventionally been centered around the diagnosis of inflammatory muscle diseases. However, with an increasing appreciation of the impact and prevalence of muscular symptoms in rheumatic diseases (1), and as a result of technological developments, recent attention has been directed toward the utility of imaging for the assessment of muscle pathology in rheumatic diseases.

The impact of muscle weakness is significant for the health of patients and is associated with disease activity (2). There is an unmet need for further understanding of more generalized muscle pathology observed in rheumatic diseases. This is required to develop effective future strategies to target this under-researched area. In addition to ultrasound and MRI, positron emission tomography combined with computed tomography (PET-CT) is increasingly used in clinical practice to aid the diagnosis of myositis, with the added advantage that this technique can screen for malignancy and evaluate related pulmonary pathologies (3, 4). This perspective will discuss recent novel imaging developments in ultrasound and MRI for the assessment of muscles in common inflammatory rheumatic diseases, with a particular focus on research applicability of shear wave elastography and quantitative MRI in improving the knowledge of muscle pathology in rheumatic diseases. The potential application of these novel techniques will be explored in the context of three common inflammatory rheumatology conditions where the muscle is of interest. The first is in myositis, a primary inflammatory condition of the muscle; the second is in glucocorticoid-induced myopathy, where patients with giant cell arteritis and polymyalgia rheumatica are at risk from the complications of prolonged high dose steroid therapy; and the third is rheumatoid arthritis where patients often complain of muscle related symptoms in addition to their joints.

MUSCLE IMAGING TECHNIQUES

Ultrasound

Due to recent innovations, ultrasonography has evolved from demonstrating mainly anatomical details to elucidating the physical properties of tissues. Although B-mode ultrasonography has been shown to be reliable in assessing muscle mass and quality (5–7), and muscle fibers during dynamic scanning (8, 9), recent interest has been directed to a new type of ultrasound called elastography (10). This technique provides a measure of the stiffness of tissue (11). The first generation machines, developed in the 1990's utilized "strain elastography," where a mechanical ultrasound pulse was generated by repeated probe compressions on the skin by the operator. The returned waves could be used to qualitatively estimate stiffness by comparing the pre- and post-compression tissue deformations. The images were represented as a color map, superimposed on a B-mode image (blue—hard, and red—soft). Shear wave elastography (SWE) has more recently been introduced to offer quantitative measurements by monitoring the velocity of the shear waves generated by strong acoustic pulses. The physics behind shear waves is complex and beyond the scope of this article, but essentially, the velocity of the shear wave increases proportionally with Young's elasticity modulus. SWE is less operator dependent than strain elastography, and offers more objective outcomes. Hence, this perspective will focus on the potential uses of SWE, which has more commonly been established for examining breast, liver, thyroid and prostate tissues (12–14).

In the musculoskeletal setting, SWE has largely been used to study tendinopathies (15, 16). More recently however, SWE has been extended to examining muscles, and has been shown to be a reliable tool to measure muscle stiffness (17–19). The technique has been used in the sports and exercise scenarios, to assess muscle injuries and the effect of exercise interventions on muscles (20, 21). Clinically, SWE of muscles, such as of the rotator cuff muscles that are commonly susceptible to tears, has been shown to inform appropriate management strategies (22). In the hospital setting, it has shown good reliability for monitoring the muscles of critically ill patients (23). Other clinical uses of SWE are in the assessment of the muscles in neuromuscular conditions including Parkinson's disease, Duchene muscular dystrophy, and in post-stroke spasticity (24–26). Insight into the potential of using SWE in assessing muscle elasticity has prompted recommendations into standardizing the technique for optimal data acquisition (27–29). It is known that muscles change with age, which is apparent in the structure and the function of the muscles (30, 31). Although some studies using SWE have shown that there is a decline in muscle stiffness with age (32–35), this observation was not corroborated by others (36–38). These studies looked at different muscles, which may have influenced the final outcomes, as it has been found that SWE findings may be muscle-dependent (39).

MRI

MRI offers the ability to examine deeper tissue structures compared to ultrasound. Although MRI can also measure the elasticity of muscles using magnetic resonance elastography (40–44), the cost of the technique is more prohibitive when compared to SWE; thus far, the utility of MRI in assessing muscle elasticity is still debatable (45).

Due to its excellent spatial and contrast resolution, MRI can evaluate a wide array of muscle pathologies including muscle injury (46) and soft tissue masses (47). MRI is beginning to have a role in the diagnosis and monitoring of muscle disease and in guiding muscle biopsy (48, 49). Whole-body MRI can help identify muscular involvement over large anatomical regions (50, 51). Aside from conventional MRI there is also an important role for quantitative MRI (qMRI) measurements, such as fat fraction, T2 measurement and diffusion tensor imaging (DTI), in muscle imaging. Quantitative MRI can provide information about tissue microstructure that may not be apparent in conventional MRI. It provides objective measurements, as opposed to a qualitative

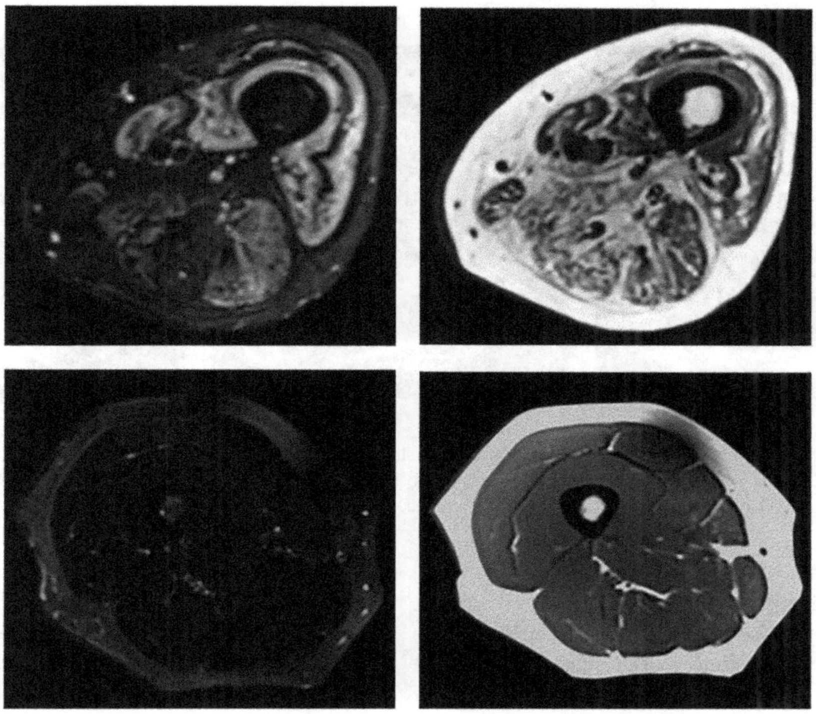

FIGURE 1 | Conventional MRI of the right thigh in **(A)** T2-STIR and **(B)** T1-weighted images of a 60-years-old male with active myositis, compared to **(C)** T2-STIR and **(D)** T1-weighted images of a 45-years-old healthy female.

assessment and has been shown to be reliable and reproducible in the muscle (52, 53).

Fat fraction measurements exploit the differences in the resonant frequencies between the MR signals of fat and water in order to generate a measurement of the proportion of fat in each voxel in the image (54). These measurements provide an objective assessment of fatty infiltration in muscle, which is a common pathology in muscle disease.

Measurements of the T2-relxation time also have applications in the muscle. T2, or the spin-spin relaxation time, is one of the fundamental contrast mechanisms in MRI. By measuring the signal at multiple echo times, measurements of T2 can be made within the muscle. Raised T2 is often interpreted as increased fluid due to edema or inflammation. However, care must be taken in the interpretation of T2. Fat can also increase T2 values and fat suppression is challenging in T2 measurements (55, 56), with some papers arguing that T2 may actually decrease with disease activity (57).

Diffusion MRI is able to measure water diffusion in the muscle. Diffusion measurements in inflamed muscle may be greater due to increased fluid in the extracellular space. Diffusion tensor imaging (DTI) allows the anisotropy of the diffusion to be assessed. As muscle is made up of long fibers, or fibrils, muscle diffusion is highly anisotropic and ordered. As muscle diameters are relatively wide, long diffusion times are necessary if the measurements are to be sensitive to restricted diffusion across the fiber. Fiber disorganization and deterioration through trauma or disease can be detected by DTI measurements, such as fractional anisotropy (FA) (26). However, the interpretation of what a change in diffusion measurement means is difficult. Fiber disorder, fiber density, fiber diameter (58, 59) and changes in extracellular water (60) can all affect diffusion parameters. There is on-going research into the use of modeling to analyse DTI acquisitions at multiple diffusion times to separate out different properties of the muscle microstructure from diffusion measurements (61–63).

In the clinical setting, qMRI of various tissues including muscles shows potential as a promising biomarker for assessing and monitoring a range of neuromuscular and musculoskeletal diseases (57, 64–68). In general, these patients show higher muscle fat fractions, smaller muscle volume, and increased T2 measures, which also correlate with muscle function (69).

MUSCLE IMAGING IN INFLAMMATORY RHEUMATIC DISEASES

Myositis

The idiopathic inflammatory myopathies (IIM) are the commonest inflammatory muscle diseases seen by rheumatologists. They are a heterogeneous group of autoimmune inflammatory muscle conditions comprising mainly of dermatomyositis and polymyositis, which present with muscle weakness, raised muscle enzymes, abnormal electromyography (EMG), abnormal muscle biopsies and myositis-related antibodies (70).

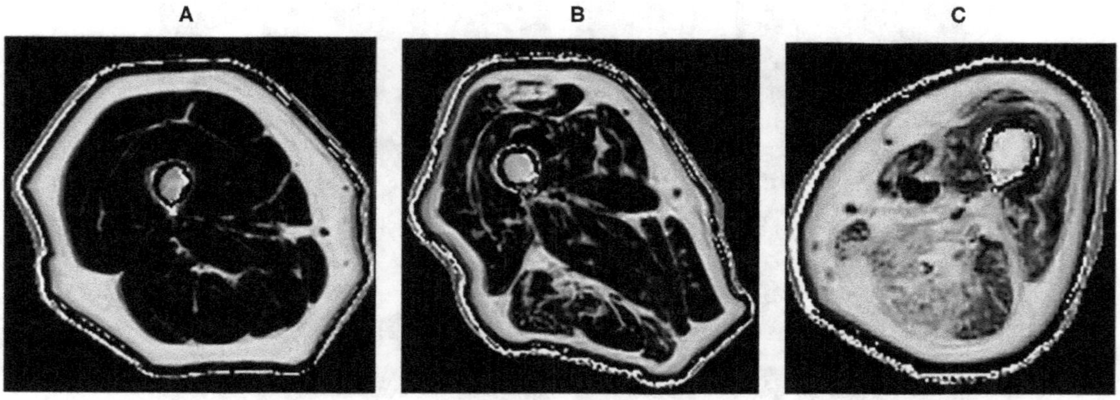

FIGURE 2 | Quantitative MRI fat fraction measurement in the quadriceps and hamstrings, respectively in the thigh in **(A)** 45-years-old healthy female with a fat fraction of 1.9 and 2.7%, respectively, **(B)** 83-years-old healthy male presenting with fatty infiltration associated with healthy aging with a fat fraction of 9.6 and 13.4%, respectively, **(C)** 60-years-old male with active myositis presenting with fatty infiltration with a fat fraction of 19.6 and 28.5%, respectively.

MRI has become an integral imaging tool in the clinical diagnosis and monitoring of disease activity of myositis due to its ability to non-invasively detect abnormal muscles and identify the most suitable site for muscle biopsies (**Figure 1**) (45, 71–74). Reassuringly, MRI findings in myositis correlate well with biopsy results (75), and whole body MRI can be more sensitive than muscle enzymes and EMG in diagnosing myositis (76). Nevertheless, the image interpretation can be subjective (77), there is no validated MRI protocol for assessing myositis (45) and MRI findings in isolation may not be specific enough for diagnostic purposes (78).

Quantitative MRI, which allows further characterization of the muscle structure at a microscopic level, can provide a more precise description of muscle pathology (55, 73, 79). It could potentially be used in longitudinal monitoring of disease (80). It has been demonstrated that T2 and fat fraction increase in myositis patients (**Figure 2**), demonstrating that MRI is sensitive enough to quantitatively detect muscle edema (55, 81) and myosteatosis (82). These measures could be used to more accurately guide muscle biopsies. This may be of greater importance in patients with low grade inflammation, where there are subtle muscle changes that might go undetected by conventional MRI. DTI measurements are sensitive to subtle changes in the muscle, and have been used to detect differences in muscle due to diseases including myositis (83). However, muscle DTI is far from standardized. The optimal methods and parameters for performing diffusion in muscle have not been established and larger studies are necessary to establish whether diffusion will be a useful tool for monitoring muscle disease in clinical practice.

One of the drawbacks of MRI as an imaging tool is its cost. Often, this is the deciding factor in choosing ultrasonography over MRI as a more feasible modality in assessing articular joints. But does this cost consideration translate to examining muscles or in patients with myositis? In addition to the more favorable cost compared to MRI, ultrasound also has a greater acceptability by patients. Although there is greater operator dependence for ultrasound, there is the possibility to apply the ultrasound information directly in the clinical setting. There is a suggestion that ultrasound elastography of muscles may be able to aid diagnosis of myositis and its follow-up (84), but the impression is that ultrasound is unlikely to replace MRI in the clinical setting in myositis just yet, because the current evidence is not strong, due to small sample sized studies that results in inconclusive findings (85).

Nevertheless, the current evidence suggests that SWE shows less muscle stiffness in myositis compared to healthy individuals (**Figure 3**), and can distinguish myositis from normal muscles (86). The loss of muscle stiffness in myositis patients was also observed using magnetic resonance elastography (87). SWE measurements also correlate with muscle strength and MRI grades of edema and atrophy (86, 88). All of these findings appear to only manifest when the muscles are under no passive or active loading.

IIM can be a very disabling condition. The potential to use promising non-invasive diagnostic and monitoring tools like qMRI and SWE could facilitate prompt diagnosis and treatment for patients. In the diagnosis of giant cell arteritis (GCA) (89), ultrasound can now reliably replace invasive temporal artery biopsies in GCA diagnosis. Similarly, the continuing development of qMRI and SWE of muscle could 1 day replace muscle biopsy in the diagnosis of IIM.

Steroid Myopathy

Glucocorticoids are powerful anti-inflammatory agents and have a variety of uses in rheumatology, most commonly as bridging therapy before other longer term treatments are started. Polymyalgia rheumatic (PMR) and the related GCA are two examples where high doses of steroids are prescribed. As a result, many often develop a proximal myopathy, without typical inflammatory laboratory markers, such as muscle enzyme abnormalities or myositis-related antibodies. These patients are often disabled by muscle weakness from the disease process. It would, therefore, be reasonable to hypothesize that, despite

A

B

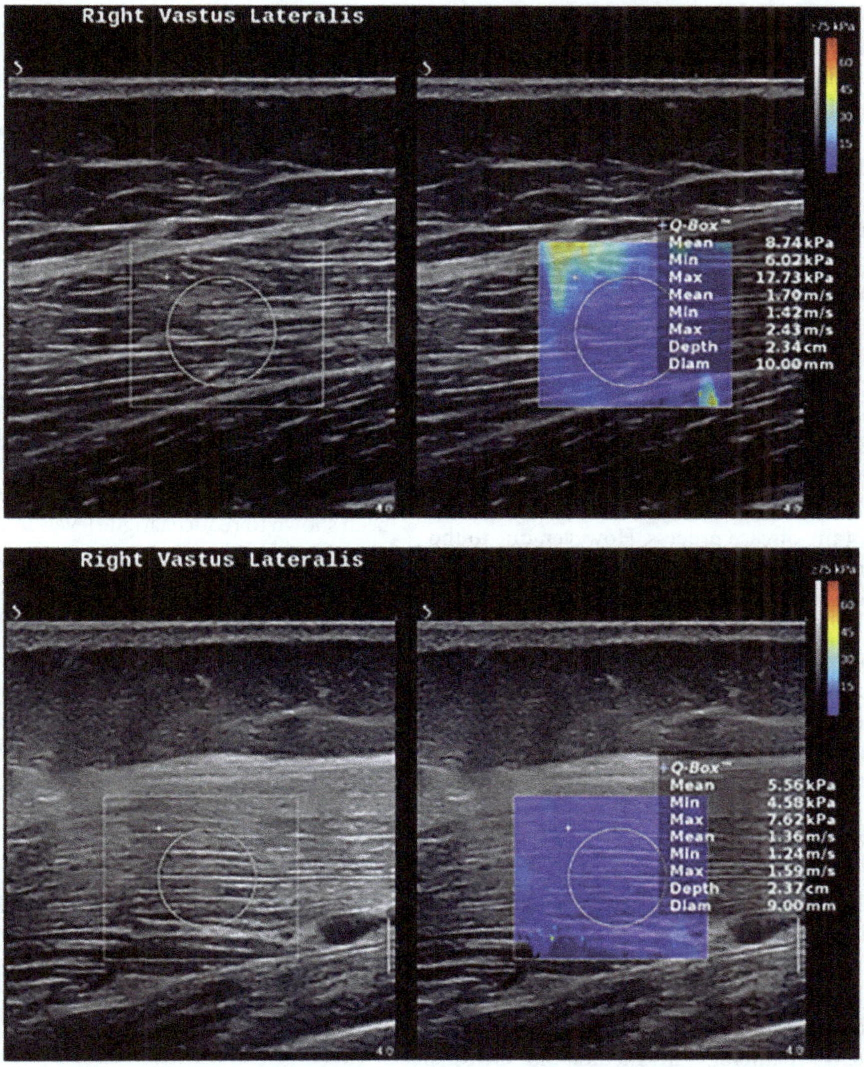

FIGURE 3 | Shear wave elastography in healthy muscles and myositis. **(A)** Shows a normal muscle stiffness (8.7 kPa) in a 50-year-old healthy female person. **(B)** Shows a low muscle stiffness (5.5 kPa) in a 49-year-old male with active polymyositis.

not demonstrating a classical myositic picture with abnormal blood markers, muscles in PMR and GCA are likely to be abnormal.

There may be a fine line between the effects of inflammation from disease (PMR and GCA) and the catabolic effects of therapy (steroids) on muscle in patients. Amongst the many adverse effects of glucocorticoids, they trigger muscle atrophy, with a particular affinity for the atrophy of fast-twitch or type II muscle fibers (90, 91). This will often present as myopathy or muscle weakness, but due to the lack of a standardized definition of glucocorticoid-induced myopathy, reporting of myopathy due to therapy in PMR and GCA can prove inconsistent (92). Therefore, the management of steroid-induced myopathy can be challenging due to the difficulty in identifying myopathy before any clinical symptoms with the current means of investigation (93).

Can imaging help in characterizing the myopathy in this group of patients? Very little research in this area has been performed. Most studies have been focused on the diagnosis of PMR and GCA and responses to steroid therapy, based mainly on joint findings (94–97). Certainly, studies have demonstrated that quantitative ultrasound was able to show muscle changes associated to chronic use of steroids, but was unable to tell if the observed changes could be due to other causes including cachexia or sarcopenia (98, 99). A recent study showed that SWE detected a higher reduction in muscle stiffness over time in GCA patients on long term glucocorticoid who were also weaker (100). However, as patients with GCA (and PMR) tend to be older, and therefore more likely to be sarcopenic, these observed muscle changes have to be interpreted cautiously. If future research shows that SWE changes could potentially be evident before patients present with signs of weakness, then we may have an imaging tool that can direct appropriate management of steroid-induced myopathy, including preventative strategies to preserve muscle function.

The fact that type II muscle fibers tend to be affected by steroid therapy suggests that techniques like MRI diffusion tensor imaging that are sensitive to changes in muscle microstructure could be potentially useful in understanding the pathogenesis of steroid-induced myopathy and its diagnosis (80, 101). Due to the inflammatory nature of PMR and GCA, T2 MRI could be able to identify the edema within the muscle itself, which could be contributing to pain and fatigue. The muscle atrophy due to the catabolic effects of glucocorticoids could be quantitatively measured to monitor muscle change over time. The challenge will be interpreting the findings and to tease out if the observed imaging changes are due to therapy (glucocorticoids), or to the inflammatory disease process. Previously, when patients with RA were treated with long term steroids, it was possible to tell when they had weaker strength compared to patients who did not receive steroid therapy (102, 103). This would have provided a useful cohort to compare imaging findings of the muscle, and changes could be attributed to the steroid therapy independent of the disease process. However, due to the complexities of modern therapy and the ethical limitations, such direct comparison studies may not be feasible. Another iatrogenic cause of myopathy is in IIM treated with glucocorticoids, which presents another challenging dilemma in differentiating between muscle changes due to therapy and that due to the inflammatory muscle disease *per se*. This proposes an unmet need for means to identify the exact cause of the myopathy to optimize management—an area for further exploration of imaging as a potential tool for this purpose.

Nevertheless, qMRI can differentiate the muscle properties between the ages and has been shown to correlate with muscle outcome measures. Therefore, it shows potential promise as a tool to help understand the varying factors that can affect muscle in rheumatic diseases (104).

Rheumatoid Arthritis

The predominant site of pathology in rheumatoid arthritis is in the joints. The articular joints are therefore the most commonly imaged structure in RA. However, there are many reasons for patients with RA to have weaker muscles, including impaired physical function and a greater tendency toward physical inactivity (105, 106). RA patients often present with lower muscle mass (107), which remains apparent in remission (105). A large proportion of RA patients report experiencing muscle problems or myopathy (108, 109). Histologically, RA is also associated with atrophy of type II muscle fibers, similar to the effects of glucocorticoids on muscle (110, 111). In addition, the pro-inflammatory state in inflammatory arthritis predisposes patients to a cachectic body composition—another reason for abnormal muscles in inflammatory arthritis (112, 113).

Despite the many causes of muscle involvement in inflammatory arthritis, there are relatively little muscle imaging data in RA. Reduced muscle strength is associated with disease activity in RA, and muscle function and physical activity are modifiable factors (2). Preliminary SWE of the muscles in RA shows some indication that muscles are less stiff compared to healthy individuals, but the results do not show statistical significance despite the fact that RA patients show reduced strength (114). The lack of differential findings from SWE studies suggests that muscle pathology in RA is less likely to be due to biomechanical properties of muscle. Quantitative MRI offers a different imaging perspective of muscle, and can provide further insight into the pathogenesis of muscle pathology in RA. Indeed, qMRI could be used to identify if rheumatic patients in remission still have muscle pathology, such as inflammation or fatty infiltration. This would identify whether effective treatment is improving muscle health, or if additional interventions, such as exercise, should be developed for a more holistic approach in patients with inflammatory arthritis.

Fatigue is a common symptom in many rheumatic conditions including inflammatory arthritis with significant impact on patients' lives (115). Although treatment including biological therapy can help improve symptoms of fatigue, they are not effective in all patients (116). Of note is that exercise has also been shown to reduce fatigue levels in RA (117); this suggests that modifying the muscles in inflammatory arthritis is a potential route to improving symptoms in patients. This is an area where the mechanism of action needs clarifying—an important cue for imaging, such as SWE and qMRI to help provide some insights.

FUTURE PERSPECTIVES AND CONCLUSIONS

The capabilities of novel imaging in muscle continue to be stretched to better understand the significance of the observations. Quantitative ultrasonographic techniques, such as muscle echo-intensity may reveal useful imaging biomarkers beyond the mechanical properties of SWE (88). The use of both SWE and qMRI in assessing muscles are relatively recent imaging advances. Due to the heterogeneous nature of muscle involvement in rheumatic diseases, a multi-parametric imaging approach may offer a clearer picture of the varying disease processes (118). Combining both techniques could result in a more powerful imaging combination that provides complementary understanding of muscle changes (119). The application of artificial intelligence (AI) in imaging in rheumatology has enhanced efficacy and efficiency in image interpretation (120). Unsurprisingly, AI in rheumatology imaging is currently confined to assessing the common joint abnormalities like joint synovitis, tenosynovitis, bone erosions and cartilage loss. Deep learning involving qMRI and SWE may accelerate the knowledge and application of these imaging techniques.

This perspective highlights that the involvement of muscle is widespread in many rheumatic diseases, which can also affect other conditions including the connective tissue diseases like systemic lupus erythematosus, Sjogren's syndrome and systemic sclerosis (1). Imaging, in particular the more recent novel techniques like SWE and qMRI, shows potential to improve the understanding of how muscle is affected in rheumatic diseases. Imaging has an important role in assessing potential interventions on preserving muscle function. Imaging has improved our knowledge of joint abnormalities, but it is now timely for a call to action for a more anatomically-holistic approach toward the understanding of the pathogenesis of rheumatic diseases, with due attention to the muscle.

AUTHOR CONTRIBUTIONS

MF and AT wrote the first draft of the manuscript. JB, RW, and AA edited and revised the manuscript. MF, JB, and AA contributed the figures. All authors revised the manuscript critically and approved the final version of the manuscript. All authors contributed to the article and approved the submitted version.

REFERENCES

1. Altabas-Gonzalez I, Perez-Gomez N, Pego-Reigosa JM. How to investigate: suspected systemic rheumatic diseases in patients presenting with muscle complaints. *Best Pract Res Clin Rheumatol.* (2019) 33:101437. doi: 10.1016/j.berh.2019.101437
2. Uutela TI, Kautiainen HJ, Hakkinen AH. Decreasing muscle performance associated with increasing disease activity in patients with rheumatoid arthritis. *PLoS ONE.* (2018) 13:e0194917. doi: 10.1371/journal.pone.0194917
3. Kubínová K, Dejthevaporn R, Mann H, Machado PM, Vencovský J. The role of imaging in evaluating patients with idiopathic inflammatory myopathies. *Clin Exp Rheumatol.* (2018) 36:74–81. Available online at: https://www.clinexprheumatol.org/abstract.asp?a=13317
4. Selva-O'Callaghan A, Gil-Vila A, Simó-Perdigó M, Trallero-Araguás E, Alvarado-Cárdenas M, Pinal-Fernandez I. PET scan: nuclear medicine imaging in myositis. *Curr Rheumatol Rep.* (2019) 21:64. doi: 10.1007/s11926-019-0864-3
5. Mourtzakis M, Parry S, Connolly B, Puthucheary Z. Skeletal muscle ultrasound in critical care: a tool in need of translation. *Ann Am Thorac Soc.* (2017) 14:1495–503. doi: 10.1513/AnnalsATS.201612-967PS
6. Scott JM, Martin DS, Ploutz-Snyder R, Caine T, Matz T, Arzeno NM, et al. Reliability and validity of panoramic ultrasound for muscle quantification. *Ultrasound Med Biol.* (2012) 38:1656–61. doi: 10.1016/j.ultrasmedbio.2012.04.018
7. Berger J, Bunout D, Barrera G, de la Maza MP, Henriquez S, Leiva L, et al. Rectus femoris (RF) ultrasound for the assessment of muscle mass in older people. *Arch Gerontol Geriatr.* (2015) 61:33–8. doi: 10.1016/j.archger.2015.03.006
8. van Hooren B, Teratsias P, Hodson-Tole EF. Ultrasound imaging to assess skeletal muscle architecture during movements: a systematic review of methods, reliability, and challenges. *J Appl Physiol.* (2020) 128:978–99. doi: 10.1152/japplphysiol.00835.2019
9. Drakonaki EE, Sudol-Szopinska I, Sinopidis C, Givissis P. High resolution ultrasound for imaging complications of muscle injury: is there an additional role for elastography? *J Ultrasonogr.* (2019) 19:137–44. doi: 10.15557/JoU.2019.0020
10. Li Y, Snedeker JG. Elastography: modality-specific approaches, clinical applications, and research horizons. *Skeletal Radiol.* (2011) 40:389–97. doi: 10.1007/s00256-010-0918-0
11. Sigrist RMS, Liau J, Kaffas AE, Chammas MC, Willmann JK. Ultrasound elastography: review of techniques and clinical applications. *Theranostics.* (2017) 7:1303–29. doi: 10.7150/thno.18650
12. Barr RG, Nakashima K, Amy D, Cosgrove D, Farrokh A, Schafer F, et al. WFUMB guidelines and recommendations for clinical use of ultrasound elastography: part 2: breast. *Ultrasound Med Biol.* (2015) 41:1148–60. doi: 10.1016/j.ultrasmedbio.2015.03.008
13. Ferraioli G, Filice C, Castera L, Choi BI, Sporea I, Wilson SR, et al. WFUMB guidelines and recommendations for clinical use of ultrasound elastography: Part 3: liver. *Ultrasound Med Biol.* (2015) 41:1161–79. doi: 10.1016/j.ultrasmedbio.2015.03.007
14. Cosgrove D, Barr R, Bojunga J, Cantisani V, Chammas MC, Dighe M, et al. WFUMB guidelines and recommendations on the clinical use of ultrasound elastography: part 4. Thyroid. *Ultrasound Med Biol.* (2017) 43:4–26. doi: 10.1016/j.ultrasmedbio.2016.06.022
15. Domenichini R, Pialat JB, Podda A, Aubry S. Ultrasound elastography in tendon pathology: state of the art. *Skeletal Radiol.* (2017) 46:1643–55. doi: 10.1007/s00256-017-2726-2
16. Dirrichs T, Quack V, Gatz M, Tingart M, Kuhl CK, Schrading S. Shear wave elastography (SWE) for the evaluation of patients with tendinopathies. *Acad Radiol.* (2016) 23:1204–13. doi: 10.1016/j.acra.2016.05.012
17. Sarabon N, Kozinc Z, Podrekar N. Using shear-wave elastography in skeletal muscle: a repeatability and reproducibility study on biceps femoris muscle. *PLoS ONE.* (2019) 14:e0222008. doi: 10.1371/journal.pone.0222008
18. Phan A, Lee J, Gao J. Ultrasound shear wave elastography in assessment of skeletal muscle stiffness in senior volunteers. *Clin Imaging.* (2019) 58:22–6. doi: 10.1016/j.clinimag.2019.06.006
19. Maslarska M, Weis C, Bode C, Hehrlein C. Shear wave elastography of peripheral muscle weakness in patients with chronic congestive heart failure. *Ultrasound Med Biol.* (2018) 44:2531–9. doi: 10.1016/j.ultrasmedbio.2018.08.011
20. Akagi R, Takahashi H. Effect of a 5-week static stretching program on hardness of the gastrocnemius muscle. *Scand J Med Sci Sports.* (2014) 24:950–7. doi: 10.1111/sms.12111
21. Zhang ZJ, Ng GYF, Lee WC, Fu SN. Increase in passive muscle tension of the quadriceps muscle heads in jumping athletes with patellar tendinopathy. *Scand J Med Sci Sports.* (2017) 27:1099–104. doi: 10.1111/sms.12749
22. Itoigawa Y, Sperling JW, Steinmann SP, Chen Q, Song P, Chen S, et al. Feasibility assessment of shear wave elastography to rotator cuff muscle. *Clin Anat.* (2015) 28:213–8. doi: 10.1002/ca.22498
23. Flatres A, Aarab Y, Nougaret S, Garnier F, Larcher R, Amalric M, et al. Real-time shear wave ultrasound elastography: a new tool for the evaluation of diaphragm and limb muscle stiffness in critically ill patients. *Crit Care.* (2020) 24:34. doi: 10.1186/s13054-020-2745-6
24. Du LJ, He W, Cheng LG, Li S, Pan YS, Gao J. Ultrasound shear wave elastography in assessment of muscle stiffness in patients with Parkinson's disease: a primary observation. *Clin Imaging.* (2016) 40:1075–80. doi: 10.1016/j.clinimag.2016.05.008
25. Lacourpaille L, Hug F, Guevel A, Pereon Y, Magot A, Hogrel JY, et al. Non-invasive assessment of muscle stiffness in patients with Duchenne muscular dystrophy. *Muscle Nerve.* (2015) 51:284–6. doi: 10.1002/mus.24445
26. Gao J, He W, Du LJ, Chen J, Park D, Wells M, et al. Quantitative ultrasound imaging to assess the biceps brachii muscle in chronic post-stroke spasticity: preliminary observation. *Ultrasound Med Biol.* (2018) 44:1931–40. doi: 10.1016/j.ultrasmedbio.2017.12.012
27. Alfuraih AM, O'Connor P, Hensor E, Tan AL, Emery P, Wakefield RJ. The effect of unit, depth, and probe load on the reliability of muscle shear wave elastography: variables affecting reliability of SWE. *J Clin Ultrasound.* (2018) 46:108–15. doi: 10.1002/jcu.22534
28. Alfuraih AM, O'Connor P, Tan AL, Hensor E, Emery P, Wakefield RJ. An investigation into the variability between different shear wave elastography systems in muscle. *Med Ultrasonogr.* (2017) 19:392–400. doi: 10.11152/mu-1113
29. Kot BC, Zhang ZJ, Lee AW, Leung VY, Fu SN. Elastic modulus of muscle and tendon with shear wave ultrasound elastography: variations with different technical settings. *PLoS ONE.* (2012) 7:e44348. doi: 10.1371/journal.pone.0044348

30. Faulkner JA, Larkin LM, Claflin DR, Brooks SV. Age-related changes in the structure and function of skeletal muscles. *Clin Exp Pharmacol Physiol.* (2007) 34:1091–6. doi: 10.1111/j.1440-1681.2007.04752.x
31. Kragstrup TW, Kjaer M, Mackey AL. Structural, biochemical, cellular, and functional changes in skeletal muscle extracellular matrix with aging. *Scand J Med Sci Sports.* (2011) 21:749–57. doi: 10.1111/j.1600-0838.2011.01377.x
32. Alfuraih AM, Tan AL, O'Connor P, Emery P, Wakefield RJ. The effect of ageing on shear wave elastography muscle stiffness in adults. *Aging Clin Exp Res.* (2019) 31:1755–63. doi: 10.1007/s40520-019-01139-0
33. Akagi R, Yamashita Y, Ueyasu Y. Age-related differences in muscle shear moduli in the lower extremity. *Ultrasound Med Biol.* (2015) 41:2906–12. doi: 10.1016/j.ultrasmedbio.2015.07.011
34. Yoshida K, Itoigawa Y, Maruyama Y, Saita Y, Takazawa Y, Ikeda H, et al. Application of shear wave elastography for the gastrocnemius medial head to tennis leg. *Clin Anat.* (2017) 30:114–9. doi: 10.1002/ca.22788
35. Sendur HN, Cindil E, Cerit MN, Kiliç P, Gültekin II, Oktar SÖ. Evaluation of effects of aging on skeletal muscle elasticity using shear wave elastography. *Eur J Radiol.* (2020) 128:109038. doi: 10.1016/j.ejrad.2020.109038
36. Eby SF, Cloud BA, Brandenburg JE, Giambini H, Song P, Chen S, et al. Shear wave elastography of passive skeletal muscle stiffness: influences of sex and age throughout adulthood. *Clin Biomech.* (2015) 30:22–7. doi: 10.1016/j.clinbiomech.2014.11.011
37. Wang CZ, Guo JY, Li TJ, Zhou Y, Shi W, Zheng YP. Age and sex effects on the active stiffness of vastus intermedius under isometric contraction. *BioMed Res Int.* (2017) 2017:9469548. doi: 10.1155/2017/9469548
38. Baumer TG, Dischler J, Davis L, Labyed Y, Siegal DS, van Holsbeeck M, et al. Effects of age and pathology on shear wave speed of the human rotator cuff. *J Orthopaedic Res.* (2018) 36:282–8. doi: 10.1002/jor.23641
39. Chodock E, Hahn J, Setlock CA, Lipps DB. Identifying predictors of upper extremity muscle elasticity with healthy aging. *J Biomech.* (2020) 103:109687. doi: 10.1016/j.jbiomech.2020.109687
40. Dresner MA, Rose GH, Rossman PJ, Muthupillai R, Manduca A, Ehman RL. Magnetic resonance elastography of skeletal muscle. *J Magn Reson Imaging.* (2001) 13:269–76. doi: 10.1002/1522-2586(200102)13:2<269::AID-JMRI1039>3.0.CO;2-1
41. Uffmann K, Maderwald S, Ajaj W, Galban CG, Mateiescu S, Quick HH, et al. *In vivo* elasticity measurements of extremity skeletal muscle with MR elastography. *NMR Biomed.* (2004) 17:181–90. doi: 10.1002/nbm.887
42. Bensamoun SF, Ringleb SI, Littrell L, Chen Q, Brennan M, Ehman RL, et al. Determination of thigh muscle stiffness using magnetic resonance elastography. *J Magn Reson Imaging.* (2006) 23:242–7. doi: 10.1002/jmri.20487
43. Zonnino A, Smith DR, Delgorio PL, Johnson CL, Sergi F. MM-MRE: a new technique to quantify individual muscle forces during isometric tasks of the wrist using MR elastography. *IEEE Int Conf Rehabil Robot.* (2019) 2019:270–5. doi: 10.1109/ICORR.2019.8779562
44. Creze M, Soubeyrand M, Yue JL, Gagey O, Maitre X, Bellin MF. Magnetic resonance elastography of the lumbar back muscles: a preliminary study. *Clin Anat.* (2018) 31:514–20. doi: 10.1002/ca.23065
45. Day J, Patel S, Limaye V. The role of magnetic resonance imaging techniques in evaluation and management of the idiopathic inflammatory myopathies. *Semin Arthritis Rheum.* (2017) 46:642–9. doi: 10.1016/j.semarthrit.2016.11.001
46. Nealon AR, Docking SI, Lucas PE, Connell DA, Koh ES, Cook JL. MRI findings are associated with time to return to play in first class cricket fast bowlers with side strain in Australia and England. *J Sci Med Sport.* (2019) 22:992–6. doi: 10.1016/j.jsams.2019.05.020
47. Crombe A, Marcellin PJ, Buy X, Stoeckle E, Brouste V, Italiano A, et al. Soft-tissue sarcomas: assessment of MRI features correlating with histologic grade and patient outcome. *Radiology.* (2019) 291:710–21. doi: 10.1148/radiol.2019181659
48. Mercuri E, Jungbluth H, Muntoni F. Muscle imaging in clinical practice: diagnostic value of muscle magnetic resonance imaging in inherited neuromuscular disorders. *Curr Opin Neurol.* (2005) 18:526–37. doi: 10.1097/01.wco.0000183947.01362.fe
49. Mercuri E, Pichiecchio A, Allsop J, Messina S, Pane M, Muntoni F. Muscle MRI in inherited neuromuscular disorders: past, present, and future. *J Magn Reson Imaging.* (2007) 25:433–40. doi: 10.1002/jmri.20804
50. Schmidt GP, Reiser MF, Baur-Melnyk A. Whole-body imaging of the musculoskeletal system: the value of MR imaging. *Skeletal Radiol.* (2007) 36:1109–19. doi: 10.1007/s00256-007-0323-5
51. Leung DG, Carrino JA, Wagner KR, Jacobs MA. Whole-body magnetic resonance imaging evaluation of facioscapulohumeral muscular dystrophy. *Muscle Nerve.* (2015) 52:512–20. doi: 10.1002/mus.24569
52. Farrow M, Grainger AJ, Tan AL, Buch MH, Emery P, Ridgway JP, et al. Normal values and test-retest variability of stimulated-echo diffusion tensor imaging and fat fraction measurements in the muscle. *Br J Radiol.* (2019) 92:20190143. doi: 10.1259/bjr.20190143
53. Schlaffke L, Rehmann R, Rohm M, Otto LAM, de Luca A, Burakiewicz J, et al. Multi-center evaluation of stability and reproducibility of quantitative MRI measures in healthy calf muscles. *NMR Biomed.* (2019) 32:e4119. doi: 10.1002/nbm.4119
54. Ma J. Dixon techniques for water and fat imaging. *J Magn Reson Imaging.* (2008) 28:543–58. doi: 10.1002/jmri.21492
55. Yao L, Yip AL, Shrader JA, Mesdaghinia S, Volochayev R, Jansen AV, et al. Magnetic resonance measurement of muscle T2, fat-corrected T2 and fat fraction in the assessment of idiopathic inflammatory myopathies. *Rheumatology.* (2015) 55:441–9. doi: 10.1093/rheumatology/kev344
56. Burakiewicz J, Hooijmans MT, Webb AG, Verschuuren J, Niks EH, Kan HE. Improved olefinic fat suppression in skeletal muscle DTI using a magnitude-based dixon method. *Magn Reson Med.* (2018) 79:152–9. doi: 10.1002/mrm.26655
57. Schlaeger S, Weidlich D, Klupp E, Montagnese F, Deschauer M, Schoser B, et al. Decreased water T2 in fatty infiltrated skeletal muscles of patients with neuromuscular diseases. *NMR Biomed.* (2019) 32:e4111. doi: 10.1002/nbm.4111
58. Scheel M, Prokscha T, von Roth P, Winkler T, Dietrich R, Bierbaum S, et al. Diffusion tensor imaging of skeletal muscle–correlation of fractional anisotropy to muscle power. *RoFo.* (2013) 185:857–61. doi: 10.1055/s-0033-1335911
59. Sinha S, Sinha U, Edgerton VR. *In vivo* diffusion tensor imaging of the human calf muscle. *J Magn Reson Imaging.* (2006) 24:182–90. doi: 10.1002/jmri.20593
60. Kermarrec E, Budzik JF, Khalil C, Le Thuc V, Hancart-Destee C, Cotten A. *In vivo* diffusion tensor imaging and tractography of human thigh muscles in healthy subjects. *AJR Am J Roentgenol.* (2010) 195:W352–6. doi: 10.2214/AJR.09.3368
61. Fieremans E, Lemberskiy G, Veraart J, Sigmund EE, Gyftopoulos S, Novikov DS. *In vivo* measurement of membrane permeability and myofiber size in human muscle using time-dependent diffusion tensor imaging and the random permeable barrier model. *NMR Biomed.* (2017) 30:3612. doi: 10.1002/nbm.3612
62. Sigmund EE, Novikov DS, Sui D, Ukpebor O, Baete S, Babb JS, et al. Time-dependent diffusion in skeletal muscle with the random permeable barrier model (RPBM): application to normal controls and chronic exertional compartment syndrome patients. *NMR Biomed.* (2014) 27:519–28. doi: 10.1002/nbm.3087
63. Malis V, Sinha U, Csapo R, Narici M, Smitaman E, Sinha S. Diffusion tensor imaging and diffusion modeling: application to monitoring changes in the medial gastrocnemius in disuse atrophy induced by unilateral limb suspension. *J Magn Reson Imaging.* (2019) 49:1655–64. doi: 10.1002/jmri.26295
64. Barendregt AM, Bray TJP, Hall-Craggs MA, Maas M. Emerging quantitative MR imaging biomarkers in inflammatory arthritides. *Eur J Radiol.* (2019) 121:108707. doi: 10.1016/j.ejrad.2019.108707
65. Maggi L, Moscatelli M, Frangiamore R, Mazzi F, Verri M, de Luca A, et al. Quantitative muscle MRI protocol as possible biomarker in Becker muscular dystrophy. *Clin Neuroradiol.* (2020). doi: 10.1007/s00062-019-00875-0. [Epub ahead of print].
66. Nunez-Peralta C, Alonso-Perez J, Llauger J, Segovia S, Montesinos P, Belmonte I, et al. Follow-up of late-onset Pompe disease patients with muscle magnetic resonance imaging reveals increase in fat replacement in skeletal muscles. *J Cachexia Sarcopenia Muscle.* (2020). doi: 10.1002/jcsm.12555. [Epub ahead of print].

67. D'Souza A, Bolsterlee B, Herbert RD. Architecture of the medial gastrocnemius muscle in people who have had a stroke: a diffusion tensor imaging investigation. *Clin Biomech.* (2020) 74:27–33. doi: 10.1016/j.clinbiomech.2020.02.004
68. Heskamp L, van Nimwegen M, Ploegmakers MJ, Bassez G, Deux JF, Cumming SA, et al. Lower extremity muscle pathology in myotonic dystrophy type 1 assessed by quantitative MRI. *Neurology.* (2019) 92:e2803–14. doi: 10.1212/WNL.0000000000007648
69. Barnard AM, Willcocks RJ, Finanger EL, Daniels MJ, Triplett WT, Rooney WD, et al. Skeletal muscle magnetic resonance biomarkers correlate with function and sentinel events in Duchenne muscular dystrophy. *PLoS ONE.* (2018) 13:e0194283. doi: 10.1371/journal.pone.0194283
70. Chinoy H, Lilleker JB. Pitfalls in the diagnosis of myositis. *Best Pract Res Clin Rheumatol.* (2020) 34:101486. doi: 10.1016/j.berh.2020.101486
71. van de Vlekkert J, Maas M, Hoogendijk JE, de Visser M, van Schaik IN. Combining MRI and muscle biopsy improves diagnostic accuracy in subacute-onset idiopathic inflammatory myopathy. *Muscle Nerve.* (2015) 51:253–8. doi: 10.1002/mus.24307
72. Pipitone N. Value of MRI in diagnostics and evaluation of myositis. *Curr Opin Rheumatol.* (2016) 28:625–30. doi: 10.1097/BOR.0000000000000326
73. Kubinova K, Mann H, Vencovsky J. MRI scoring methods used in evaluation of muscle involvement in patients with idiopathic inflammatory myopathies. *Curr opin Rheumatol.* (2017) 29:623–31. doi: 10.1097/BOR.0000000000000435
74. Connor A, Stebbings S, Anne Hung N, Hammond-Tooke G, Meikle G, Highton J. STIR MRI to direct muscle biopsy in suspected idiopathic inflammatory myopathy. *J Clin Rheumatol.* (2007) 13:341–5. doi: 10.1097/RHU.0b013e31815dca0a
75. Milisenda JC, Collado MV, Pinal-Fernandez I, Hormaza Jaramillo A, Faruch Bilfeld M, Cano MD, et al. Correlation between quantitative and semiquantitative magnetic resonance imaging and histopathology findings in dermatomyositis. *Clin Exp Rheumatol.* (2019) 37:633–40. Available online at: https://www.clinexprheumatol.org/abstract.asp?a=13003
76. Huang ZG, Gao BX, Chen H, Yang MX, Chen XL, Yan R, et al. An efficacy analysis of whole-body magnetic resonance imaging in the diagnosis and follow-up of polymyositis and dermatomyositis. *PLoS ONE.* (2017) 12:e0181069. doi: 10.1371/journal.pone.0181069
77. Filli L, Maurer B, Manoliu A, Andreisek G, Guggenberger R. Whole-body MRI in adult inflammatory myopathies: do we need imaging of the trunk? *Eur Radiol.* (2015) 25:3499–507. doi: 10.1007/s00330-015-3783-3
78. Kadoba K, Mizukawa K, Nishimura K, Murabe H. Large vessel giant cell arteritis suggested by magnetic resonance imaging of the thigh: a potential mimicker of myositis, fasciitis and skeletal muscle vasculitis. *Rheumatology (Oxford).* (2019) 58:2211. doi: 10.1093/rheumatology/kez138
79. Ran J, Ji S, Morelli JN, Wu G, Li XM. The diagnostic value of T2 maps and rs-EPI DWI in dermatomyositis. *Br J Radiol.* (2019) 92:20180715. doi: 10.1259/bjr.20180715
80. Qi J, Olsen NJ, Price RR, Winston JA, Park JH. Diffusion-weighted imaging of inflammatory myopathies: polymyositis and dermatomyositis. *J Magn Reson Imaging.* (2008) 27:212–7. doi: 10.1002/jmri.21209
81. Kim HK, Laor T, Horn PS, Racadio JM, Wong B, Dardzinski BJ. T2 mapping in Duchenne muscular dystrophy: distribution of disease activity and correlation with clinical assessments. *Radiology.* (2010) 255:899–908. doi: 10.1148/radiol.10091547
82. Gaeta M, Scribano E, Mileto A, Mazziotti S, Rodolico C, Toscano A, et al. Muscle fat fraction in neuromuscular disorders: dual-echo dual-flip-angle spoiled gradient-recalled MR imaging technique for quantification—a feasibility study. *Radiology.* (2011) 259:487–94. doi: 10.1148/radiol.10101108
83. Sigmund EE, Baete SH, Luo T, Patel K, Wang D, Rossi I, et al. MRI assessment of the thigh musculature in dermatomyositis and healthy subjects using diffusion tensor imaging, intravoxel incoherent motion and dynamic DTI. *Eur Radiol.* (2018) 28:5304–15. doi: 10.1007/s00330-018-5458-3
84. Botar-Jid C, Damian L, Dudea SM, Vasilescu D, Rednic S, Badea R. The contribution of ultrasonography and sonoelastography in assessment of myositis. *Med Ultrasonogr.* (2010) 12:120–6. Available online at: https://www.medultrason.ro/medultrason/index.php/medultrason/article/view/212
85. Berko NS, Hay A, Sterba Y, Wahezi D, Levin TL. Efficacy of ultrasound elastography in detecting active myositis in children: can it replace MRI? *Pediatr Radiol.* (2015) 45:1522–8. doi: 10.1007/s00247-015-3350-8
86. Alfuraih AM, O'Connor P, Tan AL, Hensor EMA, Ladas A, Emery P, et al. Muscle shear wave elastography in idiopathic inflammatory myopathies: a case-control study with MRI correlation. *Skeletal Radiol.* (2019) 48:1209–19. doi: 10.1007/s00256-019-03175-3
87. McCullough MB, Domire ZJ, Reed AM, Amin S, Ytterberg SR, Chen Q, et al. Evaluation of muscles affected by myositis using magnetic resonance elastography. *Muscle Nerve.* (2011) 43:585–90. doi: 10.1002/mus.21923
88. Bachasson D, Dubois GJR, Allenbach Y, Benveniste O, Hogrel JY. Muscle shear wave elastography in inclusion body myositis: feasibility, reliability and relationships with muscle impairments. *Ultrasound Med Biol.* (2018) 44:1423–32. doi: 10.1016/j.ultrasmedbio.2018.03.026
89. Ponte C, Martins-Martinho J, Luqmani RA. Diagnosis of giant cell arteritis. *Rheumatology (Oxford).* (2020) 59:iii5–16. doi: 10.1093/rheumatology/kez553
90. Schakman O, Kalista S, Barbe C, Loumaye A, Thissen JP. Glucocorticoid-induced skeletal muscle atrophy. *Int J Biochem Cell Biol.* (2013) 45:2163–72. doi: 10.1016/j.biocel.2013.05.036
91. Lofberg E, Gutierrez A, Wernerman J, Anderstam B, Mitch WE, Price SR, et al. Effects of high doses of glucocorticoids on free amino acids, ribosomes and protein turnover in human muscle. *Eur J Clin Invest.* (2002) 32:345–53. doi: 10.1046/j.1365-2362.2002.00993.x
92. Harris E, Tiganescu A, Tubeuf S, Mackie SL. The prediction and monitoring of toxicity associated with long-term systemic glucocorticoid therapy. *Curr Rheumatol Rep.* (2015) 17:513. doi: 10.1007/s11926-015-0513-4
93. Minetto MA, Rainoldi A, Jabre JF. The clinical use of macro and surface electromyography in diagnosis and follow-up of endocrine and drug-induced myopathies. *J Endocrinol Invest.* (2007) 30:791–6. doi: 10.1007/BF03350820
94. Mackie SL, Pease CT, Fukuba E, Harris E, Emery P, Hodgson R, et al. Whole-body MRI of patients with polymyalgia rheumatica identifies a distinct subset with complete patient-reported response to glucocorticoids. *Ann Rheum Dis.* (2015) 74:2188–92. doi: 10.1136/annrheumdis-2015-207395
95. McGonagle D, Pease C, Marzo-Ortega H, O'Connor P, Gibbon W, Emery P. Comparison of extracapsular changes by magnetic resonance imaging in patients with rheumatoid arthritis and polymyalgia rheumatica. *J Rheumatol.* (2001) 28:1837–41. Available online at: https://www.jrheum.org/content/28/8/1837.long
96. Mori S, Koga Y, Ito K. Clinical characteristics of polymyalgia rheumatica in Japanese patients: evidence of synovitis and extracapsular inflammatory changes by fat suppression magnetic resonance imaging. *Mod Rheumatol.* (2007) 17:369–75. doi: 10.3109/s10165-007-0595-6
97. Matteson EL, Maradit-Kremers H, Cimmino MA, Schmidt WA, Schirmer M, Salvarani C, et al. Patient-reported outcomes in polymyalgia rheumatica. *J Rheumatol.* (2012) 39:795–803. doi: 10.3899/jrheum.110977
98. Martucci MG, McIlduff CE, Shin C, Gutierrez HV, Nam JY, Greenstein P, et al. Quantitative ultrasound of muscle can detect corticosteroid effects. *Clin Neurophysiol.* (2019) 130:1460–4. doi: 10.1016/j.clinph.2019.04.709
99. Webster JM, Fenton CG, Langen R, Hardy RS. Exploring the interface between inflammatory and therapeutic glucocorticoid induced bone and muscle loss. *Int J Mol Sci.* (2019) 20:5768. doi: 10.3390/ijms20225768
100. Alfuraih AM, Tan AL, O'Connor P, Emery P, Mackie S, Wakefield RJ. Reduction in stiffness of proximal leg muscles during the first 6 months of glucocorticoid therapy for giant cell arteritis: a pilot study using shear wave elastography. *Int J Rheum Dis.* (2019) 22:1891–9. doi: 10.1111/1756-185X.13667
101. Damon BM, Froeling M, Buck AK, Oudeman J, Ding Z, Nederveen AJ, et al. Skeletal muscle diffusion tensor-MRI fiber tracking: rationale, data acquisition and analysis methods, applications and future directions. *NMR Biomed.* (2017) 30:e3563. doi: 10.1002/nbm.3563
102. Danneskiold-Samsoe B, Grimby G. Isokinetic and isometric muscle strength in patients with rheumatoid arthritis. The relationship to clinical parameters and the influence of corticosteroid. *Clin Rheumatol.* (1986) 5:459–67.
103. Rothstein JM, Delitto A, Sinacore DR, Rose SJ. Muscle function in rheumatic disease patients treated with corticosteroids. *Muscle Nerve.* (1983) 6:128–35. doi: 10.1002/mus.880060208
104. Farrow M, Biglands J, Tanner SF, Clegg A, Brown L, Hensor EMA, et al. The effect of ageing on skeletal muscle as assessed by quantitative MR imaging: an association with frailty and muscle

strength. *Aging Clin Exp Res.* (2020). doi: 10.1007/s40520-020-01530-2. [Epub ahead of print].

105. Lemmey AB, Wilkinson TJ, Clayton RJ, Sheikh F, Whale J, Jones HS, et al. Tight control of disease activity fails to improve body composition or physical function in rheumatoid arthritis patients. *Rheumatology (Oxford).* (2016) 55:1736–45. doi: 10.1093/rheumatology/kew243
106. Hanaoka BY, Ithurburn MP, Rigsbee CA, Bridges SL Jr., Moellering DR, et al. Chronic inflammation in rheumatoid arthritis and mediators of skeletal muscle pathology and physical impairment: a review. *Arthritis Care Res.* (2019) 71:173–7. doi: 10.1002/acr.23775
107. Baker JF, Von Feldt J, Mostoufi-Moab S, Noaiseh G, Taratuta E, Kim W, et al. Deficits in muscle mass, muscle density, and modified associations with fat in rheumatoid arthritis. *Arthritis Care Res.* (2014) 66:1612–8. doi: 10.1002/acr.22328
108. Ekdahl C, Andersson SI, Svensson B. Muscle function of the lower extremities in rheumatoid arthritis and osteoarthrosis. A descriptive study of patients in a primary health care district. *J Clin Epidemiol.* (1989) 42:947–54. doi: 10.1016/0895-4356(89)90159-5
109. Miro O, Pedrol E, Casademont J, Garcia-Carrasco M, Sanmarti R, Cebrian M, et al. Muscle involvement in rheumatoid arthritis: clinicopathological study of 21 symptomatic cases. *Semin Arthritis Rheum.* (1996) 25:421–8. doi: 10.1016/S0049-0172(96)80007-2
110. Brooke MH, Kaplan H. Muscle pathology in rheumatoid arthritis, polymyalgia rheumatica, and polymyositis: a histochemical study. *Arch Pathol.* (1972) 94:101–18.
111. Edstrom L, Nordemar R. Differential changes in type I and type II muscle fibres in rheumatoid arthritis. A biopsy study. *Scand J Rheumatol.* (1974) 3:155–60. doi: 10.3109/03009747409097142
112. Roubenoff R, Roubenoff RA, Cannon JG, Kehayias JJ, Zhuang H, Dawson-Hughes B, et al. Rheumatoid cachexia: cytokine-driven hypermetabolism accompanying reduced body cell mass in chronic inflammation. *J Clin Invest.* (1994) 93:2379–86. doi: 10.1172/JCI117244
113. Engvall IL, Elkan AC, Tengstrand B, Cederholm T, Brismar K, Hafstrom I. Cachexia in rheumatoid arthritis is associated with inflammatory activity, physical disability, and low bioavailable insulin-like growth factor. *Scand J Rheumatol.* (2008) 37:321–8. doi: 10.1080/03009740802055984
114. Alfuraih AM, Tan AL, O'Connor P, Emery P, Wakefield RJ. Muscle stiffness in rheumatoid arthritis is not altered or associated with muscle weakness: a shear wave elastography study. *Mod Rheumatol.* (2020) 30:617–25. doi: 10.1080/14397595.2019.1645374
115. Seifert O, Baerwald C. Impact of fatigue on rheumatic diseases. *Best Pract Res Clin Rheumatol.* (2019) 33:101435. doi: 10.1016/j.berh.2019.101435
116. Almeida C, Choy EH, Hewlett S, Kirwan JR, Cramp F, Chalder T, et al. Biologic interventions for fatigue in rheumatoid arthritis. *Cochrane Database Syst Rev.* (2016) 2016:CD008334. doi: 10.1002/14651858.CD008334.pub2
117. Azeez M, Clancy C, O'Dwyer T, Lahiff C, Wilson F, Cunnane G. Benefits of exercise in patients with rheumatoid arthritis: a randomized controlled trial of a patient-specific exercise programme. *Clin Rheumatol.* (2020) 39:1783–92. doi: 10.1007/s10067-020-04937-4
118. Bryant ND, Li K, Does MD, Barnes S, Gochberg DF, Yankeelov TE, et al. Multi-parametric MRI characterization of inflammation in murine skeletal muscle. *NMR Biomed.* (2014) 27:716–25. doi: 10.1002/nbm.3113
119. Giambini H, Hatta T, Rezaei A, An KN. Extensibility of the supraspinatus muscle can be predicted by combining shear wave elastography and magnetic resonance imaging-measured quantitative metrics of stiffness and volumetric fat infiltration: a cadaveric study. *Clin Biomech.* (2018) 57:144–9. doi: 10.1016/j.clinbiomech.2018.07.001
120. Stoel B. Use of artificial intelligence in imaging in rheumatology–current status and future perspectives. *RMD Open.* (2020) 6:e001063. doi: 10.1136/rmdopen-2019-001063

16

Innovations Developed by Patients and Informal Caregivers for Needs Associated to Rheumatic Diseases

Maria João Jacinto [1,2*], Pedro Oliveira [1,3,4] and Helena Canhão [1,5,6,7]

[1] Patient Innovation, Lisbon, Portugal, [2] Católica-Lisbon School of Business and Economics, Universidade Católica Portuguesa, Lisbon, Portugal, [3] Copenhagen Business School, Copenhagen, Denmark, [4] Nova School of Business and Economics, Universidade Nova de Lisboa, Lisbon, Portugal, [5] CHRC, Comprehensive Health Research Center, NOVA Medical School, UNL, Lisbon, Portugal, [6] EpiDoC Unit, Chronic Diseases Research Centre, Nova Medical School, Universidade Nova de Lisboa, Lisbon, Portugal, [7] National School of Public Health, Universidade Nova de Lisboa, Lisbon, Portugal

***Correspondence:**
Maria João Jacinto
maria.joao.jacinto@
patient-innovation.com

Until recently, innovation in healthcare was mainly achieved through the development of new drugs, therapies, and medical devices by big pharma and medtech companies; however, the innovative potential for this field is much broader. The patients and caregivers' role in healthcare is often associated with disease management, demand for their own illness data, and its exchange with other patients. However, the patients and caregivers' capacity to innovate to cope with limitations associated with their health condition is a growing phenomenon and starting to be supported by healthcare stakeholders to achieve a truly patient-centric system. Our previous research has shown that these uncommon innovators can develop a wide range of solutions, from simple adaptations and products to highly technological biomedical devices. In this paper, we present novel solutions developed by rheumatic patients, their caregivers, and collaborators, published on the "Patient Innovation" platform (https://patient-innovation.com/), with a focus on the innovator profile, the need that triggers the innovative process, the type of motivation behind the product, and the products developed. The most significant needs that motivate innovation are the will to increase the level of independence (71%) and to be able to perform daily routine activities (65%). In over 80% of cases, the fact that the market does not fully fulfill the needs felt during daily activities is the main motivation to innovate. It is thus concluded that there is room for innovation in rheumatic diseases with solutions developed by patients and informal caregivers that intend to solve needs that the healthcare market is not covering.

Keywords: patient innovation, user innovation, health, rheumatic diseases, disability

INTRODUCTION

Rheumatic diseases are in the group of diseases recognized earliest in the world (1), and although the most common rheumatic diseases present a high prevalence in the elderly population, rheumatic diseases affect people of all ages and currently have a great impact on patients' daily living as well as on society, as it is commonly reflected in high economic costs through a great consumption of healthcare and social resources.

Despite the critical importance of the healthcare sector for the economy and society, where average health spending reached 8.8% of gross domestic product (GDP) across the Organization for Economic Co-operation and Development (OECD) (2), current healthcare provision does not always meet patient's real and daily needs. To solve this, some patients and informal caregivers do not wait for a solution to come up in the market, and thus start developing innovative solutions to overcome limitations associated with the health condition that they face (3, 4). Von Hippel started to introduce the concept of user innovation as individuals or firms who expect to directly benefit from a product that they have created (5, 6); this concept differs from producer innovators—firms or individuals who develop novel products to benefit from selling it as a better or new product or service. Thus, when translating the concept of user innovation to the healthcare domain, patient innovators are citizens who develop useful and innovative solutions to cope with their health disorders. These patient innovations range from simple products for everyday use to unknown therapies and high-tech solutions (7). These findings suggested that patients and informal caregivers worldwide may contribute with a high number of innovative solutions with a valid need-based motivation and, if shared and adopted, can improve not only their quality of life but also the life of others with similar health conditions (8). This was the motivation for the creation of the website www.patient-innovation.com, a non-profit international, multilingual, and open platform which currently presents over 1,500 solutions developed by patients, informal caregivers, and collaborators which have been submitted or collected, medically validated, and shared.

In this paper, it is our intention to present and describe relevant innovative solutions developed by rheumatic patients, their informal caregivers, and collaborators, who decided to solve some of their everyday needs—originated by the health condition that they face—but could not find any solution in the market.

METHODS

In order to analyze innovative solutions developed by patients and informal caregivers, the '*Patient Innovation*' platform (www.patient-innovation.com) was used as its presents itself as a centralized inventory of patient-developed solutions.

The '*Patient Innovation*' platform provides the opportunity to patients and caregivers to actively engage in sharing solutions within the *Patient Innovation* community. In order to share a novel solution, the user must register on the website (the connection to *Patient Innovation* is always encrypted and personal data is only stored in high security data centers located in the European Union) and, once logged in, the user can write down his/her solutions for dealing with a condition in his/her daily life (information required: solution title, description, about the innovator, and optional images and videos). Before being published, the *Patient Innovation*'s medical team evaluates and validates (or not) the submitted solutions, by only approving the ones that are not drugs, chemicals, intake/topical substances, invasive devices, or other visibly and intrinsically dangerous proposals. Once these are online, they are available to everyone who may be interested, or can benefit from the published solutions.

The medically validated and published solutions in the '*Patient Innovation*' platform were screened, and solutions that showed features to be possible solutions for rheumatologic diseases were selected. In a first stage analysis, disease-based motivation was screened and rheumatology-based solutions were distinguished from solutions that cover rheumatologic patients' needs/symptoms but were based on other medical conditions. Through the innovation description and information available about the innovator, the type of innovator (patient, caregiver, or collaborator), sex, country, product category (the exact role/goal of the solution developed, divided into the following categories: activities of daily living, pain/therapy, hobbies, and movement), motivation (why the innovators had to develop a novel solution to cope with a limitation/need related with the health condition that they face, divided into the following categories: "the products in the market were not useful to satisfy the need," "there was not any alternative in the market," "cost of the alternatives in the market," and "other") and need to innovate (the need that made the patient, caregiver, or collaborator to innovate and create a novel product, divided into the following categories: "to be able to perform personal hygiene tasks," "to be able to perform a daily routine activity," "to increase the level of independency," "to be able to move," "to reduce pain," "to replace a lost function," "to improve therapy," and "other") were studied. The criteria used for categorization was developed by the authors based on the information available in the solutions description fields (solution title, description, about the innovator, optional images, and videos) posted on the '*Patient Innovation*' platform.

RESULTS

The '*Patient Innovation*' platform presented 1,399 medically screened and published solutions when consulted on July 8th 2020 for the purpose of this research work. From those, 101 published innovations showed features that marked them as possible solutions for rheumatologic patients; most of those solutions were developed for activities of daily living (54%), whereas for hobbies (24%), pain/therapy (15%), and movement (9%) are other significant types of products described in the platform.

Thirty-four percent (n = 34, **Table 1**) of those solutions were developed as a response to rheumatologic-based needs by patients, informal caregivers, and collaborators who face difficulties associated with this disease category. The great majority of rheumatologic-based solutions (82%) were developed in the same proportion by patients (those who develop solutions for themselves) and informal caregivers (those who develop solutions for loved ones and/or family); eighteen percent (n = 6) of the solutions were developed by collaborators (those who develop solutions for someone out of his/her family/friends circle). Fifty-four percent (n = 19) of those solutions were developed by men (46% by women) and by citizens from countries of five continents (e.g., USA, Portugal, China, Australia, and Kenya).

When analyzing the need behind the innovation process for the rheumatologic-based solutions (**Figure 1**), the most significant ones rely on efforts to increase the level of independency (71%) and to be able to perform a daily routine

TABLE 1 | Innovative solutions to cope with rheumatic diseases limitations developed by patients, informal caregivers, and collaborators published in https://patient-innovation.com/.

Product	Type of innovator	Country of origin	Rheumatologic Disease
Hair dryer adaptation for stiff upper limbs[1]	Patient	Portugal	Fibromyalgia
Home-made orthotic for foot pain[2]		USA	Arthritis
Home-made pouches for hot-cold therapy to reduce pain[3]		Canada	Arthritis
ViEx, a string-based device to reduce hand joints pain[4]		USA	Rheumatoid arthritis
Handmade toys to cope with Arthritis[5]		USA	Juvenile Arthritis
Food cutting board and knives to overcome poor hand grip[6]		New Zealand	Rheumatoid Arthritis
Tool to help with gardening without having to bend down[7]		Belgium	Arthritis
Adapted transport container for disabled people scooters[8]		Belgium	Ehlers-Danlos Syndrome
Nose-pad, a device to work in a computer/tablet using nose and lips[9]		Sweden	Arthritis
Gehrad, a walking aid device[10]		Germany	Osteoarthritis
Protective capes for wheelchair users[11]		Belgium	Ehlers-Danlos Syndrome
Sandi Gloves, an easier way to sand[12]		Australia	Arthritis
Chronically Simple, an app for chronic diseases management[13]		Canada	Ehlers-Danlos Syndrome
Fashionable walking aids[14]		UK	Fibromyalgia
Adaptor for car key turning aid to avoid wrist twisting motion[15]	Caregiver	USA	Arthritis
Accessible zipper pull[16]		USA	Arthritis
Assistive door locker[17]		USA	Arthritis
Blanket support to avoid overweighting joints and still not get cold[18]		Portugal	Arthritis
Light intensity regulator for car traveling [19]		Portugal	Arthritis
Exoskeleton glove to enhance hand movements[20]		Greece	Arthritis
Wheelchair tank to ease beach and countryside visits[21]		UK	Arthritis
Egg collector to avoid having to bend over[22]		Belgium	Myopathy
Stair-climbing wheelchair[23]		China	Arthritis
Adapted clothes to enable minimum body movement while dressing[24]		China	Osteoarthritis
Stair-climbing booster[25]		China	Arthritis
Toothpaste squeezer for people with poor grip[26]		USA	Arthritis
Orthorod, an adapted fishing pole[27]		USA	Arthritis
Swachchta Suvidha Brush, a simple slip-on floor cleaner[28]		India	Spondylosis, Arthritis
Book page turning device[29]	Collaborator	USA	Arthritis
Kitchen safety handle for limited hand strength and flexibility[30]		Taiwan	Rheumatoid Arthritis
Obi, a robotic device for autonomous feeding[31]		USA	Arthrogryposis
3D printing device to help to dress[32]		USA	Arthrogryposis Multiplex Congenita
E-Con, an all-terrain wheelchair[33]		Kenya	Arthritis
Finger support to ease finger deformities[34]		USA	Arthritis

Patient Innovation platform location (https://patient-innovation.com/xxxx/zzzz): [1]/node/502, [2]/post/654, [3]/post/920, [4]/post/1203, [5]/post/1234, [6]/post/1345, [7]/post/1365, [8]/post/1372, [9]/post/1376, [10]/post/1642, [11]/post/1648, [12]/post/1944, [13]/post/2416, [14]/post/2473, [15]/post/587, [16]/post/669, [17]/post/670, [18]/post/880, [19]/post/881, [20]/post/1204, [21]/post/1266, [22]/post/1362, [23]/post/1843, [24]/post/1845, [25]/post/1849, [26]/post/1901, [27]/post/2088, [28]/post/2355, [29]/post/861, [30]/post/1304, [31]/post/1537, [32]/post/2022, [33]/post/2039, [34]/post/2209.

activity (65%). Also, pain reduction (24%), replacing a lost function (12%), and mobility (12%) are other relevant needs found in the innovations analyzed.

Following the World Health Organization's definition for medical device (9), 32% of the solutions developed as a response to rheumatologic-based needs under analysis are framed as Class I medical devices (10), which meets the amount of pain reduction and replace a lost function as described above; still, 68% of the analyzed solutions are not framed as medical devices. However, only 15% of these rheumatologic-based solutions are approved by regulatory authorities and are currently being commercialized.

Consequently, the type of products developed by these uncommon innovators mainly rely on activities of daily living (41%), pain/therapy (24%), movement (18%), and hobbies (18%). These innovators found as their main motivation to innovate the fact that the products in the market did not fully meet a need they had (82%). Furthermore, the cost of alternative products (27%) and the inexistence of useful alternatives (9%) available in the market are also important motivations to these innovators to start developing novel solutions to cope with limitations that they face every day.

DISCUSSION

Although "innovation" is a broad term and it can be applicable in different disease's aspects, we can highlight that in the recent years "innovation" in rheumatology has widely expanded in digital health, namely through electronic health records, virtual visits, wearable technologies, and digital therapeutics which improve access, outcomes, adherence, and research (11, 12) or new

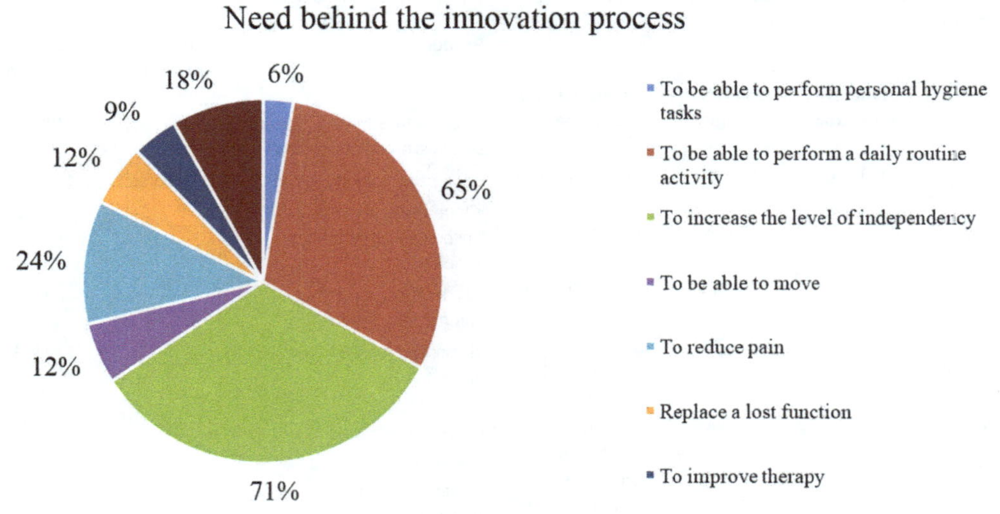

FIGURE 1 | Need behind the innovation process of rheumatologic-based innovators.

therapeutic production approaches such as biosimilars (13). Still, this paper intends to expose that there is still some room for innovation through solutions developed by patients and informal caregivers who intend to solve needs that the healthcare market is not yet covering. To do that, the authors have analyzed 34 rheumatologic-based solutions published on *Patient Innovation*'s database, 14 developed by patients and 14 by informal caregivers, which reinforces that one major source of innovation are the needs that these citizens feel in their daily lives. The fact that 54% of those solutions were developed by men (46% by women) and by citizens from countries of five continents (e.g., USA, Portugal, China, Australia, and Kenya) reflects the patient innovation process to be as global and diverse as the medical diseases themselves. The products analyzed vary from simple devices (e.g., food cutting board and knives to overcome poor hand grip) to high-tech solutions (e.g., exoskeleton glove to enhance hand movements).

Thirty-two percent of the solutions developed under analysis are framed as Class I medical devices; however, only 15% are approved by regulatory authorities and are currently being commercialized, as most of the solutions here described were developed to solve a daily life need felt by patients and informal caregivers and were not manufactured on a large scale for commercialization (at least at the analysis moment). This is a common approach for patient innovators, as this kind of uncommon inventors have only developed their novel solutions because they have a validated need that motivated them to innovate, and thus their main goal was to fulfill that need, not to profit from it. Still, there has been an increasing number of patients and informal caregivers who have been establishing their own solutions in the market as an effective way to distribute their solutions to others with similar needs (14, 15).

The authors would like to highlight the potential of platforms such as '*Patient Innovation*' and other information and communication technologies to promote an easy interaction between common citizens and healthcare professionals. Mainly, healthcare professionals and other stakeholders can use these resources to learn more about patients' real needs and the solutions that they have developed to cope with them, as well as to start including patients as consultants and their innovation process into the producer innovation processes. As innovation by patients and caregivers is still a new topic that has only started to be explored in recent years, it is important that healthcare industry representatives increase their awareness of this phenomenon and support this innovation process to achieve a more effective and cheaper product development process.

Although this work only shows a brief sample of novel solutions developed by common citizens for needs associated with rheumatic diseases, as the authors are sure that many more solutions exist developed by these uncommon inventors than the ones published in '*Patient Innovation*' platform, it is thus concluded that solutions developed by patients and informal caregivers can significantly contribute to rheumatic diseases innovations as it aims to solve needs that the healthcare market is not yet covering.

AUTHOR CONTRIBUTIONS

MJ was responsible for conceptualization, information extraction, formal analysis, methodology, writing, and edition. PO and HC were responsible for funding acquisition, project administration, resources, supervision, validation, writing, review, and editing. All authors contributed to the article and approved the submitted version.

REFERENCES

1. Sangha O. Epidemiology of rheumatic diseases. *Rheumatology (Oxford).* (2000) 39(Suppl 2):3–12. doi: 10.1093/rheumatology/39.suppl_2.3
2. Development OfEC-oa. *OECD Health Statistics.* (2020). Available online at: http://www.oecd.org/els/health-systems/health-data.htm2020
3. Oliveira P, Zejnilovic L, Canhão H, von Hippel E. Innovation by patients with rare diseases and chronic needs. *Orphanet J Rare Dis.* (2015) 10:41. doi: 10.1186/s13023-015-0257-2
4. Zejnilovic L, Oliveira P, Canhão H. Innovations by and for the patients: and how can we integrate them into the future health care system. In: Albach H, Meffert H, Pinkwart A, Reichwald R, von Eiff W, editors. *Boundaryless Hospital: Rethink and Redefine Health Care Management.* Berlin: Springer-Verlag (2016). p. 341–57.
5. von Hippel E. The dominant role of users in the scientific instrument innovation process. *Res Policy.* (1976) 5:212–39. doi: 10.1016/0048-7333(76)90028-7
6. Von Hippel E. Lead Users: a source of novel product concepts. *Manag Sci.* (1986) 32:791–805. doi: 10.1287/mnsc.32.7.791
7. Oliveira P, Canhão H. Users as service innovators: evidence from banking to healthcare. In: Lakhani K, Harhoff D, editors. *Revolutionizing Innovation.* Cambridge, MA: MIT Press (2014). 32 p.
8. Oliveira P, Zejnilovic L, Azevedo S, Rodrigues AM, Canhão H. Peer adoption and development of health innovations by patients: National Representative Study of 6204 Citizens. *J Med Internet Res.* (2019) 21:e11726. doi: 10.2196/11726
9. Organization WH. *Medical Device - Full Definition.* Available online at: https://www.who.int/medical_devices/full_deffinition/en/
10. Strålin M. *Classification of Medical Devices and Their Routes to CE Marking.* CE Check Support (2020). Available online at: https://support.ce-check.eu/hc/en-us/articles/360008712879-Classification-Of-Medical-Devices-And-Their-Routes-To-CE-Marking
11. Solomon DH, Rudin RS. Digital health technologies: opportunities and challenges in rheumatology. *Nat Rev Rheumatol.* (2020) 16:525–35. doi: 10.1038/s41584-020-0461-x
12. Rodrigues, Canhão. Innovation and digital transformation to support clinical care and prevent osteoporosis related fractures. *Acta Reumatol Port.* (2019) 44:171–2. Available online at: http://actareumatologica.pt/article_download.php?id=1408
13. Dörner T, Strand V, Cornes P, Gonçalves J, Gulácsi L, Kay J, et al. The changing landscape of biosimilars in rheumatology. *Ann Rheum Dis.* (2016) 75:974–82. doi: 10.1136/annrheumdis-2016-209166
14. Shcherbatiuk V. *Users as Developers and Entrepreneurs of Medical Treatments/Devices: The Case of Patients and their Families and Friends.* Catholic University of Portugal (2012).
15. Habicht H, Oliveira P, Shcherbatiuk V. User innovators: when patients set out to help themselves and end up helping many. *Die Unternehmung.* (2013) 66:277–94. doi: 10.5771/0042-059X-2012-3-277

17

Ultrasound Imaging in Psoriatic Arthritis: What Have We Learnt in the Last Five Years?

Sayam R. Dubash[1,2†‡], *Gabriele De Marco*[1,2†‡], *Richard J. Wakefield*[1,2‡], *Ai Lyn Tan*[1,2‡], *Dennis McGonagle*[1,2] *and Helena Marzo-Ortega*[1,2*‡]

[1] *NIHR Leeds Biomedical Research Centre, Leeds Teaching Hospitals Trust, Leeds, United Kingdom,* [2] *Leeds Institute of Rheumatic and Musculoskeletal Medicine, University of Leeds, Leeds, United Kingdom*

Correspondence:
Helena Marzo-Ortega
medhmo@leeds.ac.uk

† *These authors have contributed equally to this work*

‡**ORCID:**
Sayam R. Dubash
orcid.org/0000-0002-9303-7122
Gabriele De Marco
orcid.org/0000-0003-2406-161X
Richard J. Wakefield
orcid.org/0000-0001-5352-8683
Ai Lyn Tan
orcid.org/0000-0002-9158-7243
Helena Marzo-Ortega
orcid.org/0000-0002-9683-3407

Psoriatic arthritis (PsA) is a complex heterogeneous disease with multiple inter-related pathologies such as synovitis, enthesitis, tendinopathy, and dactylitis. Clinical assessment is limited in its detail to assess pathology, thus in recent years, ultrasound (US) has become more popular, given its high sensitivity to detect inflammatory arthritis and ability to inform clinical decisions. Although a qualitative technique, US findings can be graded semi-quantitatively for grayscale (GS) and power Doppler (PD). Synovitis is frequently present in inflammatory arthritis pathologies, and in PsA, recent evidence shows a propensity for tendon and entheseal lesions. The presence of flexor tenosynovitis and flexor tendon insertional enthesopathy at accessory pulleys is supportive of the "Deep Koebner" concept. Peri-tendinous inflammation—mutual to PsA or rheumatoid arthritis (RA), is associated with soft tissue oedema with PD signal frequently at the flexor tendon compartments in PsA. Research on enthesitis in PsA/PsO has improved understanding in subclinical and clinical PsA, explored associations with progression to PsA, and investigated links to prognosis assessment. Dactylitis is a pathognomonic PsA lesion where US has enhanced knowledge of the disease course and pathology of lesions such as: flexor tenosynovitis; synovitis; and soft tissue oedema. Increased US sensitivity has also brought innovation including promising automated ultrasound scanning techniques. So, what have we learnt in recent years and what are the unmet needs to focus future research initiatives in this disabling disease? This narrative review article assesses the neoteric evidence, bringing into context the knowledge gained and highlighting potential areas of research.

Keywords: spondyloarthritis (including psoriatic arthritis), enthesitis, dactylitis, synovitis tendon inflammation, peri-tendon inflammation, tenosynovitis, ultrasonography

INTRODUCTION

Psoriatic arthritis (PsA) is a heterogeneous disease characterized by joint, tendon, and entheseal inflammation in both the peripheral and axial skeleton. At these sites, inflammation gives rise to pain, tenderness and swelling which is either localized around a joint or more diffuse e.g., along a whole digit (dactylitis). Categorized as one of the main disorders under the umbrella term Spondyloarthritis (SpA), PsA incorporates associated extra-articular manifestations including cutaneous psoriasis (PsO), related onychodystrophy, inflammatory bowel disease and uveitis.

The musculoskeletal burden is comparable to rheumatoid arthritis (RA), with joint related damage, functional impairment and reduced quality of life over time (1).

The challenges of diagnosis in early PsA are not confined to the heterogeneity of disease, which is evident from the variety of outcome measures available (2). In contrast to RA, there are no biomarkers such as anti-citrullinated peptide antibody (ACPA) or rheumatoid factor (RF) to identify early PsA and therefore diagnosis is dependent upon identification of specific clinical features. In addition, elevation of acute phase markers such as C-reactive protein (CRP) only occurs in up to half of patients and is therefore of limited value in early PsA (3). Lastly, the absence of PsO in the presence of arthritis may lead to a label of undifferentiated arthritis. Reflecting these shortcomings, imaging has been increasingly utilized for PsA evaluation and therapy assessment.

Plain film radiographs of joints are feasible, quick to perform and low in cost, with the ability to assess progressive damage reasonably well. However, when compared to ultrasound (US) or magnetic resonance imaging (MRI), they lack sensitivity for detecting early inflammatory arthritis and associated damage (4, 5). Ultrasonography (US) has various advantages over MRI, including greater accessibility, overall reduced cost, lack of contraindications, and its availability in the clinic. However, MRI has the advantage of allowing access to sites where US has a limited acoustic window e.g., axial skeleton and all osseous based pathology. Given the mounting evidence on early treatment of active inflammation for optimal outcomes, the need for adopting sensitive imaging tools into routine practice has never been greater. The aim of this review was to evaluate the recent research literature on US use in PsA with relevance to clinical practice.

METHODS

A panel of rheumatologists undertook this project. Although no systematic search was performed as such, the Patient-Intervention-Comparison-Outcome (PICO) standard was adhered to. Intervention: the search strategy focused on scientific publications reporting on the use of US for diagnosis, management and assessment of PsA. Population: the target group included adults ($\geq$ 18 years of age) with a diagnosis of PsA of any disease duration. Specific PsA musculoskeletal manifestations explored were synovitis, dactylitis, and enthesitis. PsA-related spondylitis was not included due to unfeasible accessibility of axial skeleton structures to US imaging techniques. Comparator: the imaging techniques appraised, whenever available, were conventional radiography, computed tomography (CT), and MRI. Outcome: no pre-set outcome measures were chosen, as the panel felt that a restricted approach would narrow the focus of the review excessively. Whenever available, measures of diagnostic accuracy (sensitivity, specificity, positive/negative predictive values, and likelihood ratios) were retrieved (**Table 1**).

The search strategy encompassed clinical trials, well-designed cohorts and systematic reviews published in Pubmed from 2015 onwards and was performed by two members of the working party (SRD, GDM). Only publications in English were considered. Key papers before 2015 were included if considered relevant to the review.

RESULTS

Ultrasound for Diagnosis

Synovitis

Grayscale (GS) US findings in PsA are similar to those of RA in morphology with synovial hypertrophy, intra-articular effusion, enhanced power Doppler (PD) signal, and erosions (**Figure 1A**). However, the literature shows a trend to higher severity in RA synovitis as compared to PsA (6, 7). In these studies focussing on synovitis in PsA, US showed more prominent tendinous/entheseal involvement adjacent to synovial joints in the PsA groups (8, 9). Absence of PD signal over the hypertrophic tissues, however, did not rule out active intra-articular synovitis (6). Preliminary data suggested that the pathologic processes in the intra-articular synovia may follow - not precede- inflammation at the level of soft tissues surrounding extensor tendons in the hands (9, 10). One limitation of US, in the context of the evaluation of psoriatic polyarthritis, could be the amount of time needed to perform such investigation, as compared to clinical evaluation. However, automated US scanning techniques showed 2-fold higher sensitivity in detecting synovitis of the hands, when compared to clinical examination, and have potential for improving the current standard of care in rheumatology clinics (10).

Subclinical Synovitis: What Does it Mean?

Attribution of articular swelling to synovitis is better performed by US as compared to clinical examination, especially at a sub-clinical stage. Subclinical synovitis as detected by US is frequent in subjects with psoriasis and healthy individuals (up to 49.6% may show at least one abnormality, in at least one site investigated). Although less common, PD signal suggestive of subclinical synovitis was present in 24% of healthy subjects (11). It is interesting to note that in the healthy subjects recruited in this cross-sectional study, PD signal showed mild alteration (grading 1 out of 3) and lesions scoring 2 or 3 were uncommon or absent, respectively. Of note, PsA patients recruited in this study had subclinical synovitis more frequently, affecting more sites and with more severe PD signal alterations. Frequent findings of subclinical synovitis in healthy subjects (55%) and psoriatic patients (85%) were confirmed by another cross-sectional study (12). However, in this report, "active synovitis" (that is, the combination of synovial hypertrophy with PD signal) was found exclusively in psoriatic subjects (27.5%) (12). Histological evaluation would ideally be needed to disentangle the meaning of these imaging findings in pre-clinical PsA and in normal.

Subclinical synovitis -with or without subclinical enthesitis- at baseline is more frequent in psoriatic patients who develop PsA over a follow-up of 2 years (13). In PsA patients who are in clinical remission/minimal disease activity, US detection (using associated PD) of non-clinically noticeable synovitis is a predictor of short-term (6 months) flare (14).

TABLE 1 | References appraised and selected for inclusion.

Ultrasound for diagnosis

- Synovitis
  Records evaluated: 80;
  Records included: 6 (2 relevant references from > 5 years included)
- Subclinical synovitis
  Records evaluated: 65;
  Records included 4
- Tendon pathologies
  Records evaluated: 97;
  Records included 10 (of which 2 are also cited in "synovitis") (3 relevant references from > 5 years included)
- Entheseal pathology
  Records evaluated: 126;
  Records included 13 (of which 1 already cited in tendon pathologies) (1 relevant reference from > 5 years included)
- Dactylitis
  Records evaluated: 38;
  Records included 5 (0 references from > 5 years)
- US in differential diagnosis of PsA
  Records evaluated: 134;
  Records included 4 (of which 1 already cited in tendon)
- Limitations of US in clinical practice
  Records evaluated: 43;
  Records included 1 (0 references from > 5 years)
- Comparison of US with clinical examination and composite clinical scores
  Records evaluated: 101;
  Records included 5 (of which 1 is already cited in "dactylitis"); (1 relevant reference from > 5 years included).

Ultrasound for management

- US for management
  Records evaluated: 59;
  Records included: 2 (0 references from > 5 years)
- Monitoring of PsA
  Records evaluated: 280;
  Records included 2 (0 references from > 5 years)
- Remission assessment
  Records evaluated: 120;
  Records included 3 (of which 2 already cited in subclinical synovitis and comparison of US with clinical examination) (1 relevant reference from > 5 years included)
- Prognosis
  Records evaluated: 87;
  Records included 4 (of which 1 already cited in tendon)
- Composite US scores (joints, entheses)
  Records evaluated: 19;
  Records included 9 (of which 1 is also cited in "tendon patho ogies"), (3 relevant references from > 5 years duration).
- Guided injections
  Records evaluated: 116;
  Records included 4 (2 relevant references from >5 years).

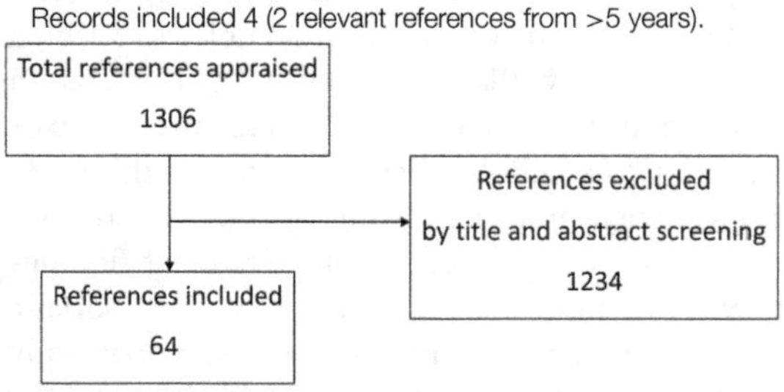

Tendon Pathologies

Tendinopathic pathologies can exist in both PsA and RA but can be difficult to attribute specifically to either disease. Benjamin et al. (15) described the concept of a "functional enthesis," an anatomical, biomechanical, and pathological feature that share fibrocartilaginous entheses proximal to regions of attachment to allow tendons or ligament to wrap around bony pulleys. It is at these sites that there is a propensity for disease in PsA which has been confirmed through US (16). Flexor tenosynovitis can be detected by high-resolution US of the hand flexor tendons as illustrated in **Figure 1B**. Peri-tendinous soft tissue oedema and PD signal have been reported in the 2nd–4th flexor tendon compartments of the dominant hand in one third of PsA vs. no RA patients (8, 17). Additionally, flexor tendon insertional enthesopathy occurs at accessory pulleys including new bone formation, significantly more common in PsA, supporting the "Deep Koebner" phenomenon (18). A much higher percentage of peritendinous extensor digitorum tendon inflammation was observed in PsA compared to RA (9). Soft tissue oedema was detected almost exclusively in PsA when the most clinically involved finger was assessed. Further, central slip enthesitis at the PIP joints was exclusively found in early PsA. Ultrasound detection of extra-synovial features and at the synovio-entheseal complex may be helpful in the differential diagnosis between early RA and early PsA (9).

There is some expert based consensus that the most useful anatomical sites for identifying disease at tendons (with sheaths) are at the hand flexor tendons, extensor tendon compartment of the wrist, and for peri-tendonitis (inflamed tendons without sheath) hand extensor tendons are favored over the feet extensor tendons (19).

Further recent studies have also added to the literature on significantly greater tendon sheath synovial thickening and tendon sheath PD signal observed in PsA compared to PsO without PsA (20). On a practical level, a previous study demonstrated greater peritendon extensor tendon inflammation at the MCP level in PsA than RA, indicating that it is a key characteristic of PsA, valuable in differential diagnosis (10). Importantly in PsA, the most recent evidence indicates that MCP swelling is actually attributable to not only synovitis, but also peri-tendonitis (**Figure 1A**), and are detectable at similar frequencies (21).

Entheseal Pathology

Enthesitis is considered characteristic of PsA and an early lesion throughout disease progression (22). The clinical assessment of the entheses can be impaired by lack of sensitivity and overlap with pain amplification syndromes (23, 24). Moreover, data suggest a disconnection between arthritis severity and enthesitis severity (25). Although recent studies found no correlation between the clinical and the US assessments of entheses in PsA there is potential for increased accuracy of enthesitis assessment using US scan (26, 27).

OMERACT proposed (28) a definition for the elementary lesions that characterize enthesopathy: (1) "hypoechogenicity at the enthesis"; (2) "thickened enthesis"; (3) "calcification/enthesophyte at enthesis"; (4) "erosion at enthesis"; (5) "Doppler signal at enthesis" (**Figures 1C–E**). Some of these lesions are structural and commonly seen in people not affected by PsA, although in PsA they tend to be more severe (29–31). Moreover, the definition of PD alterations within 2 mm from the enthesis is not accepted by the whole scientific community. Furthermore, body weight and other mechanical factors and metabolic conditions are considered confounders for enthesopathic structural lesions (17, 32). However, US-detected active enthesitis (that is, the combination of elementary lesions 1 and 5) is related to older age and higher levels of physical activity in PsA patients (33). Interestingly, inflammatory entheseal changes are commonly found in people who have psoriasis or arthralgia and psoriasis, preceding the clinical onset of PsA. In the study by Zabotti et al. (32) the presence of US evidence of enthesitis was associated with progression to PsA.

Dactylitis

The use of US has added to the understanding of pathologies involved in dactylitis that extend beyond the presence of synovitis and flexor tenosynovitis. In a recent study of dactylitis in PsA patients, joint synovitis was detected by US in 40% of dactylitic digits and was associated with longer duration of dactylitis and the asymptomatic "cold" type characterized by swelling but not pain or tenderness (34). Another study of psoriatic dactylitis identified PD at the accessory pulleys of affected digits, suggesting that these sites of mechanical stress may be more important in the disease process than previously thought (35). Moreover, flexor tenosynovitis is most prevalent in the majority of PsA imaged dactylitis and over half of patients also display subcutaneous oedema and synovitis (36). Unlike the OMERACT US definitions aforementioned for synovitis and enthesitis, no widely accepted ultrasound definition was present for dactylitis. Just recently, Zabotti et al. (37) have developed an US score for dactylitis, namely the DACTylitis glObal Sonographic score in PsA (DACTOS). Dactylitis elementary lesions were reviewed via a Delphi exercise of 12 experts to reach a consensus on scoring which resulted in moderate/excellent reliability for US scored lesions (37). Imaging scores of such may assist in the diagnosis and evaluation of the response of tissue compartments to therapies (38).

US in Differential Diagnosis in PsA

The morphological similarities between PsA synovium and that of RA leave open substantial issues related to the differential diagnosis of inflammatory arthritides. Narrowing the view on synovitis, the integration of contrast enhancement technique to US scans may assist in distinguishing across different diseases. Some evidence points to the potential of different software for quantitative analysis of the kinetic parameters of the synovial vascular perfusion pattern. In one study, this sophisticated technique has shown discriminatory ability in the assessment of RA vs. other forms of arthritis, including PsA (39). However, such advanced analysis tool would be available only in research centers for now.

Beyond synovitis, the available evidence supports the concept that PsA is mainly differentiated from RA by the involvement of non-synovial articular and peri-articular structures/tissues (17, 40). Key findings are enthesitis, peritendonitis of the extensor tendons of the hands, thickening of the pulleys of the flexor tendons of the hands, peri-tendineal dermal soft tissue oedema and bone proliferation associated with erosions (usually smaller than RA). The presence of extra-synovial features on US of the hands showed sensitivity of 68% and specificity of 88.1% for early PsA (16). Some limitations apply, since most studies were performed on limited parts of the musculoskeletal system (hands and wrists mainly). Moreover, the comparisons were made between RA, seronegative SpA and PsA (leaving out crystal-caused arthropathies, especially the chronic forms).

The Limitations of US in Clinical Practice

On a practical level, clinical examination, which is subjective and not anatomically nor pathology specific, is complemented by the high sensitivity of US to detect inflammatory and structural lesions, clearly advantageous to identify characteristic PsA-related pathologies. Despite these significant benefits, a recent systematic review reported variable diagnostic accuracy for US in PsA, in fact confirmation of a PsA diagnosis was heavily

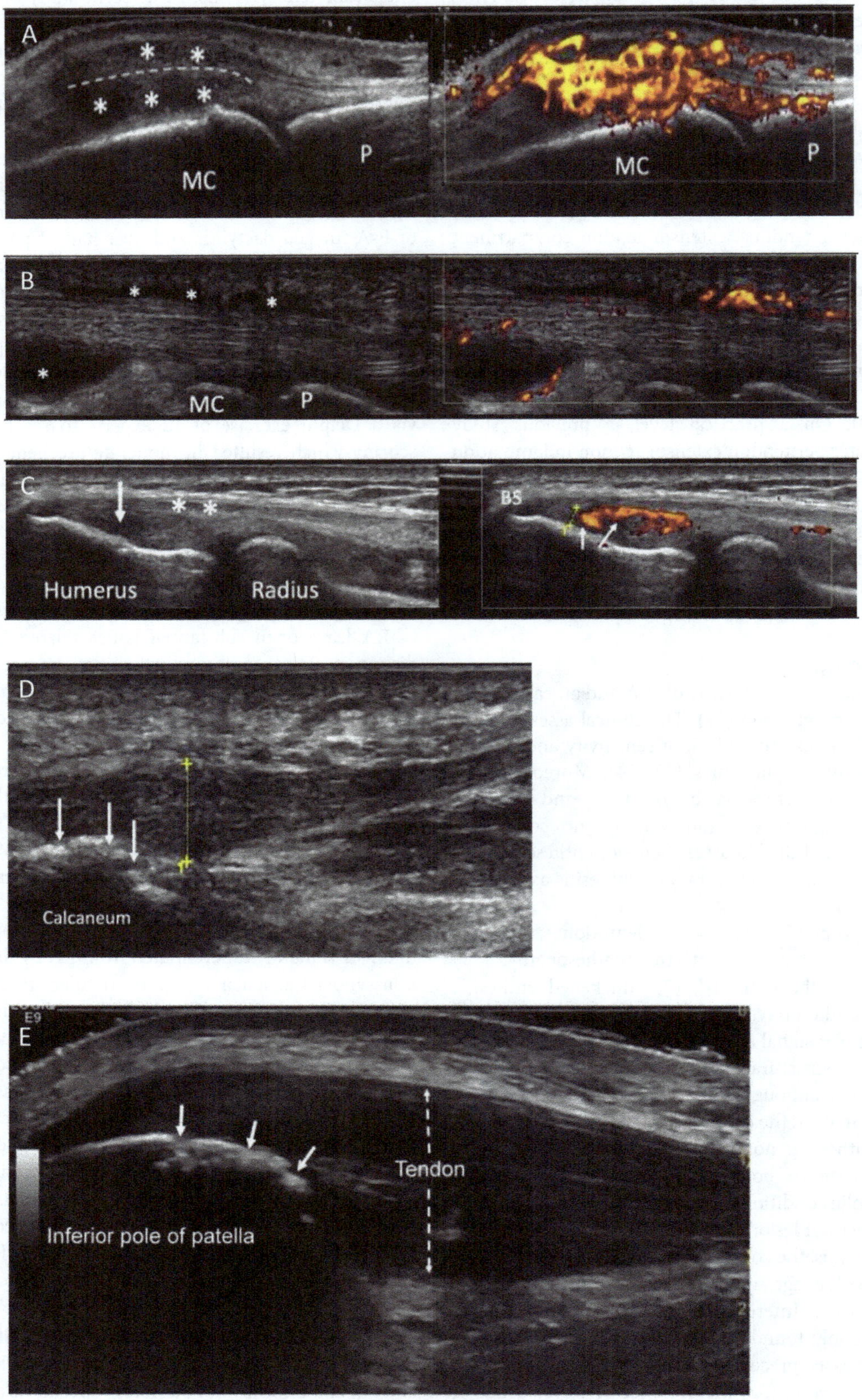

FIGURE 1 | Characteristic ultrasound appearances in Psoriatic arthritis. **(A)** Longitudinal view through a metacarpophalangeal joint with synovitis. There is gray scale

(Continued)

FIGURE 1 | thickening (*between joint and extensor tendon-dotted line) and marked increased power Doppler signal (grade 3, right image) consistent with "active" synovitis and peri-tendonitis (*above tendon). MC, metacarpal; P, phalanx. **(B)** Longitudinal view through the flexor tendon on a finger. It demonstrates fluid and synovial thickening within the tendon sheath (*). There is also marked power Doppler signal within the tendon sheath (right image). MC, metacarpal; P, phalanx. **(C)** Enthesitis of common extensor origin (CEO): Longitudinal view through the common extensor origin. Hypoechogenicity (arrow/left), loss of fibrillary pattern (*), Bone spur (BS), increased Doppler signal (small arrows/right) within 2 mm (dotted line) of bone surface. **(D)** Longitudinal view through the plantar fascia of a patient with PsA. There is thickening of the fascia (dotted yellow line measuring 8.3 mm; normal < 5 mm). Power Doppler signal is rarely seen at the plantar fascia insertion. Bone irregularity is suggestive of erosive change (arrows). **(E)** Longitudinal section through the proximal patellar tendon. The tendon is markedly thickened (dotted arrow), hypoechogenic (compared to normal tendon more distally) and has lost its fibrillary pattern. The bone surface of the patella shows bone irregularity consistent with erosive change (white arrows). This was confirmed on transverse view.

based on clinical diagnosis and classification criteria (CASPAR) (41). One should also be cognizant that the objectivity of US is dependent upon having a skilled operator for scanning and image interpretation, and a sensitive US machine/ transducer, particularly relevant for PD signal detection. Further, it is unfeasible to scan 68 joints and numerous entheses for every patient in routine clinical practice due to time constraints, therefore comprehensive US assessments of this nature occur mostly in a research setting. There are also costs to be considered involving the purchase, running, and servicing of the equipment.

Comparison of US With Clinical Examination and Composite Clinical Scores

A recent study has confirmed that in fact there is a significant association between clinical and US assessment of the large entheses when assessing Achilles and Patellar tendon origins (42). Furthermore, digital pain and tenderness in dactylitis was linked to US tenosynovitis GS ≥ 2 (34). However, large discrepancies have been reported between clinical examination and US findings for synovitis and enthesitis (43). In the same study, the DAPSA composite scores partially reflected Boolean's remission criteria and correlated with GS and PD synovitis but not the CPDAI (43). In another longitudinal study of 47 PsA patients, the SJC66, CRP, ESR, DAS28, and the physician global assessment were associated with PD, whereas the DAPSA was not (44). Therefore, the discordance between clinical examination and US synovitis needs further research. However, a recent report on clinical low disease activity (LDA) states, (determined by DAPSA, PASDAS, CPDAI, or MDA) suggests they are able to differentiate between high and low (MUDA) US determined disease activity (45). The unmet needs and suggested areas to focus US research in diagnosis and management of PsA are summarized in **Table 2**.

MANAGEMENT

Ultrasound for Management

The EULAR recommendations for the use of imaging in the diagnosis and management of SpA in clinical practice suggest that US has a place in providing "additional information" on top of clinical examination and laboratory investigation for monitoring the activity of peripheral SpA, including PsA (46). Perhaps surprising is that in RA, recent data showed a dichotomy between the relationship of the clinical TJC and SJC with US synovitis suggesting TJC is not associated with US synovitis, but data from similarly large cohorts for PsA is missing (47). The complex relationship between clinical and US examination is poorly understood in PsA and would suggest the inclusion of US can aid the assessment of disease where clinical assessment may have missed underlying occult PsA disease activity. As well as for disease monitoring, remission status, and disease activity measures, we evaluated data for the value of US in prognostication and targeted therapeutic interventions (intra-articular injections).

Monitoring of PsA

One study on PsA looking at the utility of US in the clinic showed that PD signal detected at baseline was not associated with response to treatment at 4 months [either biologic or conventional synthetic disease-modifying anti-rheumatic drugs (bDMARDs, csDMARDs, respectively)] in the routine care setting (48). These findings contrast with those from studies in RA, so Højgaard et al. (48) argued that one possible explanation could be the different presentation of the two diseases (that is, RA is more symmetric/uniform than PsA). The possibility remained that PD signal grading continuum, not merely its presence, would be more relevant for prognosis. In the TICOPA imaging substudy US inflammation scores were based on summation of GS and PD and both these features were graded 0–3. In this underpowered substudy, the US-based measure demonstrated responsiveness, was aligned to clinical outcome measures at baseline, and was aligned to the change detected by clinical outcome measures between two different time-points (49).

Remission Assessment

In PsA patients who are in clinical remission/minimal disease activity, US detection of subclinical synovitis using PD was a predictor of short-term (6 months) PsA flare (14). There is however, evidence of poor correlation between levels of clinical PsA activity (as measured by composite outcome measures) and US inflammatory findings (above all, PD signal) (50). US remission was found in 49.6% of the patients in this cross-sectional study, while clinical remission was achieved by 5.7–9.9% of the patients (depending on the composite outcome measure used). In this study, patient-reported-outcome-measures, a component of many clinical composite outcome measure, correlated with US findings worse than swollen joint count.

In another study, in 20% of PsA patients with clinically active disease (as measured by clinical composite outcome measures such as DAPSA, PASDAS, CPDAI, MDA) US assessment resulted in minimal inflammatory activity (MUDA) (43). In this study,

TABLE 2 | Unmet needs in ultrasound imaging in Psoriatic arthritis.

Topic of interest in PsA	Unmet needs: suggested research focus, by clinical phenotype	
	Psoriatic oligo/polyarthritis	**Psoriatic dactylitis**
Diagnosis:		
Sensitivity and specificity:	• PsA is frequently underdiagnosed or misdiagnosed. Can US improve the PsA diagnostic yield? • The specificity of US features to PsA is an area where further knowledge may improve clinical diagnosis given that overlapping pathologies exist between diseases. • Larger sized prospective cohorts may provide further insight into the characterisation of US features useful to differentiate different inflammatory arthritides (e.g., RA, PsA/SpA, crystal arthropathies).	• Dactylitis is a unique lesion in PsA. Yet the significance of dactylitis is still unclear in terms of the overall burden of disease in PsA. Further research on this lesion and US in PsA will drive further knowledge and understanding of this pathognomonic lesion in PsA/SpA. • The nature of dactylitis from early disease onset into chronic PsA is not fully understood. More research from large PsA cohorts may explain this further. • High sensitivity US may be useful in detection of small entheseal tissue in dactylitis research.
Synovial Synovitis:	• Disparity between clinical examination and US findings in PsA is still not well-understood. The relationship between clinical examination and US for identifying synovitis (and enthesitis below) is poorly understood and requires further research to clarify and inform clinical practice and decision making. • The large number of joints in the Psoriatic joint clinical/US assessment is time limiting and impractical in the clinic. A condensed, time-sensitive, but valid and reliable US tool that can be easily implementable is required for practicality in clinical practice and research. • More work on longitudinal PsA/PsO cohorts needed on the subject of subclinical synovitis and its prognostic value in the short and medium term (up to 5 years of follow-up).	• What is the relationship between dactylitis and synovitis? Does this differ depending upon disease course or treatment type? • Are there any ultrasound predictors that determine why some people with dactylitis may be affected by worse outcomes? • PsA cohorts with dactylitis may provide more insight into future dactylitis research. • Is there a risk from dactylitis to overall disease related affliction and treatment in early disease? • Does synovitis represent risk of dactylitis relapse/recurrence?
Extra-synovial Enthesitis:	• Discordance between clinical an US enthesitis suggests further studies may inform the differentiation between PsA and non-PsA. • Is an enthesitis US composite research score needed? If so, how many entheses should be included and which ones?	• The enthesis organ concept is highly implicated in PsA, yet we do not know whether dactylitis results in more clinical/US enthesitis? • Does dactylitis represent an intermediary lesion in the disease spectrum, developing from enthesitis and next into synovitis, or could it be a more significant clinical marker of disease severity in early PsA? These are questions that future US research may be able to answer using US at time-points in PsA evolution.
Tendon related pathologies:	• Research to improve differentiation of tendon pathologies in early PsA from RA or Palindromic rheumatism is where US may inform clinical practice. • Further research is needed on imaging of tendon pulleys and sheaths in early PsA which may hold early diagnostic value. • Identification of flexor/extensor tendons, peritendinous regions: where, when, and which should we scan? Is there a significance in terms of the disease overall burden?	• Tendon pathologies are key pathological features in dactylitis and correspond to the anatomical concept of swelling across the whole digit. Further understanding of tendinopathy in this lesion may improve targeted PsA therapy per patient based upon lesion. • Flexor tenosynovitis and flexor tendon sheath and pulley pathologies are key components of dactylitis. • Peritendon inflammation: US vs. MRI, disease course and response to therapy. • Scoring is a "hot" topic: Validation of scoring methods can permit use in research and clinical settings. • Hot and cold differentiation and active pathologies: clinical examination findings could be included to encompass the best representation of dactylitis status.
Management: US disease activity scores/composite outcome measures for monitoring	• How should overall US disease activity be measured per patient? • Which composite measure should be used?	• Isolated US vs. combined clinical and US features of dactylitis should be considered to assess dactylitis disease activity and monitor treatment response. • Clinical trials and longitudinal cohort studies may provide further clues into this arena where the data is sparse.
Disease remission:	• Clinical vs. US remission: which should be used? How should US remission/low disease activity be defined? More research in this area is needed.	
Pragmatic, additional issues:	• Advancing technologies are emerging which allow automated and simplified assessment of joints in less time. Can they be reliably and validly implemented and with cost-effectiveness?	

the pain-related items, as part of the clinical composite outcome measures, were the components conditioning higher disease activity scores. The authors postulated that the evaluation of clinical treatment targets can benefit from US evaluation.

Prognosis

In PsA patients clinically classified as oligoarthritis, US scanning has uncovered synovial hypertrophy of polyarticular distribution (51). Similar findings are relevant for the assessment of PsA prognosis. Baseline US findings of synovitis (upon GS and

PD assessment) were identified as risk factors for additional articular damage in one study (52). In this study, the presence of baseline enthesopathy/enthesitis also accounted as a risk factor for articular damage.

Another study found that 26 PsA patients who were in clinical remission had low levels of PD signal on US scan. Once csDMARD or bDMARD therapy was stopped the clinical recurrence rate of PsA was high (90%). One predictor of PsA relapse was synovial hypertrophy on US scan at the time of therapy cessation (53). Further data on the assessment of remission and prognosis are expected from the UPSTREAM study (19).

Composite US Scores

Just as there are several clinical composite scores for the assessment of PsA, US disease activity may be scored using a number of validated methods for the joints and entheses in clinical and research practice.

Joints

Two composite scores have been specifically developed to monitor disease activity in PsA: the 5TPD and PsA-Son composite scores with good sensitivity to detect inflammation and feasibility, but not yet validated in any other series (19).

Following the suit of many rheumatology clinical composite scores, Ficjan et al. (54) proposed two US scoring methods to assess inflammatory and structural PsA lesions, the PsA-Son13, (unilateral joints), and PsA-Son22 score (bilateral joints). They reported sufficient construct validity, reliability, and sensitivity to change for both scores. The reduced number of joints included may be considerably time saving, however there is potential to miss involved joints leading to a false reflection of overall disease activity, especially relevant for oligo/monoarticular phenotypes.

The "5 targets Power Doppler for Psoriatic disease" (5TDP) was based on joints, tendons, entheses, skin and nails scoring the highest expression of PD signal (55). The limitations were that the score does not consider multiple joint involvement from single joint involvement and may lead to under estimation of disease activity in polyarticular disease (55). A further drawback is that nail and skin US assessment is not commonplace in routine practice and therefore not practical outside of a research setting. Finally, it is notable that large joint involvement is frequent in PsA, therefore a tool initially developed for validation in RA, SOnography in LArge joints in Rheumatology (SOLAR), has been reported for its suitability for PsA (56).

Entheses

In a recent study, the Madrid Sonographic Enthesitis Index (MASEI), a scoring tool designed for enthesitis in SpA/PsA, failed to distinguish between enthesitis in PsA from healthy controls (57). It was found that by excluding the knee enthesis thickness and refining PD severity, marked differences could be shown between PsA patients and healthy controls, indicating that given considerable overlap of features exists between groups, setting the best discriminative thresholds for detecting pathology is imperative (57). On the contrary, a recent systematic literature review concluded that the MASEI was feasible, reliable and a valid ultrasound score for assessing enthesitis, but did not find any articles assessing MASEI as an outcome for treatment response (58). Whether clinical tenderness is derived from enthesitis or fibromyalgia can be difficult to assess, but has recently been studied using US and scored via the Glasgow enthesitis scoring system (GUESS) (59). It was found that US enthesitis was more prevalent in PsA and PsA with fibromyalgia compared to fibromyalgia alone, and clinical entheseal scores (LEI, MASES) were shown to potentially overestimate active enthesitis in fibromyalgia (59). A further preliminary enthesitis score developed in a recent GRAPPA study has reported the ability to differentiate between PsA and healthy controls (60). However, this has led to further discussion/debate on whether a further enthesitis score is actually needed, and if so, how many entheses should be included, and the suggestion that a study to prioritize differentiation of PsA from PsO and osteoarthritis/mechanical pain should be prioritized (61).

Guided Interventions (Injections)

Ultrasound provides the ability to visualize the needle for injection procedures and therefore optimize placement accuracy. There are no specific recent studies on PsA and the effectiveness of US guided routine intra-articular injections. However, previous randomized controlled trials (RCT) in inflammatory arthritis reported significantly better accuracy of joint injection by US over the blind/palpation approach (62). In the same study, the benefit of short-term outcomes could not be demonstrated. Another larger RCT of 244 patients reported superior outcomes and cost-effectiveness with US guided injection *vs.* the conventional blind/palpation technique, with an 81% reduction in injection pain, 35% reduction in pain scores and 38% increase in responder rate (63). In contrast, a large randomized trial examining the benefit of US in a clinical tight control regimen in RA (ARCTIC) did not find any significant difference in treatment efficacy between US guided and blind/palpation guided joint injections (64). There is a clear advantage of targeting pathologically active disease through US assessment prior to US guided injection given that treatment efficacy was observed when moderate PD synovitis was present, independent of whether the joint was clinically swollen (64). Given the multiple pathologies in PsA, it would seem reasonable to study targeted US injections based on region and type of pathology. Further research may clarify whether US guided joint injection for routine intra-articular joint injections can produce superior outcomes over routine blind approach, but the most recent data is limited (6).

CONCLUSIONS

Ultrasound is complementary to clinical examination by adding sensitivity and specificity to sites of disease in PsA enhancing the qualitative assessment. Several recent studies have shown added value of US in research by improving the understanding of disease. The clinical role of US for diagnosis is ever more assuring, yet there is discordance between clinical and US assessment that needs further research. Composite scoring measures remain research driven tools and are unlikely to be implemented in busy routine clinics in the near future. As US becomes more widely used, its function as a disease monitoring tool is promising, but further research is required to clarify its specific role in the clinic.

AUTHOR CONTRIBUTIONS

All authors listed have made a substantial, direct and intellectual contribution to the work, and approved it for publication.

REFERENCES

1. Gladman DD, Antoni C, Mease P, Clegg DO, Nash P. Psoriatic arthritis: epidemiology, clinical features, course, and outcome. *Ann Rheum Dis.* (2005) 64(Suppl. 2):ii14–7. doi: 10.1136/ard.2004.032482
2. Tan AL, McGonagle D. The need for biological outcomes for biological drugs in psoriatic arthritis. *J Rheumatol.* (2016) 43:3–6. doi: 10.3899/jrheum.151296
3. Bogliolo L, Crepaldi G, Caporali R. Biomarkers and prognostic stratification in psoriatic arthritis. *Reumatismo.* (2012) 64:88–98. doi: 10.4081/reumatismo.2012.88
4. Takase-Minegishi K, Horita N, Kobayashi K, Yoshimi R, Kirino Y, Ohno S, et al. Diagnostic test accuracy of ultrasound for synovitis in rheumatoid arthritis: systematic review and meta-analysis. *Rheumatology.* (2018) 57:49–58. doi: 10.1093/rheumatology/kex036
5. Wiell C, Szkudlarek M, Hasselquist M, Møller JM, Vestergaard A, Nørregaard J, et al. Ultrasonography, magnetic resonance imaging, radiography, and clinical assessment of inflammatory and destructive changes in fingers and toes of patients with psoriatic arthritis. *Arthritis Res Ther.* (2007) 9:1–13. doi: 10.1186/ar2327
6. Zabotti A, Bandinelli F, Batticciotto A, Scirè CA, Iagnocco A, Sakellariou G. Musculoskeletal ultrasonography for psoriatic arthritis and psoriasis patients: a systematic literature review. *Rheumatology.* (2017) 56:1518–32. doi: 10.1093/rheumatology/kex179
7. Vreju AF, Chisalau BA, Parvanescu CD, Barbulescu A, Rogoveanu O, Firulescu S, et al. High frequency ultrasonography of the hand in rheumatoid arthritis, psoriatic arthritis, gout and osteoarthritis patients. *Curr Heal Sci J.* (2016) 42:35–9. doi: 10.12865/CHSJ.42.01.05
8. Fournié B, Margarit-Coll N, Champetier de Ribes TL, Zabraniecki L, Jouan A, Vincent V, et al. Extrasynovial ultrasound abnormalities in the psoriatic finger. Prospective comparative power-doppler study versus rheumatoid arthritis. *Jt Bone Spine.* (2006) 73:527–31. doi: 10.1016/j.jbspin.2006.01.019
9. Zabotti A, Salvin S, Quartuccio L, De Vita S. Differentiation between early rheumatoid and early psoriatic arthritis by the ultrasonographic study of the synovio-entheseal complex of the small joints of the hands. *Clin Exp Rheumatol.* (2016) 34:459–65.
10. Gutierrez M, Filippucci E, Salaffi F, Di Geso L, Grassi W. Differential diagnosis between rheumatoid arthritis and psoriatic arthritis: the value of ultrasound findings at metacarpophalangeal joints level. *Ann Rheum Dis.* (2011) 70:1111–4. doi: 10.1136/ard.2010.147272
11. Tang Y, Yang Y, Xiang X, Wang L, Zhang L, Qiu L. Power doppler ultrasound evaluation of peripheral joint, entheses, tendon, and bursa abnormalities in psoriatic patients: a clinical study. *J Rheumatol.* (2018) 45:811–7. doi: 10.3899/jrheum.170765
12. Zuliani F, Zabotti A, Errichetti E, Tinazzi I, Zanetti A, Carrara G, et al. Ultrasonographic detection of subclinical enthesitis and synovitis: a possible stratification of psoriatic patients without clinical musculoskeletal involvement. *Clin Exp Rheumatol.* (2019) 37:593–9.
13. Elnady B, El Shaarawy NK, Dawoud NM, Elkhouly T, Desouky DES, ElShafey EN, et al. Subclinical synovitis and enthesitis in psoriasis patients and controls by ultrasonography in Saudi Arabia; incidence of psoriatic arthritis during two years. *Clin Rheumatol.* (2019) 38:1627–35. doi: 10.1007/s10067-019-04445-0
14. Ruta S, Marin J, Felquer MLA, Ferreyra-Garrot L, Rosa J, García-Monaco R, et al. Utility of power doppler ultrasound-detected synovitis for the prediction of short-term flare in psoriatic patients with arthritis in clinical remission. *J Rheumatol.* (2017) 44:1018–23. doi: 10.3899/jrheum.161347
15. Benjamin M, McGonagle D. The enthesis organ concept and its relevance to the spondyloarthropathies. *Adv Exp Med Biol.* (2009) 649:57–70. doi: 10.1007/978-1-4419-0298-6_4
16. Zabotti A, Errichetti E, Zuliani F, Quartuccio L, Sacco S, Stinco G, et al. Early psoriatic arthritis versus early seronegative rheumatoid arthritis: role of dermoscopy combined with ultrasonography for differential diagnosis. *J Rheumatol.* (2018) 45:648–54. doi: 10.3899/jrheum.170962
17. Tinazzi I, McGonagle D, Zabotti A, Chessa D, Marchetta A, Macchioni P. Comprehensive evaluation of finger flexor tendon entheseal soft tissue and bone changes by ultrasound can differentiate psoriatic arthritis and rheumatoid arthritis. *Clin Exp Rheumatol.* (2018) 36:785–90.
18. Tinazzi I, McGonagle D, Aydin SZ, Chessa D, Marchetta A, Macchioni P. "Deep Koebner" phenomenon of the flexor tendon-associated accessory pulleys as a novel factor in tenosynovitis and dactylitis in psoriatic arthritis. *Ann Rheum Dis.* (2018) 77:922–5. doi: 10.1136/annrheumdis-2017-212681
19. Zabotti A, Piga M, Canzoni M, Sakellariou G, Iagnocco A, Scirè CA, et al. Ultrasonography in psoriatic arthritis: which sites should we scan? *Ann Rheum Dis.* (2018) 77:1537–8. doi: 10.1136/annrheumdis-2018-213025
20. Tang Y, Cheng S, Yang Y, Xiang X, Wang L, Zhang L, et al. Ultrasound assessment in psoriatic arthritis (PsA) and psoriasis vulgaris (non-PsA): which sites are most commonly involved and what features are more important in PsA? *Quant Imaging Med Surg.* (2020) 10:86–95. doi: 10.21037/qims.2019.08.09
21. Macía-Villa C, Falcao S, Gutierrez M, Medina J, Hammer HB, De Miguel E. What is metacarpophalangeal joint swelling in psoriatic arthritis? Ultrasound findings and reliability assessment. *Clin Exp Rheumatol.* (2018) 36:896–9. doi: 10.1136/annrheumdis-2017-eular.1437
22. McGonagle D, Gibbon W, Emery P. Classification of inflammatory arthritis by enthesitis. *Lancet.* (1998) 352:1137–40. doi: 10.1016/S0140-6736(97)12004-9
23. Kaeley GS, Eder L, Aydin SZ, Gutierrez M, Bakewell C. Enthesitis: a hallmark of psoriatic arthritis. *Semin Arthritis Rheum.* (2018) 48:35–43. doi: 10.1016/j.semarthrit.2017.12.008
24. Macchioni P, Salvarani C, Possemato N, Gutierrez M, Grassi W, Gasparini S, et al. Ultrasonographic and clinical assessment of peripheral enthesitis in patients with psoriatic arthritis, psoriasis, and fibromyalgia syndrome: the ULISSE study. *J Rheumatol.* (2019) 46:904–11. doi: 10.3899/jrheum.171411
25. Florescu A, Vere CC, Florescu LM, Muşetescu AE, Bondari A, Ciurea PL. Clinical and ultrasound assessment of enthesis in psoriatic arthritis in a romanian cohort. *Curr Heal Sci J.* (2018) 44:347–51. doi: 10.12865/CHSJ.44.04.04
26. Yamada Y, Inui K, Okano T, Mandai K, Mamoto K, Koike T, et al. Ultrasound assessment, unlike clinical assessment, reflects enthesitis in patients with psoriatic arthritis. *Clin Exp Rheumatol.* (2020). [Epub ahead of print].
27. Michelsen B, Diamantopoulos AP, Soldal DM, Hammer HB, Kavanaugh A, Haugeberg G. Achilles enthesitis defined by ultrasound is not associated with clinical enthesitis in patients with psoriatic arthritis. *RMD Open.* (2017) 3:1–5. doi: 10.1136/rmdopen-2017-000486
28. Balint P, Terslev L, Aegerter P, Bruyn G, Chary-Valckenaere I, Gandjbakhch F, et al. Reliability of a consensus-based ultrasound definition and scoring for enthesitis in spondyloarthritis and psoriatic arthritis: an OMERACT US initiative. *Ann Rheum Dis.* (2018) 77:1730–5. doi: 10.1136/annrheumdis-2018-213609
29. Wervers K, Luime JJ, Tchetverikov I, Gerards AH, Kok MR, Appels CWY, et al. Comparison of disease activity measures in early psoriatic arthritis in usual care. *Rheumatology.* (2019) 58:2251–9. doi: 10.1093/rheumatology/kez215

30. Arslan Alhussain F, Kasapoglu Gunal E, Kurum E, Bakirci S, Ozturk AB, McGonagle D, et al. Greater magnitude of entheseal microdamage and repair in psoriatic arthritis compared with ankylosing spondylitis on ultrasound. *Rheumatology.* (2019) 58:299–303. doi: 10.1093/rheumatology/key238
31. Yumusakhuylu Y, Kasapoglu-Gunal E, Murat S, Kurum E, Keskin H, Icagasioglu A, et al. A preliminary study showing that ultrasonography cannot differentiate between psoriatic arthritis and nodal osteoarthritis based on enthesopathy scores. *Rheumatology.* (2016) 55:1703–4. doi: 10.1093/rheumatology/kew218
32. Zabotti A, Mcgonagle DG, Giovannini I, Errichetti E, Zuliani F, Zanetti A, et al. Transition phase towards psoriatic arthritis: clinical and ultrasonographic characterisation of psoriatic arthralgia. *RMD Open.* (2019) 5:1067. doi: 10.1136/rmdopen-2019-001067
33. Wervers K, Herrings I, Luime JJ, Tchetverikov I, Gerards AH, Hazes JMW, et al. Association of physical activity and medication with enthesitis on ultrasound in psoriatic arthritis. *J Rheumatol.* (2019) 46:1290–4. doi: 10.3899/jrheum.180782
34. Girolimetto N, Macchioni P, Tinazzi I, Costa L, Peluso R, Tasso M, et al. Predominant ultrasonographic extracapsular changes in symptomatic psoriatic dactylitis: results from a multicenter cross-sectional study comparing symptomatic and asymptomatic hand dactylitis. *Clin Rheumatol.* (2019) 39:1157–65. doi: 10.1007/s10067-019-04683-2
35. Tinazzi I, McGonagle D, Macchioni P, Aydin SZ. Power Doppler enhancement of accessory pulleys confirming disease localization in psoriatic dactylitis. *Rheumatology.* (2019) 59:1–5. doi: 10.1093/rheumatology/kez549
36. McGonagle D, Tan AL, Watad A, Helliwell P. Pathophysiology, assessment and treatment of psoriatic dactylitis. *Nat Rev Rheumatol.* (2019) 15:113–22. doi: 10.1038/s41584-018-0147-9
37. Zabotti A, Sakellariou G, Tinazzi I, Batticciotto A, Canzoni M, Carrara G, et al. Clinical science novel and reliable DACTylitis global sonographic (DACTOS) score in psoriatic arthritis. *Ann Rheum Dis.* (2020) 1–7. doi: 10.1136/annrheumdis-2020-217191
38. Kaeley GS, Eder L, Aydin SZ, Gutierrez M, Bakewell C. Dactylitis: a hallmark of psoriatic arthritis. *Semin Arthritis Rheum.* (2018) 48:263–73. doi: 10.1016/j.semarthrit.2018.02.002
39. Rizzo G, Raffeiner B, Coran A, Ciprian L, Fiocco U, Botsios C, et al. Pixel-based approach to assess contrast-enhanced ultrasound kinetics parameters for differential diagnosis of rheumatoid arthritis. *J Med Imaging.* (2015) 2:034503. doi: 10.1117/1.JMI.2.3.034503
40. Sapundzhieva T, Karalilova R, Batalov A. Hand ultrasound patterns in rheumatoid and psoriatic arthritis: the role of ultrasound in the differential diagnosis. *Rheumatol Int.* (2020) 40:837–48. doi: 10.1007/s00296-020-04559-8
41. Sakellariou G, Scirè CA, Adinolfi A, Batticciotto A, Bortoluzzi A, Sedie AD, et al. Differential diagnosis of inflammatory arthropathies by musculoskeletal ultrasonography : a systematic literature review. *Front Med.* (2020) 7:141. doi: 10.3389/fmed.2020.00141
42. Aydin SZ, Bakirci S, Kasapoglu E, Castillo-Gallego C, Arslan Alhussain F, Ash ZR, et al. The relationship between physical examination and ultrasonography of large entheses of the achilles tendon and patellar tendon origin. *J Rheumatol.* (2019) 47:1026–30. doi: 10.3899/jrheum.190169
43. Husic R, Gretler J, Felber A, Graninger WB, Duftner C, Hermann J, et al. Disparity between ultrasound and clinical findings in psoriatic arthritis. *Ann Rheum Dis.* (2014) 73:1529–36. doi: 10.1136/annrheumdis-2012-203073
44. Pukšić S, Bolton-King P, Sexton J, Michelsen B, Kvien TK, Berner Hammer H. DAPSA and ultrasound show different perspectives of psoriatic arthritis disease activity: results from a 12-month longitudinal observational study in patients starting treatment with biological disease-modifying antirheumatic drugs. *RMD Open.* (2018) 4:e000765. doi: 10.1136/rmdopen-2018-000765
45. Bosch P, Husic R, Ficjan A, Gretler J, Lackner A, Graninger WB, et al. Evaluating current definitions of low disease activity in psoriatic arthritis using ultrasound. *Rheumatology.* (2019) 58:2212–20. doi: 10.1093/rheumatology/kez237
46. Mandl P, Navarro-Compán V, Terslev L, Aegerter P, Van Der Heijde D, D'Agostino MA, et al. EULAR recommendations for the use of imaging in the diagnosis and management of spondyloarthritis in clinical practice. *Ann Rheum Dis.* (2015) 74:1327–39. doi: 10.1136/annrheumdis-2014-206971
47. Hammer HB, Michelsen B, Sexton J, Haugen IK, Provan SA, Haavardsholm EA, et al. Swollen, but not tender joints, are independently associated with ultrasound synovitis: results from a longitudinal observational study of patients with established rheumatoid arthritis. *Ann Rheum Dis.* (2019) 78:1179–85. doi: 10.1136/annrheumdis-2019-215321
48. Højgaard P, Ellegaard K, Nielsen SM, Christensen R, Guldberg-Møller J, Ballegaard C, et al. Pain mechanisms and ultrasonic inflammatory activity as prognostic factors in patients with psoriatic arthritis: a prospective cohort study. *Arthritis Care Res.* (2019) 71:798–810. doi: 10.1002/acr.23693
49. Helliwell PS, Coates LC, Chew NS, Lettieri G, Moverley AR, Freeston JE, et al. Comparing psoriatic arthritis low-field magnetic resonance imaging, ultrasound and clinical outcomes: data from the TICOPA trial. *J Rheumatol.* (2019). doi: 10.3899/jrheum.181385. [Epub ahead of print].
50. Michelsen B, Diamantopoulos AP, Hammer HB, Soldal DM, Kavanaugh A, Haugeberg G. Ultrasonographic evaluation in psoriatic arthritis is of major importance in evaluating disease activity. *Ann Rheum Dis.* (2016) 75:2108–13. doi: 10.1136/annrheumdis-2015-208806
51. Østergaard M, Eder L, Christiansen SN, Kaeley GS. Imaging in the diagnosis and management of peripheral psoriatic arthritis—The clinical utility of magnetic resonance imaging and ultrasonography. *Best Pract Res Clin Rheumatol.* (2016) 30:624–37. doi: 10.1016/j.berh.2016.08.012
52. El Miedany Y, El Gaafary M, Youssef S, Ahmed I, Nasr A. Tailored approach to early psoriatic arthritis patients: clinical and ultrasonographic predictors for structural joint damage. *Clin Rheumatol.* (2015) 34:307–13. doi: 10.1007/s10067-014-2630-2
53. Araujo EG, Finzel S, Englbrecht M, Schreiber DA, Faustini F, Hueber A, et al. High incidence of disease recurrence after discontinuation of disease-modifying antirheumatic drug treatment in patients with psoriatic arthritis in remission. *Ann Rheum Dis.* (2015) 74:655–60. doi: 10.1136/annrheumdis-2013-204229
54. Ficjan A, Husic R, Gretler J, Lackner A, Graninger WB, Gutierrez M, et al. Ultrasound composite scores for the assessment of inflammatory and structural pathologies in psoriatic arthritis (PsASon-Score). *Arthritis Res Ther.* (2014) 16:476. doi: 10.1186/s13075-014-0476-2
55. Gutierrez M, Di geso L, Salaffi F, Bertolazzi C, Tardella M, Filosa G, et al. Development of a preliminary US power Doppler composite score for monitoring treatment in PsA. *Rheumatology.* (2012) 51:1261–8. doi: 10.1093/rheumatology/kes014
56. Schäfer VS, Fleck M, Kellner H, Strunk J, Sattler H, Schmidt WA, et al. Evaluation of the novel ultrasound score for large joints in psoriatic arthritis and ankylosing spondylitis: six month experience in daily clinical practice. *BMC Musculoskelet Disord.* (2013) 14:2–6. doi: 10.1186/1471-2474-14-358
57. Wervers K, Vis M, Rasappu N, van der Ven M, Tchetverikov I, Kok MR, et al. Modification of a sonographic enthesitis score to differentiate between psoriatic arthritis and young healthy volunteers. *Scand J Rheumatol.* (2018) 47:291–4. doi: 10.1080/03009742.2017.1393695
58. Macía-Villa C, De Miguel E. Updating the use of the madrid sonographic enthesis index (MASEI): a systematic review of the literature. *Rheumatology.* (2020) 59: 1031–40. doi: 10.1093/rheumatology/kez356
59. Fiorenza A, Bonitta G, Gerratana E, Marino F, Sarzi-Puttini P, Salaffi F, et al. Assessment of enthesis in patients with psoriatic arthritis and fibromyalgia using clinical examination and ultrasound. *Clin Exp Rheumatol.* (2020) 38:31–9.
60. Tom S, Zhong Y, Cook R, Aydin SZ, Kaeley G, Eder L. Development of a preliminary ultrasonographic enthesitis score in psoriatic arthritis - GRAPPA ultrasound working group. *J Rheumatol.* (2019) 46:384–90. doi: 10.3899/jrheum.171465
61. D'Agostino MA, Coates LC. The role of ultrasound in psoriatic arthritis - do we need a score? *J Rheumatol.* (2019) 46:337–9. doi: 10.3899/jrheum.181044
62. Cunnington J, Marshall N, Hide G, Bracewell C, Isaacs J, Platt P, et al. A randomized, double-blind, controlled study of ultrasound-guided

corticosteroid injection into the joint of patients with inflammatory arthritis. *Arthritis Rheum.* (2010) 62:1862–9. doi: 10.1002/art.27448

63. Sibbitt WL, Band PA, Chavez-Chiang NR, DeLea SL, Norton HE, Bankhurst AD. A randomized controlled trial of the cost-effectiveness of ultrasound-guided intraarticular injection of inflammatory arthritis. *J Rheumatol.* (2011) 38:252–63. doi: 10.3899/jrheum.100866
64. Nordberg LB, Lillegraven S, Aga AB, Sexton J, Lie E, Hammer HB, et al. The impact of ultrasound on the use and efficacy of intraarticular glucocorticoid injections in early rheumatoid arthritis: secondary analyses from a randomized trial examining the benefit of ultrasound in a clinical tight control regimen. *Arthritis Rheumatol.* (2018) 70:1192–9. doi: 10.1002/art.40494

18

The Impact of Serum Anti-Neutrophil Cytoplasmic Antibody on Clinical Characteristics and Outcomes in Pediatric-Onset Systemic Lupus Erythematosus Patients

Chun-Chun Gau [1,2,3], *Min-Hua Tseng* [4], *Chao-Yi Wu* [1], *Huang-Yu Yang* [5] *and Jing-Long Huang* [1,6*]

[1] *Division of Allergy, Asthma, and Rheumatology, Department of Pediatrics, Chang Gung Memorial Hospital and Chang Gung University College of Medicine, Taoyuan, Taiwan,* [2] *Division of Pediatric General Medicine, Department of Pediatrics, Chang Gung Memorial Hospital and Chang Gung University College of Medicine, Taoyuan, Taiwan,* [3] *Department of Pediatrics, Chang Gung Memorial Hospital at Keelung, Keelung, Taiwan,* [4] *Division of Nephrology, Department of Pediatrics, Chang Gung Memorial Hospital and Chang Gung University College of Medicine, Taoyuan, Taiwan,* [5] *Department of Nephrology, Chang Gung Memorial Hospital, College of Medicine, Chang Gung University, Taoyuan, Taiwan,* [6] *Department of Pediatrics, New Taipei Municipal TuCheng Hospital, Chang Gung Memorial Hospital and Chang Gung University, New Taipei City, Taiwan*

***Correspondence:**
Jing-Long Huang
long@adm.cgmh.org.tw

Background: Systemic lupus erythematosus (SLE), an autoimmune disease, is characterized by the overproduction of autoantibodies. Anti-neutrophil cytoplasmic antibodies (ANCAs) have been recognized in SLE for decades. To date, their association with SLE disease activity, especially in pediatric-onset SLE (pSLE) patients, is limited.

Methods: We conducted a retrospective case-control study of pSLE patients with ANCAs from 2010 to 2020. Clinical characteristics, laboratory data, renal histological features, treatment and outcomes were analyzed.

Results: A total of 70 pediatric-onset SLE patients (9 ANCA-positive vs. 61 ANCA-negative) with a median age of 12.23 years (age ranging from 4 years to 18 years) at diagnosis were enrolled. Among patients with ANCAs, MPO-ANCA was found in seven and PR3-ANCA in two of those cases. Patients with ANCAs had a tendency to have hematuria compared with those without ANCAs (66 vs. 24.6%, respectively; $p = 0.026$). Of the 70 SLE patients, 8 with ANCAs and 44 without ANCAs underwent renal biopsies. Patients with ANCAs (25%, 2/8) were more likely to lack the typical full-house pattern in their renal immunofluorescence (IF) staining.

Conclusion: pSLE patients with ANCAs tend to have hematuria and an absence of typical IF histology. However, patients with and without ANCAs showed no difference in their clinical presentations and treatment outcomes.

Keywords: anti-neutrophil cytoplasmic antibody, pediatric-onset systemic lupus erythematosus, lupus nephritis, hematuria, children

BACKGROUND

Systemic lupus erythematosus (SLE), a prototype of autoimmune disease with systemic involvement, is characterized by the breakdown of self-tolerance and various autoantibody production. Pediatric-onset SLE (pSLE) accounts for 15–20% of all cases and usually presents with a more aggressive clinical phenotype compared with adult-onset SLE. Although pediatric and adult lupus patients share similar clinical manifestations, lupus nephritis (LN) among the pediatric-onset population has been suggested to be different from the adult-onset form in its abrupt onset and relatively poor response to treatment (1).

Anti-neutrophil cytoplasmic antibodies (ANCAs) are a group of autoantibodies directed against cytoplasmic antigens within human neutrophils and monocytes and have been detected in patients with small vessel vasculitis and inflammatory disease (2–4). In fact, vasculitis is a common manifestation in lupus patients, and the presence of ANCAs related to clinical presentation, including interstitial lung disease, chronicity index and histopathology of lupus nephritis, has been flourishingly reported in adult lupus patients in this 5-year study (5–9). However, the association of ANCAs with pediatric-onset SLE has not been well-reviewed and has limited the discussion on the association between ANCA presence and clinical characteristics (10, 11). To date, the impact of ANCAs on renal manifestations, disease severity and clinical outcome among pediatric SLE patients remains to be elucidated.

The aim of this study was to investigate the impact of ANCAs on clinical manifestations, organ involvement and outcomes in pediatric-onset lupus patients.

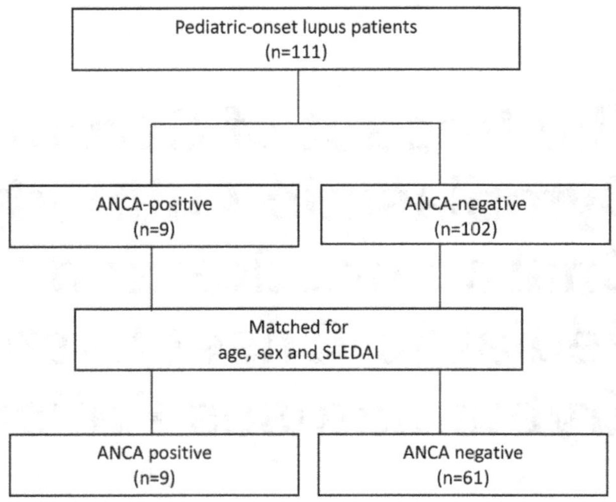

FIGURE 1 | Flow chart of patient collection and categorization.

METHODS

This retrospective case-control study was approved by the Ethics Committee on Human Studies at Chang Gung Memorial Hospital in Taiwan, R.O.C. (IRB 201601678A3C501). Informed consent was obtained from the patients and their parents, and all methods including chart review were performed in accordance with the relevant regulations.

Subjects

One hundred and eleven SLE patients diagnosed according to the 1997 SLE American College of Rheumatology criteria from 2010 to 2020 were recruited from a tertiary hospital (12). Patients with disease onset before the age of 18 who received regular clinical follow-up every 1–3 months for more than 6 months were enrolled (**Figure 1**). Nine patients with ANCAs were identified. Sixty-one patients without ANCAs were consecutively enrolled in the control group after adjustment for age, sex, and SLE disease activity index (SLEDAI) score (13).

Clinical and Laboratory Characteristics and Outcome

The SLE-related laboratory data, including renal function (creatinine data and urinary analysis), hematology including lymphopenia (white blood count <4,000/mm^3 more than twice), leukopenia (lymphocyte count <4,000/mm^3 more than two times), hemolytic anemia with reticulocytosis and thrombocytopenia (platelet count <1,000.00/mm^3 in the absence of drug use), complement C3 and C4, anti-nuclear antibody (ANA), and anti-double stranded DNA antibody (anti-dsDNA Ab), were collected, and clinical manifestations noted within the previous 10 years, including mucocutaneous presentation (malar rash, photosensitivity, discoid rash or oral ulcer), cardiovascular systems (myocarditis, pericardial effusion or pericarditis), non-erosive arthritis, pulmonary manifestations (hemoptysis or abnormality on image by radiologists) and neurological disorder (neuritis, seizure or psychosis), at presentation and follow up were recorded. Proteinuria was defined as daily protein excretion more than 4 mg/m^2/h, 500 mg per 24 h or more than 3+ on urinalysis based on the 1997 American College of Rheumatology revised criteria (12). Hematuria was diagnosed as more than five red blood cells per high-power field. The demographic data, medications and outcomes, including acute kidney injury, chronic renal failure and all-cause mortality were also analyzed during the follow-up. Hypocomplementemia was defined as a C3 level less than the lower limit (90 mg/dl) or a C4 level less than the lower limit (10 mg/dl). Disease activity, quantified by the SLEDAI-2K score, was also calculated (13). Acute kidney injury was defined as a serum creatinine level more than 0.3 mg/ dl within 48 h or serum creatine more than 1.5 times that of the baseline value within the prior seven days (14). Furthermore, we utilized the bedside Schwartz equation to estimate the measured glomerular filtration rate (mGFR, ml/min/1.73 m^2) status, and chronic kidney disease (CKD) was assessed at 6 months after the administration of proper treatment: stage 1, mGFR>90; stage 2, 89>mGFR>60; stage 3, 59>mGFR>30; stage 4, 29> mGFR>15 and stage 5, mGFR<15 (15, 16).

Renal Histopathology

Fifty-two of the patients (8 positive and 44 negative for ANCAs) underwent renal biopsy due to nephritis. The histological studies, including light microscopy, immunofluorescence (IF) and electron microcopy studies, were reviewed by a pathologist who was an expert in renal diseases. The full-house pattern, which is the histological hallmark of lupus nephritis as described in the 2012 Systemic Lupus International Collaborating Clinics criteria based on their proposed classification of systemic lupus erythematosus, was defined as the presence of IgG, IgA, IgM, C1q and C3 on IF staining (12). Lupus nephritis, activity and chronicity were classified according to the International Society of Nephrology/Renal Pathology Society (17).

TABLE 1 | Clinical Data of Lupus patients with Anti-neutrophil cytoplasmic antibodies (ANCA) at the first diagnosis.

	1	2	3	4	5	6	7	8	9
Onset age (year)	14	11	13	13	14	15	14	10	12
Follow-up duration (months)	195	124	124	19	81	53	21	99	228
Sex	Female	Female	Female	Male	Female	Female	Female	Female	Female
Laboratory data at presentation									
ANA (Normal range < 1:80)	-	+	+	+	+	+	+	+	+
Anti-dsDNA antibodies*(Normal range <130 WHO unit/mL)	83.5	35.6	490.1	49.1	195.3	47	351.6	40.5	221.3
ANCA, p-ANCA (Normal range < 5 IU/ml)	6.1	11.8	11	134.7	134	146	146	-	-
ANCA, c-ANCA (Normal range <3 IU/ml)	-	-	-	-	-	-	-	5.7	3.3
Hypocomplementemia/ (Normal range C3 >90 or C4>10 mg/dl)	+	+	+	+	-	+	+	+	+
Urine protein	Negative	18.2mg/m^2/h	12.8 mg/m^2/h	79.8 mg/m^2/h	30mg/dl	77.6 mg/m^2/h	718 24 mg/m^2/h	118.7 mg/m^2/h	1+
Hematuria	-	+	+	+	+	-	+	+	-
Serum albumin (Normal range 2.8–5.4 g/dl)	-	4.6	2.86	3.09	3.79	3.86	2.9	3.25	4.8
Serum creatinine** (Normal range 0.2–1.0 mg/dl)	-	0.47	0.34	0.91	0.65	0.49	5.39	0.36	0.51
Renal pathology									
Light microscopy	-	LN III	Cast nephropathy	LN IV	LN V	LN V	LN V	LN IV	LN IV
Full house	-	+	(IgG 1+)	+	(IgG 3+)	+	+	+	+
Organ involvement at presentation									
Kidney	-	+	+	+	+	+	+	+	+
Hematology	+	-	+	+	+	-	+	+	+
Dermatology	-	+	-	+	-	-	-	+	+
Joints	+	+	-	-	-	-	-	-	-
Heart	-	-	+	-	-	-	-	-	-
Neurology	-	-	-	-	-	+	-	-	-
Pulmonary	-	-	-	+	-	-	-	-	-
Treatment									
Steroid	+	+	+	+	+	+	+	+	+
Azathioprine	+	-	+	-	-	+	-	–	+
HCQ	+	+	+	-	-	-	-	+	+
MMF	-	+	-	+	+	+	+	-	-
Others	-	Cyclosporine, Cyclophosphamide	-	Plasma exchange	Cyclosporine	-	Plasma exchange	Cyclophosphamide	-
Outcome									
Persistent hematuria	-	-	-	+	+	-	-		-
Chronic kidney disease (stage)	-	-	-	2	1	1	3	1	-

LN, lupus nephritis; HCQ, hydroxychloroquine; MMF, mycophenolic acid.

**Anti-double stranded DNA (dsDNA) antibodies (WHO unit/mL), **serum creatinine (mg/dl) at biopsy.*

+Case 1 did not have the indication for renal biopsy.

Measurement of Serum ANCAs

Serum ANCA levels were routinely checked at presentation, every clinic visit and follow-up for all enrolled patients during the follow-up. Serum ANCA levels were measured by an enzyme-linked immunosorbent assay (ELISA), and an anti-MPO antibody level >5.0 U/ml and anti-PR3 antibody level >3.0 U/ml were defined as positive findings according to the manufacturer's instructions (Pharmacia Diagnostic AB, Uppsala, Sweden). In addition, defining ANCA positivity according to the ELISA method for MPO and PR3 (not as immunofluorescence assay testing positive) is an important issue, while it has been suggested that the p-ANCA pattern in the immunofluorescence test could be misinterpreted due to the interference of ANA (6, 18).

Statistical Analyses

Data were analyzed using Student's *t* test to compare the means between two groups of continuous data. The chi-square test or Fisher's exact test (if any value was <5 in all comparisons) was used for categorical data to assess differences in clinical characteristics and evaluate the result of renal biopsy, medication and outcomes. Moreover, 95% confidence intervals were applied. Statistical analysis was performed with SPSS Statistics version 22.0.0 (SPSS Inc., Chicago, United States), and a *p*-value <0.05 was considered indicative of statistical significance.

RESULTS

Demographic and Clinical Manifestations of pSLE Patients With ANCAs

As shown in **Table 1**, nine patients (one male and eight females) with a mean age of 12.6 ± 1.5 years (ranging from 10 to 15 years) and ANCA positivity were enrolled over 10 years. Seven and two patients had anti-MPO antibody and anti-PR3 antibody, respectively. Eight patients had proteinuria or hematuria at the initial presentation and underwent renal biopsy. Two patients had biopsy-proven membranous glomerulopathy and cast nephropathy without full-house deposition on IF staining. Seven, four, two and one patient had hematological presentations, mucocutaneous lesions, arthritis and serositis, respectively. The cases with high ANCA levels (ANCA level >100) had severe extra-renal presentations; specifically, case 4 had pulmonary hemorrhage and case 6 had vestibulocochlear neuritis. Four patients (cases 4, 5, 6, and 7) with high serum ANCA levels of more than 100 IU/ml had acute kidney injury at presentation and reached chronic kidney disease during follow up. After 6 month treatment, two patients had persistent hematuria.

Comparison of pSLE Patients With and Without ANCAs

Demographic Data

Sixty-one pSLE patients were enrolled in the control group. As shown in **Table 2**, there were no differences between patients with and without ANCAs with respect to sex (88.9 vs. 90.2% were female), age at diagnosis (12.93 ± 3.28 vs. 13.02 ± 1.63 years old) or follow-up duration (98.73 ± 68.43 vs. 132.16 ± 73.14 months).

TABLE 2 | Clinical characteristics of pediatric-onset SLE patients with and without anti-neutrophil cytoplasmic antibodies (ANCAs).

	ANCA-positive (*n* = 9)	ANCA-negative (*n* = 61)	*P*-value
Female (%)	8 (88.9%)	55 (90.2%)	0.905
Onset age (year)	12.93 ± 3.28	13.02 ± 1.63	0.937
Follow-up (months)	98.73 ± 68.43	132.16 ± 73.14	0.368
SLEDAI^{+} at presentation	12.11 ± 6.92	12.95 ± 7.11	0.314
Laboratory data at presentation			
C3 (g/L)	66.49 ± 29.67	54.31 ± 35.51	0.334
C4 (g/L)	11.86 ± 7.32	9.75 ± 7.54	0.449
Anti-dsDNA antibodies (unit/mL)	178.68 ± 156.60	240.76 ± 150.78	0.948
Creatinine (mg/dL)	1.16 ± 1.62	0.68 ± 0.43	0.059
WBC (10^6/L)	6255.56 ± 4143.40	5417.54 ± 2930.88	0.455
Platelets (10^6/L)	189.78 ± 93.03	180.51 ± 113.32	0.817
Hemoglobin (g/L)	9.86 ± 2.75	11.30 ± 2.91	0.168
Proteinuria (%)	4 (50%)	41 (67.2%)	0.435
Hematuria (%)	6 (66.6%)	15 (24.6%)	0.026*
Renal histology			
Activity	8.25 ± 2.63	7.28 ± 4.39	0.64
Chronicity	0.5 ± 1.00	2.30 ± 2.48	0.11
Treatment at presentation and during follow-up, numbers			
Prednisolone (%)	9 (100%)	61(100%)	N/A
Azathioprine (%)	5 (55.6%)	44 (72.1%)	0.128
Cyclophosphamide (%)	3 (33.3%)	23 (37.7%)	1.000
Mycophenolic acid (%)	3 (33.3%)	31 (50.8%)	0.479
Hydroxychloroquine (%)	6 (66.7%)	43 (70.5%)	1.000
Cyclosporine (%)	1 (11.1%)	12 (19.7%)	1.000
Rituximab (%)	0 (0%)	3 (4.9%)	1.000
Outcome, numbers			
Acute kidney injury (%)	1 (11.1%)	3 (4.9%)	0.538
Chronic renal disease (%)	5 (55.6%)	29 (47.5%)	0.970
End-stage renal disease (%)	0 (0%)	4 (6.6%)	0.143
Death (%)	0 (0%)	1 (1.7%)**	0.696

$^{+}$ *SLEDAI, SLE disease activity index; **Died of sepsis, *p < 0.05.*

Laboratory Characteristics

There were no significant differences in serological characteristics, including complement, anti-dsDNA antibody, serum creatinine, white blood cell count, platelet count and hemoglobin, between patients with and without ANCAs at the time of diagnosis. However, patients with ANCAs had a higher rate of initial hematuria than those without ANCAs (62.5 vs. 24.6%, respectively; $p = 0.026$), as shown in **Table 2**.

Organs Involved

As shown in **Figure 2**, skin, cardiovascular and joint involvements were the most common manifestations in patient with ANCA. Only patients without ANCAs had gastrointestinal organ damage. However, there was no significant difference in organ involvement between the two groups.

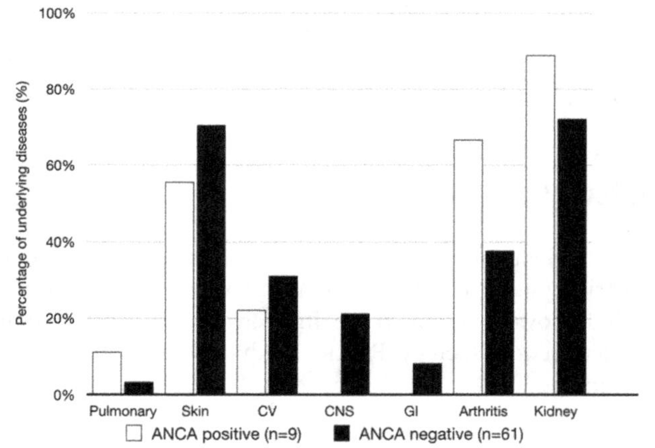

FIGURE 2 | Organ systems involved in the patients with and w ithout ANCAs during the follow-up were investigated. CV, cardiovascular; GI, gastrointestinal.

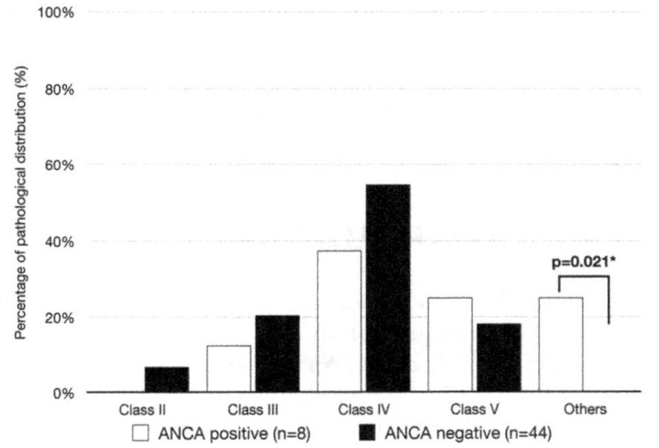

FIGURE 3 | Patients with biopsy with ISN classes of lupus nephritis in the ANCA-positive and ANCA-negative groups. A significant difference was observed in the ANCA-positive group, but the classic full-house deposition was absent (p-value <0.05).

Renal Histology

The lack of typical full-house IF staining was revealed in two patients with ANCAs but not in patients without ANCAs (25 vs. 0%, $p = 0.021$). In patients with ANCAs, the histological features were class IV glomerulonephritis (3, 37.5%), class V glomerulonephritis (2, 25%), class I glomerulonephritis (1, 12.5%) and nephritis with an absence of glomerulonephritis (2, 25%). As shown in **Figure 3**, in the 44 lupus patients without ANCAs, class IV was also the most prevalent histopathology (24, 54.5%), followed by class II, class III and class IV glomerulonephritis (3, 6.8%; 9, 20.4%; 9,18.2%; respectively).

Treatment

As shown in **Table 2**, all of the patients received steroid treatment. Immunosuppressants, including azathioprine and hydroxychloroquine, were used if there was hematological or mucocutaneous involvement. For the patients with biopsy-proven proliferative lupus nephritis, intravenous cyclophosphamide or mycophenolic acid (MMF) was administered. In addition, rituximab and cyclosporin were administered in cases of poor response to each of these drugs. There were no obvious differences between patients with or without ANCAs.

Outcomes

During the observation period, in the ANCA group, one patient had acute kidney injury and five had chronic kidney disease after 6 months of treatment, while three patients had acute kidney injury and twenty-nine had chronic kidney disease in the non-ANCA group, which did not correspond to a significant difference. Of the patients without ANCAs, four needed hemodialysis, and one died due to sepsis during follow up. In contrast to the patients without ANCAs, none of the nine patients with ANCAs progressed to renal failure or death during the follow-up period. However, no significant difference in mortality between patients with and without ANCAs was found.

DISCUSSION

This was the first longitudinal study that analyzed the impact of ANCAs on pSLE patients clinical implications. Our results indicate that the positive ANCA titers in pSLE cases are significantly associated with hematuria. In cases with positive ANCAs, two distinct histopathologies and atypical presentation without the full-house pattern of deposition in IF staining were discovered. Furthermore, in the case analysis, obvious renal manifestation as hematuria was noted in positive ANCA cases, and some patients with a high ANCA level also had pulmonary hemorrhage and neurological manifestations. Therefore, we focused on determining the renal association of hematuria and IF staining.

During the Hill et al. clinical follow-up, patients with ANCA-associated vasculitis had persistent hematuria (17). In addition, Mahoney et al. noted that persistent hematuria may be observed in ANCA vasculitis in adults, but it is not related to recurrence (19). In adult lupus patients with ANCAs, however, Pyo et al. reported no increased incidence of hematuria (5). To date, only two studies have mentioned the clinical presentation in pSLE with ANCAs, but neither studied the clinical manifestations of hematuria (10, 20). As indicated by Wang et al., the ANCA was thought to relate to neutrophil extracellular trap (NET) formation, which caused cell death and provided a novel source of autoantigens that resulted in poor renal outcome of lupus patients (21). Additionally, in our study, we found that pediatric-onset SLE patients may be prone to renal damage, which is considered to be related to ANCAs with hematuria.

The typical renal histopathological presentation of patients with ANCA-associated systemic vasculitis includes necrotizing vasculitis. According to previous reports, crescentic glomerulonephritis and global sclerosing were the most common renal histopathologies among patients with ANCA-associated renal vasculitis (22). In addition, Turner-Stokes et al. found a high frequency of lupus class IV-S lupus nephritis in ANCA-positive adult patients (8). Furthermore, recent studies confirmed that ANCA-associated vasculitis is related to the chronicity index in adults (5). However, there was no significant difference in treatment outcome or disease severity (8). After reviewing these 8 cases with ANCA-associated LN, we did not find evidence of differences in outcomes, treatment, crescent formation, classification or chronicity index in pSLE patients in the presence or absence of ANCAs. However, while examining the deposition of immunofluorescence, the renal biopsy samples lacked the full-house pattern present in the two pSLE patients with ANCAs. Although the relationship between the mechanism of ANCA vasculitis and lupus needs further investigation, the early recognition of ANCAs in pSLE patients may result in favorable and appropriate outcomes in contrast to the results of a previous study. However, this may contribute to a faster and more intensive treatment for patients with than without ANCAs.

In a review of laboratory data, Su et al. found that ANCA-positive patients with new-onset adult SLE may have higher serum creatinine levels than ANCA-negative patients (9). However, the laboratory data or renal histopathological presentation were never reviewed in pSLE patients with ANCA. In our study, although not statistically significant, the serum creatinine of patients with ANCAs was higher than that of patients without ANCAs in our study. However, the lack of significance may be due to the small number of subjects in this case or the quicker intervention than that received by the adult lupus nephritis patients.

Furthermore, as is already known, a positive ANCA titer may be related to interstitial lung disease (7). Yu et al. conducted a study on lupus patients with ANCAs that indicated no obvious difference in mucocutaneous, gastrointestinal and arthritis aspects but indicated a propensity for lupus myocarditis (23). An evidence study indicated that lupus patients with ANCAs are more likely to have severe neurological presentations, including psychosomatic manifestations (24). In a Faure-Fontenla study, pSLE patients with positive ANCA did not have evidence of vasculitis-associated features or specific organ involvement (10). This is also in accordance with research reporting no obvious extra-renal characteristics.

These were some limitations of our study. One is the small population due to the low prevalence [16% prevalence of ANCA in patients with lupus nephritis (21)] in pSLE patients, which may mask the possibility of complications, and we had to select appropriate control cases with the same disease severity for analysis. Furthermore, although the treatment may have selection bias, we treated our patients according to the current standard protocol (25).

CONCLUSION

Currently, hematuria and the lack of a full house were found in pediatric lupus patients with ANCA, and patients with or without ANCAs showed no difference in their clinical presentations and treatment outcomes. Further study is warranted to verify our findings.

ETHICS STATEMENT

The studies involving human participants were reviewed and approved by This retrospective case-control study was approved by the Ethics Committee on Human Studies at Chang Gung Memorial Hospital in Taiwan, R.O.C. (IRB 201601678A3C501). Informed consent was obtained from the patients and their parents. Written informed consent to participate in this study was provided by the participants' legal guardian/next of kin.

AUTHOR CONTRIBUTIONS

C-CG, M-HT, C-YW, H-YY, and J-LH: study conception and design. C-CG: acquisition of data and drafting the article. C-CG, M-HT, C-YW, and H-YY: analysis and interpretation of data. M-HT and C-YW: revising the article. All authors have finally approved the submitted version to be published.

ACKNOWLEDGMENTS

The authors would like to thank Yu-Ching Chou, Ph.D., in the School of Public Health, National Defense Medical Center, for his statistical analysis suggestions and Jhao-Jhuang Ding, MD, in the Department of Pediatrics, Tri-Service General Hospital, National Defense Medical Center, Taipei, Taiwan, for the critical review of the manuscript.

REFERENCES

1. Aggarwal A, Srivastava P. Childhood onset systemic lupus erythematosus: how is it different from adult SLE? *Int J Rheum Dis.* (2015) 18:182–91. doi: 10.1111/1756-185x.12419
2. Kirito Y, Yamamoto D, Uchiyama T. Proteinase 3-antineutrophil cytoplasmic antibody-positive ulcerative colitis presenting with abducens neuropathy. *BMJ Case Rep.* (2017) 2017:bcr2016218353. doi: 10.1136/bcr-2016-218353
3. Mahler M, Damoiseaux J, Ballet V, Dillaerts D, Bentow C, Cohen Tervaert JW, et al. PR3-anti-neutrophil cytoplasmic antibodies (ANCA) in ulcerative colitis. *Clin Chem Lab Med.* (2017) 56:e27–e30. doi: 10.1515/cclm-2017-0346
4. Olbjorn C, Cvancarova Smastuen M, Thiis-Evensen E, Nakstad B, Vatn MH, Perminow G. Serological markers in diagnosis of pediatric inflammatory bowel disease and as predictors for early tumor necrosis factor blocker therapy. *Scand J Gastroenterol.* (2017) 52:414–9. doi: 10.1080/00365521.2016.1259653

5. Pyo JY, Jung SM, Song JJ, Park YB, Lee SW. ANCA positivity at the time of renal biopsy is associated with chronicity index of lupus nephritis. *Rheumatol Int.* (2019) 39:879–84. doi: 10.1007/s00296-019-04263-2
6. Weinstein A. ANCA in lupus nephritis. *Lupus.* (2018) 27:522. doi: 10.1177/0961203317734925
7. Alba MA, Flores-Suarez LF, Henderson AG, Xiao H, Hu P, Nachman PH, et al. Interstital lung disease in ANCA vasculitis. *Autoimmun Rev.* (2017) 16:722–9. doi: 10.1016/j.autrev.2017.05.008
8. Turner-Stokes T, Wilson HR, Morreale M, Nunes A, Cairns T, Cook HT, et al. Positive antineutrophil cytoplasmic antibody serology in patients with lupus nephritis is associated with distinct histopathologic features on renal biopsy. *Kidney Int.* (2017) 92:1223–31. doi: 10.1016/j.kint.2017.04.029
9. Su F, Xiao W, Yang P, Chen Q, Sun X, Li T. Anti-neutrophil cytoplasmic antibodies in new-onset systemic lupus erythematosus. *An Bras Dermatol.* (2017) 92:466–9. doi: 10.1590/abd1806-4841.20175476
10. Faure-Fontenla MA, Rodriguez-Suarez RS, Arias-Velasquez R, Garcia-Gonzalez JE. Antineutrophil cytoplasmic antibodies in systemic lupus erythematosus in childhood. *J Rheumatol.* (1999) 26:2480–1.
11. Bakkaloglu A, Topaloglu R, Saatci U, Ozdemir S, Ozen S, Bassoy Y, et al. Antineutrophil cytoplasmic antibodies in childhood systemic lupus erythematosus. *Clin Rheumatol.* (1998) 17:265–7.
12. Petri M, Orbai AM, Alarcón GS, Gordon C, Merrill JT, Fortin PR, et al. Derivation and validation of the Systemic Lupus International Collaborating Clinics classification criteria for systemic lupus erythematosus. *Arthritis Rheum.* (2012) 64:2677-86. doi: 10.1002/art.34473
13. Bombardier C, Gladman DD, Urowitz MB, Caron D, Chang CH. Derivation of the SLEDAI. A disease activity index for lupus patients. The Committee on Prognosis Studies in SLE. *Arthritis Rheum.* (1992) 35:630–40.
14. Khwaja A. KDIGO clinical practice guidelines for acute kidney injury. *Nephron Clin Pract.* (2012) 120:c179–84. doi: 10.1159/000339789
15. Schwartz GJ, Haycock GB, Edelmann CM Jr, Spitzer A. A simple estimate of glomerular filtration rate in children derived from body length and plasma creatinine. *Pediatrics.* (1976) 58:259–63.
16. K/DOQI clinical practice guidelines for chronic kidney disease: evaluation, classification, and stratification. *Am J Kidney Dis.* (2002) 39(2 Suppl 1):S1–266.
17. Hill GS, Delahousse M, Nochy D, Tomkiewicz E, Remy P, Mignon F, et al. A new morphologic index for the evaluation of renal biopsies in lupus nephritis. *Kidney Int.* (2000) 58:1160–73. doi: 10.1046/j.1523-1755.2000.00272.x
18. Sobral S, Ramassur K, Apsley E, Isenberg D. Do anti-neutrophil cytoplasmic antibodies play a role in systemic lupus erythematosus (SLE) patients? Analysis of the University College Hospital SLE cohort. *Lupus.* (2018) 27:343–4. doi: 10.1177/0961203317724218
19. Mahoney SL, Nachman PH. Persistent hematuria in ANCA vasculitis: ominous or innocuous? *Clin J Am Soc Nephrol.* (2018) 13:201–2. doi: 10.2215/cjn.14101217
20. Bobek D, Vukovic J, Malenica B, Bojanic K, Rukavina I, Jelusic M. Anti-neutrophil cytoplasmic antibody positivity in five children with systemic lupus erythematosus–what is the importance of this finding? *Acta Dermatovenerol Croat.* (2014) 22:264–70.
21. Wang Y, Huang X, Cai J, Xie L, Wang W, Tang S, et al. Clinicopathologic characteristics and outcomes of lupus nephritis with antineutrophil cytoplasmic antibody: a retrospective study. *Medicine.* (2016) 95:e2580. doi: 10.1097/MD.0000000000002580
22. Cordova-Sanchez BM, Mejia-Vilet JM, Morales-Buenrostro LE, Loyola-Rodriguez G, Uribe-Uribe NO, Correa-Rotter R. Clinical presentation and outcome prediction of clinical, serological, and histopathological classification schemes in ANCA-associated vasculitis with renal involvement. *Clin Rheumatol.* (2016) 35:1805–16. doi: 10.1007/s10067-016-3195-z
23. Yu YW, Liu ZR, Xie D, Chen SX, Li HY. [Clinical significance of antineutrophil cytoplasmic antibodies in patients with lupus nephritis]. *Nan fang yi ke da xue xue bao = J South Med Univ.* (2006) 26:833–6.
24. Martinez-Morillo M, Lopez R, Ibernon M, Olive A. [Renal p-ANCA vasculitis in patients with systemic lupus erythematosus]. *Med Clin.* (2011) 137:379–80. doi: 10.1016/j.medcli.2010.10.004
25. Bertsias G, Ioannidis JP, Boletis J, Bombardieri S, Cervera R, Dostal C, et al. EULAR recommendations for the management of systemic lupus erythematosus. Report of a Task Force of the EULAR Standing Committee for International Clinical Studies Including Therapeutics. *Ann Rheum Dis.* (2008) 67:195–205. doi: 10.1136/ard.2007.070367

19

Innovative Imaging Technique for Visualization of Vascularization and Established Methods for Detection of Musculoskeletal Inflammation in Psoriasis Patients

Michaela Köhm [1,2,3], Lukas Zerweck [3,4], Phuong-Ha Ngyuen [3,4], Harald Burkhardt [1,2,3,5] and Frank Behrens [1,2,3,5]*

[1] Division of Rheumatology, Goethe-University Frankfurt, Frankfurt, Germany, [2] Clinical Research, Fraunhofer Institute for Molecular Biology and Applied Ecology IME, Branch for Translational Medicine and Pharmacology TMP, Frankfurt, Germany, [3] Fraunhofer Cluster of Excellence Immune-Mediated Diseases CIMD, Frankfurt, Germany, [4] Fraunhofer Institute for Applied Information Technology FIT, St. Augustin, Germany, [5] Centre of Innovative Diagnostics and Therapeutics Rheumatology/Immunology CIRI, Frankfurt, Germany

***Correspondence:**
Michaela Köhm
michaela.koehm@ime.fraunhofer.de

Psoriasis (PsO) is one of the common chronic inflammatory skin diseases. Approximately 3% of the European Caucasian population is affected. Psoriatic arthritis (PsA) is a chronic immune-mediated disease associated with PsO characterized by distinct musculoskeletal inflammation. Due to its heterogeneous clinical manifestations (e.g., oligo- or polyarthritis, enthesitis, dactylitis, and axial inflammation), early diagnosis of PsA is often difficult and delayed. Approximately 30% of PsO patients will develop PsA. The responsible triggers for the transition from PsO only to PsA are currently unclear, and the impacts of different factors (e.g., genetic, environmental) on disease development are currently discussed. There is a high medical need, recently unmet, to specifically detect those patients with an increased risk for the development of clinically evident PsA early to initiate sufficient treatment to inhibit disease progression and avoid structural damage and loss of function or even intercept disease development. Increased neoangiogenesis and enthesial inflammation are hypothesized to be early pathological findings in PsO patients with PsA development. Different disease states describe the transition from PsO to PsA. Two of those phases are of value for early detection of PsA at-risk patients to prevent later development of PsA as changes in biomarker profiles are detectable: the subclinical phase (soluble and imaging biomarkers detectable, no clinical symptoms) and the prodromal phase (imaging biomarkers detectable, unspecific musculoskeletal symptoms such as arthralgia and fatigue). To target the unmet need for early detection of this at-risk population and to identify the subgroup of patients who will transition from PsO to PsA, imaging plays an important role in characterizing patients precisely. Imaging techniques such as ultrasound (US), magnetic resonance imaging (MRI), and computerized tomography (CT) are advanced techniques to detect sensitively inflammatory changes or changes in bone structure. With the use of these techniques, anatomic structures involved in inflammatory processes can be identified. These techniques are complemented by fluorescence optical imaging as a sensitive method for detection of changes in vascularization, especially in longitudinal measures. Moreover, high-resolution peripheral quantitative CT (HR-pQCT) and dynamic contrast-enhanced MRI (DCE-MRI) may give the advantage to identify PsA-related early characteristics in PsO patients reflecting transition phases of the disease.

Keywords: psoriasis, psoriatic arthritis, early detection, imaging, musculoskeletal inflammation

INTRODUCTION

Psoriasis (PsO) is one of the common chronic inflammatory skin diseases. Approximately 3% of the European Caucasian population is affected. Psoriatic arthritis (PsA) is a chronic immune-mediated disease associated with PsO characterized by distinct musculoskeletal inflammation. Due to its heterogeneous clinical manifestations (e.g., oligo- or polyarthritis, enthesitis, dactylitis, and axial inflammation), and the fact that only classification criteria are available [ClASsification for Psoriatic ARthritis (CASPAR) criteria], early diagnosis of PsA is often difficult to set and frequently delayed. Approximately 30% of PsO patients will develop PsA in their lifetime. Moreover, many patients develop a destructive form of arthritis with substantial morbidity and disability (1). Reasons for the transition from PsO to PsA are currently unclear as well as their impact on disease development. It is currently discussed that different factors such as genetic and/or clinical–demographic risk factors (e.g., nail PsO, PsO severity and type) may promote PsA development and its progression. Risk factors are observed in different epidemiologic studies, but there seems to be as well a heterogeneous profile for different factors identified (2).

The underlying molecular mechanisms for the transition from PsO to PsA are still poorly defined but better understood due to the use of biologic treatments addressing different target molecules for both PsO and PsA. Similar to the predictive value of anti-citrullinated peptide antibodies (ACPAs) for the development of rheumatoid arthritis (RA) in patients with arthralgia, the medical condition of PsO as an underlying disease describes an at-risk population to develop PsA. There is a high medical need, recently unmet, to identify early those patients with an increased risk for PsA development and first signs of musculoskeletal inflammatory changes for clinically evident PsA development. Only by early detection, sufficient treatments to inhibit disease progression and avoid structural damage and loss of function can be initiated. Moreover, here, the interception of PsA may be targeted with sufficient treatment when initiated in a very early stage of the PsO patients at risk for PsA development (principle of disease interception). However, ~50% of patients with PsO present with subclinical imaging enthesopathy, and only a subgroup of them will develop PsA (3). So, even as the evidence of signs for musculoskeletal inflammation being found by use of sensitive imaging technique may be of high value to identify the at-risk collective, the technique must also be appropriate to differentiate between disease-related changes of PsA to predict progression from PsO to clinically manifested PsA. Therefore, there is a need for a specific biomarker panel including either soluble molecular markers and/or sensitive imaging markers to solve this challenge. Different imaging techniques are available with various modes to identify inflammation or inflammatory changes and heterogeneous impact for sensitive detection of signs for very early musculoskeletal inflammatory changes.

THE TRANSITION FROM PSORIASIS TO PSORIATIC ARTHRITIS

PsA mostly develops in patients with established PsO; only in 15% of patients PsO occurs in parallel or after PsA development (4). The incidence of PsA with PsO onset increases with time, reaching ~20% after 30 years (5). Nail, scalp, and inverse PsO and its severity are identified as potential clinical factors for increased risk for PsA development (4). In focusing on comorbidities, obesity is identified as a strong risk factor for PsA development (6), with an additional link of the magnitude of body mass index (BMI) and PsA risk (7). For genetic background, a first-degree relative with arthritis contributes to the risk (8). Moreover, arthralgia mainly in female PsO patients is a strong predictor for PsA development (9). This finding was confirmed by Zabotti et al. (10) in 2019 in a longitudinal study.

Scher et al. (2) recently proposed three clinically inconspicuous stages after PsO onset and before the clinical presentation of PsA: (a) a preclinical phase characterized by aberrant activation of the immune system which may originate from the skin, intestinal mucosa, or the entheses; (b) the subclinical PsA phase with the detection of soluble biomarkers and imaging findings without clinical symptoms; (c) the prodromal phase of PsA in which patients report unspecific symptoms such as arthralgia and fatigue without objective detection of signs of musculoskeletal inflammation with synovitis and/or enthesitis in physical examination (**Figure 1**).

So, the subclinical and prodromal phases are linked by changes that might be detectable by established biomarkers or a specific biomarker profile including imaging techniques predicting later clinical development of PsA. In the clinical care setting, patients will mainly be presented to a specialist rheumatologist in the prodromal phase, when clinical symptoms

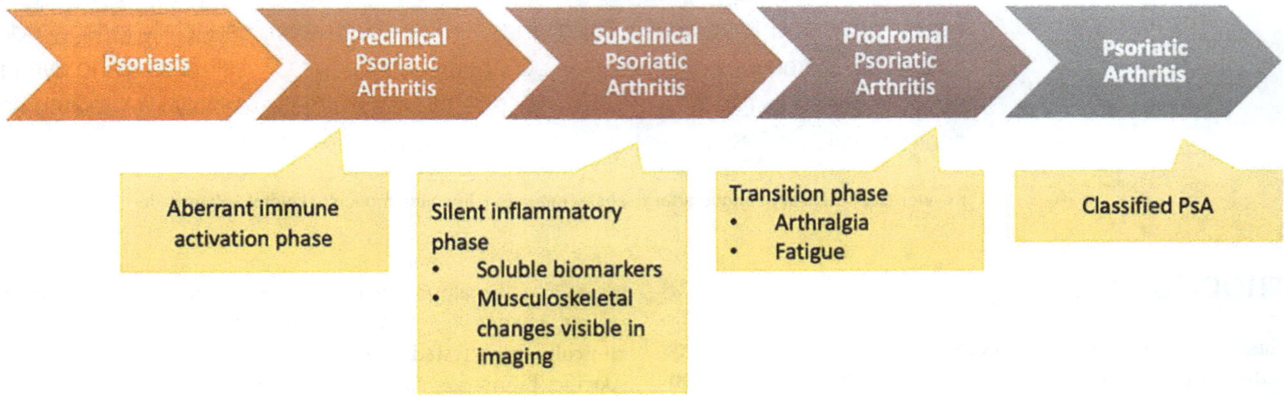

FIGURE 1 | Transition model from psoriasis to psoriatic arthritis [adapted from Scher et al. (2)].

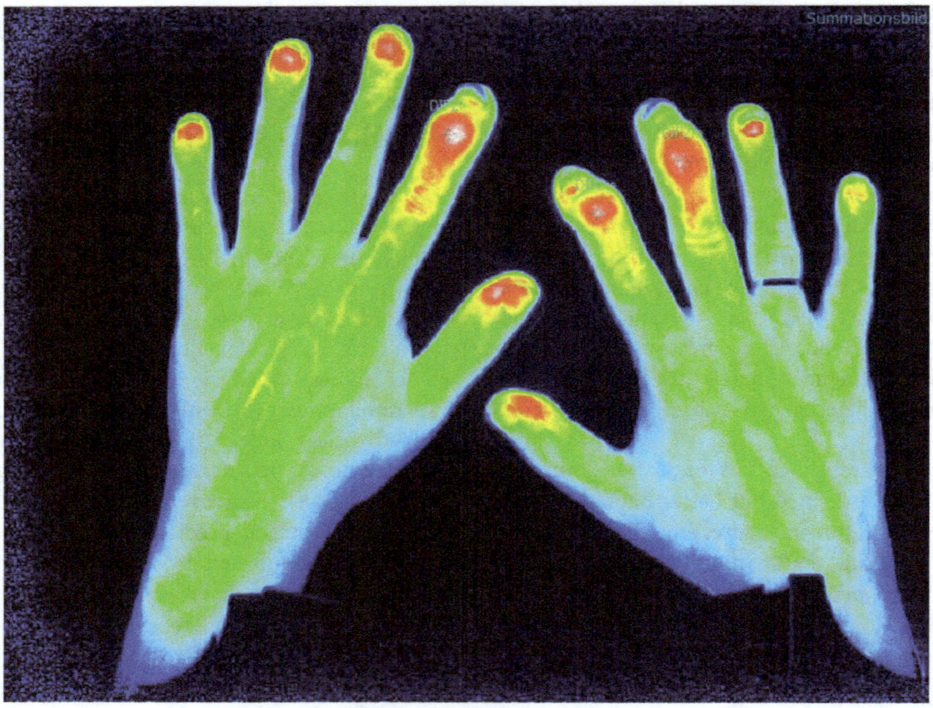

FIGURE 2 | Fluorescence optical imaging (FOI) assessment with detection of distal interphalangeal (DIP) arthritis.

such as arthralgia and fatigue occur. The subclinical identification of PsA will be necessary for dermatologists or general practitioners (GPs) to select the patients being presented to the rheumatologist or change treatment strategy.

In both scenarios, the biomarker to detect either patient in the subclinical or prodromal phase must be sensitive for detection of musculoskeletal inflammatory changes but also specific to identify those changes as PsA-related and highly predictive for later development of clinically evident PsA. Imaging studies of early PsA suggest that inflammatory enthesopathy is an early sign that is presented in PsA development (11). However, as shown in longitudinal studies, ~50% of patients with PsO that present with subclinical imaging enthesopathy will develop clinically manifested PsA (3).

IMAGING TECHNIQUES FOR THE DETECTION OF EARLY CHANGES IN ANGIOGENESIS AND MUSCULOSKELETAL INFLAMMATION

Different imaging techniques are available in clinical routine care to determine inflammatory musculoskeletal changes and increase in angiogenesis (**Table 1**). Different vascular and musculoskeletal compartments can be assessed and rated in focus on changes in vascularization, the severity of inflammation, disease manifestation, and disease state. Fluorescence optical imaging (FOI) is an indocyanine green (ICG)-tailored imaging technique that visualizes changes in micro-vascularization of the hands. FOI is a well-tolerated and fast method that seems sensitive for the detection of signs of inflammation and their changes over time. Nevertheless, it is limited by the rate of skin texture responsible for the penetration depth of the measurement system. Imaging of bone structure, entheses, and synovia is of high importance for classification of disease state and disease activity. By use of ultrasonography (US), changes in synovial and enthesial structure in early inflammation can be detected as it is commonly used but restricted by the experience of the observer and assessment algorithm. Moreover, by the use of US, changes of vascularization in the synovia and the enthesial structures can be easily evaluated using Doppler mode presenting as a sensitive marker for inflammation. Magnetic resonance imaging (MRI) is used to assess the presence of bone marrow edema, enthesitis, and changes in vascularization as early and disease activity indicators of inflammation of the joints, entheses, and spine. X-ray and computerized tomography (CT) can be used to assess structural damage in two and three dimensions. Innovative methods, such as high-resolution peripheral quantitative CT (HR-pQCT), can visualize pathophysiological processes and the morphological consequences at the bones even in the early stages of the disease. Moreover, techniques such as dual-energy CT (DECT) with iodine mapping may be helpful in discrimination of early arthritis.

Fluorescence Optical Imaging

Increase in micro-vascularization is identified as an early marker for PsA and of higher value than in other inflammatory joint diseases such as RA and may be a parameter to distinguish PsO from PsA in the subclinical phase of transition (12). FOI is an innovative imaging technique which detects changes in micro-vascularization of the hands as the camera system is only available for the hands by now. The method is tailored to indocyanine green injection which is a tolerable color agent used in different medical indication fields. The assessment lasts 360 s (one picture per second), and after measurement, the ICG kinetic profile is used for the (manual) assessment (**Figure 2**).

First studies to validate FOI were performed by assessment of its ability to detect synovitis/arthritis compared to the US and MRI examination (sensitivity 76%, specificity 94%) (13). Thuermel et al. (14) compared different disease states of synovitis between FOI and MRI findings. It was shown that mild synovitis was discriminated poorly by both FOI and MRI (81.6 vs. 86.8%), but with worsening of severity of synovitis, the potential for the discriminative ability increased in both methods with high correlation (moderate synovitis false positive in 12.5 vs. 16% for FOI and severe synovitis false positive in 0.7 vs. 2.4% for FOI). Additionally, Hirano et al. (15) confirmed the correlation of FOI measurement in the assessment of synovitis compared to US examination.

TABLE 1 | Overview of imaging techniques available for diagnosis of psoriatic arthritis (PsA) in psoriasis (PsO) patients and their advantages and disadvantages.

Technique	Advantage	Disadvantage
X-Ray	• Bone structure can be assessed (late changes)	• (Availability) • Radiation • Sensitivity for early changes: only structural changes to be detected • Only one structure per examination
Computerized tomography (CT)	• Bone structure can be assessed in 3 dimensions and related to anatomically structures (late changes)	• Availability • Sensitivity for early changes: only structural changes to be detected • Radiation • Only one structure per examination
High-resolution peripheral quantitative CT (HR-pQCT)	• Sensitivity: early structural changes can be detected	• Availability • Radiation • Only one structure per examination
Scintigraphy	• Availability • Whole body scan for increased metabolism (related to inflammation)	• Application of radioactive tracer • Poor specificity
^{18}F-FDG PET	• Whole body scan for increased metabolism (related to inflammation)	• Availability • Tolerability • Poor specificity
Ultrasound (US)	• Availability • Tolerability • Scan of all anatomically related structures possible • Doppler function: increase in vascularisation	• Time consuming when used in all joints and msk structures • Rater dependent (experience)
Magnetic Resonance Imaging (MRI)	• Scan of all anatomically related structures possible • Bone structure and metabolism	• Availability • Tolerability (contrast agent) • Only one structure per examination
Whole Body MRI (WB-MRI)	• Scan of whole body in one examination • Bone structure and metabolism	• Availability • Tolerability (contrast agent)
Dynamic contrast enhanced MRI (DCE-MRI)	• Scan of all anatomically related structures possible • Bone structure and metabolism • Quantification of inflammation	• Availability • Tolerability (contrast agent) • Only one structure per examination
Fluorescence-optical imaging (FOI)	• Availability • Tolerability • displays changes in micro vascularisation of the hands	• Only hands • Depth of measure limited • Rater dependent for (maunal) assessment

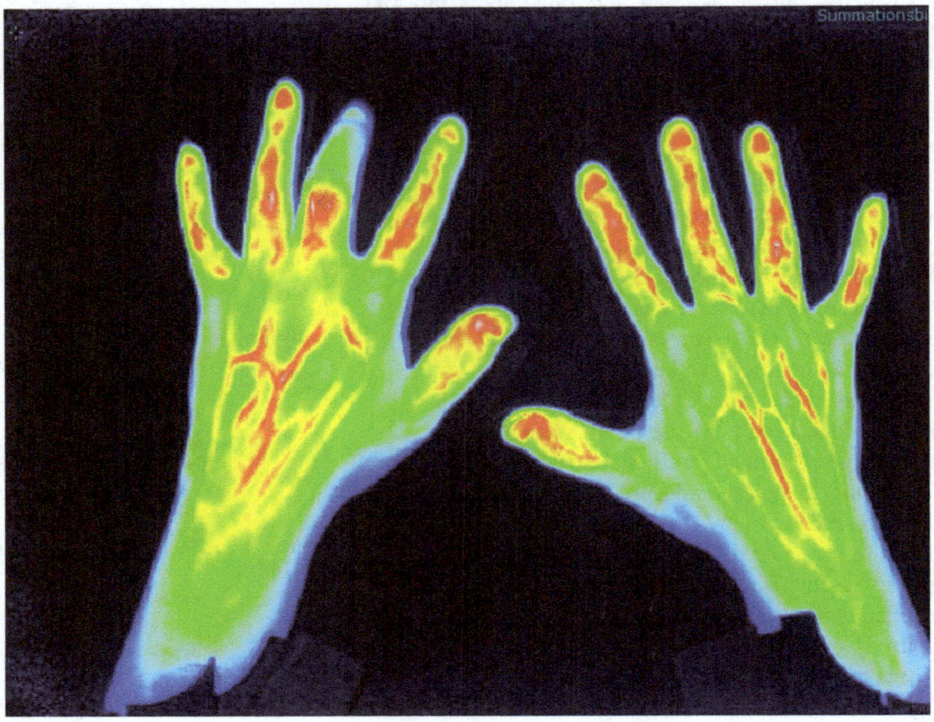

FIGURE 3 | Fluorescence optical imaging (FOI) assessment of arthritis/tendinitis in the hands.

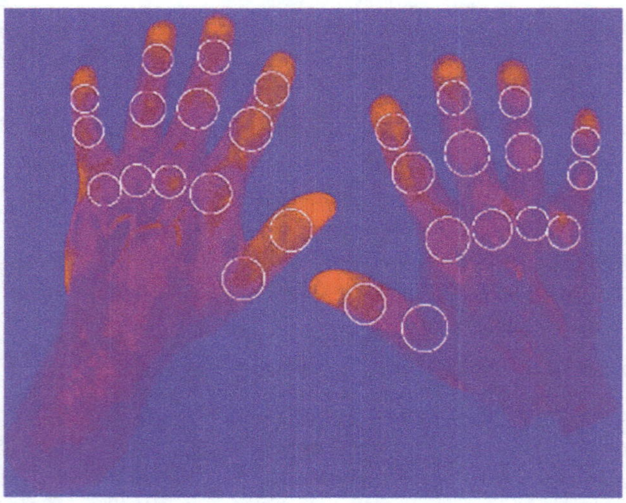

FIGURE 4 | Example: Nine clusters, maximum slope.

The different morphologic patterns can be identified in PsA patients that might be specific for the disease (**Figure 3**): in 94% of patients with clinically manifested PsA, a triangular increase of the color agent is detected at distal interphalangeal (DIP) joints (compared to 21% of RA patients), in 21% of PsA patients, a "green nail" sign was detectable (compared to 3% in RA patients), with a specificity of 87% and a sensitivity of 28% (16).

In the XCITING study, FOI was performed in patients with PsO and at risk for PsA development (nail PsO, musculoskeletal complaints within the last 6 months). In ~46% of the patients, FOI showed an increase of micro-vascularization defined as related to subclinical PsA (with the determination of inflammatory changes in MRI in 37%). Here, longitudinal data will show how many of those patients develop PsA in a 24-month follow-up period (17) to indicate its potential to select the at-risk population of PsO patients with later overt PsA. Therefore, FOI might be a promising imaging technique with little limitations (injection of the tolerable color agent, manual reading with the need of an experienced reader) and high advantages (fast performance, high sensitivity) to be of value in early detection in the transition from PsO to PsA.

Objective Joint Evaluation Based on Fluorescence Optical Imaging

FOI is assessed with the use of a manual assessment algorithm published by Werner et al. (13). To use FOI for the screening of PsO patients for changes in vascularization suspect for PsA, an objective assessment method is needed to allow fast assessment of the images with an automated algorithm. Therefore, methods to automate the assessment of the fluorescence intensities are in development.

To visualize the micro-vascularization of the hands with the FOI technique, a time-dependent data set of 360 images is

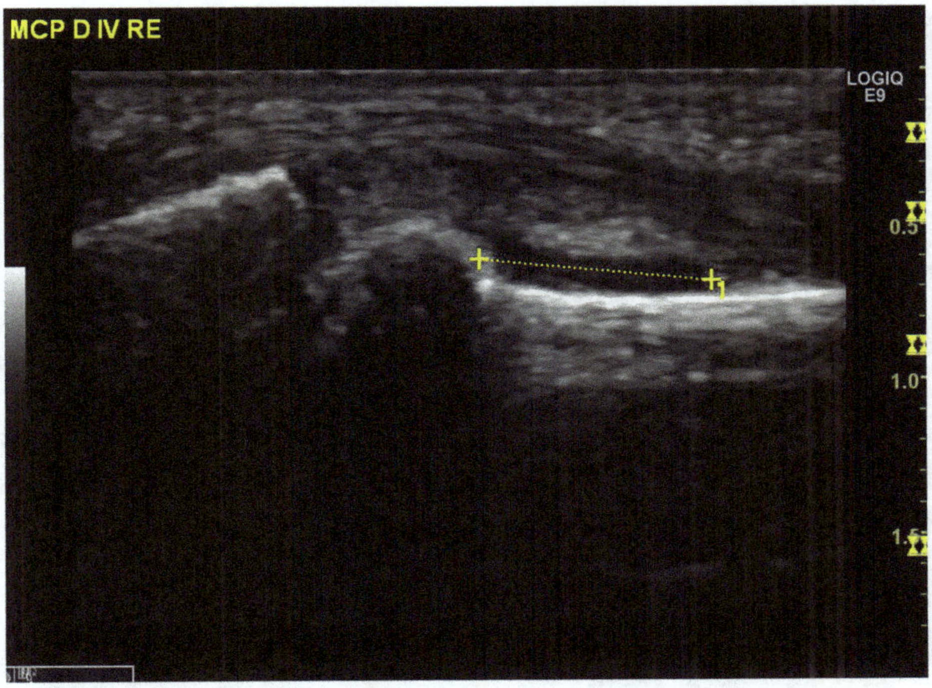

FIGURE 5 | Ultrasound assessment of synovitis metacarpophalangeal joint digit IV (MCP D IV).

acquired. Each image shows the current state of the proceeding distribution of the contrast agent ICG. To objectively evaluate the status of the subject's joints individually, the microvascularization at each joint position is evaluated.

To represent the status of each joint, several scores are calculated, representing different characteristics of the microvascularization. In the first step, each pixel (680 512) is represented by a time series containing 360 values. For each time series, three different features are extracted: the amplitude, the mean value during the signal increasing time, and the maximal gradient. Then, each of the three sets is clustered by k-means clustering, with $k \in \{3\ ,5,\ 7,9\}$. Furthermore, each pixel is assigned a shade of red–blue, where the brightest (red) corresponds to the highest cluster indicating highest dynamics and the darkest to the lowest indicating the smallest dynamics (**Figure 4**).

Therefore, 12 heatmaps (three features 4 ks) are generated. Finally, scores for the defined joint areas are calculated based on the assigned cluster values, number of pixels in the joint area and the number of clusters k.

Applying this newly developed method to 271 clinical examination (CE) labeled patients with 6,426 healthy joints and 1,162 affected joints (tender, swollen, or both) results in a clear distinction between the scores for healthy and affected labeled joints. The summarized results for $k = 9$ are visualized in **Table 2**.

TABLE 2 | Resulting scores for $k = 9$ for all 271 patients.

Statistic value \ Feature	Amplitude		Mean		Slope	
	Healthy	**Affected**	**Healthy**	**Affected**	**Healthy**	**Affected**
Average	0.503	0.528	0.486	0.509	0.395	0.414
Median	0.496	0.532	0.482	0.505	0.389	0.415

Ultrasound

Ultrasound (US) is used to identify structural and inflammatory changes in the joints and the musculoskeletal system (**Figures 5–7**). In different clinical studies, it has been demonstrated that US examination is more sensitive than radiography (18). The US is more sensitive than clinical examination for the assessment of inflammatory and structural changes in inflammatory arthritis, including PsA, and particularly synovitis, enthesitis, tenosynovitis, and bursitis (19, 20). Besides, US results are comparable to those of MRI, except for the detection of bone marrow edema. The reproducibility and low cost of US examination provide advantages compared to MRI for early PsA detection (21). However, a complete US examination of all joints, entheses, tendons, and bursae is extremely time-consuming and infeasible. Moreover, US examination is assessor related and depends on the experience of the rater.

As it was shown that inflammatory enthesopathy is a subclinical sign in the transition from PsO to PsA, the US may be a sensitive and feasible method to detect early inflammatory changes at entheses. Savage et al. (22) showed that subclinical enthesopathy and associated osteitis are present in patients with PsO but without arthritis, for which clinical examination is ineffective. And 49.3% of the PsO patients included had

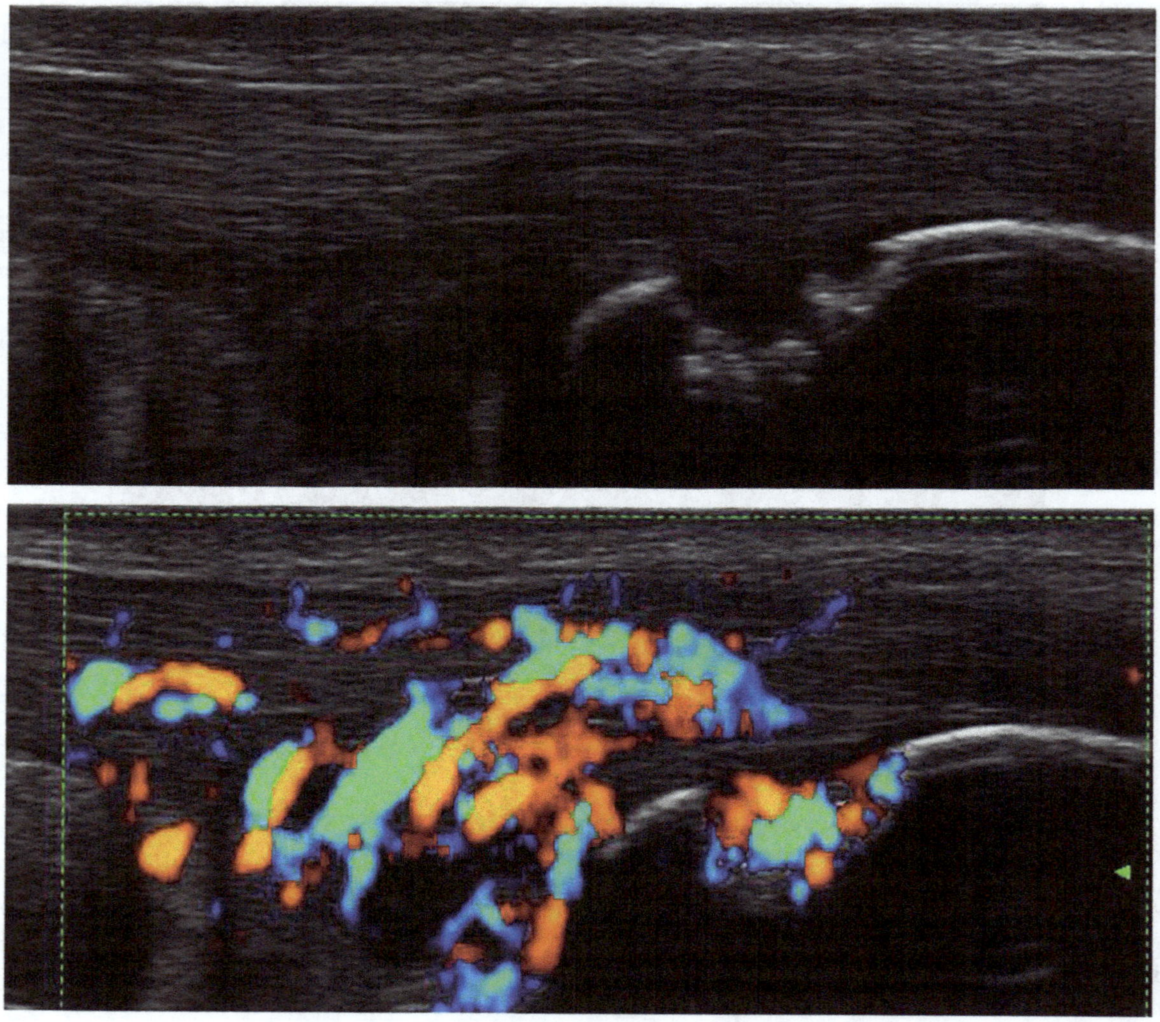

FIGURE 6 | Ultrasound assessment. Tendinitis of the Achilles tendon with the formation of osteophytes and power Doppler activity.

no evidence of clinically manifested PsA but showed at least one sonographic inflammatory abnormality that fulfilled the OMERACT definition of enthesopathy. These findings support the assumption that even in PsO, changes at the enthesial sites are detectable. It is necessary to assess in longitudinal how many of those patients developed overt PsA to specify these findings for risk stratification.

Magnetic Resonance Imaging

MRI is a very sensitive method for visualization of musculoskeletal structures that are involved in inflammatory processes. There are only little data on the detection of early PsA as the main studies on the detection of early arthritis were performed for the indication field of RA (23). With the use of MRI, arthritis, synovitis, tenosynovitis, periarticular inflammation, bone marrow edema, erosions, and bone proliferation can be sensitively visualized and anatomically classified. Limitations of MRI examination are the need of long examination times with illustration of only a single anatomic structure per examination and the need of contrast agent (tolerability). Definitions of disease-specific abnormalities are provided by the OMERACT working group, whereas enthesial disease criteria are only recently published (24). For inflammation and structural changes, T1-weighted sequences in two planes are performed (signal mainly reflecting fat content and a contrast agent), supplemented with a T2-weighted, fat-suppressed sequence or short tau inversion recovery (STIR) sequence (signal mainly reflecting water content). Performance of additional T1-weighted sequences (after intravenous gadolinium-containing contrast agent; **Figure 8**) with or without fat suppression assists in the assessment of tissue inflammation in peripheral joints. Use of contrast agent is needed for illustration of synovitis and tenosynovitis but not for detection of erosions, bony proliferation, and bone marrow edema (24).

Differences between PsA and other inflammatory diseases classified by MRI are reported. In PsA, enthesitis is not related to a focal inflammation but to a wider "synovio-enthesal complex"

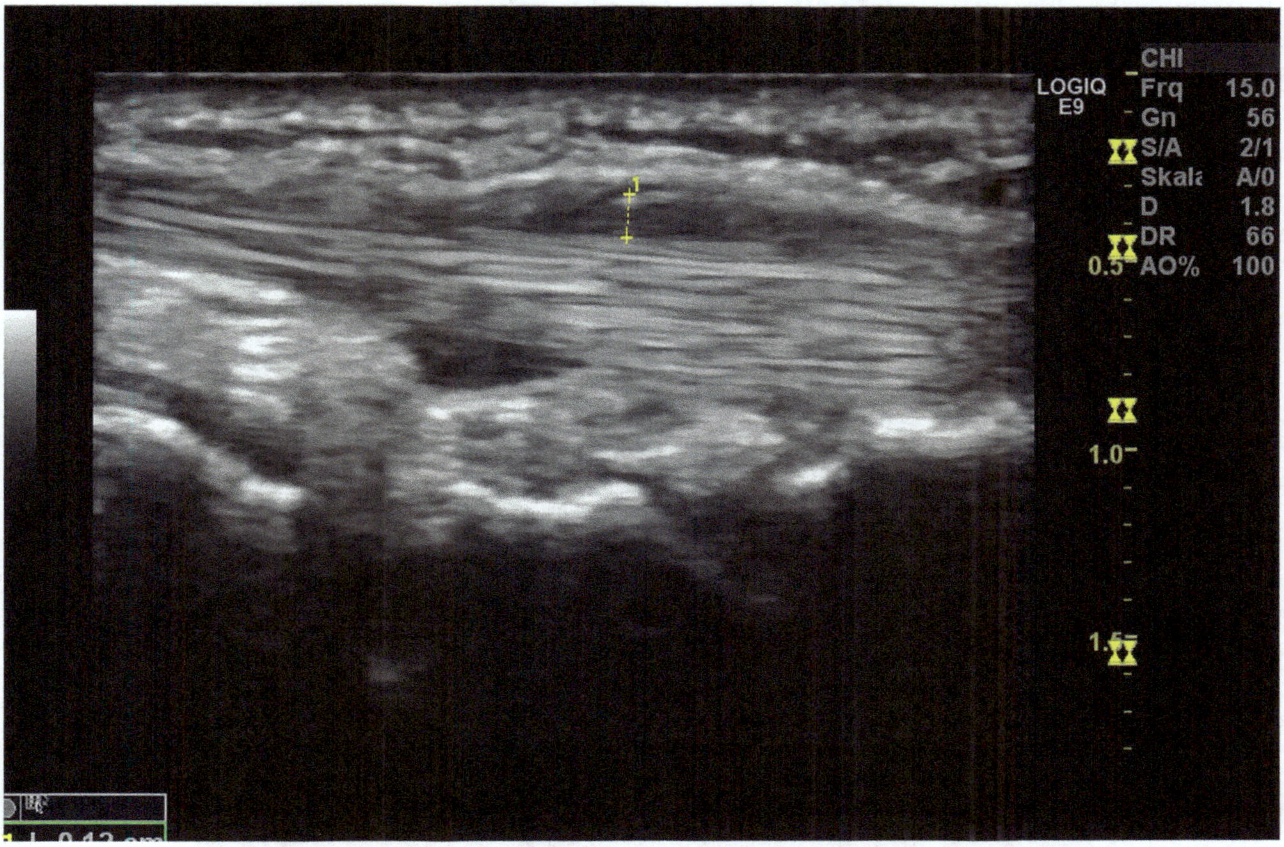

FIGURE 7 | Ultrasound assessment of flexor tendinitis.

(25), including adjacent tendons, periosteum, fibrocartilage, synovium, and bone at the attachment sites. Whereas, MRI findings such as synovitis, enthesitis, tenosynovitis, and bone marrow edema that appear frequently in PsA are not disease-specific and appear in any other inflammatory joint disease, PsA is characterized by more prevalent diaphyseal bone marrow and/or enthesitis, soft tissue inflammation, extracapsular inflammation, and involvement of primarily flexor tendons in contrast to extensor tendons in RA (26). Erosions are often located close to the collateral ligaments in contrast to osteoarthritis where they are frequently found centrally (27). In comparison to RA, in PsA, periostitis is found more frequent than erosions (28).

Assessments in PsO patients without evident arthritis revealed subclinical inflammation in both joints and entheses. Moreover, it was found that PsO patients with subclinical inflammation in MRI and arthralgia had a high risk (55.5%) for the later development of PsA, whereas patients without arthralgia had a low risk (15.3%) for PsA development (29). The specific pattern is recently not defined to detect PsO patients in subclinical development of PsA.

New methods of MRI such as whole-body MRI (WB-MRI) and dynamic contrast-enhanced MRI (DCE-MRI) are used in the research of PsO and PsA discrimination and prediction of PsA development. DCE-MRI allows semiautomated quantification of inflammation based on the measurement of contrast enhancement pattern over time in the selected region of interest. A recent report reports differences in RA and PsA in the pattern of enhancement of the synovial membrane with higher inflamed tissue in RA but a higher degree of inflammation in PsA (30). WB-MRI assessment indicated agreement between enthesitis on clinical scores and MRI results in PsA patients, suggesting value in detecting subclinical inflammation and the total burden of inflammation (31, 32).

Conventional X-Ray and Computerized Tomography

Conventional radiographic imaging methods such as x-ray (**Figure 9**) or conventional CT are often used to detect changes in bone structure in progressive PsA after clinical detection of inflammation by assessment of swollen or tender joints (33). The sensitivity for the detection of early changes in PsO patients at risk for PsA development is poor as only pronounced changes in bone structure are detectable being evident and often found only in a late stage of the disease.

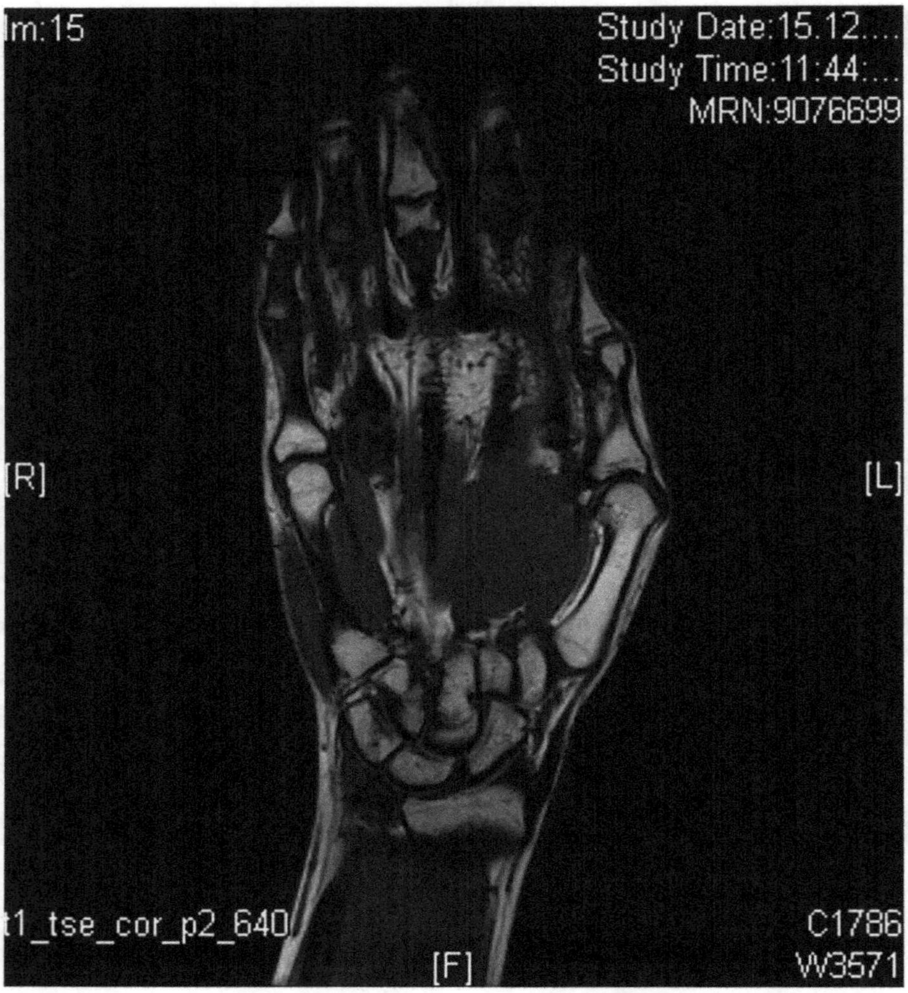

FIGURE 8 | MRI of the left hand without signs of inflammation (T1 sequence).

Innovative Techniques Using Computerized Tomography Methods

Innovative methods, such as high-resolution peripheral quantitative CT (HR-pQCT) are available to sensitively detect early changes in bone metabolism in PsO patients compared to PsA and other joint diseases. Bone erosions can be detected early in the disease state of PsA (34), and the severity of erosions depends on its articular type and its activity (inflammation) status (35). Bone erosions in PsA pathophysiology result from an accumulation of osteoclasts in the joints, which is promoted by pro-inflammatory cytokines (36). Anabolic bone changes in PsA are mainly based on new bone formation. These changes typically occur at insertion sites of tendons to bone. Enthesial inflammation is a key process in PsA and most likely triggered by mechanical stress (37). Bone structure responses at the inflamed enthesial sites result in the formation of enthesophytes. An HR-pQCT-based study showed that the formation of enthesophytes are pronounced in PsA but are not found in rheumatoid arthritis (38). Furthermore, a more recent study revealed that enthesophytes occur early in patients with PsO without joint involvement, suggesting that their formation reflects a common process in PsO and PsA (39). In another study from Simon et al. (40), bone structure, number erosions, and enthesophytes were compared between different patient cohorts (PsO, PsA, and healthy controls) to measure a discriminative potential. Data on the extent of bone erosions and enthesophytes were collected and correlated to different categories of age, duration of PsO, and duration of PsA. Additionally, demographic and disease-specific data, including physical function [Health Assessment Questionnaire (HAQ)], were collected. A total of 203 patients were analyzed (101 with PsA, 55 with PsO, and 47 as healthy controls). Patients with PsA had a significantly higher number with a higher extent of erosions and enthesophytes compared to patients with PsO and healthy controls. Patients with PsO and healthy controls did not differ in number and extent of erosions, while enthesophytes were more frequent in patients with PsO

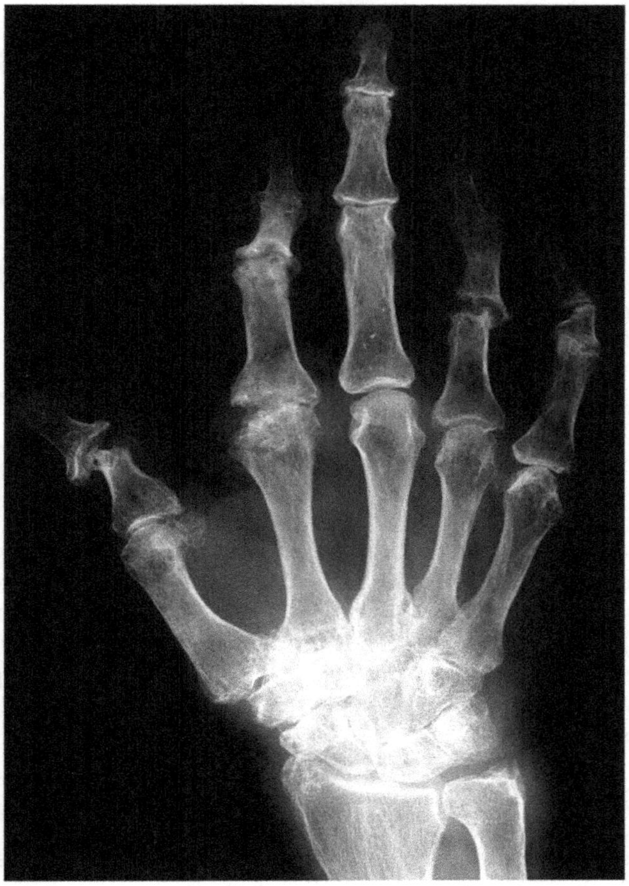

FIGURE 9 | Plain x-ray of the right hand with arthritis mutilans.

than in healthy controls. Bone erosions, but not enthesophytes, showed strong age dependency in all three groups. In contrast, enthesophytes were mostly influenced by the duration of PsO and PsA and, in contrast to bone erosions, were associated with poorer physical function, as measured by HAQ. Unfortunately, data on the association between the risk collective of PsO patients who develop PsA are currently missing but under examination. The longitudinal change will give more insights into the potential of HR-pQCT as an imaging method predicting PsA development in PsO patients.

Besides HR-pQCT, dual-energy CT (DECT) with iodine mapping to improve iodine contrast resolution may be a sensitive method to discriminate early inflammatory arthritis (41) but restricted in longitudinal measurement by radiation rate. Only a few studies were performed by now showing potential for early discrimination, but further studies are needed to confirm the findings in larger cohorts and over time.

Scintigraphy

Bone scintigraphy is an established method displaying an increase of metabolism of the tracer as a sign for abnormal metabolism rates, e.g., in the inflammatory state. It is used to detect inflammatory changes in the whole body, especially if other imaging techniques are not available. It has poor specificity and is limited by the use of the radioactive isotopes (tracers). In PsA, it was used in different cohorts to detect subclinical signs of inflammation in PsO patients without evident clinical PsA. The results were compared to the findings in US examination and clinical examination (42). It was revealed that a significantly higher number of joints were verified by the US to have increased uptake of tracer compared to clinical examination (34).

Fluorine-18-Labeled Fluorodeoxyglucose Positron Emission Tomography

Fluorine-18-labeled fluorodeoxyglucose positron emission tomography (^{18}F-FDG-PET) is a very sensitive imaging method for detection of changes in metabolism, e.g., inflammation-dependent early musculoskeletal changes indicating PsA-related changes. Takata et al. (43) performed a clinical study in PsO patients without clinically manifested PsA compared to PsA patients with long-lasting clinical overt PsA. Eighteen PsO and 28 PsA patients were enrolled for examination by positron emission tomography/computerized tomography (PET/CT) using ^{18}F-FDG. In the PsA cohort, ^{18}F-FDG accumulation was identified in all affected joints, illustrating its reliability in correlation to clinical examination sensitivity. In the PsO cohort, asymptomatic enthesitis was detected in six out of 18 PsO patients (33%), demonstrating its high sensitivity in the detection of inflammation at the entheses.

IMAGING TECHNIQUES FOR SENSITIVE AND SPECIFIC DETECTION OF EARLY PSORIATIC ARTHRITIS IN DIFFERENT TRANSITION PHASES

The transition from PsO to PsA contains different phases (preclinical, subclinical, and prodromal). In only two of those phases, early changes in soluble biomarkers/imaging can be detected (subclinical phase) or first unspecific clinical symptoms (e.g., arthralgia and fatigue) occur (prodromal phase). These two phases may be useful in early discrimination of the PsO patients at risk to develop overt PsA to prevent its occurrence (**Figure 10**).

In the transition model, the subclinical phase includes early musculoskeletal inflammatory changes in PsO patients without musculoskeletal complaints. In this phase of the disease, MRI, HR-pQCT, and high-frequency ultrasonography might have the highest potential to distinguish inflammatory changes in the defined at-risk-population with the limitation of the specificity to be PsA-related. By a combination of these techniques, patients are deeply characterized in focus on first musculoskeletal inflammatory changes and early changes in bone structure/bone metabolism. This characterization is completed by the use of FOI to generate additional information on early changes in vascularization as signs of increased angiogenesis, reported as an early marker in PsA progress (12). In different clinical studies within this special patient population, it was shown that in a high proportion of asymptomatic PsO patients, enthesial inflammation was detectable (44). Moreover, Simon

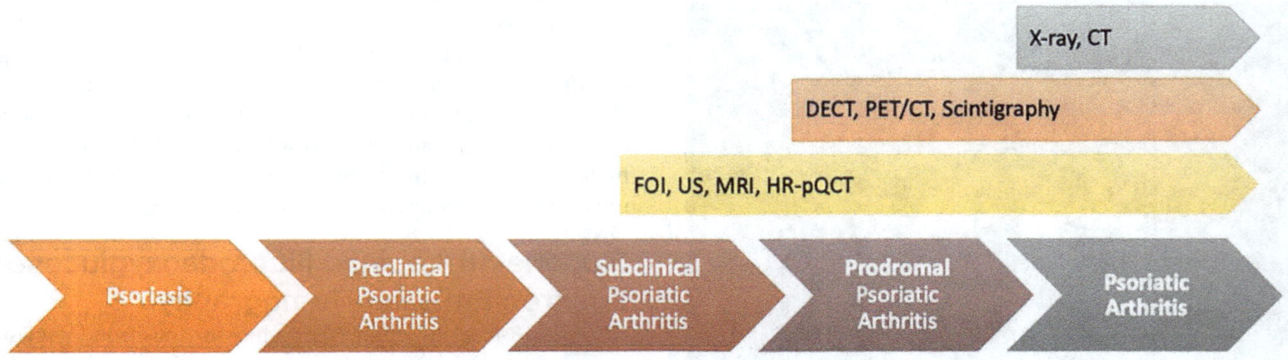

FIGURE 10 | Value of different imaging techniques to find unspecific musculoskeletal changes in psoriasis (PsO) patients with the transition phases from PsO to psoriatic arthritis (PsA).

et al. (40) showed that by the use of HR-pQCT, the number of enthesophytes was significantly higher in asymptomatic PsO patients than in healthy controls. Moreover, the duration of skin disease influenced the number of enthesophytes (45). Nevertheless, only a part of those patients will develop clinical overt PsA afterwards. The potential of imaging biomarker to detect the specific at-risk population is poor. Additionally, clinical definitions adapted from other inflammatory diseases such as the criteria for subclinical inflammation in RA are not usable in PsA as by its use, half of the asymptomatic PsO patients are classified as subclinical PsA, but only part of them will develop PsA later. So, within this phase is a high need of clear classification and characterization of patients to define the correct at-risk population for PsA development, maybe by a combination of different biomarkers (e.g., combination with soluble biomarkers, e.g., on miRNA base, biomarkers for comorbid conditions that were shown to occur early in the disease process or different imaging techniques). Beside the definition of the biomarker set, its usability must be high to be implemented into clinical routine care.

The prodromal phase of the disease is classified as unspecific clinical symptoms such as arthralgia and/or fatigue combined with the occurrence of inflammatory changes in imaging. A recent study showed that, in this phase, tenosynovitis was the most significant contributor to the reported musculoskeletal symptoms (PsO vs. PsO with arthralgia vs. PsA). In the US, in a high proportion of patients, tenosynovitis especially of the flexor tendon of the hands was detected (in 29.5% of the arthralgia patients compared to 5.3% in the PsO group) (10), whereas active enthesitis and synovitis did not reach a significant difference. In the longitudinal part of the study, in the US, determined enthesitis was the only US feature linked to the future evolution of PsA. Faustini et al. (29) confirmed this link between subclinical inflammation detected and PsA, highlighting that patients with synovitis detected by MRI and arthralgia had 55.5% likelihood to develop PsA within 1 year. In the IVEPSA (Interception in very early PsA) study, psoriatic patients with inflammatory arthralgia without joint swelling and with concomitant predictors of PsA [i.e., Psoriasis Area and Severity Index (PASI) >6 or scalp PsO or nail involvement] were treated with anti-interleukin (IL)-17 for a disease interception. Baseline MRI investigation of the dominant hand revealed at least one inflammatory lesion in 83% of patients, highlighting synovitis as the most prevalent (66.7%), followed by tenosynovitis (55.6%) (46).

DISCUSSION

PsO is one of the common chronic inflammatory skin diseases, affecting ~3% of the European Caucasians. PsA is a chronic immune-mediated disease associated with PsO characterized by distinct musculoskeletal inflammation. Due to its heterogeneous clinical manifestations (e.g., oligo- and polyarthritis, enthesitis, dactylitis, and axial inflammation), early diagnosis of PsA is often difficult and delayed. PsO patients are of high risk for PsA development as ~30% of PsO patients will be affected by (chronic) musculoskeletal inflammation.

The main events for the transition from PsO to PsA are currently unclear: the combination of genetic and clinical-demographic risk factors (e.g., nail PsO, PsO severity, and type) may promote PsA development and its progression. The underlying molecular mechanisms for the transition from PsO to PsA are still poorly defined. The increase of neoangiogenesis (12) and the development of enthesitis is hypothesized to be a primary manifestation in PsA, detectable early using imaging and clinical examination in patients developing later overt PsA (22).

Different phases were defined to describe the transition from PsO to PsA (2). Three phases are named between PsO and overt PsA of which two have high relevance to be detectable in the at-risk population with the use of sensitive biomarkers such as sensitive imaging techniques: the subclinical phase (detection of soluble biomarkers, e.g., on miRNA base and early musculoskeletal inflammation such as synovio-enthesitis detected in imaging but missing related clinical symptoms) and the prodromal phase (detection of musculoskeletal inflammation in imaging techniques and unspecific clinical symptoms such as fatigue and arthralgia).

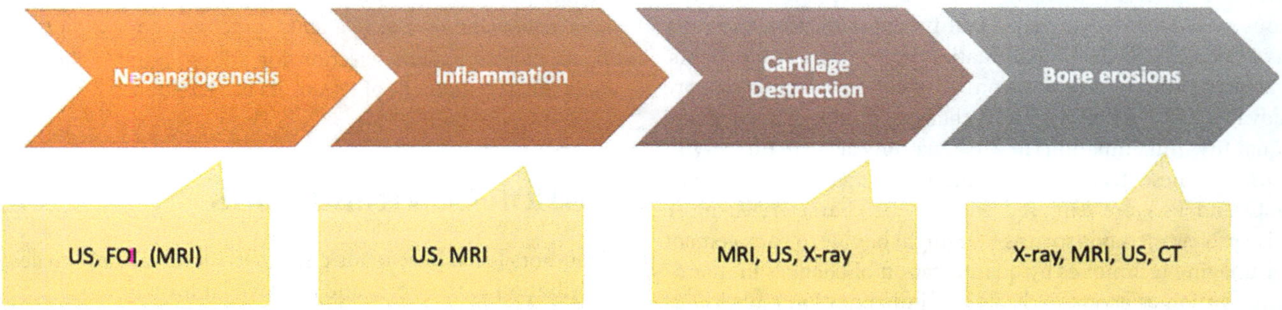

FIGURE 11 | Different disease activity characteristics with the ability of imaging methods to be measured adequately.

The potential of the available imaging techniques to detect patients in one of these two phases differs widely as all of these techniques characterize different pathophysiologic states of the inflammatory process that might have the highest value by being combined for deep characterization of the patients (**Figure 11**).

Besides sensitivity and specificity in the detection of anatomical and pathophysiological changes by use of advanced imaging techniques, standardized assessment tools are needed to bring innovative imaging methods in context to the suspected indications and process results to enable detection of coherence between saliences and the underlying disease. Technological advances should be integrated into assessment algorithms to use its full potential to be beneficial in the detection of at-risk patients especially in context to PsO and PsA patients.

FOI as an ICG-tailored imaging technique visualizes changes in micro-vascularization of the hands (13). It is a well-tolerated and fast method that seems sensitive for detection of early signs of inflammation related to changes in angiogenesis. Early changes of micro-vascularization may be indicators for early signs of inflammation of the joints and tendons as neoangiogenesis was identified as a symptom associated with musculoskeletal inflammation in PsA differently to other arthritides (47). Due to its mechanism, the detection of changes in micro-vascularization may be of value to define a very early disease state of PsA in the subclinical phase of transition when clinical signs such as arthralgia are missing. With its high sensitivity to detect changes, it is of value to be used in longitudinal observation. These aspects should be investigated in further studies as it gives an advantage to easily screen PsO patients without symptoms but defined risk profile early. Automated measurement of the fluorescence signals gives an objective assessment of the state and its changes over time when used in longitudinal assessments.

MRI and US are the recent widely used methods for sensitive detection of inflammation in the joints and musculoskeletal structures (entheses, bursa, tendons). Bone marrow edema, enthesitis, and changes in vascularization as early indicators of inflammation of the joints, entheses, and spine in the subclinical and prodromal phases can be visualized with high sensitivity by both (23). The US has the benefit of its availability as well as of its possibility to detect changes in synovial and enthesial structure in early inflammation. Changes of vascularization in the synovia and the enthesial structures can be easily evaluated using Doppler mode presenting as a sensitive marker for inflammation (subclinical and prodromal phase) (44). Structures of interest can be associated with anatomica structures, and due to their tolerability, longitudinal status can be measured easily.

HR-pQCT, developed from CT technique, might be of high value to detect early changes in bone metabolism and structure in PsO and PsA patients (compared to other inflammatory diseases), but the value for discrimination of PsO or PsO transient to PsA is recently not clear. Simon et al. (40) showed that in PsO and PsA patients, the formation of enthesophytes is pronounced compared to RA and healthy controls, but the differentiation of those findings between PsO in early PsA state is poor. Longitudinal data are missing to evaluate within this group. Dual-energy CT might be as well a very sensitive method to discriminate between PsO/PsA disease state, but its performance and repeatability are limited to radiation and validity.

Established methods such as x-ray or CT are not sensitive enough to detect early inflammatory changes of the musculoskeletal disease but changes in bone structure.

PET/CT and scintigraphy have established methods with a focus on metabolism and its changes in the inflammatory disease state. Both methods are limited by their poor specificity but sensitive to illustrate changes early and with focus on the whole body not restricted by use in one region of interest.

For US, MRI, and HR-pQCT, the relevance of the early findings of enthesophytes (HR-pQCT) or detection of enthesopathy (MRI, US) as signs for early musculoskeletal inflammation without clinical symptoms (subclinical phase) in PsO patients is still unclear. In a longitudinal study, it was found that although these findings were detectable in 50% of the PsO patients, only a part of them developed overt PsA later in their disease state (40, 45). So, these imaging findings are not specific for the definition of high risk for PsA development and must be completed by a multifactorial characterization of the patient profile, e.g., using data on the comorbid condition, clinical data, and data of soluble biomarker (in the investigation).

The potential of these imaging techniques increases in the prodromal phase when clinical symptoms appear, even if they are non-specific. Here, the at-risk population is enriched, and the combination of both imaging findings and arthralgia predicts the development of PsA significantly.

Overall, different imaging techniques are available with various methods to sensitively quantify vascularization and early signs of musculoskeletal inflammation in PsO and PsA patients. Advanced methods adapted from conventional techniques are of advantage to illustrate early changes in bone metabolism or quantify inflammation in the anatomical structure. With the use of these techniques, pathophysiological backgrounds of PsO and PsA are explored and can be characterized more precisely. New methods such as FOI might be able to complement other imaging techniques by quantification of changes in micro-vascularization as a very early sign of inflammation (subclinical PsA without clinical symptoms). Nevertheless, by now, it is not possible to specifically discriminate between PsO patients and those who will develop PsA by solely using imaging as a biomarker. So, further studies are needed to explore the impact of different characteristics/biomarkers (e.g., clinical data, comorbid condition, soluble/molecular biomarkers, different imaging techniques) and their impact in predicting PsA to characterize the at-risk patients precisely and explore their impact of PsO patient selection for a longitudinal follow-up to assess the development of PsA or its interception.

AUTHOR CONTRIBUTIONS

All authors listed have made a substantial, direct and intellectual contribution to the work, and approved it for publication.

ACKNOWLEDGMENTS

We would like to thank the participating patients and study center personnel.

REFERENCES

1. Ritchlin CT, Colbert RA, Gladman DD. Psoriatic Arthritis. *N Engl J Med.* (2017) 376:2095–6. doi: 10.1056/NEJMra1505557
2. Scher JU, Ogdie A, Merola JF, Ritchlin C. Preventing psoriatic arthritis: focusing on patients with psoriasis at increased risk of transition. *Nat Rev Rheumatol.* (2019) 15:153–66. doi: 10.1038/s41584-019-0175-0
3. Zabotti A, Tinazzi I, Aydin SZ, McGonagle D. From psoriasis to psoriatic arthritis: insights from imaging on the transition to psoriatic arthritis and implications for arthritis prevention. *Curr Rheumatol Rep.* (2020) 22:24. doi: 10.1007/s11926-020-00891-x
4. Gladman DD, Antoni C, Mease P, Clegg DO, Nash P. Psoriatic arthritis: epidemiology, clinical features, course, and outcome. *Ann Rheum Dis.* (2005) 64(Suppl. 2):ii14–7. doi: 10.1136/ard.2004.032482
5. Christophers E, Barker JN, Griffiths CE, Dauden E, Milligan G, Molta C, et al. The risk of psoriatic arthritis remains constant following initial diagnosis of psoriasis among patients seen in European dermatology clinics. *J Eur Acad Dermatol Venereol.* (2010) 24:548–54. doi: 10.1111/j.1468-3083.2009.03463.x
6. Eder L, Haddad A, Rosen CF, Lee KA, Chandran V, Cook R, et al. The incidence and risk factors for psoriatic arthritis in patients with psoriasis: a prospective cohort study. *Arthritis Rheumatol.* (2016) 68:915–23. doi: 10.1002/art.39494
7. Love TJ, Zhu Y, Zhang Y, Wall-Burns L, Ogdie A, Gelfand JM, et al. Obesity and the risk of psoriatic arthritis: a population-based study. *Ann Rheum Dis.* (2012) 71:1273–7. doi: 10.1136/annrheumdis-2012-201299
8. Myers A, Kay LJ, Lynch SA, Walker DJ. Recurrence risk for psoriasis and psoriatic arthritis within sibships. *Rheumatology.* (2005) 44:773–6. doi: 10.1093/rheumatology/keh589
9. Eder L, Polachek A, Rosen CF, Chandran V, Cook R, Gladman DD. The development of psoriatic arthritis in patients with psoriasis is preceded by a period of nonspecific musculoskeletal symptoms: a prospective cohort study. *Arthritis Rheumatol.* (2017) 69:622–9. doi: 10.1002/art.39973
10. Zabotti A, McGonagle DG, Giovannini I, Errichetti E, Zuliani F, Zanetti A, et al. Transition phase towards psoriatic arthritis: clinical and ultrasonographic characterisation of psoriatic arthralgia. *RMD Open.* (2019) 5:e001067. doi: 10.1136/rmdopen-2019-001067
11. McGonagle D, Gibbon W, Emery P. Classification of inflammatory arthritis by enthesitis. *Lancet.* (1998) 352:1137–40. doi: 10.1016/S0140-6736(97)12004-9
12. Veale DJ, Fearon U. What makes psoriatic and rheumatoid arthritis so different? *RMD Open.* (2015) 1:e000025. doi: 10.1136/rmdopen-2014-000025
13. Werner SG, Langer HE, Ohrndorf S, Bahner M, Schott P, Schwenke C, et al. Inflammation assessment in patients with arthritis using a novel *in vivo* fluorescence optical imaging technology. *Ann Rheum Dis.* (2012) 71:504–10. doi: 10.1136/annrheumdis-2010-148288
14. Thuermel K, Neumann J, Jungmann PM, Schaffeler C, Waldt S, Heinze A, et al. Fluorescence optical imaging and 3T-MRI for detection of synovitis in patients with rheumatoid arthritis in comparison to a composite standard of reference. *Eur J Radiol.* (2017) 90:6–13. doi: 10.1016/j.ejrad.2017.02.016
15. Hirano F, Yokoyama-Kokuryo W, Yamazaki H, Tsutsumino M, Sakai R, Satoh S, et al. Comparison of fluorescence optical imaging, ultrasonography and clinical examination with magnetic resonance imaging as a reference in active rheumatoid arthritis patients. *Immunol Med.* (2018) 41:75–81. doi: 10.1080/13497413.2018.1481578
16. Wiemann O, Werner SG, Langer HE, Backhaus M, Chatelain R. The "green nail" phenomenon in ICG-enhanced fluorescence optical imaging - a potential tool for the differential diagnosis of psoriatic arthritis. *J Dtsch Dermatol Ges.* (2019) 17:138–47. doi: 10.1111/ddg.13747
17. Koehm M, Rossmanith T, Langer HE, Backhaus M, Burmester GR, Wassenberg S, et al. Detection of clinical signs of arthritis and subclinical evidence of inflammation in psoriasis patients with risk for arthritis: value of clinical examination, ultrasound and fluorescence-optical imaging - results from the Prospective Multicentre Xciting Study [abstract]. *Arthritis Rheumatol.* (2017) 69 (Suppl. 10).
18. Wiell C, Szkudlarek M, Hasselquist M, Moller JM, Vestergaard A, Norregaard J, et al. Ultrasonography, magnetic resonance imaging, radiography, and clinical assessment of inflammatory and destructive changes in fingers and toes of patients with psoriatic arthritis. *Arthritis Res Ther.* (2007) 9:R119. doi: 10.1186/ar2327
19. Weiner SM, Jurenz S, Uhl M, Lange-Nolde A, Warnatz K, Peter HH, et al. Ultrasonography in the assessment of peripheral joint involvement in psoriatic arthritis : a comparison with radiography, MRI and scintigraphy. *Clin Rheumatol.* (2008) 27:983–9. doi: 10.1007/s10067-008-0835-y
20. Dougados M, Jousse-Joulin S, Mistretta F, d'Agostino MA, Backhaus M, Bentin J, et al. Evaluation of several ultrasonography scoring systems for synovitis and comparison to clinical examination: results from a prospective multicentre study of rheumatoid arthritis. *Ann Rheum Dis.* (2010) 69:828–33. doi: 10.1136/ard.2009.115493
21. Coates LC, Hodgson R, Conaghan PG, Freeston JE. MRI and ultrasonography for diagnosis and monitoring of psoriatic arthritis. *Best Pract Res Clin Rheumatol.* (2012) 26:805–22. doi: 10.1016/j.berh.2012.09.004
22. Savage L, Goodfield M, Horton L, Watad A, Hensor E, Emery P, et al. Regression of peripheral subclinical enthesopathy in therapy-naive patients treated with ustekinumab for moderate-to-severe chronic plaque psoriasis: a

fifty-two-week, prospective, open-label feasibility study. *Arthritis Rheumatol.* (2019) 71:626–31. doi: 10.1002/art.40778

23. McQueen F, Lassere M, Ostergaard M. Magnetic resonance imaging in psoriatic arthritis: a review of the literature. *Arthritis Res Ther.* (2006) 8:207. doi: 10.1186/ar1934
24. Ostergaard M, McQueen F, Wiell C, Bird P, Boyesen P, Ejbjerg B, et al. The OMERACT psoriatic arthritis magnetic resonance imaging scoring system (PsAMRIS): definitions of key pathologies, suggested MRI sequences, and preliminary scoring system for PsA Hands. *J Rheumatol.* (2009) 36:1816–24. doi: 10.3899/jrheum.090352
25. McGonagle D, Aydin SZ, Tan AL. The synovio-entheseal complex and its role in tendon and capsular associated inflammation. *J Rheumatol Suppl.* (2012) 89:11–4. doi: 10.3899/jrheum.120233
26. Narvaez J, Narvaez JA, de Albert M, Gomez-Vaquero C, Nolla JM. Can magnetic resonance imaging of the hand and wrist differentiate between rheumatoid arthritis and psoriatic arthritis in the early stages of the disease? *Semin Arthritis Rheum.* (2012) 42:234–45. doi: 10.1016/j.semarthrit.2012.03.016
27. Braum LS, McGonagle D, Bruns A, Philipp S, Hermann S, Aupperle K, et al. Characterisation of hand small joints arthropathy using high-resolution MRI–limited discrimination between osteoarthritis and psoriatic arthritis. *Eur Radiol.* (2013) 23:1686–93. doi: 10.1007/s00330-012-2739-0
28. Schoellnast H, Deutschmann HA, Hermann J, Schaffler GJ, Reittner P, Kammerhuber F, et al. Psoriatic arthritis and rheumatoid arthritis: findings in contrast-enhanced MRI. *AJR Am J Roentgenol.* (2006) 187:351–7. doi: 10.2214/AJR.04.1798
29. Faustini F, Simon D, Oliveira I, Kleyer A, Haschka J, Englbrecht M, et al. Subclinical joint inflammation in patients with psoriasis without concomitant psoriatic arthritis: a cross-sectional and longitudinal analysis. *Ann Rheum Dis.* (2016) 75:2068–74. doi: 10.1136/annrheumdis-2015-208821
30. Cimmino MA, Barbieri F, Boesen M, Paparo F, Parodi M, Kubassova O, et al. Dynamic contrast-enhanced magnetic resonance imaging of articular and extraarticular synovial structures of the hands in patients with psoriatic arthritis. *J Rheumatol Suppl.* (2012) 89:44–8. doi: 10.3899/jrheum.120242
31. Poggenborg RP, Eshed I, Ostergaard M, Sorensen IJ, Moller JM, Madsen OR, et al. Enthesitis in patients with psoriatic arthritis, axial spondyloarthritis and healthy subjects assessed by "head-to-toe" whole-body MRI and clinical examination. *Ann Rheum Dis.* (2015) 74:823–9. doi: 10.1136/annrheumdis-2013-204239
32. Poggenborg RP, Pedersen SJ, Eshed I, Sorensen IJ, Moller JM, Madsen OR, et al. Head-to-toe whole-body MRI in psoriatic arthritis, axial spondyloarthritis and healthy subjects: first steps towards global inflammation and damage scores of peripheral and axial joints. *Rheumatology.* (2015) 54:1039–49. doi: 10.1093/rheumatology/keu439
33. Siannis F, Farewell VT, Cook RJ, Schentag CT, Gladman DD. Clinical and radiological damage in psoriatic arthritis. *Ann Rheum Dis.* (2006) 65:478–81. doi: 10.1136/ard.2005.039826
34. Scarpa R, Cuocolo A, Peluso R, Atteno M, Gisonni P, Iervolino S, et al. Early psoriatic arthritis: the clinical spectrum. *J Rheumatol.* (2008) 35:137–41.
35. Queiro-Silva R, Torre-Alonso JC, Tinture-Eguren T, Lopez-Lagunas I. A polyarticular onset predicts erosive and deforming disease in psoriatic arthritis. *Ann Rheum Dis.* (2003) 62:68–70. doi: 10.1136/ard.62.1.68
36. Ritchlin CT, Haas-Smith SA, Li P, Hicks DG, Schwarz EM. Mechanisms of TNF-α- and RANKL-mediated osteoclastogenesis and bone resorption in psoriatic arthritis. *J Clin Invest.* (2003) 111:821–31. doi: 10.1172/JCI200316069
37. McGonagle D, Lories RJ, Tan AL, Benjamin M. The concept of a "synovio-entheseal complex" and its implications for understanding joint inflammation and damage in psoriatic arthritis and beyond. *Arthritis Rheum.* (2007) 56:2482–91. doi: 10.1002/art.22758
38. Finzel S, Englbrecht M, Engelke K, Stach C, Schett G. A comparative study of periarticular bone lesions in rheumatoid arthritis and psoriatic arthritis. *Ann Rheum Dis.* (2011) 70:122–7. doi: 10.1136/ard.2010.132423
39. Simon D, Faustini F, Kleyer A, Haschka J, Englbrecht M, Kraus S, et al. Analysis of periarticular bone changes in patients with cutaneous psoriasis without associated psoriatic arthritis. *Ann Rheum Dis.* (2016) 75:660–6. doi: 10.1136/annrheumdis-2014-206347
40. Simon D, Kleyer A, Faustini F, Englbrecht M, Haschka J, Berlin A, et al. Simultaneous quantification of bone erosions and enthesiophytes in the joints of patients with psoriasis or psoriatic arthritis - effects of age and disease duration. *Arthritis Res Ther.* (2018) 20:203. doi: 10.1186/s13075-018-1691-z
41. Fukuda T, Umezawa Y, Asahina A, Nakagawa H, Furuya K, Fukuda K. Dual energy CT iodine map for delineating inflammation of inflammatory arthritis. *Eur Radiol.* (2017) 27:5034–40. doi: 10.1007/s00330-017-4931-8
42. Raza N, Hameed A, Ali MK. Detection of subclinical joint involvement in psoriasis with bone scintigraphy and its response to oral methotrexate. *Clin Exp Dermatol.* (2008) 33:70–3. doi: 10.1111/j.1365-2230.2007.02581.x
43. Takata T, Taniguchi Y, Ohnishi T, Kohsaki S, Nogami M, Nakajima H, et al. (18)FDG PET/CT is a powerful tool for detecting subclinical arthritis in patients with psoriatic arthritis and/or psoriasis vulgaris. *J Dermatol Sci.* (2011) 64:144–7. doi: 10.1016/j.jdermsci.2011.08.002
44. Zabotti A, Bandinelli F, Batticciotto A, Scire CA, Iagnocco A, Sakellariou G. Musculoskeletal ultrasonography for psoriatic arthritis and psoriasis patients: a systematic literature review. *Rheumatology.* (2017) 56:1518–32. doi: 10.1093/rheumatology/kex179
45. Naredo E, Moller I, de Miguel E, Batlle-Gualda E, Acebes C, Brito E, et al. High prevalence of ultrasonographic synovitis and enthesopathy in patients with psoriasis without psoriatic arthritis: a prospective case-control study. *Rheumatology.* (2011) 50:1838–48. doi: 10.1093/rheumatology/ker078
46. Kampylafka E, Simon D, d'Oliveira I, Linz C, Lerchen V, Englbrecht M, et al. Disease interception with interleukin-17 inhibition in high-risk psoriasis patients with subclinical joint inflammation-data from the prospective IVEPSA study. *Arthritis Res Ther.* (2019) 21:178. doi: 10.1186/s13075-019-1957-0
47. Cantatore FP, Maruotti N, Corrado A, Ribatti D. Angiogenesis dysregulation in psoriatic arthritis: molecular mechanisms. *Biomed Res Int.* (2017) 2017:5312813. doi: 10.1155/2017/5312813

20

Risk of Systemic Lupus Erythematosus in Patients With Anti-Phospholipid Syndrome

Hsin-Hua Chen[1,2,3,4,5], *Ching-Heng Lin*[1,4,6,7] *and Wen-Cheng Chao*[8,9,10*]

[1] Department of Medical Research, Taichung Veterans General Hospital, Taichung, Taiwan, [2] Division of Allergy, Immunology and Rheumatology, Department of Internal Medicine, Taichung Veterans General Hospital, Taichung, Taiwan, [3] Institute of Biomedical Science and Rong Hsing Research Centre for Translational Medicine, Chung Hsing University, Taichung, Taiwan, [4] Department of Industrial Engineering and Enterprise Information, Tunghai University, Taichung, Taiwan, [5] Institute of Public Health and Community Medicine Research Center, National Yang-Ming University, Taipei, Taiwan, [6] Department of Healthcare Management, National Taipei University of Nursing and Health Sciences, Taipei, Taiwan, [7] Department of Public Health, College of Medicine, Fu Jen Catholic University, New Taipei City, Taiwan, [8] Department of Critical Care Medicine, Taichung Veterans General Hospital, Taichung, Taiwan, [9] Department of Computer Science, Tunghai University, Taichung, Taiwan, [10] Department of Automatic Control Engineering, Feng Chia University, Taichung, Taiwan

***Correspondence:**
Wen-Cheng Chao
cwc081@hotmail.com

Objective: To investigate the association between anti-phospholipid syndrome (APS) and the risk of newly diagnosed systemic lupus erythematosus (SLE).

Methods: We used 2003–2013 data derived from Taiwan's National Health Insurance Research Database to conduct this nationwide, population-based. We identified AS patients newly diagnosed between 2005 to 2013 as the study group and applied age-sex matched (1:20) and propensity score-matched (PSM) (1:2) non-SLE individuals as controls. The association between APS and risk of incident SLE was determined by calculating hazard ratios (HRs) with 95% confidence intervals (CIs) using Cox proportional hazard regression analysis.

Results: We identified 1,245 patients with APS as well as 24,900 age- and sex-matched non-APS controls and 727 APS patients as well as 1,454 PSM non-APS controls. We found that the risk for incident SLE in the APS group was 80.70 times higher than the non-APS group, and the association remained robust after PSM (HR, 28.55; 95% CI, 11.49–70.91). The increased risk for SLE in patients with APS mainly existed within 5 years after the diagnosis of APS. The sensitivity analyses found that the risk for SLE in patients with APS was consistent excluding patients with ITP/AIHA and using distinct definitions of SLE.

Conclusion: The present population-based study revealed a robust association between SLE risk and recent APS and highlights the need for vigilance of SLE-associated symptoms in patients who had been diagnosed with APS.

Keywords: anti-phospholipid syndrome, systemic lupus erythematosus, autoimmune diseases, risk, propensity matching

INTRODUCTION

Systemic lupus erythematosus (SLE) can manifest with haematological and vascular abnormalities prior to the diagnosis of SLE, and recent studies including our study have found an increased risk for SLE in patients with haematological abnormalities, including immune thrombocytopenia (ITP) and autoimmune hemolytic anaemia (AIHA) (1, 2). However, clinical evidence with regards to the association between vascular abnormalities and SLE remains sparse.

Anti-phospholipid syndrome (APS), characterised by obstetric morbidities and/or arterial/venous thrombosis, has been highly implicated with SLE. APS and SLE are two closely correlated autoimmune diseases with overlapped clinical and biological characteristics (3–5). Approximately 30% of APS has been reported to be associated with SLE (6, 7). Cervera et al. conducting a 10-year-follow-up study among 1,000 patients with APS in 13 European countries, reported that 36.2% of APS was associated with SLE (7). Furthermore, the anti-phospholipid antibodies were found in ~40% of patients with SLE (6, 8). Additionally, SLE-associated APS was found to be more likely to have thrombocytopenia than patients with primary APS (7, 9). Therefore, APS appears to be associated with the development of SLE, and we hence aim to investigate the association between APS and incident SLE. In the present study, we used a nationwide population-based database and propensity matching to address the strength and time-course of association between APS and the development of SLE.

MATERIALS AND METHODS

Ethics Statement

The Institutional Review Board of Taichung Veterans General Hospital in Taiwan approved the present study (approval number: CE17100B). The requirement for informed consent was waived due to that the data in the present study were anonymised before analyses.

Data Sources

The data used in this study were derived from the National Health Insurance Database (NHID). The Taiwan National Health Research Institutes (NHRI) collected and maintained the enrollment files and original reimbursement claims data from the National Health Insurance (NHI) administration, and then released them to the NHID. The database includes the stored medical claims from 1997 to 2013 for nearly 99% of the 23.74 million Taiwanese residents. Diagnosis of inpatients and outpatients based on the International Classification of Diseases, Ninth Revision, Clinical Modification (ICD-9-CM), clinical examinations, prescriptions, and medical expenses are recorded in this database, which can be used to study the incidence and correlation of diseases. However, the NHIRD lacked laboratory data and some personal information such as smoking, drinking, body weight, and body length.

Study Design and Participants

This retrospective study was designed to address the association between anti-phospholipid syndrome (APS) and incident systemic lupus erythematosus (SLE), and the flow-chart is illustrated in **Figure 1**. The study population was a nationwide population from the period between 2003 and 2013 (n = 23,280,949), and we identified patients who had one inpatient or three outpatient visits with a diagnosis of APS between 2003 and 2012 as APS cases (n = 2,976). The index date was defined as the date on which APS was first diagnosed in the hospital. The exclusion criteria included the following: (1) index date before 2005 (n = 295); (2) diagnosis of SLE before the index date (n = 1,361); (3) death during hospitalisation (n = 3); and (4) missing data regarding region of residence or insured amount (n = 21). A total of 1,296 APS patients met the aforementioned inclusion criteria and were defined as the APS cases in this study. As for the control group, we enrolled individuals who had at least one ambulatory visit during 2005–2012 and applied the following exclusion criteria. (1) an APS diagnosis from 2003 to 2013 (n = 267), (2) an SLE diagnosis before the index date (n = 2,978), and (3) missing data about region of residence or insured amount (n = 13,104). A total of 874,316 individuals were eligible for analyses as the control group. We used age-sex matching and propensity matching in this study. We matched the APS group and the control group at a ratio of 1:20 for sex, age, and year of the index date. After matching, there were 1,245 patients in the APS group and 24,900 individuals in the non-APS group. Moreover, we aimed to reduce the impact of bias and confounding variables on the incidence of SLE through propensity-score matching (PSM), which was conducted at a ratio of 1:2 for sex, age, index date, and selected comorbidities. In the propensity-matched subjects, we identified 727 APS patients and 1,454 control individuals without APS.

Outcome and Relevant Variables

The ICD-9-CM code of 710.0 was used to identify SLE patients, and ICD-9-CM code of 289.8 was applied for APS. The main outcome of this study was a diagnosis of the above code and at least one hospitalisation or three outpatient visits in a year. We considered baseline comorbidities associated with the risk of developing SLE, including human immunodeficiency virus infection (ICD-9-CM codes 042–044, V08), hyperthyroidism (ICD-9-CM code 242), thyroiditis (ICD-9-CM code 245), diabetes mellitus (ICD-9-CM code 250), hyperlipidemia (ICD-9-CM codes 272.0–272.4), affective psychosis (ICD-9-CM code 296), hypertension (ICD-9-CM codes 401–405), coronary artery disease (ICD-9-CM codes 410–414), vasculitis (ICD-9-CM code 443.0), cerebral vascular accident (ICD-9-CM codes 430–438), chronic obstructive pulmonary disease (ICD-9-CM codes 490–496), asthma (ICD-9-CM code 493), inflammatory bowel disease (ICD-9-CM codes 555–556), pancreatitis (ICD-9-CM codes 577.0 and 577.1), chronic liver diseases (ICD-9-CM codes 571 and 573), chronic kidney disease (ICD-9-CM code 585), rheumatoid arthritis (ICD-9-CM code 714.0), systemic sclerosis (ICD-9-CM code 710.1), Sjogren's syndrome (ICD-9-CM code 710.2), ankylosing spondylitis (ICD-9-CM code 720.0), and osteoporosis (ICD-9-CM code 733). Comorbidities

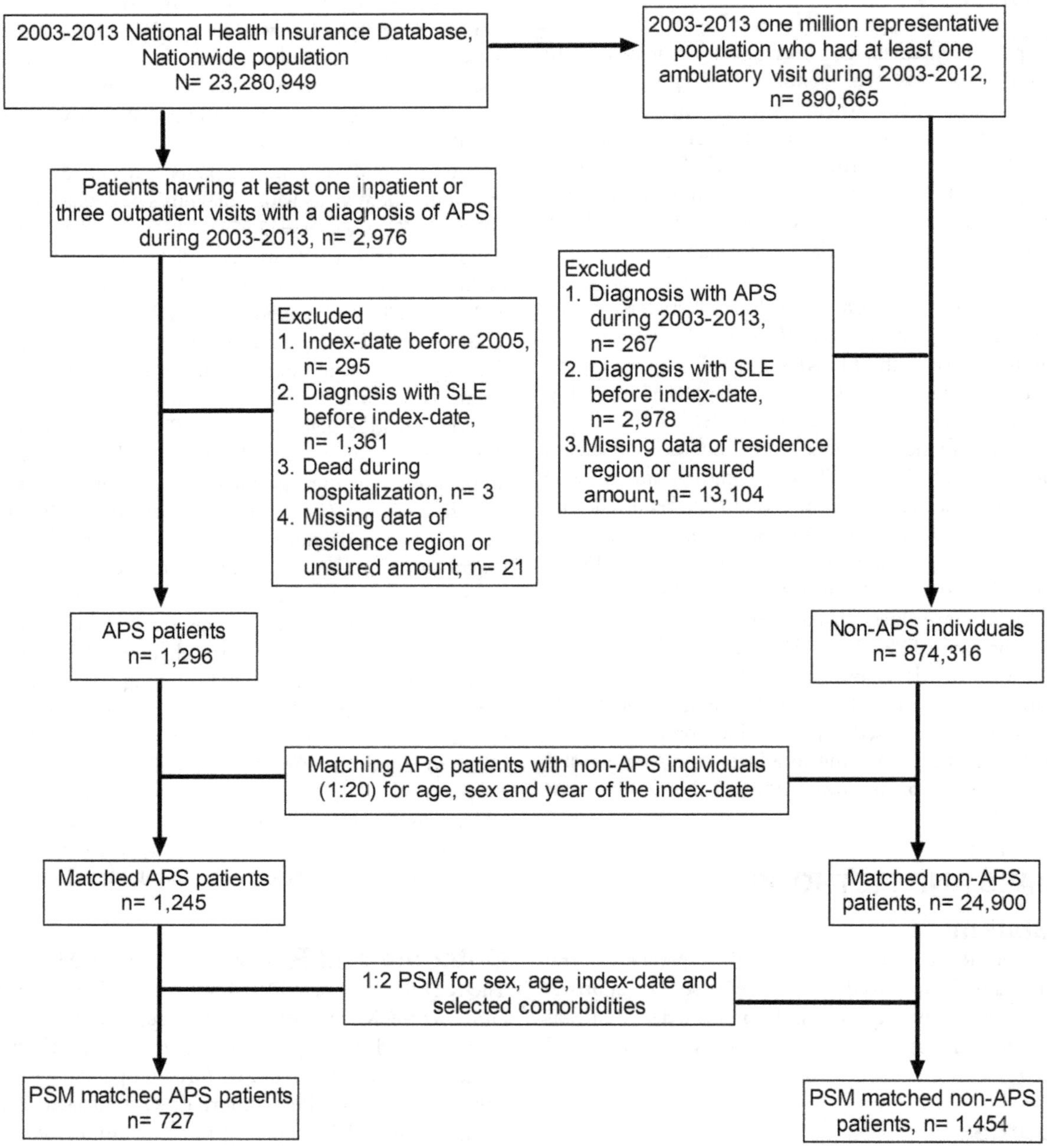

FIGURE 1 | Flow chart of the study design. APS, anti-phospholipid syndrome; SLE, systemic lupus erythematosus; PSM, propensity score matching.

were identified as diseases diagnosed within 1 year before the index date.

Statistical Analysis

Following matching, we assessed the balance of baseline characteristics in the populations using the absolute standardised difference (ASD). A high degree of balance was reflected by an ASD < 0.1. We counted follow-up person-months and the number of persons diagnosed with SLE, calculated the incidence of SLE (per 100,000 person-months), and estimated the crude relative risk with its 95% confidence interval using Poisson regression. Multivariate Cox proportional hazard regression analysis was then used to estimate the adjusted HR (aHR) for SLE. Four different models were used to investigate the effects of APS exposure and covariates on aHR of SLE, including APS exposure alone, demographic variables, medical utilisation and comorbidities, and a conditional Cox model with APS exposure alone was performed in propensity score-matched populations. Sensitivity analysis was used to estimate the risk of SLE in APS exposure patients who were in age-matched and sex-matched populations under different SLE definitions. Kaplan-Meier curves were generated on the cumulative incidence of SLE in the APS and non-APS groups. The differences between the curves were evaluated using the Log-rank test. In all our studies,

$p < 0.05$ was considered statistically significant. All statistical analyses were performed using the Statistical Analysis Software Version 9.4 (SAS Institute Inc., NC, USA).

RESULTS

Characteristics of the Study Population

We used the 2003–2013 Taiwanese National Health Insurance Database (NHIRD) to identify 1,296 patients with newly diagnosed APS between 2005 and 2012. We then selected age- and sex-matched (1:20) non-APS subjects, and 1,245 patients with APS as well as 24,900 non-APS controls were eligible for analyses. Furthermore, we selected a comparison group through propensity-score matching (PSM) (1:2) for age, sex, comorbidities, and potential confounders including ITP and AIHA. In the propensity-matched subjects, we enrolled 727 APS patients and 1,454 PSM-matched non-APS controls to address the risk for SLE in patients with APS (**Figure 1**). **Table 1** summaries the baseline characteristics of enrolled subjects with APS and control individuals selected by age-sex matching (1:20) as well as propensity score matching (1:2) (See **Supplementary Dataset** for details).

Comparison of the Risk for SLE in Subjects With and Without APS

We compared the incidence rate of SLE in patients with and without APS. In the age- and sex-matched subjects, we found a higher incidence rate of SLE (289.79 per 100,000 person-months) in patients with APS compared with the incidence rate of SLE (2.742 per 100,000 person-months) in patients without APS. Similar distinct incident SLE between APS and non-APS controls was found in the propensity-matched subjects, and the incidence rate of SLE in patients with and without APS was 254.15 per 100,000 person-months and 8.19 per 100,000 person-months, respectively (**Table 2**). After adjustment of the potential confounders, including comorbidities, urbanisation level, history of thromboembolism, pregnancy morbidities, autoimmune hemolytic anaemia, and immune thrombocytopenia, we found that APS was independently associated with incident SLE (HR 80.70; 95% CI 51.37–126.77) (**Table 2, Supplementary Table 1**). In the propensity-matched subjects, the association between APS and incident SLE remained robust using the conditional Cox regression model (HR 28.55; 95% CI 11.19–70.91). Furthermore, we used Kaplan-Meier plot to demonstrate the time-course of newly diagnosed SLE in patients with and without APS. We found an increased risk for SLE in patients with APS than those without APS and SLE mainly diagnosed within 5 years after the diagnosis of APS (**Figure 2**).

Sensitivity Analyses

We performed sensitivity analyses through using distinct definitions of SLE based on SLE treatment and excluding patients who might have secondary APS from non-APS controls (**Table 3**). We defined SLE by stringent criteria by management with systemic corticosteroid and disease-modifying antirheumatic drugs (DMARDs), and adjHR was 81.12 (95% CI 51.27–128.37) in incident SLE underwent systemic corticosteroid and 82.46 (95% CI 48.82–139.28) in incident SLE underwent DMARDs. The strength of association was consistent with the association between APS and incident SLE without stringent criteria by management (adjHR 80.70, 95% CI 51.37–126.77). Moreover, to mitigate the potential confounding effect of secondary APS on the association between APS and SLE, we hence excluded patients with autoimmune diseases, inflammatory bowel disease, autoimmune hemolytic anaemia and idiopathic thrombocytopenia from the non-APS controls. We found that the association between APS and incident SLE remained consistent after exclusion patient who might has secondary APS (adjHR 88.90; 95% CI 55.21–143.12). Collectively, using a population-based database and propensity matching, we found that patients with APS had a significantly higher risk for SLE compared with those in non-APS controls.

DISCUSSION

In the present nationwide population-based study, we aimed to address the association between APS and incident SLE using age-sex matching and propensity matching. We identified that diagnosis with APS was highly associated with an increased risk for SLE, and the SLE mainly diagnosed within 5 years after the diagnosis of APS. These findings highlight the essential need of vigilance for SLE in patients diagnosed with APS.

APS is highly associated with SLE and may affect the outcome in patients with SLE (10–12). Unlike SLE, which is the prototypical autoimmune disease with a wide range of anti-nuclear antibodies and clinical presentations, APS mainly manifested with thrombotic events and a positive anti-phospholipid antibody (13). Therefore, there is a crucial need to explore the risk of incident SLE in patients with APS. In line with our findings, Freire et al., using an APS cohort with 80 APS patients, reported that 17.5% (14/80) of patients with primary APS evolved into SLE within 5.2 ± 4 years (14). Given that thrombotic event mainly managed by non-rheumatologists, the aforementioned evidence highlight the need for collaboration with the rheumatologist for subtle signs of SLE, particularly in the first few years after the diagnosis of APS.

Anti-phospholipid syndrome (APS) is characterised by vascular thrombosis, including venous and arterial thrombosis (6). Intriguingly, Zuily et al. recently conducted a hierarchical cluster analysis using 30 data points among 497 anti-phospholipid antibody-positive patients in the Alliance for Clinical Trials and International Networking (APS ACTION) registry and reported three main phenotypes, including female patients without autoimmune diseases but with venous thrombosis (36.0%, 179/497), female patients with SLE, thrombocytopaenia and haemolytic anaemia (36.2%, 180/497), and older men with arterial thrombosis and cardiovascular manifestations (27.8%, 138/497) (15). The aforementioned finding highlights the high correlation between SLE and hametological abnormalitie as shown in recent studies including our previous study and the present study (1, 2), and we further specified the risk and time-course of incident SLE in APS patients. Additionally, in line with the finding of Zuily et al. we

TABLE 1 | Baseline characteristics in the APS and non-APS groups.

	Before PSM (1:20 age–sex matching)			1:2 PSM		
	Non-APS $n = 24,900$	APS $n = 1,245$	ASD	Non-APS $n = 1,454$	APS $n = 727$	ASD
Sex			0.000			0.000
Female	19,400 (77.9)	970 (77.9)		1,094 (75.2)	547 (75.2)	
Male	5,500 (22.1)	275 (22.1)		360 (24.8)	180 (24.8)	
Age (years)			0.000			0.079
<30	3,960 (15.9)	198 (15.9)		262 (18.0)	140 (19.3)	
30–45	11,680 (46.9)	584 (46.9)		570 (39.2)	299 (41.1)	
45–65	6,720 (27.0)	336 (27.0)		438 (30.1)	216 (29.7)	
≥65	2,540 (10.2)	127 (10.2)		184 (12.7)	72 (9.9)	
Urbanisation			0.204			0.070
Urban	8,036 (32.3)	531 (42.7)		647 (44.5)	303 (41.7)	
Suburban	12,041 (48.4)	524 (42.1)		626 (43.1)	319 (43.9)	
Rural	4,823 (19.4)	190 (15.3)		181 (12.4)	105 (14.4)	
Low income#	15,463 (62.1)	741 (59.5)	0.053	935 (64.3)	466 (64.1)	0.004
Length of hospital stay*			0.598			0.054
0 day	21,448 (86.1)	774 (62.2)		983 (67.6)	503 (69.2)	
1–6 days	2,191 (8.8)	197 (15.8)		210 (14.4)	112 (15.4)	
≥7 days	1,261 (5.1)	274 (22.0)		261 (18)	112 (15.4)	
Comorbidities†						
No comorbidities	19,314 (77.6)	373 (30.0)	<0.001	775 (53.3)	373 (51.3)	0.131
Comorbidities 1–2	4,190 (16.8)	585 (47)		470 (32.3)	264 (36.3)	
Comorbidities ≥3	1,396 (5.6)	287 (23.1)		209 (14.4)	90 (12.4)	
Rheumatoid arthritis	86 (0.3)	82 (6.6)	0.346	54 (3.7)	32 (4.4)	0.035
Sjogren's syndrome	56 (0.2)	236 (19.0)	0.671	6 (0.4)	10 (1.4)	0.102
Systemic sclerosis	0 (0.0)	18 (1.4)	NA	0 (0.0)	0 (0.0)	
Vasculitis	5 (0.02)	25 (2.0)	0.199	4 (0.3)	2 (0.3)	0.000
Hypertension	2,973 (11.9)	205 (16.5)	0.130	266 (18.3)	118 (16.2)	0.055
Diabetes mellitus	1,431 (5.7)	82 (6.6)	0.035	103 (7.1)	45 (6.2)	0.036
Hyperlipidemia	1,429 (5.7)	136 (10.9)	0.188	191 (13.1)	85 (11.7)	0.044
Thromboembolism	1,129 (4.5)	234 (18.8)		207 (14.2)	97 (13.3)	
Coronary artery disease	717 (2.9)	76 (6.1)	0.156	89 (6.1)	45 (6.2)	0.003
Cerebral vascular accident	467 (1.9)	112 (9.0)	0.318	148 (10.2)	52 (7.2)	0.108
Pulmonary embolism	5 (0.02)	34 (2.7)	0.234	0 (0)	1 (0.1)	NA
Venous thromboembolism	19 (0.1)	45 (3.6)	0.265	6 (0.4)	5 (0.7)	0.037
Portal vein thrombosis	1 (0.004)	4 (0.3)	0.079	1 (0.1)	0 (0)	NA
Arterial embolism and thrombosis	25 (0.1)	16 (1.3)	0.143	6 (0.4)	3 (0.4)	0.000
Pregnancy morbidity	40 (0.2)	90 (7.2)		19 (1.3)	5 (0.7)	
Spontaneous abortion	3 (0.01)	11 (0.9)	0.131	0 (0.0)	0 (0.0)	
Habitual abortion	9 (0.04)	71 (5.7)	0.344	0 (0.0)	0 (0.0)	
Pre-eclampsia/eclampsia	23 (0.1)	11 (0.9)	0.114	15 (1.0)	4 (0.6)	0.054
Abortion	5 (0.02)	4 (0.3)	0.073	4 (0.3)	1 (0.1)	0.030
Infertility	155 (0.6)	178 (14.3)	0.539	93 (6.4)	51 (7.0)	0.025
Raynaud's syndrome	5 (0.02)	25 (2.0)	0.199	4 (0.3)	2 (0.3)	0.000
Thromboangiitis obliterans	2 (0.01)	6 (0.5)	0.096	0 (0.0)	1 (0.1)	NA
Osteoporosis	299 (1.2)	57 (4.6)	0.203	34 (2.3)	21 (2.9)	0.034
Asthma	438 (1.8)	44 (3.5)	0.111	50 (3.4)	25 (3.4)	0.000
Chronic obstructive pulmonary disease	968 (3.9)	90 (7.2)	0.146	109 (7.5)	49 (6.7)	0.029
Chronic kidney disease	147 (0.6)	18 (1.4)	0.085	25 (1.7)	12 (1.7)	0.005
Chronic liver diseases	812 (3.3)	87 (7.0)	0.170	82 (5.6)	44 (6.1)	0.018

(Continued)

TABLE 1 | Continued

	Before PSM (1:20 age–sex matching)			1:2 PSM		
	Non-APS n = 24,900	APS n = 1,245	ASD	Non-APS n = 1,454	APS n = 727	ASD
Hyperthyroidism	215 (0.9)	35 (2.8)	0.145	29 (2.0)	18 (2.5)	0.033
Thyroiditis	35 (0.1)	80 (6.4)	0.358	17 (1.2)	13 (1.8)	0.051
Pancreatitis	32 (0.1)	18 (1.4)	0.149	19 (1.3)	8 (1.1)	0.019
Affective psychosis	181 (0.7)	38 (3.1)	0.171	36 (2.5)	16 (2.2)	0.018
Ankylosing spondylitis	22 (0.1)	46 (3.7)	0.267	2 (0.1)	4 (0.6)	0.071
Inflammatory bowel disease	58 (0.2)	7 (0.6)	0.052	9 (0.6)	4 (0.6)	0.009
Human immunodeficiency virus	13 (0.1)	0 (0.0)	NA	0 (0.0)	0 (0.0)	
Autoimmune hemolytic anaemia	2 (0.01)	24 (1.9)	0.197	0 (0.0)	0 (0.0)	
Immune thrombocytopenia	1 (0.004)	35 (2.8)	0.240	0 (0.0)	0 (0.0)	
APS treatment at baseline						
No drug administration		165 (13.3)			143 (19.7)	
Antiplatelet/anticoagulant only		91 (7.3)			55 (7.6)	
Hydroxychloroquine/corticosteroid +/– Antiplatelet/anticoagulant		989 (79.4)			529 (72.8)	

#Insured income lower than median income (21,900 New Taiwan dollars).
**Length of hospital stay is defined by hospitalisation days within 2 years of the index date.*
†Comorbidities are comorbidities identified within 2 years before the index date.
APS treatment is treatment received within 6 months after diagnosis with APS.
PSM, propensity score-matching; APS, anti-phospholipid syndrome; ASD, absolute standardised difference.

TABLE 2 | Incidence of SLE in the study groups before and after PSM.

	Before PSM (1:20 age–sex matching)		1:2 PSM	
	Non-APS	APS	Non-APS	APS
n	24,900	1,245	1,454	727
Follow-up person-months	1,057,555	43,480	61,051	25,576
SLE	29	126	5	65
Incidence rate* (95% CI)	2.742 (2.739–2.745)	289.79 (289.63–289.95)	8.19 (8.17–8.21)	254.15 (253.95–254.34)
Crude relative risk (95% CI)	Reference	105.68 (70.58–158.24)	Reference	31.03 (12.50–77.06)
Adjusted hazard ratio (95% CI)	Reference	80.70 (51.37–126.77)†	Reference	28.55 (11.49–70.91)‡

**Incidence rate, per 10,000 person-months.*
SLE, systemic lupus erythematosus; PSM, propensity score-matching; APS, anti-phospholipid syndrome; CI, confidence interval.
†,‡Definition of length of hospital day and comorbidities window.

also found that venous thromboembolism (adjHR 2.67, 95% CI 1.34–5.32) and portal vein thrombosis (adjHR 4.78, 95% CI 1.06–21.53), instead of arterial and cardiovascular thrombosis, was independently associated with incident SLE in patients with APS (**Supplementary Table 1**).

Indeed, mechanisms underlie evolution into over SLE in patients with APS remain a research niche. The development of SLE involves a gradual loss of tolerance to self-antigens, followed by an autoantibodies production (16). Genetic susceptibility and environmental exposure, have been implicated with the development of SLE (17–20). Distinct Human leukocyte antigen-DRB1 and -DQB1 allele was reported to be associated with APS with and without SLE, and more studies are required to elucidate the genetic basis of APS-SLE (17, 21, 22). A number of environmental factors, including diet, medication, pollutant, vaccination and microbial infection, and complex gene-environment interaction have been implicated with the development of autoimmunity (20). Currently, hypercoagulation has been increasingly reported in patients with coronavirus COVID-19 infection (23). Given that COVID-19 infection and SLE are both implicated with dysregulated immune responses, such as type I interferon pathway, there are increasing studies to address the correlation among autoimmune disease, hypercoagulation and COVID-19 infection (24–27). These evidence highlight the substantial needs for studies to clarify the underlying biological mechanism for the development of SLE in patients with APS.

SLE is associated with ITP and APS; however, it is somehow difficult to delineate APS and ITP among patients

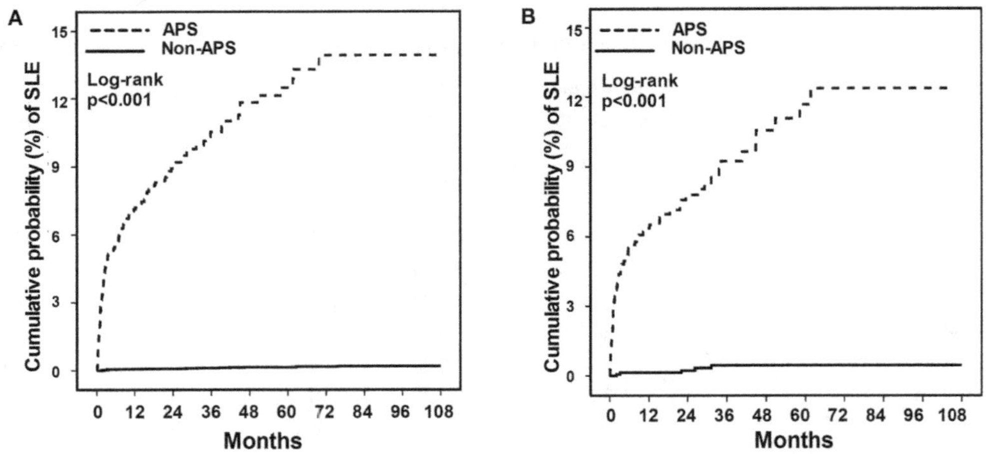

FIGURE 2 | The cumulative incidence of SLE for patients with and without APS. **(A)** age- and sex-matched population. **(B)** Propensity score-matched population. APS, anti-phospholipid syndrome; SLE, systemic lupus erythematosus.

TABLE 3 | Sensitivity analysis in the estimation of the SLE risk for APS exposure in age-matched and sex-matched populations.

Scenario	Definition of SLE event	aHR* (95%CI)
1	At least three outpatient visits or 1 admission within 1 year by rheumatologist (main finding)	80.70 (51.37–126.77)
2	Scenario 1+ treated with systemic corticosteroids or DMARDs (including HCQ or azathioprine)	81.12 (51.27–128.37)
3	Scenario 1+ treated with DMARDs (including HCQ or azathioprine)[†]	82.46 (48.82–139.28)
4	Exclusion of patients with rheumatoid arthritis, Sjogren's syndrome, systemic sclerosis, vasculitis, thyroiditis, ankylosing spondylitis, inflammatory bowel disease, human immunodeficiency virus, AIHA, ITP at baseline (excluding secondary APS)	88.90 (55.21–143.12)

aHR of AIHA exposure on the risk of SLE, the covariates including age group, sex, urbanisation, low income, length of hospital stay, and comorbidities listed in* ***Table 1**.*
[†]The treatment of SLE was identified within 6 months after first diagnosis of SLE.
SLE, systemic lupus erythematosus; APS, anti-phospholipid syndrome; aHR, adjusted HR; DMARD, disease modifying antirheumatic drugs; HCQ, hydroxychloroquine; AIHA, autoimmune hemolytic anemias; ITP, immune thrombocytopenia.

with thrombocytopenia (28). In one population-based study aiming to address the association between ITP and SLE, Zhu et al. reported that patients with ITP were more likely to have APS compared with those without ITP (2.77 vs. 0.02%, $p < 0.05$) (1). Thrombocytopenia is a cardinal haematological manifestation of APS, but the presence of thrombocytopenia, the main manifestation in patients with ITP, does not exclude the risk for the development of thrombosis (28). In the present study, we found a consistent association between APS and incident SLE using regression adjusted with ITP diagnosis and excluded patients with ITP. Therefore, APS should be an independent risk factor for incident SLE.

There are limitations in this study. First, the lack of laboratory data to validate the diagnosis of SLE in the claim database. However, we have conducted sensitivity analyses and used stringent criteria with concomitant management with systemic corticosteroid and DMARDs, and the strength of association between APS and incident is consistent. Therefore, the concern regarding the diagnosis of SLE should be at least partly mitigated. Second, the diagnosis of APS without laboratory data should also be a concern. Given that APS is relatively a specific diagnosis in patients with thromboembolism, we think that the diagnosis of APS with one inpatient or three outpatient visits could mainly be underestimated, instead of overestimated, in the present study. The strength of the study was the use of nationwide, population-based database to minimise the risk of selection and participation bias although clinical features and laboratory data, including anti-nuclear antibody and APS profiles, are not available in NHIRD. Third, the undiagnosed SLE in the diagnosis of APS could also be a concern, and we believe this concern somehow indicates the needs for collaboration with the rheumatologist in the management of patients with APS. Fourth, the finding of the present study should be further validated in another independent cohort.

CONCLUSION

In conclusion, using a population-based study, we demonstrate a high risk of developing SLE among APS patients, in particular during the first 5 years after APS diagnosis. These findings highlight the substantial need for close monitoring for SLE among patients with APS. More studies are warranted to explore factors including genetic and environmental factors leading to SLE in patients with APS.

ETHICS STATEMENT

This study was approved by the Institutional Review Board of Taichung Veterans General Hospital in Taiwan (approval number: CE17100B). Written informed consent for participation was not required for this study in accordance with the national legislation and the institutional requirements.

AUTHOR CONTRIBUTIONS

H-HC and W-CC conceptualised the research and drafted the manuscripts. H-HC, C-HL, and W-CC acquired and interpreted the data. All authors have read and approved the final manuscript.

REFERENCES

1. Zhu FX, Huang JY, Ye Z, Wen QQ, Wei JC. Risk of systemic lupus erythematosus in patients with idiopathic thrombocytopenic purpura: a population-based cohort study. *Ann Rheum Dis.* (2020) 79:793–99. doi: 10.1136/annrheumdis-2020-217013
2. Mo HY, Wei JCC, Chen XH, Chen HH. Increased risk of systemic lupus erythematosus in patients with autoimmune haemolytic anaemia: a nationwide population-based cohort study. *Ann Rheum Dis.* (2020) 80:403–4. doi: 10.1136/annrheumdis-2020-219328
3. Tincani A, Andreoli L, Chighizola C, Meroni PL. The interplay between the antiphospholipid syndrome and systemic lupus erythematosus. *Autoimmunity.* (2009) 42:257–9. doi: 10.1080/08916930902827918
4. Belizna C, Stojanovich L, Cohen-Tervaert JW, Fassot C, Henrion D, Loufrani L, et al. Primary antiphospholipid syndrome and antiphospholipid syndrome associated to systemic lupus: are they different entities? *Autoimmun Rev.* (2018) 17:739–45. doi: 10.1016/j.autrev.2018.01.027
5. Shoenfeld Y, Meroni PL, Toubi E. Antiphospholipid syndrome and systemic lupus erythematosus: are they separate entities or just clinical presentations on the same scale? *Curr Opin Rheumatol.* (2009) 21:495–500. doi: 10.1097/BOR.0b013e32832effdd
6. Giannakopoulos B, Krilis SA. The pathogenesis of the antiphospholipid syndrome. *N Engl J Med.* (2013) 368:1033–44. doi: 10.1056/NEJMra1112830
7. Cervera R, Serrano R, Pons-Estel GJ, Ceberio-Hualde L, Shoenfeld Y, de Ramon E, et al. Morbidity and mortality in the antiphospholipid syndrome during a 10-year period: a multicentre prospective study of 1000 patients. *Ann Rheum Dis.* (2015) 74:1011–8. doi: 10.1136/annrheumdis-2013-204838
8. Tarr T, Lakos G, Bhattoa HP, Szegedi G, Shoenfeld Y, Kiss E. Primary antiphospholipid syndrome as the forerunner of systemic lupus erythematosus. *Lupus.* (2007) 16:324–8. doi: 10.1177/0961203307077993
9. Unlu O, Erkan D, Barbhaiya M, Andrade D, Nascimento I, Rosa R, et al. The impact of systemic lupus erythematosus on the clinical phenotype of antiphospholipid antibody-positive patients: results from the antiphospholipid syndrome alliance for clinical trials and international clinical database and repository. *Arthritis Care Res.* (2019) 71:134–41. doi: 10.1002/acr.23584
10. Meroni PL, Tsokos GC. Editorial: systemic lupus erythematosus and antiphospholipid syndrome. *Front Immunol.* (2019) 10:199. doi: 10.3389/fimmu.2019.00199
11. Ruiz-Irastorza G, Egurbide MV, Ugalde J, Aguirre C. High impact of antiphospholipid syndrome on irreversible organ damage and survival of patients with systemic lupus erythematosus. *Arch Intern Med.* (2004) 164:77–82. doi: 10.1001/archinte.164.1.77
12. Torricelli AK, Ugolini-Lopes MR, Bonfa E, Andrade D. Antiphospholipid syndrome damage index (DIAPS): distinct long-term kinetic in primary antiphospholipid syndrome and antiphospholipid syndrome related to systemic lupus erythematosus. *Lupus.* (2020) 29:256–62. doi: 10.1177/0961203320901598
13. Agmon-Levin N, Shoenfeld Y. The spectrum between antiphospholipid syndrome and systemic lupus erythematosus. *Clin Rheumatol.* (2014) 33:293–5. doi: 10.1007/s10067-014-2486-5
14. Freire PV, Watanabe E, dos Santos NR, Bueno C, Bonfa E, de Carvalho JF. Distinct antibody profile: a clue to primary antiphospholipid syndrome evolving into systemic lupus erythematosus? *Clin Rheumatol.* (2014) 33:349–53. doi: 10.1007/s10067-013-2472-3
15. Zuily S, Clerc-Urmes I, Bauman C, Andrade D, Sciascia S, Pengo V, et al. Cluster analysis for the identification of clinical phenotypes among antiphospholipid antibody-positive patients from the APS ACTION registry. *Lupus.* (2020) 29:961203320940776. doi: 10.1177/0961203320940776
16. Leffers HCB, Lange T, Collins C, Ulff-Moller CJ, Jacobsen S. The study of interactions between genome and exposome in the development of systemic lupus erythematosus. *Autoimmun Rev.* (2019) 18:382–92. doi: 10.1016/j.autrev.2018.11.005
17. Rullo OJ, Tsao BP. Recent insights into the genetic basis of systemic lupus erythematosus. *Ann Rheum Dis.* (2013) 72 (Suppl. 2):ii56–61. doi: 10.1136/annrheumdis-2012-202351
18. Armstrong DL, Zidovetzki R, Alarcon-Riquelme ME, Tsao BP, Criswell LA, Kimberly RP, et al. GWAS identifies novel SLE susceptibility genes and explains the association of the HLA region. *Genes Immun.* (2014) 15:347–54. doi: 10.1038/gene.2014.23
19. Ceccarelli F, Perricone C, Borgiani P, Ciccacci C, Rufini S, Cipriano E, et al. Genetic factors in systemic lupus erythematosus: contribution to disease phenotype. *J Immunol Res.* (2015) 2015:745647. doi: 10.1155/2015/745647
20. Kamen DL. Environmental influences on systemic lupus erythematosus expression. *Rheum Dis Clin North Am.* (2014) 40:401–12, vii. doi: 10.1016/j.rdc.2014.05.003
21. Kapitany A, Tarr T, Gyetvai A, Szodoray P, Tumpek J, Poor G, et al. Human leukocyte antigen-DRB1 and -DQB1 genotyping in lupus patients with and without antiphospholipid syndrome. *Ann N Y Acad Sci.* (2009) 1173:545–51. doi: 10.1111/j.1749-6632.2009.04642.x
22. Ortiz-Fernandez L, Sawalha AH. Genetics of antiphospholipid syndrome. *Curr Rheumatol Rep.* (2019) 21:65. doi: 10.1007/s11926-019-0869-y
23. Helms J, Tacquard C, Severac F, Leonard-Lorant I, Ohana M, Delabranche X, et al. High risk of thrombosis in patients with severe SARS-CoV-2 infection: a multicenter prospective cohort study. *Intensive Care Med.* (2020) 46:1089–98. doi: 10.1007/s00134-020-06062-x
24. Novelli L, Motta F, De Santis M, Ansari AA, Gershwin ME, Selmi C. The JANUS of chronic inflammatory and autoimmune diseases onset during COVID-19 - a systematic review of the literature. *J Autoimmun.* (2020) 117:102592. doi: 10.1016/j.jaut.2020.102592
25. Xourgia E, Tektonidou MG. Type I interferon gene expression in antiphospholipid syndrome: pathogenetic,

clinical and therapeutic implications. *J Autoimmun.* (2019) 104:102311. doi: 10.1016/j.jaut.2019.102311

26. Kamel MH, Yin W, Zavaro C, Francis JM, Chitalia VC. Hyperthrombotic milieu in COVID-19 patients. *Cells.* (2020) 9:2392. doi: 10.3390/cells9112392
27. Talarico R, Aguilera S, Alexander T, Amoura Z, Antunes AM, Arnaud L, et al. The impact of COVID-19 on rare and complex connective tissue diseases: the experience of ERN ReCONNET. *Nat Rev Rheumatol.* (2021) 17:177–84. doi: 10.1038/s41584-020-00565-z
28. Artim-Esen B, Diz-Kucukkaya R, Inanc M. The significance and management of thrombocytopenia in antiphospholipid syndrome. *Curr Rheumatol Rep.* (2015) 17:14. doi: 10.1007/s11926-014-0494-8

21

Multi-Modal Imaging to Assess the Interaction Between Inflammation and Bone Damage Progression in Inflammatory Arthritis

Justin J. Tse[1,2], *Scott C. Brunet*[1,2,3], *Peter Salat*[1,2], *Glen S. Hazlewood*[2,4], *Cheryl Barnabe*[2,4] *and Sarah L. Manske*[1,2,3]*

[1] Department of Radiology, Cumming School of Medicine, University of Calgary, Calgary, AB, Canada, [2] Cumming School of Medicine, McCaig Institute for Bone and Joint Health, University of Calgary, Calgary, AB, Canada, [3] Biomedical Engineering Graduate Program, Schulich School of Engineering, University of Calgary, Calgary, AB, Canada, [4] Division of Rheumatology, Department of Medicine, Cumming School of Medicine, University of Calgary, Calgary, AB, Canada

***Correspondence:**
Sarah L. Manske
smanske@ucalgary.ca

Combining results from multiple imaging techniques (i.e., multi-modal imaging) through image registration can result in the better characterization of joint tissue characteristics. In the context of inflammatory arthritis conditions, high-resolution peripheral quantitative computed tomography (HR-pQCT) provides excellent bone contrast while magnetic resonance imaging (MRI) provides superior contrast and resolution of soft tissue and inflammatory characteristics. Superimposing these imaging results upon each other provides a robust characterization of the joint. In a preliminary study of nine rheumatoid arthritis (RA) participants in clinical remission, we acquired HR-pQCT and MR images of their 2nd and 3rd metacarpophalangeal (MCP) joints at two timepoints 6 months apart. We present the benefits of a multi-modal imaging approach, in which we demonstrate the ability to localize regions of inflammation with subtle changes in bone erosion volume. Using HR-pQCT and MRI to visualize bone damage and inflammation, respectively, will improve our understanding of the impact that subclinical inflammation has on bone damage progression, and demonstrating if bone repair occurs where inflammation is resolved. The presented multi-modal imaging technique has the potential to study the progression of bone damage in relation to inflammation that otherwise would not be possible with either imaging technique alone. The multi-modal image registration technique will be helpful to understanding the development and pathogenesis of RA-associated bone erosions. Additionally, multi-modal imaging may provide a technique to probe the tissue-level changes that occur as a result of treatment regimes.

Keywords: high resolution peripheral quantitative computed tomography (HR-pQCT), magnetic resonance imaging, multi-modal imaging, image registration, rheumatoid arthritis, subclinical inflammation

MULTI-MODAL IMAGING: UTILIZING EACH INDIVIDUAL IMAGING MODALITY'S STRENGTHS

Inflammatory arthritis conditions are complex in pathophysiology and affect many joint tissues. Imaging plays an important role in the diagnosis, treatment evaluation and understanding of pathophysiological processes. Every imaging modality has its own strengths and weaknesses for tissue and disease assessment, due to their differing abilities to provide tissue contrast, spatial resolution, and access to joints of interest. In the context of inflammatory arthritis, conventional radiography provides 2-dimensional (2D) planar, projection images of structural damage (i.e., joint space narrowing, erosions, and osteophytes) of bony features. Computed tomography (CT) provides 3-dimensional (3D) views, resulting in greater contrast and spatial resolution to visualize the same bony features; however, this is at the expense of greater radiation exposure depending on the joints of interest and their proximity to radiation-sensitive tissues and organs. High-resolution peripheral quantitative computed tomography (HR-pQCT) is a CT modality adapted for imaging extremities and provides significantly enhanced contrast, superior spatial resolution of bony features, and reduced radiation dose when compared to conventional whole-body CT. While originally introduced to image the distal tibia and distal radius, applications of HR-pQCT have extended to include the hand, wrist and knee joints (1–3). HR-pQCT allows for the resolution of individual trabeculae (4), and the ability to quantitatively evaluate joint properties. Semi-automated techniques have been developed to assess periarticular bone mineral density and microarchitecture, joint space width as well as erosion volume (5–8). An overview of these techniques is provided in a review by Klose-Jensen et al. (9) in this special issue.

In contrast to HR-pQCT's excellent spatial resolution of bone, ultrasound and magnetic resonance imaging (MRI) have superior contrast and resolution of soft tissue and can detect features of inflammation. While ultrasound can acquire multiplanar images and facilitate the identification and grading of superficial bony features (10, 11), this imaging technique is limited in its application for analysis below the cortical surface and only provides images several centimeters below the probe (12). However, the presence of a power doppler signal identifies sites of active synovial inflammation without exogenous contrast enhancement. On the other hand, MRI facilitates the 3D visualization of internal features such as bone marrow edema but requires the administration of an intravenous gadolinium contrast agent for the accurate differentiation of inflammatory signals from fluid signals. An additional benefit of MRI is that a semi-quantitative assessment of inflammatory arthritis can be evaluated with MR images using validated scoring systems such as the RA MRI scoring system (RAMRIS) (13, 14) and the psoriatic arthritis MRI scoring system (15).

To date, most multi-modal imaging studies examine each imaging modality independently from one another. However, the 3D multiplanar image acquisition from CT and MRI can facilitate the superimposition of images after accurate image co-registration and transformation, providing complementary information (e.g., bone image from CT, synovitis and inflammation from MRI) to better characterize the entire joint.

IMAGE REGISTRATION

A strategy to visualize and understand bone damage in inflammatory arthritis within a patient is to align and superimpose images acquired from longitudinal time points or multiple imaging modalities using a computational tool known as image registration. We present a brief overview of image registration as a technique that can be used for joint-based imaging on HR-pQCT and MRI datasets.

Image registration is a computational process which iteratively searches for the best alignment based on common information within two or more images. The "best" alignment is defined by metrics such as mutual information or the cross-correlation coefficient (16, 17). The cross-correlation coefficient is typically used when measuring the similarity between image registration of images from the same modality, while mutual information is preferred for multi-modal images. The actual image registration can be performed in a *rigid* or *non-rigid* fashion. *Rigid* image registration aligns the anatomy within the images, without changing the shapes, by a series of rotations and translations. *Rigid* registration is particularly useful when aligning images from the same individual where differences in overall bone shape and size are not expected but the position may differ; acquired either at different times from the same modality, or from multiple modalities at the same time. In contrast, *non-rigid* or *deformable* image registration may allow for local image deformations to facilitate their registration. This technique is beneficial to align images from different individuals to either compare differences in shape or define a common region of interest across multiple individuals, or from the same individual when differences in anatomical shape or size exist between the images.

An initial guess of the translations and rotations is typically required to initialize the registration; this can be accomplished by identifying anatomical landmarks on each image, or by using physical properties of the image such as the center of mass. An optimization algorithm then iteratively searches for the most appropriate transformation (i.e., translations and rotations) to reorient and optimally fit one image onto another image (18), until no further improvement in the alignment metric is detected.

Assessing Longitudinal Changes and Bone Remodeling With HR-pQCT

As previously mentioned, *rigid* image registration is ideal to align baseline and follow-up images from the same participant on the same imaging modality—ensuring the same region-of-interest is evaluated at both timepoints and improve reproducibility (19, 20). In the context of erosion assessment, image registration allows for a careful comparison of bone changes at the site of the erosion that occur over time (20, 21). Specifically, recent developments have applied image-based bone remodeling algorithms (22) to sensitively assess change in erosion volume over time by aligning, registering, and subtracting baseline from follow-up images (21, 23). *Rigid* image registration is particularly well-suited for follow-up imaging because the gross morphological features remain relatively constant over the time frames typically studied (e.g., 6 months to 2 years), and new structural damage is small relative to the overall size and shape of the bone. However, the main barriers to accurate measures of bone remodeling using this technique are patient motion during the scan time and slow bone remodeling rates, as thickness changes must exceed the true spatial resolution of the scanner at $\sim$100 µm (4). While we have demonstrated good performance of this algorithm in rheumatoid arthritis patients with relatively slow rates of bone changes, performance suffers if significant patient motion is present in the baseline or follow-up images (23).

Multi-Modal Image Registration

The main advantage of imaging the same individual with a different imaging modality is the ability to simultaneously study different tissue characteristics (i.e., CT for bone and MRI for synovitis and inflammation). As intensity values between imaging modalities represent different tissues, we use mutual information to align images from multiple modalities (24, 25). This technique identifies and matches common clusters of regions between the two images; for example, homogeneous regions of one image will be mapped to a homogeneous region in a second image (17).

USING HR-pQCT AND MRI TO INVESTIGATE THE ROLE OF INFLAMMATION IN BONE DAMAGE PROGRESSION

Rationale

Timely, target-driven therapeutic intervention with disease modifying medications is currently an effective mechanism to achieve clinical remission in rheumatoid arthritis (RA). Clinical remission is typically defined by a combination of low tender and swollen joint count, patient reported outcomes, and inflammatory biomarkers in RA patients. However, many patients classified as in clinical remission, with an absence of painful, tender or swollen joints on clinical exam, have evidence of "sub-clinical inflammation" present on MRI or ultrasound (26). Unfortunately, a subset of these patients continue to have worsening radiographic damage scores and progressive disability (27, 28). Cross-sectional evidence of patients in remission with inflammation, visualized on ultrasound, showed an altered trabecular bone mineral density as measured by HR-pQCT when compared with those with no subclinical inflammation (29). While acute inflammation plays an important role in bone repair (30), the significance of sustained subclinical inflammation on bone changes over time is unknown. Therefore, we present a pilot study in which we combined imaging modalities for soft tissue and inflammation (MRI) and bone (HR-pQCT) to determine whether we could provide important pathophysiological information on bone damage progression that is not possible with either imaging modality alone.

Methods

In a preliminary study of nine RA participants recruited based on physician-classified clinical remission, we acquired HR-pQCT (XtremeCTII, Scanco Medical, Brüttisellen, Switzerland) images of the 2nd and 3rd metacarpophalangeal (MCP) joints and MR images (1.5T Optima MR430s, GE Healthcare) of 2nd to 5th MCP joints of the same hand at baseline and 6-month follow-up. The combination of HR-pQCT and a 6-month follow-up was selected because previous research has demonstrated that bone changes may be detected with HR-pQCT as early as three- to 6-months (31); thus, HR-pQCT would provide the resolution necessary to image these changes. MR sequences included T1-weighted sequence with and without fat saturation using the Dixon method in the coronal and axial plane as well as a short tau inverted recovery (STIR) sequence in the coronal plane, and a repeat of T1-weighted sequences after administration of gadolinium contrast. Approval for all procedures was obtained from the Conjoint Health Research Ethics Board at the University of Calgary (REB17-0188).

Three-dimensional (3D) volumetric joint space width (JSW; volume, minimum, maximum, and mean) was quantified on HR-pQCT images (5). Erosion volume was quantified on HR-pQCT images at baseline and follow-up using the Medical Image Analysis Framework [MIAF, University of Erlangen; (6)]. A radiologist (PS) scored bone marrow edema, synovitis and erosions on MR images using the RAMRIS scoring system (13). A multi-modal image registration technique was adapted and employed to register and transform the MR image to be overlaid with the HR-pQCT image at each timepoint (32) (**Supplementary Figure 1**). On HR-pQCT images, a trained observer (SB) followed Study grouP for x-trEme Computed Tomography in Rheumatoid Arthritis (SPECTRA) guidelines for the definition of a bone erosion (33): a cortical break observed in two consecutive slices and two orthogonal planes. Bone marrow edema and erosion volume changes were confirmed by visual inspection after superimposition of HR-pQCT and MRI images.

Statistical analysis was completed using R (v3.4.3) in RStudio v1.1.423. To examine group-level time effects, the Wilcoxon rank sum test was used for clinical outcomes and RAMRIS scores, while a non-parametric marginal model for longitudinal designs [nparLD package in R (34)] was used for total erosion volume and JSW. Significance was observed if $p < 0.05$. Changes in erosion volume and JSW at the individual joint level were evaluated against the least significant change (LSC) (35), which was calculated based on previous scan-rescan reproducibility work (36). Using the LSC criteria, participants were classified in one of three groups for each outcome measure: a significant decrease, stable, or a significant increase (20). Results are presented as median and interquartile range (IQR) unless otherwise indicated.

Results

Clinical Outcomes

The nine participants (4 females and 5 males) in clinical remission [DAS28CRP 1.75 (1.63–2.6)], ESR 7 (3–11), CRP

3.4 (1.1–4.2), were 62 (59–63) years old, and had been diagnosed with RA for 7.8 (5.1–8.0) years. All participants were being treated with conventional disease-modifying anti-rheumatic drugs (DMARDs; methotrexate, sulfasalazine, and/or hydroxychloroquine), six with biologic DMARDs (3 with adalimumab, 1 golimumab, 1 abatacept, 1 rituximab), 1 with denosumab (a biologic non-DMARD) and 1 with 2.5 mg bi-daily prednisone.

Group level results are presented for those in clinical remission only. Over the 6-month follow-up, there was a significant improvement in patient global assessment (−1 improvement on a 1–10 scale, IQR −2 to 0, $p = 0.03$). There were trends toward further improvements in DAS28 (−0.42 IQR −0.82 to −0.03, $p = 0.07$), Jebsen Taylor Hand Function test z-score (−0.8 IQR −1.2 to −0.3, $p = 0.08$), HAQ score (−0.12, IQR −0.50 to −0.26, $p = 0.09$), the self-reported Disabilities of the Arm, Shoulder, and Hand questionnaire (DASH, −7.5, IQR −11.4 to 0, $p = 0.08$) and pain (−1 improvement on a 1–10 scale, IQR −2 to 0, $p = 0.06$).

HR-pQCT Outcomes

The analysis for JSW and erosions was performed on the acquired HR-pQCT of the 2nd and 3rd MCP joints; however, for both analyses, the same two participants were excluded due to motion (4 joints) and 2 additional joints from two separate participants could not be segmented accurately. Therefore, a total of 12 joints were analyzed across 7 participants. At the group level, there were no significant changes over time in any of the joint space outcomes ($p > 0.05$). When compared with the LSC, the joint space parameters remained stable except for one patient who showed a decrease in minimum joint space width (−0.42 mm) in one joint.

Across the 12 joints from 7 participants, 19 erosions were found to range in size from 0.19 mm^3 to 93.11 mm^3. Ten erosions were identified at the 2nd MCP, and 9 erosions identified at the 3rd MCP. At the group level, there were no significant changes in the total erosion volume per joint ($p = 0.11$). When compared against the LSC, 5 patients had erosion volumes that stayed stable in 10 joints, one patient had a decrease in total erosion volume (−2.3 mm^3) in one joint, and one participant had an increase in erosion volume (+2.1 mm^3) in one joint. These changes can be visualized with longitudinal image registration (**Figure 2**).

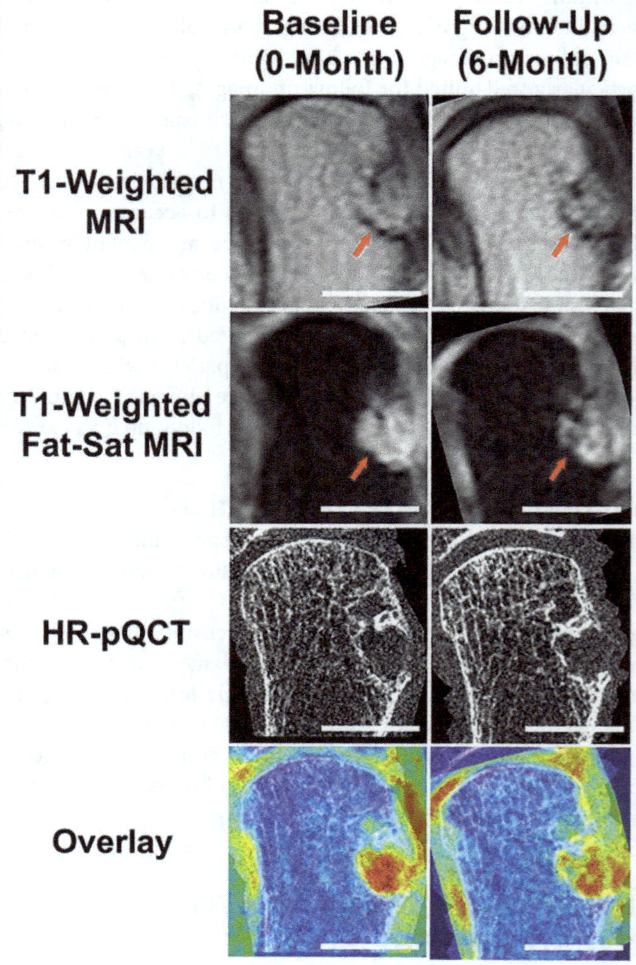

FIGURE 1 | Results demonstrating the benefits of multi-modal imaging. Using MRI and RAMRIS scoring, this RA participant was noted to have a dramatic increase in bone erosion score during their 6-month follow-up, when compared to their baseline score. The post-contrast (Gd) T1-weighted MRI visually displays a larger erosion in the follow-up image (note red arrows). Through accurate image co-registration and overlay, we can observe that the increase in bone erosion score may be due to the differences in positioning during acquisition. While the post-contrast, fat-saturated T1-weighted MRIs display a difference in intensities, the HR-pQCT demonstrates an almost identical erosion size. The Overlay demonstrates the addition of the T1-weighted MRI overlaid with the respective, co-registered HR-pQCT scans. Scalebars represent 1 cm.

MRI Outcomes

The RAMRIS total score across MCP joints 2–5 for all 9 patients in clinical remission was 3.0 (1–6) for synovitis, 2.0 (1–2) for bone marrow edema, and 2 (2–4) for erosions at baseline. At follow-up the mean total scores were 5 (3–6) for synovitis, 2 (1–5) for bone marrow edema, and 3 (2–6) for erosions. There were no significant differences ($p > 0.05$) in RAMRIS scores between baseline and follow-up for synovitis, edema, or erosions.

When looking at the 2nd and 3rd MCPs only, at baseline, 1 joint had no evidence of synovitis while 9 joints had a synovitis score of 1 (mild), and 8 joints had a synovitis score of 2 (moderate). Over the 6-month period, 9 joints were scored as stable, 5 joints had an increase of 1, 1 joint had an increase of 2, and 3 joints had a decrease in synovitis.

For bone edema at baseline in the 2nd and 3rd MCPs, 10 joints had no edema at either the proximal phalange or distal metacarpal, and 8 joints had an edema score of 1 (which represents a volume of bone infiltration between 1 and 33% by the edema). Over the 6-month period, 11 joints had stable bone edema status, while 5 joints showed an increase in edema, and 2 joints showed a decrease in edema.

For the baseline erosions scored on MRI, 9 participants had evidence of erosions on the 2nd MCP. Eight of these had an erosion score of 1 (1–10% of bone covered by erosion) and one bone had an erosion score of 2 (11–20% bone covered

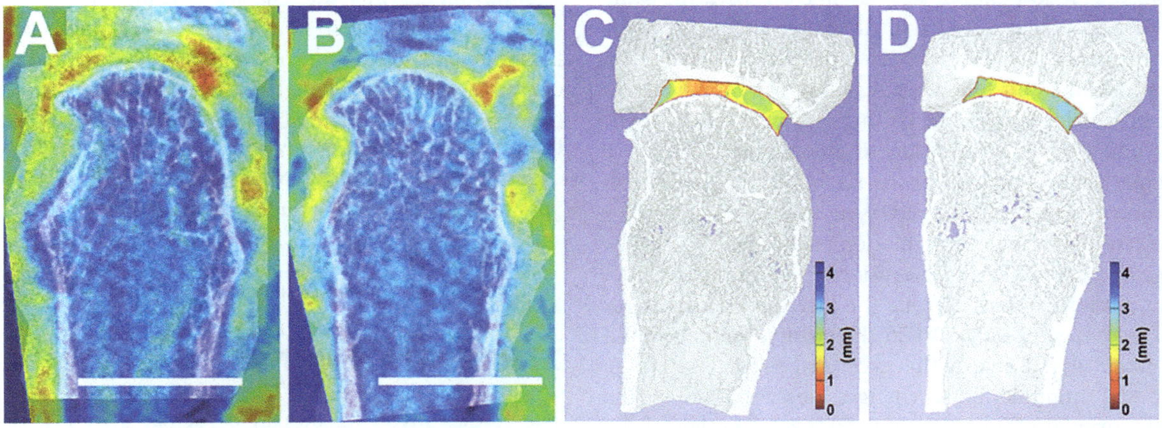

FIGURE 2 | Accurate image co-registration between a selected individual's baseline, 0-month **(A)**, and follow-up, 6-month **(B)** facilitated the overlay between their MRI and HR-pQCT. This image co-registration allows for the consistent analysis of the same areas-of-interest between timepoints. Additionally, joint space width changes from baseline **(C)** to follow-up **(D)** are compared. White scalebars represent 1 cm.

by erosion). For the 3rd MCP, 4 participants had evidence of erosions with 3 having a score of 1, and 1 participant having a score of 2. Over the 6-month period, 12 joints had stable erosion scores on MRI while 2 joints showed decreases and 4 joints showed increases.

Relationship Between MRI and HR-pQCT Outcomes

One participant with no evidence of bone marrow edema or synovitis near the site of the erosion underwent a significant decrease in erosion volume, assessed by HR-pQCT, over the 6-month follow-up. This was also consistent with a decrease in MRI erosion score. In contrast, all participants who presented with MRI-evidence of inflammation within the joints maintained no change in erosion volume over the 6-month follow-up, similarly to those in clinical remission.

At the group level, baseline bone marrow edema was not associated with increased erosion volume, however the participant with the largest increase in erosion volume also demonstrated progression in the bone marrow edema score. In addition, more participants had changes in erosion severity when evaluated by MRI than by HR-pQCT (**Figure 1**).

One participant had a significant decrease in minimum JSW (**Figure 2**). This participant had a synovitis score of 2 at baseline which decreased over 6-months, but also demonstrated a decrease in ESR, a moderate EULAR DAS28 response, and a large decrease in HAQ and pain.

DISCUSSION

We have presented the benefits of a multi-modal imaging approach through our ability to now localize how synovitis and bone marrow edema affect bone damage in RA patients. This was achieved by using accurate image registration, to facilitate improved reproducibility by adjusting for differences in positioning between scans and accurately mapping soft tissues and inflammation onto bone. In addition, we observed discordances in erosion changes assessed by HR-pQCT and MRI. The higher spatial resolution of the HR-pQCT images, combined with longitudinal registration allowed us to detect bone changes with greater sensitivity and reproducibility (19, 37, 38)—emphasizing the utility of multi-modal imaging approaches to fully understand all the tissue types involved in the progression of a disease.

While we have shown the utility of HR-pQCT for research purposes, its applicability as routine imaging in clinical studies remains unknown. Motion artifact due to patient motion during acquisitions can result in missing data. While we implemented an overlapping stacking process, which significantly reduced the need to discard scans due to motion artifact, rather than eliminating the artifact, this process simply smoothed the data (36). Currently, we have begun exploring implementing established motion correction algorithms that will increase the usability of acquired data (39, 40). Additionally, recent research has shown that the current SPECTRA defined bone erosion definition may result in the under-estimation of the number of bone erosions, when compared to histological evaluation (41). It should be noted that while we propose the implementation of HR-pQCT to measure disease progress in the research setting, the extra scanning will unavoidably increase radiation dose to the patient; however, a single HR-pQCT scan is < 20 μSv, which equates to a third of the radiation dose one would receive on a transcontinental flight. Regardless, the impact of the multi-modal imaging and in-depth erosion evaluation measures on clinical outcomes needs to be determined. Thus, a larger sample size, further in-depth analysis, and multiple reader assessments will be required to better understand how individual erosions changed over the time points.

Despite these limitations, the finding of more erosion changes in RAMRIS scores than HR-pQCT was surprising. Two of the joints with erosion progression on MRI had an erosion that was identified at follow-up but not baseline on MRI; the same erosions were identified but at both times on HR-pQCT. This discrepancy may be the result of differences in positioning on the MRI at baseline and follow-up resulting in the inability to see the small erosion at baseline or the improved sensitivity of HR-pQCT as a tool for erosion identification. Also, there were scans that met our motion scoring criteria, but within the volume of the erosion on HR-pQCT there was motion that appeared to hinder the erosion volume segmentation on HR-pQCT. Finally, an increase of 1 for the RAMRIS erosion equates to only a 10% increase in erosion volume. Despite the increased sensitivity of HR-pQCT, a change of only 10% in the erosion volume would generally not result in a change that exceeds the LSC.

Despite the minimal bone changes observed across the participants over multiple time-points, likely explained by the patients' low disease activity, short follow-up period and sample size, we have presented the benefits of a multi-modal imaging approach that can be utilized to simultaneously visualize, localize, and characterize how synovitis and bone marrow edema may affect bone damage in RA patients. The combination of HR-pQCT and MRI to visualize bone damage and inflammation, respectively, provides the ability to probe mechanistic questions about whether bone loss occurs via an inside-out or outside-in approach (38, 42, 43), as well as how local inflammatory signals lead to bone erosion progression. This multi-modal imaging approach will improve our understanding of the role of both clinical levels of inflammation in arresting bone repair in inflammatory arthritis and the impact that subclinical inflammation has on bone damage progression. In addition, it will allow us to probe the pathophysiological processes that occur at the tissue level in the development and progression of bone damage, and the mechanisms by which treatments halt or repair bone damage, further increasing our understanding of the etiology and pathophysiology of diseases.

Overall, multi-modal imaging can be combined synergistically with functional and biochemical imaging. Examples of other applications include combining CT with positron emission tomography (PET). PET/CT using 2-deoxy-2[18F]fluoro-d-glucose (FDG) to visualize glucose metabolism has been has recently been used to investigate increased glycolysis due to inflammation in inflammatory arthritis, demonstrating correlations between metabolic markers identified with PET and clinical diseases activity in rheumatoid arthritis (44), and between PET activity score and inflammation score on MRI in patients with sacroiliitis in spondylarthropathy (45). Further, PET uptake predicts radiographic progression in RA (46). PET-MRI techniques are also emerging to investigate musculoskeletal disease, which allow linkage of bone metabolic activity with high levels of soft tissue contrast (47, 48), demonstrating that sites of synovitis and tenosynovitis identified on MRI are linked to increased FDG uptake.

Multi-modal imaging enables investigation of underlying tissue pathology using non-invasive techniques. Advances in hardware and software have enabled unprecedented spatial and contrast resolution. Combined with image registration and other image processing techniques, multi-modal imaging provides the great potential to study the mechanisms underlying tissue changes in inflammatory arthritis that otherwise would not be possible with any single imaging technique alone.

ETHICS STATEMENT

The studies involving human participants were reviewed and approved by Conjoint Health Research Ethics Board at the University of Calgary. The patients/participants provided their written informed consent to participate in this study.

AUTHOR CONTRIBUTIONS

PS, GH, CB, and SM contributed conception and design of the study. SB, CB, and SM acquired the data. SB and JT performed data analysis. JT and SM drafted the manuscript. All authors contributed to manuscript revision, read, and approved the submitted version.

ACKNOWLEDGMENTS

We would like to thank the Rheum4U Investigators and Team for assistance with recruitment, our imaging technicians Anne Cooke, Stephanie Kwong and Irene Pauchard for image acquisition, and Shaheer Chishti for assistance with image processing.

SUPPLEMENTARY MATERIAL

Supplementary Figure 1 | Workflow for MRI-HR-pQCT image registration. **(A)** The T1-weighted MRI and HR-pQCT images are landmarked using common anatomy and the T1-weighted image is registered to the HR-pQCT image space. **(B)** The transformation is then applied to the contrast enhanced fat-saturated MRI image and **(C)** overlaid with the HR-pQCT image. A color map can be applied to visualize areas of inflammation (red) in relationship to the bone damage.

Supplementary Table 1 | Overall demographic parameters outlining our participants (top), and changes in their patient- and clinical-reported outcomes after 6-months (bottom). DAS, Disease Activity Score; ESR, Erythrocyte

Sedimentation Rate; CRP, C-Reactive Protein; JTHF, Jebsen-Taylor Hand Function Test; HAQ, Health Assessment Questionnaire; DASH, Disabilities of the Arm, Shoulder, and Hand. Values are reported as mean (range) unless reported otherwise [i.e., mean (IQR)].

Supplementary Table 2 | Reported outcomes from HR-pQCT and MRI displaying the changes in erosions and joint space width, as calculated from HR-pQCT, and RAMRIS score (i.e., synovitis, bone marrow edema, and erosions) as calculated from MRI. Values are reported as mean (IQR) unless noted otherwise.

REFERENCES

1. Boutroy S, Bouxsein ML, Munoz F, Delmas PD. *In vivo* assessment of trabecular bone microarchitecture by high-resolution peripheral quantitative computed tomography. *J Clin Endocrinol Metab.* (2005) 90:6508–15. doi: 10.1210/jc.2005-1258
2. Burghardt AJ, Lee CH, Kuo D, Majumdar S, Imboden JB, Lin TM, et al. Quantitative *in vivo* HR-pQCT imaging of 3D wrist and metacarpophalangeal joint space width in rheumatoid arthritis. *Ann Biomed Eng.* (2013) 41:2553–64. doi: 10.1007/s10439-013-0871-x
3. Kroker A, Zhu Y, Manske SL, Barber R, Mohtadi N, Boyd SK. Quantitative *in vivo* assessment of bone microarchitecture in the human knee using HR-pQCT. *Bone.* (2017) 97:43–8. doi: 10.1016/j.bone.2016.12.015
4. Manske SL, Zhu Y, Sandino C, Boyd SK. Human trabecular bone microarchitecture can be assessed independently of density with second generation HR-pQCT. *Bone.* (2015) 79:213–21. doi: 10.1016/j.bone.2015.06.006
5. Stok KS, Burghardt AJ, Boutroy S, Peters MPH, Manske SL, Stadelmann V, et al. Consensus approach for 3D joint space width of metacarpophalangeal joints of rheumatoid arthritis patients using high-resolution peripheral quantitative computed tomography. *Quanti Imaging Med Surg.* (2020) 10:314–25. doi: 10.21037/qims.2019.12.11
6. Topfer D, Finzel S, Museyko O, Schett G, Engelke K. Segmentation and quantification of bone erosions in high-resolution peripheral quantitative computed tomography datasets of the metacarpophalangeal joints of patients with rheumatoid arthritis. *Rheumatology.* (2014) 53:65–71. doi: 10.1093/rheumatology/ket259
7. Peters M, de Jong J, Scharmga A, van Tubergen A, Geusens P, Loeffen D, et al. An automated algorithm for the detection of cortical interruptions and its underlying loss of trabecular bone; a reproducibility study. *BMC Med imaging.* (2018) 18:13. doi: 10.1186/s12880-018-0255-7
8. Kocijan R, Finzel S, Englbrecht M, Engelke K, Rech J, Schett G. Decreased quantity and quality of the periarticular and nonperiarticular bone in patients with rheumatoid arthritis: a cross-sectional HR-pQCT study. *J Bone Mineral Res.* (2014) 29:1005–14. doi: 10.1002/jbmr.2109
9. Klose-Jensen R, Tse JJ, Keller KK, Barnabe C, Burghardt AJ, Finzel S, et al. High-resolution peripheral quantitative computed tomography for bone evaluation in inflammatory rheumatic disease. *Front Med Rheumatol.* (2020) 7:337. doi: 10.3389/fmed.2020.00337
10. Ohrndorf S, Halbauer B, Martus P, Reiche B, Backhaus TM, Burmester GR, et al. detailed joint region analysis of the 7-joint ultrasound score: evaluation of an arthritis patient cohort over one year. *Int J Rheumatol.* (2013) 2013:493848. doi: 10.1155/2013/493848
11. Backhaus M, Ohrndorf S, Kellner H, Strunk J, Backhaus TM, Hartung W, et al. Evaluation of a novel 7-joint ultrasound score in daily rheumatologic practice: a pilot project. *Arthritis Rheum.* (2009) 61:1194–201. doi: 10.1002/art.24646
12. Ihnatsenka B, Boezaart AP. Ultrasound: basic understanding and learning the language. *Int J Shoulder Surg.* (2010) 4:55–62. doi: 10.4103/0973-6042.76960
13. Ostergaard M, Peterfy C, Conaghan P, McQueen F, Bird P, jbjerg B, et al. OMERACT rheumatoid arthritis magnetic resonance imaging studies. Core set of MRI acquisitions, joint pathology definitions, and the OMERACT RA-MRI scoring system. *J Rheumatol.* (2003) 30:1385–6.
14. Østergaard M, Peterfy CG, Bird P, Gandjbakhch F, Glinatsi D, Eshed I, et al. The OMERACT rheumatoid arthritis Magnetic Resonance Imaging (MRI) scoring system: updated recommendations by the OMERACT MRI in arthritis working group. *J Rheumatol.* (2017) 44:1706–12. doi: 10.3899/jrheum.161433
15. Ostergaard M, McQueen F, Wiell C, Bird P, Boyesen P, Ejbjerg B, et al. The OMERACT psoriatic arthritis magnetic resonance imaging scoring system (PsAMRIS): definitions of key pathologies, suggested MRI sequences, and preliminary scoring system for PsA hands. *J Rheumatol.* (2009) 36:1816–24. doi: 10.3899/jrheum.090352
16. Klein S, Staring M, Murphy K, Viergever MA, Pluim JP. elastix: a toolbox for intensity-based medical image registration. *IEEE Trans Med Imaging.* (2010) 29:196–205. doi: 10.1109/TMI.2009.2035616
17. Mattes D, Haynor D, Vesselle H, Lewellyn T, Eubank W. Nonrigid multimodality image registration. *Med Imaging.* (2001) 4322:1–12. doi: 10.1117/12.431046
18. Alam F, Rahman SU, Khusro S, Ullah S, Khalil A. Evaluation of medical image registration techniques based on nature and domain of the transformation. *J Med Imaging Rad Sci.* (2016) 47:178–93. doi: 10.1016/j.jmir.2015.12.081
19. Ellouz R, Chapurlat R, van Rietbergen B, Christen P, Pialat JB, Boutroy S. Challenges in longitudinal measurements with HR-pQCT: evaluation of a 3D registration method to improve bone microarchitecture and strength measurement reproducibility. *Bone.* (2014) 63:147–57. doi: 10.1016/j.bone.2014.03.001
20. Topfer D, Gerner B, Finzel S, Kraus S, Museyko O, Schett G, et al. Automated three-dimensional registration of high-resolution peripheral quantitative computed tomography data to quantify size and shape changes of arthritic bone erosions. *Rheumatology.* (2015) 54:2171–80. doi: 10.1093/rheumatology/kev256
21. Peters M, van den Bergh JP, Geusens P, Scharmga A, Loeffen D, Weijers R, et al. Prospective follow-up of cortical interruptions, bone density, and micro-structure detected on HR-pQCT: a study in patients with rheumatoid arthritis and healthy subjects. *Calcif. Tissue Int.* (2019) 104:571–81. doi: 10.1007/s00223-019-00523-2
22. Christen P, Muller R. *In vivo* visualisation and quantification of bone resorption and bone formation from time-lapse imaging. *Curr Osteoporos Rep.* (2017) 15:311–17. doi: 10.1007/s11914-017-0372-1
23. Brunet SC, Bhatla JL, Lemay S, Pauchard Y, Salat P, Barnabe C, et al. The utility of multi-stack alignment and 3D longitudinal image registration to assess bone remodeling in rheumatoid arthritis patients from second generation HR-pQCT scans. *BMC Med Imaging.* (2019) 20:1–20. doi: 10.21203/rs.2.14575/v3
24. Studholme C, Hill DLG, Hawkes DJ. An overlap invariant entropy measure of 3D medical image alignment. *Pattern Recognit.* (1999) 32:71–86. doi: 10.1016/S0031-3203(98)00091-0
25. Maes F, Collignon A, Vandermeulen D, Marchal G, Suetens P. Multimodality image registration by maximization of mutual information. *IEEE Trans Med Imaging.* (1997) 16:187–98. doi: 10.1109/42.563664
26. Brown AK, Quinn MA, Karim Z, Conaghan PG, Peterfy CG, Hensor E, et al. Presence of significant synovitis in rheumatoid arthritis patients with disease-modifying antirheumatic drug-induced clinical remission: evidence from an imaging study may explain structural progression. *Arthritis Rheumat.* (2006) 54:3761–73. doi: 10.1002/art.22190
27. Brown AK, Conaghan PG, Karim Z, Quinn MA, Ikeda K, Peterfy GC, et al. An explanation for the apparent dissociation between clinical remission and continued structural deterioration in rheumatoid arthritis. *Arthritis Rheumat.* (2008) 58:2958–67. doi: 10.1002/art.23945
28. Forslind K, Svensson B. MRI evidence of persistent joint inflammation and progressive joint damage despite clinical remission during treatment of early rheumatoid arthritis. *Scand J Rheumatol.* (2016) 45:99–102. doi: 10.3109/03009742.2015.1070902
29. Kong S, Locrelle H, Amouzougan A, Denarie D, Collet P, Pallot-Prades B, et al. Remaining local subclinical joint inflammation is associated with deteriorated metacarpeal head bone microarchitecture in rheumatoid arthritis patients low disease activity. *Joint Bone Spine.* (2018) 85:569–72. doi: 10.1016/j.jbspin.2017.11.010
30. Claes L, Recknagel S, Ignatius A. Fracture healing under healthy and inflammatory conditions. *Nat Rev Rheumatol.* (2012) 8:133–43. doi: 10.1038/nrrheum.2012.1

31. Shimizu T, Choi HJ, Heilmeier U, Tanaka M, Burghardt AJ, Gong J, et al. Assessment of 3-month changes in bone microstructure under anti-TNFα therapy in patients with rheumatoid arthritis using high-resolution peripheral quantitative computed tomography (HR-pQCT). *Arthritis Res Ther.* (2017) 19:222. doi: 10.1186/s13075-017-1430-x
32. Kroker A, Besler BA, Bhatla JL, Shtil M, Salat P, Mohtadi N, et al. Longitudinal effects of acute anterior cruciate ligament tears on peri-articular bone in human knees within the first year of injury. *J Orthop Res.* (2019) 37:2325–36. doi: 10.1002/jor.24410
33. Barnabe C, Toepfer D, Marotte H, Hauge EM, Scharmga A, Kocijan R, et al. Definition for rheumatoid arthritis erosions imaged with high resolution peripheral quantitative computed tomography and interreader reliability for detection and measurement. *J Rheumatol.* (2016) 43:1935–40. doi: 10.3899/jrheum.160648
34. Noguchi K, Gel Y, Brunner E, Konietschke F. nparLD: an R software package for the nonparametric analysis of longitudinal data in factorial experiments. *J Stat Softw.* (2012) 50:1–23. doi: 10.18637/jss.v050.i12
35. Shepherd JA, Lu Y. Ageneralized least significant change for individuals measured on different DXA systems. *J Clin Densitom.* (2007) 10:249–58. doi: 10.1016/j.jocd.2007.05.002
36. Brunet SC, Finzel S, Engelke K, Boyd SK, Barnabe C, Manske SL. Bone changes assessed with High-Resolution peripheral Quantitative Computed Tomography (HR-pQCT) in early inflammatory arthritis: a 12-month cohort study. *Joint Bone Spine.* (in press). doi: 10.1016/j.jbspin.2020.07.014
37. Nishiyama KK, Pauchard Y, Nikkel LE, Iyer S, Zhang C, McMahon DJ, et al. Longitudinal HR-pQCT and image registration detects endocortical bone loss in kidney transplantation patients. *J Bone Mineral Res.* (2015) 30:554–61. doi: 10.1002/jbmr.2358
38. Schett G, Gravallese E. Bone erosion in rheumatoid arthritis: mechanisms, diagnosis and treatment. *Nat Rev Rheumatol.* (2012) 8:656–64. doi: 10.1038/nrrheum.2012.153
39. Sisniega A, Thawait GK, Shakoor D, Siewerdsen JH, Demehri S, Zbijewski W. Motion compensation in extremity cone-beam computed tomography. *Skelet Radiol.* (2019) 48:1999–2007. doi: 10.1007/s00256-019-03241-w
40. Sisniega A, Stayman JW, Yorkston J, Siewerdsen JH, Zbijewski W. Motion compensation in extremity cone-beam CT using a penalized image sharpness criterion. *Phys Med Biol.* (2017) 62:3712–34. doi: 10.1088/1361-6560/aa6869
41. Scharmga A, Keller KK, Peters M, van Tubergen A, van den Bergh JP, van Rietbergen B, et al. Vascular channels in metacarpophalangeal joints: a comparative histologic and high-resolution imaging study. *Sci Rep.* (2017) 7:8966. doi: 10.1038/s41598-017-09363-2
42. Jimenez-Boj E, Nobauer-Huhmann I, Hanslik-Schnabel B, Dorotka R, Wanivenhaus AH, Kainberger J, et al. Bone erosions and bone marrow edema as defined by magnetic resonance imaging reflect true bone marrow inflammation in rheumatoid arthritis. *Arthritis Rheumat.* (2007) 56:1118–24. doi: 10.1002/art.22496
43. van den Bergh J, Geusens P. Bone erosions in rheumatoid arthritis. *Rheumatology.* (2013) 53:4–5. doi: 10.1093/rheumatology/ket358
44. Raynor WY, Jonnakuti VS, Zirakchian Zadeh M, Werner TJ, Cheng G, Zhuang H, et al. Comparison of methods of quantifying global synovial metabolic activity with FDG-PET/CT in rheumatoid arthritis. *Int J Rheum Dis.* (2019) 22:2191–8. doi: 10.1111/1756-185X.13730
45. Raynal M, Bouderraoui F, Ouichka R, Melchior J, Morel O, Blum A, et al. Performance of (18)F-sodium fluoride positron emission tomography with computed tomography to assess inflammatory and structural sacroiliitis on magnetic resonance imaging and computed tomography, respectively, in axial spondyloarthritis. *Arthritis Res Ther.* (2019) 21:119. doi: 10.1186/s13075-019-1903-1
46. Suto T, Yonemoto Y, Okamura K, Okura C, Kaneko T, Kobayashi T, et al. Predictive factors associated with the progression of large-joint destruction in patients with rheumatoid arthritis after biologic therapy: a *post-hoc* analysis using FDG-PET/CT and the ARASHI (assessment of rheumatoid arthritis by scoring of large-joint destruction and healing in radiographic imaging) scoring method. *Mod Rheumatol.* (2017) 27:820–7. doi: 10.1080/14397595.2016.1266132
47. Kogan F, Broski SM, Yoon D, Gold GE. Applications of PET-MRI in musculoskeletal disease. *J Magn Reson Imaging.* (2018) 48:27–47. doi: 10.1002/jmri.26183
48. Miese F, Scherer A, Ostendorf B, Heinzel A, Lanzman RS, Kropil P, et al. Hybrid 18F-FDG PET-MRI of the hand in rheumatoid arthritis: initial results. *Clin Rheumatol.* (2011) 30:1247–50. doi: 10.1007/s10067-011-1777-3

22

Cartilage Degradation in Psoriatic Arthritis is Associated with Increased Synovial Perfusion as Detected by Magnetic Resonance Imaging

Daniel B. Abrar [1†], Christoph Schleich [1†], Anja Müller-Lutz [1], Miriam Frenken [1], K. Ludger Radke [1], Stefan Vordenbäumen [2], Matthias Schneider [2], Benedikt Ostendorf [2] and Philipp Sewerin [2]*

[1] *Department of Diagnostic and Interventional Radiology, Medical Faculty, University Dusseldorf, Düsseldorf, Germany,*
[2] *Department and Hiller Research Unit for Rheumatology, UKD, Heinrich Heine University Düsseldorf, Düsseldorf, Germany*

Correspondence:
Philipp Sewerin
philipp.sewerin@med.uni-duesseldorf.de

† These authors have contributed equally to this work

Objective: Even though cartilage loss is a known feature of psoriatic arthritis (PsA), research is sparse on its role in the pathogenesis of PsA and its potential use for disease detection and monitoring. Using delayed gadolinium-enhanced magnetic resonance imaging of cartilage (dGEMRIC) and dynamic contrast-enhanced MRI (DCE MRI), research has shown that early cartilage loss is strongly associated with synovial inflammation in rheumatoid arthritis (RA). The aim of this study was to determine if acute inflammation is associated with early cartilage loss in small finger joints of patients with PsA.

Methods: Metacarpophalangeal (MCP), proximal interphalangeal (PIP), and distal interphalangeal (DIP) joints of 17 patients with active PsA were evaluated by high-resolution 3 Tesla dGEMRIC and DCE MRI using a dedicated 16-channel hand coil. Semi-quantitative and quantitative perfusion parameters were calculated. Images were analyzed by two independent raters for dGEMRIC indices, PsA MRI scores (PsAMRIS), total cartilage thickness (TCT), and joint space width (JSW).

Results: We found significant negative correlations between perfusion parameters (except K_{ep}) and dGEMRIC indices, with the highest value at the MCP joints (K_{Trans}: $\tau = -0.54$, $p = 0.01$; K_{ep}: $\tau = -0.02$, $p = 0.90$; IAUC: $\tau = -0.51$, $p = 0.015$; Initial Slope: $\tau = -0.54$, $p = 0.01$; Peak: $\tau = -0.67$, $p = 0.002$). Heterogeneous correlations were detected between perfusion parameters and both, total PsAMRIS and PsAMRIS synovitis sub-scores. No significant correlation was seen between any perfusion parameter and JSW and/or TCT.

Conclusion: As examined by DCE MRI and dGEMRIC, there is a potential association between early cartilage loss and acute synovial inflammation in small finger joints of PsA patients.

Keywords: psoriatic arthritis, magnetic resonance imaging, dGEMRIC, cartilage, compositional imaging

INTRODUCTION

Psoriatic arthritis (PsA) is a chronic autoimmune disease that ultimately leads to joint destruction and functional disability (1). As in rheumatoid arthritis (RA), early diagnosis and treatment are pivotal for a better clinical outcome (2, 3). Therefore, treat-to-target (T2T) strategies have been introduced for the treatment of PsA (4, 5). Even though magnetic resonance imaging is not yet included in the classification criteria for PsA (CASPAR), it becomes increasingly important for the early detection and monitoring of disease-related joint changes (6–8). In 2009, the Outcome Measures in Rheumatology Clinical Trials (OMERACT) working group introduced a semi-quantitative PsA MRI score (PsAMRIS) that evaluates metacarpophalangeal (MCP), proximal (PIP), and distal interphalangeal joints concerning the osteodestructive (bone erosion), osteoproliferative (bone proliferation), and acute inflammatory (synovitis, flexor tenosynovitis, periarticular inflammation) features of PsA (9). Several studies have shown that the degree of synovial contrast enhancement in arthritic joints can be quantified by dynamic contrast-enhanced MRI (DCE MRI), and hence, have found a strong correlation between the synovitis sub-score of PsAMRIS and RA MRI score (RAMRIS) and DCE MRI parameters (10–12). Furthermore, elevated synovial perfusion assessed by DCE MRI reflects histological findings of acute synovitis (13). Even though cartilage damage is a known feature of PsA, research is sparse on its value in the pathogenesis and the disease course (14). That is why it is not included in the PsAMRIS as opposed to its RA equivalent (15). Several studies using delayed gadolinium-enhanced MRI of cartilage (dGEMRIC) have shown that early cartilage loss in RA is associated with the severity of synovitis (10, 16). dGEMRIC is a histologically validated and robust method that depicts proteoglycan loss in cartilage by measurement of fixed-charge density (17, 18). Proteoglycans have negatively charged side chains that allow for the inversely proportional penetration of similarly negatively charged contrast agent molecules (e.g., gadolinium) following intravenous administration. Consequently, proteoglycan depletion leads to an accumulation of gadolinium ions in degenerated cartilage.

However, the placement of region of interests in small joints is difficult using conventional MRI or with high-resolution MRI surface coils. We, therefore, used a 16-channel high-resolution hand coil to allow for an improved evaluation of smaller joints.

Herein, we set out to evaluate if there was any association between acute inflammation and early cartilage loss in small finger joints of patients with PsA.

METHODS

Study Population

Seventeen patients with PsA (mean age 53.7 ± 11.6; minimum/maximum 26/72 years, male/female 9/8) fulfilling the CASPAR criteria, mean disease duration 4 ± 3.6 years, and suffering from peripheral joint involvement of at least two MCP joints and dactylitis of at least one finger were prospectively recruited for the "Analysis of the DActylic Melange" (ADAM) research initiative. All patients had failed methotrexate (MTX) monotherapy and were escalated to etanercept therapy after a baseline MRI scan. Patient recruitment took place in the Department of Rheumatology from 06/ 2015 to 01/ 2017. The same study population has been included in a different study. However, this study has been published as a pre-print only (19).

The study was approved by the local ethics committee (study number: 4962R, "Analysis of the Dactylitic Melange (ADAM): Defining the morphological components of dactylitis in psoriatic arthritis and their responsiveness to etanercept therapy). Written and informed consent was obtained from all patients before initiation of the study. The Disease Activity Score 28 (DAS 28) was 2.42 ± 0.72 (range 1.8–4.3, median 2.2). C-reactive protein (CRP) levels were 0.87 ± 1.35 mg/dl (range 0.1–5.8 mg/dl, median 0.3 mg/dl).

MR Imaging

A 3T MRI scanner (Magentom Skyra, Siemens Healthineers, Erlangen, Germany) and a dedicated 16-channel hand coil (3T Tim Coil [receive only], Siemens Healthineers, Erlangen, Germany) was used for all patients. Patients were imaged in the prone position with their arm extended overhead ("superman position" with palm facing down).

The imaging protocol included coronal T1-weighted turbo spin echo (TSE) sequences before and after intravenous injection of an ionic gadolinium-based contrast agent (Gd-DOTA$^-$ [Dotarem, Guerbet Villepinte, France] in double dose, 0.4 mmol/kg bodyweight). The intravenous injection was carried out by an injection pump followed by a saline chaser. Also, non-contrast enhanced, fat-saturated T2-weighted/short tau inversion recovery (STIR) as well as post-contrast fat-saturated T1-weighted sequences in at least two different orthogonal planes were obtained.

Compositional MRI using the dGEMRIC technique of the MCP, PIP, and DIP joints 2–5 was performed 40 min after intravenous contrast-agent administration. To this end, we used a flip-angle three-dimensional gradient-echo (GE) imaging (FLASH) sequence with two excitation flip angles (5° and 26°) as in previously published studies of our institute (17, 20, 21). 40 sagittal slices were acquired perpendicular to the joint surface. Total acquisition time was 2.25 min.

For perfusion imaging, a dynamic T1-weighted GE turbo FLASH sequence and two T1-weighted GE 3D-FLASH sequences with two different flipangles were acquired; the contrast agent was injected 20 s after sequence initiation. Total acquisition time was 7.20 min. B_1 shimming was applied to maximize image quality.

The detailed sequence parameters were as follows:

Coronal T1 turbo spin echo (TSE) (TR/TE 862/27 ms; flip angle 150°; slice thickness 2.5 mm; field of view 140 × 140 mm; imaging matrix: 512 × 512; pixel size 0.3 × 0.3 mm), coronal STIR (TR/TE, 5560/31 ms; flip angle 120°; slice thickness 2.5 mm; 8.0; slice thickness 3.0 mm; field of view 140 × 140 mm; imaging matrix: 448 × 312; pixel size 0.3 × 0.3 mm), sagittal proton density (PD) TSE fat-saturated (TR/TE 3150/47 ms, flip angle 150°, slice thickness 2.5 mm, field of view 60 × 150 mm; imaging matrix: 448 × 182; pixel size 0.3 × 0.3 mm), transversal T2 TSE fat-saturated (TR/TE 5693.8/89 ms, flip angle 180°, slice thickness 3.0 mm, field of view 160 × 160 mm; imaging matrix: 512 × 358; pixel size 0.3 × 0.3 mm), transversal T1 SE fat-saturated after intravenous (iv) contrast administration (TR/TE 807/16 ms; flip angle 90°; slice thickness 3.0 mm; field of view 130 × 130 mm; imaging matrix: 384 × 288; pixel size 0.3 × 0.3 mm), coronal T1 TSE after iv contrast (TR/TE 862/27 ms; flip angle 150°; slice thickness 2.5 mm; field of view 140 × 140 mm; imaging matrix: 512 × 512; pixel size 0.3 × 0.3 mm), 3D FLASH GE (TR/TE 5.8/1.9 ms; flip angle 5/26°; slice thickness 3.0 mm; field of view 65 × 110 mm; imaging matrix: 384 × 228; pixel size 0.3 × 0.3 mm) and T1 GE Turbo FLASH (TR/TE 5.8 / 1.9 ms; flip angle 5°; slice thickness 3.0 mm; field of view 140 × 140 mm; imaging matrix: 128 × 96; pixel size 1.1 × 1.1 mm).

Image Analysis

MR images were independently read and analyzed by two radiologists (DBA and CS, trained in musculoskeletal imaging with 3 and 8 years experience) and one rheumatologist (PS, trained in musculoskeletal imaging with 8 years of experience) according to the OMCERACT PsAMRIS guidelines (9). In addition, joint space width (JSW; minimal distance in mm between the proximal and distal bone surface) and total cartilage thickness (TCT; sum of the proximal and distal cartilage layer) were measured for each MCP, PIP and DIP joint of finger 2–5. Measurements were performed perpendicular to the subchondral bone in the medial part of the joint using the inbuilt digital caliper tool of the picture archiving and communication system (PACS, Sectra Workstation IDS7, Sectra AB, Linköping, Sweden) on sagittal PDw images.

Perfusion in the MCP, PIP, and DIP joints of finger 2-5 was evaluated with quantitative and semi-quantitative analysis using The DCE Tool (The DCE Tool for ClearCanvas 2.0 SP1, http://thedcetool.com) as described in previously published studies of our institute (10). The quantitative analysis of this tool is based upon the Tofts model (22). Perfusion analysis requires the knowledge of T1 relaxation times. Therefore, the T1w GE 3D FLASH sequence with variable flip angles was used for a pixel-based calculation of the T1 time. For this calculation we applied the following formula:

$$T1\left(x,y,z\right)=\frac{\mathrm{TR}}{\ln\left[\frac{\sin(\alpha1)\cos(\alpha2)-Q(x,y,z)\sin(\alpha2)\cos(\alpha1)}{\sin(\alpha1)-Q\left(x,y,z\right)\sin(\alpha2)}\right)}$$

where

$$Q\left(x,y,z\right)=\frac{S\alpha1\left(x,y,z\right)}{S\alpha2\left(x,y,z\right)}$$

And $S_{\alpha 1}$ (x, y, z) and $S_{\alpha 2}$ (x, y, z) are the corresponding pixel intensities to flip angles α_1 and α_2. Then, the T1 relaxation was used for the perfusion analysis.

A region of interest (ROI) was placed on the radial and ulnar side of each joint by one reader (DBA). After ROI placement a second reader (CS) confirmed the optimal placement before each measured signal intensity was used to determine a corresponding concentration time curve using the following formula:

$$C_{GD}\ (t)=\frac{\mathrm{S}\ (t)-\mathrm{S}_0}{\mathrm{S}_0 T_{10} R}$$

where T_{10} is the native T1 time, $R = 4.5\ s^{-1}\ mM^{-1}$ is the relaxivity of the contrast agent, S is the average signal intensity in the ROI and S_0 is the average signal intensity in the ROI in absence of the contrast agent. This Tofts model requires the knowledge of the arterial input function (AIF). AIF can be calculated individually from the blood signal or, alternatively, a population average can be used (22). In this study, we used an analytically described AIF population average that can be used at any temporal resolution (22).

The following perfusions parameters were calculated:

Perfusion parameters are displayed and explained in **Table 1**: K_{Trans}, k_{ep} (quantitative parameters) and IAUC (integral of the signal curve over time), initial slope and peak (semiquantitative parameters).

For compositional analyses of cartilage quality with dGEMRIC, motion correction was applied using STROKETOOL (Digital Image Solutions, Frechen, Germany, http://www.digitalimagesolutions.de) for all images to reduce movement artifacts. This tool has been validated for dGEMRIC analyses of the finger joints and corrects for patient motion between the measurements using a dedicated image registration method (23).

Readers were allowed to adjust the window settings as required to guarantee optimal visualization of the intra- and periarticular structures for ROI placement. T1 maps were analyzed by first defining regions-of-interest (ROIs) on the central sagittal slice. ROI outlines comprising the full thickness of the proximal and distal portion of the articular cartilage of MPC, PIP and DIP joints of finger 2-5 were manually defined on the morphological images of the 3D T1-weighted FLASH sequence with the flip angle of 5° for dGEMRIC. Particular care was taken to exclude artifacts and surrounding structures such as synovial fluid and cortical bone. Consequently, four ROIs were set per digit (i.e., metacarpal, base of proximal phalanx, apex of proximal phalanx, and base of intermediate phalanx) and 16 ROIs per patient (i.e., four ROIs of four digits) and visually checked by the second and third reader to confirm that only cartilage was included. Next, ROIs were copied to the corresponding slices of the color-coded T1 parameter maps. Further analyses involved the pixel-wise calculation post-contrast T1 values as before (17, 24, 25). More specifically, the T1 maps representing the spatially resolved dGEMRIC indices were analyzed in terms of the ROIs as defined above the mean dGEMRIC indices [ms] were recorded. All images were analyzed by two readers (DBA and CS, radiologists) who were blinded for patients' data.

Statistical Analysis

All statistical analyses were performed using SPSS software (IBM, version 22, Armonk, NY, USA). For descriptive analysis mean,

TABLE 1 | Description of quantitative and semi-quantitative perfusion parameters. IAUC: initial area under the curve.

Quantitative parameters		**Semi-quantitative parameters**		
K_{Trans}	**k_{ep}**	**IAUC**	**Initial slope**	**Peak**
Transfer constant between EES and blood plasma	KTrans/Ve, V_e: relative volume of EES	Integral of the signal curve over time starting at the onset time (t_{onset}) of the bolus	Slope of the signal curve determined by linear regression within the initial seconds after onset	Maximal signal enhancement

EES, extravascular extracellular space.

standard deviation, minimum, and maximum were calculated. Due to the small sample size and the heterogeneity of our data, non-normal distribution was assumed. For comparison of means, Kruskal-Wallis test and a *post-hoc* Bonferroni test were performed. Correlation analysis was performed between each dGEMRIC indices, total PsAMRIS and all its sub-scores and TCT using the Kendall–Tau correlation coefficient. p-values < 0.05 were considered to be significant.

RESULTS

Descriptive Analysis of dGEMRIC Indices, Perfusion Parameters, JSW, and TCT at MCP and PIP Joints

The descriptive analysis (mean, standard deviation, and range) of dGEMRIC values, quantitative (K_{Trans}, K_{ep}) and semi-quantitative (IAUC, initial slope, peak) perfusion parameters, JSW, and TCT of MCP, PIP, and DIP joints and overall are displayed in **Table 2**.

Perfusion and dGEMRIC maps are shown in **Figure 1**.

Correlation Between Perfusion Parameters and JSW, TCT, Total PsAMRIS, Synovitis Sub-score, dGEMRIC Indices, CRP-Levels, and DAS 28

The correlation between perfusion parameters and JSW, TCT, total PsAMRIS, synovitis sub-score, DAS 28, and dGEMRIC indices is illustrated in **Table 3**.

There was no significant correlation between any perfusion parameter and JSW or TCT, neither overall nor at any joint level (MCP, PIP, DIP).

Overall, there was a significant negative correlation between dGEMRIC indices and all perfusion parameters except k_{ep}. The strongest correlation was found at the MCP joint level.

No significant correlation was seen between any perfusion parameter and overall PsAMRIS and/or synovitis sub-score at the MCP joints and overall. For PIP joints, we found a significant correlation for the parameter peak and total PsAMRIS ($\tau = 0.44, p = 0.032$) and for the parameters IAUC and peak and the synovitis sub-score ($\tau = 0.41, p = 0.042$; $\tau = 0.451, p = 0.032$). At the DIP level, there was a significant correlation between the perfusions parameters K_{Trans}, IAUC, initial slope, and peak and the total PsAMRIS ($\tau = 0.54, p = 0.07$; $\tau = 0.48, p = 0.018$; $\tau = 0.46, p = 0.024$; $\tau = 0.43, p = 0.032$). Further, no significant correlations were found between perfusion parameters and DAS 28 as well as serum CRP levels.

The negative correlations between dGEMRIC values and the quantitative parameter K_{Trans} and the semi-quantitative parameter peak at the MCP joint level are depicted in **Figure 2**.

DISCUSSION

Cartilage degradation is a known feature of PsA that can reliably be assessed by dGEMRIC (26). However, as opposed to RA, research is sparse on the role of cartilage in the pathogenesis of PsA. DCE MRI is a valid tool for the evaluation of inflammation in a given joint that has been validated for many types of arthritis (11, 12). In this study, we set out to investigate the relationship between joint inflammation and cartilage loss measured by DCE MRI and dGEMRIC.

We found a significant negative correlation of dGEMRIC indices and quantitative and semi-quantitative perfusion parameters, wherein MCP and PIP joints showed the highest values. The exact reason for the missing correlations at the DIP joints remain unclear, but might be due to a constitutively different proteoglycan content of cartilage along the finger joints or a higher loss of proteoglycans at MCP and PIP than at DIP joints in this specific population of PsA patients. This indicates that molecular cartilage loss is associated with inflammatory joint changes in patients with established PsA, and hence, high inflammation of joints leads to cartilage damage. These findings concur with previous research on cartilage loss, synovial inflammation and perfusion parameters in patients with early RA (10, 16, 20). Since biochemical MRI detects molecular cartilage degradation preceding structural damage, it might be applicable as a monitoring tool for very early disease-related joint changes in PsA.

The association of perfusion parameters and PsAMRIS (sub-scores) has not yet been evaluated. Previous studies on RA showed that perfusion parameters highly correlated with RAMRIS and histological synovitis in affected patients (10, 13, 27–29). As opposed to these findings, we found heterogeneous correlations of perfusion parameters and total PsAMRIS, as well as the synovitis sub-score in PsA patients. DCE MRI is known to indicate the severity of inflammation at a given joint; that is why one could have expected a strong association between perfusion parameters and PsAMRIS. However, previous research using DCE MRI has partially shown that PsA and RA can differ regarding the degree of their synovial enhancement, despite indistinguishable appearances on non-dynamic MRI (30, 31).

TABLE 2 | Descriptive analysis (mean, standard deviation (SD) and range (maximum, minimum) of quantitative and semi-quantitative perfusion parameters, delayed Gadolinium Enhanced Magnetic Resonance Imaging of Cartilage (dGEMRIC) indices, joint space width (JSW), and total cartilage thickness (TCT) of finger 2–5 at the metacarpophalangeal (MCP), proximal interphalangeal (PIP), and distal interphalangeal (DIP) joint region and overall.

		K trans ml/g per min	K ep 1/min	IAUC mM/l per s	Initial slope mM/l per s	Peak mM/l per s	dGEMRIC in ms	TCT in mm	JSW in mm
MCP	Mean	0.06	0.18	3.08	0.0023	0.15	542.65	1.15	1.5
	SD	0.04	0.13	2.46	0.002	0.10	130.34	0.26	0.17
	Max	0.14	0.53	8.45	0.007	0.36	828.03	1.59	1.83
	Min	0.02	0.03	0.81	0.0004	0.05	340.4	0.73	1.27
PIP	Mean	0.05	0.17	2.90	0.002	0.15	411.92	0.71	1.02
	SD	0.03	0.13	2.01	0.002	0.08	104.46	0.18	0.24
	Max	0.12	0.65	7.59	0.006	0.31	639.6	1.11	1.49
	Min	0.008	0.04	0.58	0.0004	0.04	237.18	0.38	0.69
DIP	Mean	0.06	0.21	3.72	0.003	0.16	352.86	0.57	0.8
	SD	0.04	0.15	2.72	0.002	0.08	98.75	0.2	0.18
	Max	0.17	0.68	9.96	0.009	0.29	585.03	0.79	1.19
	Min	0.01	0.06	0.43	0.0003	0.04	184.35	0	0.55
Overall	Mean	0.06	277.32	3.11	0.003	0.15	436.30	0.77	1.07
	SD	0.03	802.71	1.88	0.002	0.07	110.09	0.2	0.18
	Max	0.12	3141.11	7.67	0.006	0.30	670.98	1.13	1.44
	Min	0.01	0.04	0.57	0.0004	0.05	253.98	0.40	0.75
	MCP vs PIP	0.359	0.591	0.864	0.531	1.00	**0.019**	**0.029**	**<0.001**
p-value	MCP vs DIP	0.724	0.803	0.558	0.818	0.848	**0.001**	**0.02**	**0.007**
	PIP vs DIP	0.079	0.918	0.874	0.896	0.848	0.491	0.566	0.116

Mean values of each parameter were compared with a Kruskal-Wallis test and a post-hoc Bonferroni test. P-values <0.05 were considered significant and are given in bold type.

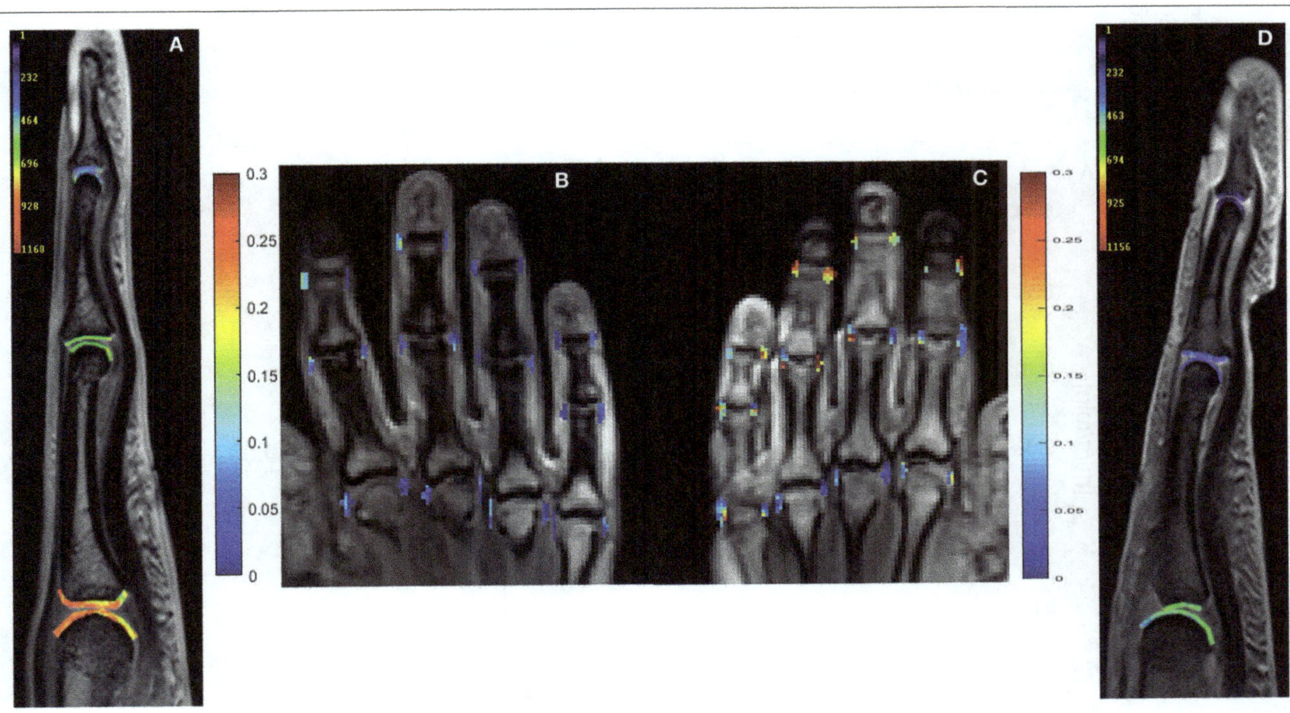

FIGURE 1 | Delayed Gadolinium Enhanced Magnetic Resonance Imaging of Cartilage (dGEMRIC) maps (ms, third digit) and perfusion maps (peak parameter) of metacarpophalangeal (MCP), proximal interphalangeal (PIP), and distal interphalangeal (DIP) joints in 26-year-old male **(A,B)** and a 59-year-old female **(C,D)** with PsA. Lower dGEMRIC values are illustrated in **(D)**, indicating more proteoglycan loss than in **(A)**. Higher peak values are depicted in **(C)**, indicating a higher severity of synovitis than in **(B)**. Peak parameter is illustrated in mM/l per second, dGEMRIC indices in ms.

TABLE 3 | Kendall Tau correlation τ between quantitative and semi-quantitative perfusion parameters and dGEMRIC indices, total Psoriatic arthritis magnetic resonance imaging score (PsAMRIS), PsAMRIS sub-score "synovitis."

		K_{Trans}		K_{ep}		IAUC		Initial slope		Peak	
		τ	p	τ	p	τ	p	τ	p	τ	p
Overall	JSW	0.1	0.35	−0.1	0.33	0.05	0.64	0.02	0.84	0.04	0.69
	TCT	0.03	0.8	−0.12	0.26	0	0.97	−0.12	0.91	−0.12	0.91
	dGEMRIC	−0.27	**0.014**	−0.29	**0.008**	−0.29	**0.008**	0.32	**0.004**	−0.26	**0.02**
	PsAMRIS	−0.44	0.826	−0.27	0.188	0.09	0.661	0.13	0.51	0.18	0.38
	Synovitis	0.17	0.409	−0.12	0.545	0.26	0.205	0.26	0.205	0.35	0.088
	DAS 28	0.19	0.335	−0.04	0.854	0.27	0.169	0.014	0.952	0.32	0.108
MCP	JSW	0.2	0.3	−0.01	0.96	0.03	0.87	0.03	0.87	0.12	0.55
	TCT	−0.21	0.3	−0.17	0.41	−0.25	0.2	−0.25	0.2	−0.25	0.2
	dGEMRIC	−0.54	**0.01**	−0.02	0.90	−0.51	**0.015**	−0.54	**0.01**	−0.67	**0.002**
	PsAMRIS	0.02	0.912	−0.16	0.44	0.09	0.657	0.14	0.375	0.23	0.268
	Synovitis	0.11	0.612	−0.04	0.866	0.16	0.463	0.23	0.284	0.3	0.159
	DAS28	0.24	0.459	−0.03	0.939	0.22	0.5	0.28	0.385	0.22	0.489
PIP	JSW	0.07	0.73	−0.03	0.88	0.11	0.59	0.17	0.41	0.17	0.41
	TCT	0.12	0.55	−0.06	0.77	0.15	0.43	0.22	0.27	0.22	0.27
	dGEMRIC	−0.43	**0.03**	0.07	0.7	−0.39	0.055	−0.51	**0.015**	−0.51	**0.015**
	PsAMRIS	0.34	0.089	0.02	0.920	0.34	0.089	0.26	0.205	0.44	**0.032**
	Synovitis	0.39	0.053	0.14	0.476	0.41	**0.042**	0.31	0.142	0.45	**0.032**
	DAS28	0.18	0.568	0.05	0.886	0.2	0.536	0.12	0.708	0.22	0.489
DIP	JSW	−0.1	0.62	−0.1	0.62	−0.03	0.87	−0.01	0.96	−0.25	0.21
	TC	−0.05	0.78	−0.1	0.62	0.01	0.96	0.03	0.87	−0.17	0.41
	dGEMRIC	−0.26	0.22	0.1	0.63	−0.18	0.39	−0.15	0.46	−0.08	0.71
	PsAMRIS	0.54	**0.007**	0.10	0.621	0.48	**0.018**	0.46	**0.024**	0.43	**0.032**
	Synovitis	0.22	0.294	−0.01	0.956	0.17	0.407	0.15	0.473	0.21	0.294
	DAS28	−0.06	0.848	0.01	0.901	−0.04	0.901	−0.12	0.722	0.07	0.829

Disease Activity Score 28 (DAS 28), JSW and TCT of finger 2–5 at the MCP, PIP, and DIP joint level and overall. p-values < 0.05 were considered significant and are written in bold type.

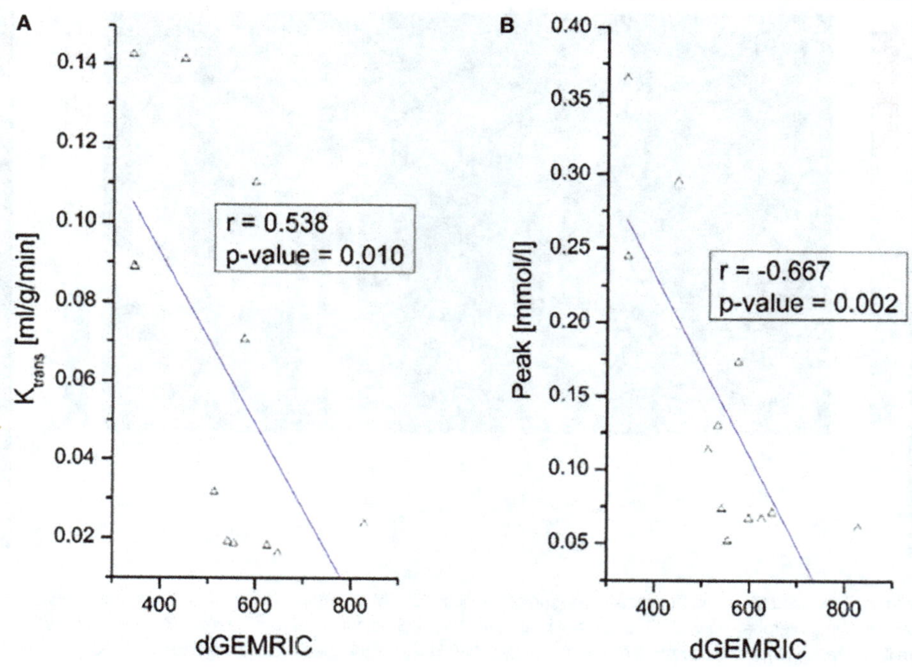

FIGURE 2 | Correlation between dGEMRIC indices and perfusion parameters K_{Trans} **(A)** and peak **(B)** of finger 2–5 at the MCP joint level.

Also, the synovial involvement of PsA histologically differs from RA regarding the extent of inflammation, synovial thickness, and blood supply (31–33). These differences of synovial changes are potentially due to the different pathogenesis of both entities, with RA being primarily a synovial and PsA being an entheseal-driven disease (34, 35). Therefore, the visual degree of synovitis using PsAMRIS could be over- or underrepresenting synovitis measured by DCE MRI, possibly due to a disease-specific type of synovial involvement. Further, for PsAMRIS scoring, we used coronal and transversal planes, wherein for DCE MRI, we only considered radial and ulnar ROI in coronal slices, which could also contribute to heterogeneous correlations of perfusion parameters and synovitis sub-scores. Additionally, the heterogeneity between MCP, PIP, and DIP joints could be explained by the known circumstances that the state of diffusion equilibrium is reached faster in smaller compared to larger joints (36).

Further, no significant correlations were found between perfusion parameters and clinical disease activity as measured by DAS 28. Previous studies have shown that MRI is more sensitive than clinical scores at the detection of joint inflammation (37, 38). Some studies even demonstrated an radiological progression despite clinical remission and postulated a "silent progression" (39–41). That is why, the lacking correlation of imaging features and clinical data could be due to the superior sensitivity of MRI, especially since a high-field MRI scanner and a dedicated hand-coil have been used resulting in high-resolution imaging.

Our Study Has Limitations

Firstly, our study population of PsA patients had a small sample size. That is why our results should only be considered exploratory and need confirmation by further research with larger populations.

Secondly, we did not use a synovial and cartilage biopsy as a means of validation regarding the extent of synovitis and the cartilage composition. However, previous studies have already histologically validated both DCE MRI and dGEMRIC data (13, 42).

In conclusion, there is a potential association between early cartilage loss and acute synovial inflammation in small finger joints of PsA patients.

ETHICS STATEMENT

The studies involving human participants were reviewed and approved by Ethics committee of the Heinrich-Heine University. The patients/participants provided their written informed consent to participate in this study.

AUTHOR CONTRIBUTIONS

DA: acquisition and analysis and interpretation of data. Draft and design of the work. PS: design and conception of the study. Analysis and interpretation of data. Draft and design of the work. Revision of the work. BO, MS, SV, and KR: analysis and interpretation of data. Draft and design of the work. Revision of the work. MF and AM-L: interpretation and analysis of data. Draft and design of the work. Revision of the work. CS: conception and design of the study. Interpretation and analysis of data. Draft and design of the work. Revision of the work. All authors read and approved the final manuscript. All authors contributed to the article and approved the submitted version.

FUNDING

DA was supported by the local research committee of the medical faculty. PS and SV received funding from Pfizer Germany with the Pfizer GIP Inflammation Germany Research Initiative 2014. PS and BO received funding from AbbVie Deutschland GmbH & Co. KG for the Delayed Gadolinium-enhanced MR Imaging of Cartilage—A pilot study to measure the effect of Adalimumab plus MTX vs. Placebo plus MTX on cartilage in early RA patients (CAR-ERA) Study. PS received a grant from the German Bundesministerium für Bildung und Forschung (BMBF), ArthroMark (01EC1009).

ACKNOWLEDGMENTS

We thank Mrs. Erika Rädisch for conducting all MRI studies.

REFERENCES

1. Sewerin P, Brinks R, Schneider M, Haase I, Vordenbäumen S. Prevalence and incidence of psoriasis and psoriatic arthritis. *Ann Rheum Dis.* (2019) 78:286–7. doi: 10.1136/annrheumdis-2018-214065
2. Coates LC, Navarro-Coy N, Brown SR, Brown S, McParland L, Collier H, et al. The TICOPA protocol (TIght COntrol of Psoriatic Arthritis): a randomised controlled trial to compare intensive management versus standard care in early psoriatic arthritis. *BMC Musculoskelet Disord.* (2013) 14:101. doi: 10.1186/1471-2474-14-101
3. Singh JA, Guyatt G, Ogdie A, Gladman DD, Deal C, Deodhar A, et al. Special article: 2018 American College of Rheumatology/National psoriasis foundation guideline for the treatment of psoriatic arthritis. *Arthritis Care Res.* (2019) 71:2–29. doi: 10.1002/art.40726
4. Coates LC. Treating to target in psoriatic arthritis. *Curr Opin Rheumatol.* (2015) 27:107. doi: 10.1097/BOR.0000000000000140
5. Coates LC, Lubrano E, Perrotta FM, Emery P, Conaghan PG, Helliwell PS. What should be the primary target of "treat to target" in psoriatic arthritis? *J Rheumatol.* (2019) 46:38–42. doi: 10.3899/jrheum.180267
6. Tillett W, Costa L, Jadon D, Wallis D, Cavill C, McHugh J, et al. The ClASsification for Psoriatic ARthritis (CASPAR) criteria–a retrospective feasibility, sensitivity, and specificity study. *J Rheumatol.* (2012) 39:154–6. doi: 10.3899/jrheum.110845
7. Coates LC, Conaghan PG, D'Agostino MA, Wit M de, FitzGerald O, Kvien TK, et al. Remission in psoriatic arthritis-where are we now? *Rheumatology.* (2018) 57:1321–31. doi: 10.1093/rheumatology/kex344
8. Yue J, Wu D, Tam L-S. The role of imaging in early diagnosis and prevention of joint damage in inflammatory arthritis. *Expert Rev Clin Immunol.* (2018) 14:499–511. doi: 10.1080/1744666X.2018.1476849

9. Ostergaard M, McQueen F, Wiell C, Bird P, Bøyesen P, Ejbjerg B, et al. The OMERACT psoriatic arthritis magnetic resonance imaging scoring system (PsAMRIS): definitions of key pathologies, suggested MRI sequences, and preliminary scoring system for PsA Hands. *J Rheumatol.* (2009) 36:1816–24. doi: 10.3899/jrheum.090352
10. Müller-Lutz A, Schleich C, Sewerin P, Gross J, Pentang G, Wittsack H-J, et al. Comparison of quantitative and semiquantitative dynamic contrast-enhanced MRI with respect to their correlation to delayed gadolinium-enhanced MRI of the cartilage in patients with early rheumatoid arthritis. *J Comput Assist Tomogr.* (2015) 39:64–9. doi: 10.1097/RCT.0000000000000164
11. Schwenzer NF, Kötter I, Henes JC, Schraml C, Fritz J, Claussen CD, et al. The role of dynamic contrast-enhanced MRI in the differential diagnosis of psoriatic and rheumatoid arthritis. *AJR Am J Roentgenol.* (2010) 194:715–20. doi: 10.2214/AJR.09.2671
12. Cimmino MA, Barbieri F, Boesen M, Paparo F, Parodi M, Kubassova O, et al. Dynamic contrast-enhanced magnetic resonance imaging of articular and extraarticular synovial structures of the hands in patients with psoriatic arthritis. *J Rheumatol Suppl.* (2012) 89:44–8. doi: 10.3899/jrheum.120242
13. Vordenbäumen S, Schleich C, Lögters T, Sewerin P, Bleck E, Pauly T, et al. Dynamic contrast-enhanced magnetic resonance imaging of metacarpophalangeal joints reflects histological signs of synovitis in rheumatoid arthritis. *Arthritis Res Ther.* (2014) 16:452. doi: 10.1186/s13075-014-0452-x
14. Bhattaram P, Chandrasekharan U. The joint synovium: A critical determinant of articular cartilage fate in inflammatory joint diseases. *Semin Cell Dev Biol.* (2017) 62:86–93. doi: 10.1016/j.semcdb.2016.05.009
15. Østergaard M, Peterfy CG, Bird P, Gandjbakhch F, Glinatsi D, Eshed I, et al. The OMERACT rheumatoid arthritis magnetic resonance imaging (MRI) scoring system: updated recommendations by the OMERACT MRI in arthritis working group. *J Rheumatol.* (2017) 44:1706–12. doi: 10.3899/jrheum.161433
16. Herz B, Albrecht A, Englbrecht M, Welsch GH, Uder M, Renner N, et al. Osteitis and synovitis, but not bone erosion, is associated with proteoglycan loss and microstructure damage in the cartilage of patients with rheumatoid arthritis. *Ann Rheum Dis.* (2014) 73:1101–6. doi: 10.1136/annrheumdis-2012-202850
17. Miese F, Buchbender C, Scherer A, Wittsack H-J, Specker C, Schneider M, et al. Molecular imaging of cartilage damage of finger joints in early rheumatoid arthritis with delayed gadolinium-enhanced magnetic resonance imaging. *Arthritis Rheum.* (2012) 64:394–9. doi: 10.1002/art.33352
18. van Tiel J, Kotek G, Reijman M, Bos PK, Bron EE, Klein S, et al. Is T1ρ mapping an alternative to delayed gadolinium-enhanced MR imaging of cartilage in the assessment of sulphated glycosaminoglycan content in human osteoarthritic knees? An *in vivo* validation study. *Radiology.* (2016) 279:523–31. doi: 10.1148/radiol.2015150693
19. Abrar DB, Schleich C, Brinks R, Vordenbäumen S, Frenken M, Goertz C, et al. Is a simplified version of PsAMRIS (sPsAMRIS) a potential tool for therapy monitoring in established psoriatic arthritis? *Res Square [Preprint].* (2019). doi: 10.21203/rs.2.14892/v1
20. Sewerin P, Schleich C, Brinks R, Müller-Lutz A, Fichter F, Eichner M, et al. Assessing associations of synovial perfusion, cartilage quality, and outcome in rheumatoid arthritis using dynamic contrast-enhanced magnetic resonance imaging. *J Rheumatol.* (2020) 47:15–9. doi: 10.3899/jrheum.180832
21. Sewerin P, Schleich C, Brinks R, Müller-Lutz A, Fichter F, Eichner M, et al. Synovial perfusion assessed by dynamic contrast-enhanced MRI is associated to treatment response, remission, and cartilage quality in rheumatoid arthritis. *J Rheumatol.* (2019). doi: 10.3899/jrheum.180832. [Epub ahead of print].
22. Tofts PS. T1-weighted DCE imaging concepts: modelling, acquisition and analysis. *MAGNETOM Flash.* (2010) 2010:30–9.
23. Miese F, Kröpil P, Ostendorf B, Scherer A, Buchbender C, Quentin M, et al. Motion correction improves image quality of dGEMRIC in finger joints. *Eur J Radiol.* (2011) 80:e427–31. doi: 10.1016/j.ejrad.2011.01.006
24. Miese FR, Ostendorf B, Wittsack H-J, Reichelt DC, Mamisch TC, Zilkens C, et al. Metacarpophalangeal joints in rheumatoid arthritis: delayed gadolinium-enhanced MR imaging of cartilage–a feasibility study. *Radiology.* (2010) 257:441–7. doi: 10.1148/radiol.10100459
25. Sewerin P, Müller-Lutz A, Abrar DB, Odendahl S, Eichner M, Schneider M, et al. Prevention of the progressive biochemical cartilage destruction under methotrexate therapy in early rheumatoid arthritis. *Clin Exp Rheumatol.* (2019) 37:179–85.
26. Sewerin P, Schleich C, Vordenbäumen S, Ostendorf B. Update on imaging in rheumatic diseases: cartilage. *Clin Exp Rheumatol.* (2018) 36 Suppl 114:139–44.
27. Hodgson R, Grainger A, O'Connor P, Barnes T, Connolly S, Moots R. Dynamic contrast enhanced MRI of bone marrow oedema in rheumatoid arthritis. *Ann Rheum Dis.* (2008) 67:270–2. doi: 10.1136/ard.2007.077271
28. Boesen M, Kubassova O, Bouert R, Axelsen MB, Ostergaard M, Cimmino MA, et al. Correlation between computer-aided dynamic gadolinium-enhanced MRI assessment of inflammation and semi-quantitative synovitis and bone marrow oedema scores of the wrist in patients with rheumatoid arthritis–a cohort study. *Rheumatology.* (2012) 51:134–43. doi: 10.1093/rheumatology/ker220
29. Wojciechowski W, Tabor Z, Urbanik A. Assessing synovitis based on dynamic gadolinium-enhanced MRI and EULAR-OMERACT scores of the wrist in patients with rheumatoid arthritis. *Clin Exp Rheumatol.* (2013) 31:850–6.
30. Sudoł-Szopińska I, Pracoń G. Diagnostic imaging of psoriatic arthritis. Part II: magnetic resonance imaging and ultrasonography. *J Ultrason.* (2016) 16:163–74. doi: 10.15557/JoU.2016.0018
31. Narváez J, Narváez JA, Albert M de, Gómez-Vaquero C, Nolla JM. Can magnetic resonance imaging of the hand and wrist differentiate between rheumatoid arthritis and psoriatic arthritis in the early stages of the disease? *Semin Arthritis Rheum.* (2012) 42:234–45. doi: 10.1016/j.semarthrit.2012.03.016
32. Sankowski AJ, Lebkowska UM, Cwikła J, Walecka I, Walecki J. Psoriatic arthritis. *Pol J Radiol.* (2013) 78:7–17. doi: 10.12659/PJR.883763
33. Sudoł-Szopińska I, Płaza M, Pracoń G. Selected issues in diagnostic imaging of spondyloarthritides: psoriatic arthritis and juvenile spondyloarthritis. *Reumatologia.* (2016) 54:310–7. doi: 10.5114/reum.2016.64908
34. McGonagle D, Hermann K-GA, Tan AL. Differentiation between osteoarthritis and psoriatic arthritis: implications for pathogenesis and treatment in the biologic therapy era. *Rheumatology.* (2015) 54:29–38. doi: 10.1093/rheumatology/keu328
35. Schett G, Coates LC, Ash ZR, Finzel S, Conaghan PG. Structural damage in rheumatoid arthritis, psoriatic arthritis, and ankylosing spondylitis: traditional views, novel insights gained from TNF blockade, and concepts for the future. *Arthritis Res Ther.* (2011) 2011:S4. doi: 10.1186/1478-6354-13-S1-S4
36. Peterfy CG. MR imaging. *Baillieres Clin Rheumatol.* (1996) 10:635–78. doi: 10.1016/S0950-3579(96)80055-0
37. Østergaard M, Hansen M, Stoltenberg M, Jensen KE, Szkudlarek M, Pedersen-Zbinden B, et al. New radiographic bone erosions in the wrists of patients with rheumatoid arthritis are detectable with magnetic resonance imaging a median of two years earlier. *Arthritis Rheum.* (2003) 48:2128–31. doi: 10.1002/art.11076
38. Ejbjerg BJ, Vestergaard A, Jacobsen S, Thomsen HS, Østergaard M. The smallest detectable difference and sensitivity to change of magnetic resonance imaging and radiographic scoring of structural joint damage in rheumatoid arthritis finger, wrist, and toe joints: a comparison of the OMERACT rheumatoid arthritis magnetic resonance imaging score applied to different joint combinations and the Sharp/van der Heijde radiographic score. *Arthritis Rheum.* (2005) 52:2300–6. doi: 10.1002/art.21207
39. Møller-Bisgaard S, Hørslev-Petersen K, Ejbjerg BJ, Boesen M, Hetland ML, Christensen R, et al. Impact of a magnetic resonance imaging-guided treat-to-target strategy on disease activity and progression in patients with rheumatoid arthritis (the IMAGINE-RA trial): study protocol for a randomized controlled trial. *Trials.* (2015) 16:178. doi: 10.1186/s13063-015-0693-2
40. Sewerin P, Vordenbaeumen S, Hoyer A, Brinks R, Buchbender C, Miese F, et al. Silent progression in patients with rheumatoid arthritis: is DAS28 remission an insufficient goal in RA? Results from the German Remission-plus cohort. *BMC Musculoskelet Disord.* (2017) 18:163. doi: 10.1186/s12891-017-1528-y

41. Hetland ML, Stengaard-Pedersen K, Junker P, Østergaard M, Ejbjerg BJ, Jacobsen S, et al. Radiographic progression and remission rates in early rheumatoid arthritis - MRI bone oedema and anti-CCP predicted radiographic progression in the 5-year extension of the double-blind randomised CIMESTRA trial. *Ann Rheum Dis.* (2010) 69:1789–95. doi: 10.1136/ard.2009.125534
42. Schmaranzer F, Arendt L, Liechti EF, Nuss K, Rechenberg B von, Kircher PR, et al. Do dGEMRIC and T2 imaging correlate with histologic cartilage degeneration in an experimental ovine FAI model? *Clin Orthop Relat Res.* (2019) 477:990–1003. doi: 10.1097/CORR.0000000000000593

23

High Prevalence of Ultrasound Verified Enthesitis in Patients With Inflammatory Bowel Disease With or Without Spondylarthritis

Rusmir Husic[1], Angelika Lackner[1], Patrizia Katharina Kump[2], Christoph Högenauer[2], Winfried Graninger[1] and Christian Dejaco[1,3]*

[1] Department of Rheumatology and Immunology, Medical University Graz, Graz, Austria, [2] Department of Gastroenterology and Hepatology, Medical University Graz, Graz, Austria, [3] Department of Rheumatology, Hospital of Brunico (Südtiroler Sanitätsbetrieb-Azienda Sanitaria dell'Alto Adige), Brunico, Italy

***Correspondence:**
Christian Dejaco
christian.dejaco@gmx.net

Specialty section:
This article was submitted to Rheumatology, a section of the journal Frontiers in Medicine

Background: Inflammatory bowel disease (IBD) is closely associated with spondylarthritis (SpA) and enthesitis, as an important feature of SpA, is a common extraintestinal manifestation of IBD. Enthesitis may be clinically silent in a high proportion of patients with IBD without clinical signs or a diagnosis of SpA.

Objectives: The aim of this study was to compare the prevalence of ultrasound (US) verified enthesitis in IBD patients with and without SpA, with patients with irritable bowel syndrome (IBS) and healthy subjects (HC) serving as controls.

Methods: IBD patients with or without SpA, patients with IBS and HC were prospectively recruited and clinically assessed. Ultrasound examination was performed at 14 entheses. The ultrasound abnormalities were scored according to the Madrid Ankylosing Spondylitis Enthesitis Index (MASEI).

Results: We included 33 IBD patients without SpA, 14 IBD patients with SpA, 26 IBS patients and 18 HC. Higher MASEI scores were found in patients with IBD without SpA [median 21.0 range (8.0–53.0)] and IBD associated SpA [33.0 (8–50)] than in IBS patients [10.5 (0–42.0)-$p < 0.001$ for both comparison] and HC [12.0 (2.0–38.0)-$p < 0.01$]. PD, enthesophytes and erosions were more common in patients with IBD with or without SpA as compared to IBS patients and HC. IBD patients with SpA compared to IBD without SpA demonstrated significant higher prevalence of erosion and structural irregularity and consequently significant higher MASEI ($p < 0.05$ for all comparison).

Conclusions: Ultrasound verified enthesitis is more common in patients with IBD with or without SpA as compared to patients with IBS or HC.

Keywords: enthesitis, spondyloarthropathies, inflammatory bowel diseases, ultrasound, power Doppler ultrasonography

INTRODUCTION

Enthesitis is defined as inflammation of the insertion of tendons, ligaments, and capsules into bone (1). There are some observations suggesting that repeated mechanical overload or excessive irritation of entheses may lead to enthesal inflammation and given that lower limbs are exposed to higher mechanical load, this might explain why enthesitis primarily involves the lower limbs in patients with spondylarthritis (SpA).

Enthesitis is considered to be the initial lesion in SpA that only secondarily involves bone and synovial tissue leading to spondylitis and arthritis (2). The detection of enthesitis at early stages of SpA might be an interesting window of opportunity to treat patients with this disease.

There is a close link between intestinal disease and SpA. We know that 15% of inflammatory bowel disease (IBD) patients develop peripheral SpA and 36% suffer from sacroilitis (3). Besides, subclinical intestinal inflammation has been identified in up to 60–70% of patients with axial SpA (4, 5). Other patients with IBD might present subclinical or abortive forms of SpA which might only later evolve in clinically manifest SpA.

The prevalence of sub-clinical entheseal involvement in IBD patients, detected with ultrasound, seems to be more common in IBD patients compared to the healthy controls and in sum there is no difference between IBD and SpA (6, 7).

Ultrasound has been used to detect subclinical enthesitis, mainly in lower limbs of patients with SpA (8–10). In patients with psoriasis, another disease that is closely related to SpA and where a proportion of patients develop clinical manifestations of SpA, a high prevalence of subclinical enthesitis was detected by imaging. In psoriasis, it has even been observed that ultrasound verified enthesitis predicted the later development of psoriatic arthritis (11, 12). In patients with IBD, reports about the prevalence and the possible predictive value of subclinical enthesitis are scarce despite the known link between axial, articular, and intestinal inflammation.

The aim of the present study was to investigate the prevalence of enthesitis using sonography in patients with IBD without associated SpA and to compare them to patients with IBD associated SpA, irritable bowel syndrome (IBS) and healthy subjects (HC).

METHODS

We prospectively recruited 47 IBD patients: 33 patients had no clinical symptoms or history of SpA [i.e., no axial, articular, or enthesal pain and 14 patients with confirmed SpA fulfilling the ASAS classification criteria (13)]. All patients fulfilled the diagnostic criteria for IBD (14, 15). As controls, we recruited 26 consecutive IBS patients who all fulfilled the Rome criteria for IBS (16) and 18 HC. All patients and controls gave written informed consent to participate in the study, and the study was approved by the institutional ethics committee (Prot. Number: 23-432 ex 10/11).

Clinical Assessment

Demographics, level of regular sport activity (defined as sport or physical activity at least once a week) and body mass index (BMI) were determined in all participants. All patients with IBD underwent routine clinical and laboratory examinations and assessment of IBD activity using the Crohn's disease activity index (CDAI) for patients with Crohn's disease and the partial Mayo score for ulcerative colitis (17, 18). The Bath Ankylosing Spondylitis Disease Activity Index (BASDAI) was determined in all IBD patients (19). Clinical examination of entheses was conducted in all study participants by a rheumatologist blinded to ultrasound results. Enthesitis was defined as tenderness or swelling at clinical examination at the following sites: entheses of the common extensor tendon at lateral epicondyle, distal insertion of the triceps into the olecranon, quadriceps insertion into the upper pole of the patella, patellar tendon insertion into the lower pole of the patella and into the tibial anterior tuberosity, insertion of the Achilles tendon as well as the insertion of plantar aponeurosis into calcaneal bone.

Ultrasound Protocol

Ultrasound examination was performed by one of two investigators blinded to clinical results (CD or RH). In total 14 entheses were examined in every subject: bilateral triceps, lateral epicondyles, distal insertion of quadriceps, proximal and distal insertion of patellar tendon, distal insertion of Achilles tendon and plantar fascia using an Esaote MyLab Twice ultrasound device with 18-MHz linear array transducer (20). B-mode and Power Doppler (PD) sonography was performed in a darkened room in which the temperature was held constant at 20°C. PD-settings were standardized accordingly: frequency 9.1 MHz, pulse repetition frequency 750 Hz and medium persistence. The PD-gain was optimized by increasing gain until noise appeared and then reduced just enough to suppress the noise.

The following abnormalities were scored according to the Madrid Ankylosing Spondylitis Enthesitis Index (MASEI) as appropriate: Power Doppler (PD) changes, enthesophytes, erosions, enthesal thickening, bursitis, and structural abnormalities (21, 22). According to (MASEI): Structure was considered pathological (score = 1) if there was a loss of fibrillar pattern, hypoechoic aspect, or fusiform thickening of the entheses. Erosions were defined as a cortical breakage with a step-down contour defect at the attachment of entheses at bone and graded with 0 = absent or 3 = present. Fascia and tendon thickness were measured at the point of maximum thickness on the bony insertion and graded with 0 = normal or 1 = thickened according to the reference values published previously. Enthesophytes were defined as calcifications at the entheses insertion into bone and graded with 0 = absent, 1 = small calcification, 2 = clear presence of enthesophyte/calcification, 3 = large calcifications or ossifications (see **Figure 1**). PD-signals within entheses were scored with 0 = absent or 3 = present. Bursitis was investigated at the level of distal patellar tendon (infrapatellar bursitis) and at the level of Achilles tendon. Bursitis was defined as a well-circumscribed anechoic or hypoechoic area at the site of an anatomical bursa and which was compressible by the transducer. The total (MASEI) score ranges from 0 to 136 for

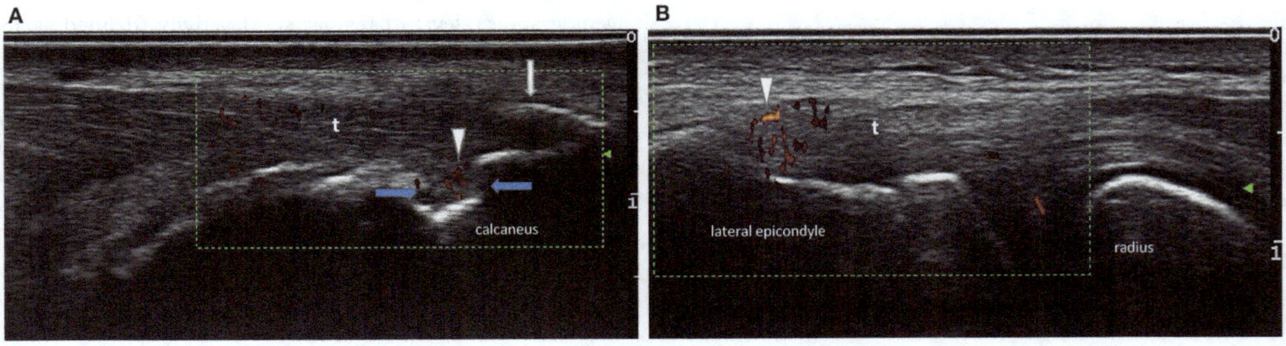

FIGURE 1 | Examples of ultrasound findings. **(A)** Longitudinal scan of a achilles tendon revealing active PD signal (arrows heads), enthesophyt (white arrow), erosion on insertion (blue arrow), **(B)** longitudinal scan of tendon insertion on lateral epicondyl with PD signal (arrow heads), t-tendon.

both sides of 12 entheses. In order to calculate the difference of separate ultrasound findings between the groups we calculated a modified MASEI. The MASEI was modified toward the inclusion of the lateral epicondyle given that this site is incorporated in clinical enthesitis scores such as the Leeds Enthesitis Index (LEI) and because previous studies demonstrated a high prevalence of enthesitis at this site in SpA patients (23–26). For this modified score, only the presence =1 or absence = 0 of each abnormality was counted in order to avoid the higher weighting of PD and erosions (presence of any lesions adds three points to the total score) er of enthesophytes (semiquantitative scale of 0–3) as compared to other lesions.

Statistical Analysis

Statistical analysis was performed using SPSS v22. Descriptive statistics were used to summarize the data. Independent groups of quantitative data were compared with the Student's *T*-Test (parametric) or the Mann-Whitney *U*-test (non-parametric distribution), as appropriate. Correlations analysis was conducted using Pearson *r* (parametric) or Spearman-Rho test (non-parametric data), as appropriate. All statistical analyses were performed using IBM SPSS Statistics (v23.0). Inter-reader agreement between ultrasound examiners was tested in seven patients, in which entheses were scanned by both investigators, and by using the Intra-class correlation coefficient (ICC).

RESULTS

Patients' characteristics are depicted in **Table 1**. A greater proportion of the recruited IBD patients ($n = 47$) were male, however we did not observe any gender-based difference of clinical activity of IBD or the MASEI score within the IBD group. The disease duration of IBD showed no significant correlation with IBD activity or with MASEI score. Crohn disease (CD) and Ulcerative colitis (UC) patients yielded the same frequency of therapy with TNFi, Azathioprine or Masalazine. One (7.1%) patient with CD associated SpA and 6 (18.2%) CD patients showed a CDAI score above 150.

In all examined entheses (n = 1,274, all groups), the most common ultrasound abnormalities were enthesophyte/calcification [n = 397 (31%)], structural irregularity [n = 372 (29%)], increased thickness [n = 303 (24%)], bursitis [n = 101 (8%)], erosions [n = 95 (7%)], and positive PD [n = 58 (5%)].

At least one positive PD-signal was observed in nine (64%) patients with IBD and SpA, in 22 (67%) patients with IBD without SpA, in five (19%) patients with IBS and in four (22%) HC. A highest prevalence of PD was observed at lateral epicondyle [39 entheses (67% of all PD positive enthesis)] followed by distal insertion of patellar tendon [n = 7 (12%)]. A presence of positive PD at lateral epicondyle did not yield significant difference in group IBD with or without SpA but it was significantly higher compared to IBS and HC ($p < 0.01$). The distribution of PD positive enthesitis among the sites investigated was similar in healthy controls. In patients with IBS, however, lateral epicondyle was more commonly involved than the other enthesis ($p < 0.05$). Comparing prevalence of PD signs at other entheses yielded no difference between groups. There was no difference between involvements of left or right sites.

At least one erosion was observed in 11 (79%, group IBD and SpA), 18 (55 %, group IBD without SpA), 10 (39%, group IBS) patients and 2 (11%) HC. The erosions were found more frequently with comparable distribution in the following enthesis: distal insertion of patellar tendon [22 erosions (23% of all erosions)], triceps tendon [n = 19 (20%)] and Achilles tendon [n = 18 (19%)]. Bursitis was most frequently observed in distal insertion of patellar tendon 65 (36% out examined enthesis) and in achileon 29 (16% out examined enthesis). Enthesophytes were most commonly observed in the achilleon, followed by lateral epicondyle, triceps tendon, and distal insertion of patellar tendon.

Higher MASEI scores were found in patients with IBD without SpA [median 21.0 range (8.0–53.0)] and IBD associated SpA [33.0 (8–50)] than in IBS patients [10.5 (0–42.0)-$p < 0.001$ for both comparison] and HC [12.0 (2.0–38.0)-$p < 0.01$ for both comparisons]. The MASEI score was significantly higher in IBD with SpA compared to IBD without SpA ($p < 0.05$). Only one patient with IBS did not reveal any US abnormalities according to the MASEI score.

As shown in the **Table 2**, all separate ultrasound findings were significantly higher in IBD patients with or without SpA than IBS and HC. The modified MASEI score in IBD

TABLE 1 | Clinical characteristics of IBD patients and controls.

	IBD without SpA $n = 33$	IBD with SpA $n = 14$	IBS $n = 26$	HC $n = 18$
Male, n (%)	22 (66.7%)	10 (71.4%)	7 (26.9%) $p < 0.05$*	5 (27.8%) $p < 0.05$*
IBD type	CD $n = 27$ UC $n = 6$	CD $n = 8$ UC $n = 6$		
Age years‡	44 (19–62)	45 (21–56)	41 (18–65)	43 (21–58)
Disease duration of IBD in years‡	10 (1–30)	7.5 (1–21)		
ESR‡	9 (1–45)	10 (3–25)	–	–
CRP‡	3.5 (0.6–39.2)	3 (0.1–41.0)	–	–
Anti-TNF therapy, n (%)	15 (45)	10 (71.4)	–	–
Azathioprin / Mesalazin, n (%)	9 (27) / 7 (21)	1 (7) / 2 (14)		
BASDAI‡	2.99 (0.3–7.1)	3.5(1.4–5.9)	–	–
CDAI†	87.3 (55.5)	84.9 (50.2)		
Partial Mayo score†	4 (1–7)	3.1 (0–5)		
BMI‡	24.9 (17.3–34.1)	24.3 (18.8–38.1)	23.6 (16.3–33.2)	22.5 (19.1–31.2)
Sport activity, n (%)	13 (39)	6 (43)	19 (73.1)	10 (56)
HLA B 27 positive	-	10 (71%)		

‡Median (range); †mean (standard deviation); BASDAI, Bath Ankylosing Spondylitis Disease Activity Index; BMI, Body Mass Index; CDAI, Crohn's Disease Activity Index; CD, Crohn disease; UC, Ulcerative colitis; CRP, C-reactive protein (normal values 0–5 mg/L); ESR, erythrocyte sedimentation rate (normal values 1–10 mm/1st h); MASEI, Madrid Ankylosing Spondylitis Enthesitis Index; Sport activity defined as sport or physical activity at least once a week; IBD with/without SpA inflammatory bowel disease with or without Spondylarthritis; IBS, irritable bowel syndrome; HC, healthy subjects.
**$p < 0.05$ compared to IBD patients without and with SpA.*

with SpA [median 29.5 range (9–51)] und IBD without SpA [median 22.0 range (9–39)] did not show significant difference between each other but it was significantly higher compared to IBS [median 10.5 range (2–32)] and HC [median 11.5 (5–33)]. Patients with IBD and SpA demonstrated significantly more erosions ($p < 0.001$) and structural abnormalities ($p < 0.05$) compared to patients with IBD.

No association was found between clinical IBD activity (CDAI and partial Mayo score) and MASEI, nor between clinical IBD activity and erosion-, PD- and enthesophyte subscores. We found no influence on the enthesitis scores by any current therapy or regular sport activities. Out of 25 patients with ongoing TNFi therapy 16 (64%) received Infliximab, eight (32%) Adalimumab and one (4%) Etanercept. We observed no significant difference in the MASEI score between patients receiving the different TNF inhibitors ($p = 0.75$). Besides, we found significant, moderate correlation of BMI with MASEI in the IBS group ($r = 0.453$, $p < 0.05$) and HC ($r = 0.538$, $p < 0.05$).

TABLE 2 | Distribution of ultrasound findings in IBD patients and control population (IBS and HC).

	Enthesophyte	Structure	Thickness	Bursitis	Erosion	PD
IBD with SpA	7 (0–13)	9 (3–14)	6 (0–9)	1.5 (1.6)	3 (0–4)	1 (0–3)
IBD without SpA	6 (2–14)	6 (0–13)**	4 (0–8)	2 (0–3)	1 (0–4)**	1 (0–2)
IBS	3 (0–12)*	0 (0–9)*	1 (0–12)*	0 (0–3)*	0.5 (0–2)*	0 (0–2)*
HC	4 (0–12)*	1.5 (0–7)*	1.8 (1.9)*	1 (0–4)*	0 (0–2)*	0 (0–3)*

PD, Power Doppler; Structure, pathological structure of the enthesis; IBD with/without SpA, inflammatory bowel disease with or without spondylarthritis; IBS, irritable bowel syndrome; HC, healthy subjects.
Data indicate the median (range) ultrasound score for each abnormalities IBD /IBS per patient or control subjects. Statistical differences were tested with the Wilcoxon test.
**$p < 0.05$ compared to IBD patients without or with SpA.*
***$p < 0.05$ compared to IBD patient with SpA.*

Reliability Exercise

The inter-reader agreement for the MASEI was good, revealing an ICC of 0.89 (0.52–0.98).

DISCUSSION

In the present study we demonstrated that ultrasound verified enthesitis is higher in patients with IBD with or without SpA in comparison to IBS patients and HC. All components of enthesitis were more common in both IBD subgroups.

The most interesting finding of our study is that PD, a sign of active inflammation of entheses, was equally present in patients with IBD with or without associated SpA. Structural changes of entheses including erosions, tended to be higher in IBD with SpA. This also accounted for the higher MASEI score in the latter group. All changes were more common in IBD than in IBS and HC. This indicates that active inflammation of entheses is a common extra-intestinal manifestation in IBD, independent of clinical symptoms of enthesitis (and SpA) as well as IBD activity. Subclinical enthesitis might precede or even predict the development of clinical manifest SpA, as has been the case in psoriasis, but future follow-up studies are required to clarify this issue (11). Structural changes might be the consequence of previous active enthesitis and seem to be linked more closely to clinical features of SpA than PD, but are also independent of current IBD activity.

In our study the prevalence of PD positive enthesis in IBD patients (64%) was higher than reported by Bandinelli at al. who found a positive PD only in 16% IBD patients (6). Possible explanations for the difference are the use of a highly-sensitive 18-MHz linear array transducer in our study compared to a 10-MHz used by Bandinelli. Furthermore, the extensor tendon at lateral epicondyle was frequently a PD positive enthesis in our study and this site was not examined in the Bandinelli study. After the exclusion of lateral epicondyle from the calculation, the distribution of vascularity in IBD patient was in line with other studies like from Rovicso et al. (7). The prevalence of PD and entheseal thickening in IBS and HC in our study was comparable with the data of prevalence of such abnormalities in healthy subjects (27).

The occurrence of a new PsA in a group of patients with asymptomatic enthesitis and in psoriasis was 4.3% during a 2-year observation (12). In CED, 17–39% of patients develop clinically manifest SpA during the course of the disease, however, how many of these cases have asymptomatic enthesitis or other subclinical musculoskeletal manifestation preceding the clinical onset of SpA is unknown and can only be clarified by prospective follow-up studies (28). Our data, however, suggest that the presence of erosion might help in distinguishing between subclinical and definitive SpA in patients with IBD.

Another unresolved issue is the interpretation of clinical and imaging signs of enthesitis in patients with SpA and SpA-related diseases. We know from the present and previous studies that clinical and ultrasound examination of enthesitis only partially overlap. While pain (spontaneous and by palpation) is the most frequent symptom of enthesitis and is also part of the ASAS classification criteria for SpA, it is neither sensitive nor specific for enthesitis, particularly when deep tendon insertions like the plantar facia are affected (29). Nevertheless, little is known about the clinical impact of imaging verified subclinical enthesitis: data is limited on whether patients will develop clinical manifestations of enthesitis later, or if subclinical enthesitis provokes structural damage, or whether it has an impact on the future functionality or quality of life. Further, the response of subclinical, imaging verified enthesitis on anti-inflammatory therapy is unknown. Currently, it is not necessary to treat subclinical enthesitis in IBD patients. Follow-up studies are needed to address these open issues.

While the MASEI included retrocalcaneal and infrapatellar bursitis in the score, bursitis is not considered an elementary lesion of enthesitis according to OMERACT. The OMERACT experts were of the opinion, that bursae are not part of the enthesitis complex and that inflammation affects them only at a later stage of enthesitis when it extends toward the tendon and peri-tendinous structures (30).

While in Rheumatoid arthritis, MSK ultrasound is mainly used to investigate the presence of synovial inflammation, in PsA and SpA it is also applied to investigate enthesitis. Ultrasound verified synovitis in RA predicted the progression of bone erosions and occurrence of a clinical relapse even in the absence of clinical inflammation (31). Whether ultrasound verified synovitis has a similar predictive value in PsA and SpA is unclear. Earlier studies in SpA and PsA demonstrated that ultrasound verified enthesitis does not correlate with clinical signs of enthesitis (20). We previously observed that enthesophytes but neither PD nor clinical tenderness at entheses were linked with radiographic enthesal progression (32). Whether similar result could be found in SpA and whether clinically quiescent but sonographically active enthesitis would predict future clinical worsening are questions that only future research can clarify.

The main strength of our study is the inclusion of IBD patients with and without SpA as well as IBS patients as a relevant control group. While low-grade intestinal inflammation and other factors contribute to the pathophysiology of IBS, there is a clear difference in terms of extra-intestinal enthesal inflammation in comparison to IBD patients, as our data clearly demonstrates. Whether the presence of subclinical enthesitis might also be used for diagnostic purposes (i.e., to differentiate between IBD and IBS patients, needs to be evaluated further). We also took into account the possible influence of external factors such as sport and BMI on the level of enthesitis, however no relevant association was observed in our IBD group.

The main limitations of our study are the limited sample size and the absence of follow-up data which would have been important to analyse the relevance of subclinical enthesitis for future outcomes as stated above. Other limitations are the relatively low level of clinical activity (concerning the intestine) of IBD patients, as well as the heterogeneity of them in regard to disease duration and treatment. All these factors, however, had no influence on the level of ultrasound verified enthesitis in our analyses.

In conclusion, ultrasound verified enthesitis components are more common in patients with IBD with or without SpA as compared to patients with IBS or HC.

ETHICS STATEMENT

The studies involving human participants were reviewed and approved by Ethikkommission der Medizinischen Universität Graz. The patients/participants provided their written informed consent to participate in this study.

AUTHOR CONTRIBUTIONS

RH, CD, PK, and CH substantially contributed to study conception and design, acquisition of data, and analysis and interpretation of data. AL was involved in planning, acquisition of data, and supervised the work. RH and CD wrote the paper. All the authors revised the paper and approved the final version of the article to be published.

ACKNOWLEDGMENTS

The content of this manuscript has been presented in part at the EULAR 2015, SAT0628 High Prevalence of Ultrasound Verified Enthesitis in Patients with Inflammatory Bowel Disease with or without Spondylarthritis, Annals of the Rheumatic Diseases 2015;74:888–889.

REFERENCES

1. McGonagle D, Khan MA, Marzo-Ortega H, O'Connor P, Gibbon W, Emery P. Enthesitis in spondyloarthropathy. *Curr Opin Rheumatol.* (1999) 11:244–50. doi: 10.1097/00002281-199907000-00004
2. McGonagle D, Gibbon W, Emery P. Classification of inflammatory arthritis by enthesitis. *Lancet.* (1998) 352:1137–40. doi: 10.1016/S0140-6736(97)12004-9
3. Turkcapar N, Toruner M, Soykan I, Aydintug OT, Cetinkaya H, Duzgun N, et al. The prevalence of extraintestinal manifestations and HLA association in patients with inflammatory bowel disease. *Rheumatol Int.* (2006) 26:663–8. doi: 10.1007/s00296-005-0044-9
4. Harbord M, Annese V, Vavricka SR, Allez M, Acosta MB de, Boberg KM, et al. The first european evidence-based consensus on extra-intestinal manifestations in inflammatory bowel disease. *J Crohn's Colitis.* (2016) 10:239–54. doi: 10.1093/ecco-jcc/jjv213
5. Mielants H, Veys EM, Cuvelier C, De Vos M, Goemaere S, De Clercq L, et al. The evolution of spondyloarthropathies in relation to gut histology. III. Relation between gut and joint. *J Rheumatol.* (1995) 22:2279–84.
6. Bandinelli F, Milla M, Genise S, Giovannini L, Bagnoli S, Candelieri A, et al. Ultrasound discloses entheseal involvement in inactive and low active inflammatory bowel disease without clinical signs and symptoms of spondyloarthropathy. *Rheumatology.* (2011) 50:1275–9. doi: 10.1093/rheumatology/keq447
7. Rovisco J, Duarte C, Batticcioto A, Sarzi-Puttini P, Dragresshi A, Portela F, et al. Hidden musculoskeletal involvement in inflammatory bowel disease: a multicenter ultrasound study. *BMC Musculoskelet Disord.* (2016) 17:1–7. doi: 10.1186/s12891-016-0932-z
8. Lehtinen A, Taavitsainen M, Leirisalo-Repo M. Sonographic analysis of enthesopathy in the lower extremities of patients with spondylarthropathy. *Clin Exp Rheumatol.* (1994) 12:143–8.
9. Kiris A, Kaya A, Ozgocmen S, Kocakoc E. Assessment of enthesitis in ankylosing spondylitis by power Doppler ultrasonography. *Skeletal Radiol.* (2006) 35:522–8. doi: 10.1007/s00256-005-0071-3
10. Gisondi P, Tinazzi I, El-Dalati G, Gallo M, Biasi D, Barbara LM, et al. Lower limb enthesopathy in patients with psoriasis without clinical signs of arthropathy: a hospital-based case-control study. *Ann Rheum Dis.* (2008) 67:26–30. doi: 10.1136/ard.2007.075101
11. El Miedany Y, El Gaafary M, Youssef S, Ahmed I, Nasr A. Tailored approach to early psoriatic arthritis patients: clinical and ultrasonographic predictors for structural joint damage. *Clin Rheumatol.* (2015) 34:307–13. doi: 10.1007/s10067-014-2630-2
12. Elnady B, El Shaarawy NK, Dawoud NM, Elkhouly T, Desouky DES, ElShafey EN, et al. Subclinical synovitis and enthesitis in psoriasis patients and controls by ultrasonography in Saudi Arabia; incidence of psoriatic arthritis during 2 years. *Clin Rheumatol.* (2019) 38:1627–35. doi: 10.1007/s10067-019-04445-0
13. Rudwaleit M, van der Heijde D, Landewé R, Akkoc N, Brandt J, Chou CT, et al. The Assessment of SpondyloArthritis International Society classification criteria for peripheral spondyloarthritis and for spondyloarthritis in general. *Ann Rheum Dis.* (2011) 70:25–31. doi: 10.1136/ard.2010.133645
14. Gomollón F, Dignass A, Annese V, Tilg H, Van Assche G, Lindsay JO, et al. 3rd European evidence-based consensus on the diagnosis and management of crohn's disease 2016: part 1: diagnosis and medical management. *J Crohns Colitis.* (2017) 11:3–25. doi: 10.1093/ecco-jcc/jjw168
15. Magro F, Gionchetti P, Eliakim R, Ardizzone S, Armuzzi A, Barreiro-de Acosta M, et al. Third European evidence-based consensus on diagnosis and management of ulcerative colitis. Part 1: definitions, diagnosis, extra-intestinal manifestations, pregnancy, cancer surveillance, surgery, and ileo-anal pouch disorders. *J Crohns Colitis.* (2017) 11:649–70. doi: 10.1093/ecco-jcc/jjx008
16. Longstreth GF, Thompson WG, Chey WD, Houghton La, Mearin F, Spiller RC. Functional bowel disorders. *Gastroenterology.* (2006) 130:1480–91. doi: 10.1053/j.gastro.2005.11.061
17. Best WR, Becktel JM, Singleton JW, Kern FJ. Development of a Crohn's disease activity index. National Cooperative Crohn's Disease Study. *Gastroenterology.* (1976) 70:439–44. doi: 10.1016/S0016-5085(76)80163-1
18. Moss AC, Farrell RJ. Infliximab for induction and maintenance therapy for ulcerative colitis. *Gastroenterology.* (2006) 131:1649–51. doi: 10.1053/j.gastro.2006.09.039
19. Garrett S, Jenkinson T, Kennedy LG, Whitelock H, Gaisford P, Calin A. A new approach to defining disease status in ankylosing spondylitis: the Bath Ankylosing Spondylitis Disease Activity Index. *J Rheumatol.* (1994) 21:2286–91.
20. Husic R, Gretler J, Felber A, Graninger WB, Duftner C, Hermann J, et al. Disparity between ultrasound and clinical findings in psoriatic arthritis. *Ann Rheum Dis.* (2014) 73:1529–36. doi: 10.1136/annrheumdis-2012-203073
21. Balint PV, Kane D, Wilson H, McInnes IB, Sturrock RD. Ultrasonography of entheseal insertions in the lower limb in spondyloarthropathy. *Ann Rheum Dis.* (2002) 61:905–10. doi: 10.1136/ard.61.10.905
22. Miguel E de, Cobo T, Mun S, Naredo E, Uso J, Acebes JC. Validity of enthesis ultrasound assessment in spondyloarthropathy. *Ann Rheum Dis.* (2009) 68:169–74. doi: 10.1136/ard.2007.084251
23. Healy PJ, Helliwell PS. Measuring clinical enthesitis in psoriatic arthritis: assessment of existing measures and development of an instrument specific to psoriatic arthritis. *Arthritis Rheum.* (2008) 59:686–91. doi: 10.1002/art.23568
24. Ficjan A, Husic R, Gretler J, Lackner A, Graninger WB, Gutierrez M, et al. Ultrasound composite scores for the assessment of inflammatory and structural pathologies in Psoriatic Arthritis (PsASon-Score). *Arthritis Res Ther.* (2014) 16:1–13. doi: 10.1186/s13075-014-0476-2
25. Mouterde G, Aegerter P, Correas J-M, Breban M, D'Agostino M-A. Value of contrast-enhanced ultrasonography for the detection and quantification of enthesitis vascularization in patients with spondyloarthritis. *Arthritis Care Res.* (2014) 66:131–8. doi: 10.1002/acr.22195
26. Tom S, Zhong Y, Cook R, Aydin SZ, Kaeley G, Eder L. Development of a preliminary ultrasonographic enthesitis score in psoriatic arthritis—GRAPPA ultrasound working group. *J Rheumatol.* (2019) 46:384–90. doi: 10.3899/jrheum.171465
27. Di Matteo A, Filippucci E, Cipolletta E, Martire V, Jesus D, Musca A, et al. How normal is the enthesis by ultrasound in healthy subjects? *Clin Exp Rheumatol.* (2020) 38:472–8.
28. Peluso R, Di Minno MND, Iervolino S, Manguso F, Tramontano G, Ambrosino P, et al. Enteropathic spondyloarthritis: from diagnosis to treatment. *Clin Dev Immunol.* (2013) 2013:631408. doi: 10.1155/2013/631408
29. Klauser AS, Wipfler E, Dejaco C, Moriggl B, Duftner C, Schirmer M. Diagnostic values of history and clinical examination to predict ultrasound signs of chronic and acute enthesitis. *Clin Exp Rheumatol.* (2008) 26:548–53.
30. Balint PV, Terslev L, Aegerter P, Bruyn GAW, Chary-Valckenaere I, Gandjbakhch F, et al. Reliability of a consensus-based ultrasound definition and scoring for enthesitis in spondyloarthritis and psoriatic arthritis: an OMERACT US initiative. *Ann Rheum Dis.* (2018) 77:1730–5. doi: 10.1136/annrheumdis-2018-213609
31. Brown AK, Quinn MA, Karim Z, Conaghan PG, Peterfy CG, Hensor E, et al. Presence of significant synovitis in rheumatoid arthritis patients with disease-modifying antirheumatic drug-induced clinical remission: evidence from an imaging study may explain structural progression. *Arthritis Rheum.* (2006) 54:3761–73. doi: 10.1002/art.22190
32. Lackner A, Heber D, Bosch P, Adelsmayr G, Duftner C, Ficjan A, et al. Ultrasound verified enthesophytes are associated with radiographic progression at entheses in psoriatic arthritis. *Rheumatology.* (2020) 28:1–5. doi: 10.1093/rheumatology/keaa028

24

Automatic Quantification of Interstitial Lung Disease From Chest Computed Tomography in Systemic Sclerosis

Alysson Roncally S. Carvalho[1,2,3*], *Alan R. Guimarães*[2], *Flávio R. Sztajnbok*[4], *Rosana Souza Rodrigues*[5,6], *Bruno Rangel Antunes Silva*[7], *Agnaldo José Lopes*[7], *Walter Araujo Zin*[3], *Isabel Almeida*[8] *and Manuela Maria França*[9]

[1] *Department of Radiology, Medical School, Centro Hospitalar Universitário do Porto (CHUP), Instituto de Ciências Biomédicas Abel Salazar (ICBAS), Porto University, Porto, Portugal,* [2] *Laboratory of Pulmonary Engineering, Biomedical Engineering Program, Alberto Luiz Coimbra Institute of Post-Graduation and Research in Engineering, Universidade Federal do Rio de Janeiro, Rio de Janeiro, Brazil,* [3] *Laboratory of Respiration Physiology, Carlos Chagas Filho Institute of Biophysics, Universidade Federal do Rio de Janeiro, Rio de Janeiro, Brazil,* [4] *Division of Pediatric Rheumatology, State University of Rio de Janeiro, Rio de Janeiro, Brazil,* [5] *Department of Radiology, Universidade Federal do Rio de Janeiro, Rio de Janeiro, Brazil,* [6] *IDOR - D'Or Institute for Research and Education, Rio de Janeiro, Brazil,* [7] *Graduate Program in Medical Sciences, School of Medical Sciences, State University of Rio de Janeiro, Rio de Janeiro, Brazil,* [8] *Clinical Immunology Unit, Deptartment of Medicine, Centro Hospitalar Universitário do Porto (CHUP), Instituto de Ciências Biomédicas Abel Salazar (ICBAS), Porto University, Porto, Portugal,* [9] *Radiology Department, Centro Hospitalar Universitário do Porto (CHUP), Instituto de Ciências Biomédicas Abel Salazar (ICBAS), Porto University, Porto, Portugal*

Correspondence:
Alysson Roncally S. Carvalho
roncally.carvalho@gmail.com

Background: Interstitial lung disease (ILD) is a common complication in patients with systemic sclerosis (SSc), and its diagnosis contributes to early treatment decisions.

Purposes: To quantify ILD associated with SSc (SSc-ILD) from chest CT images using an automatic quantification method based on the computation of the weight of interstitial lung opacities.

Methods: Ninety-four patients with SSc underwent CT, forced vital capacity (FVC), and carbon monoxide diffusion capacity (DL_{CO}) tests. Seventy-three healthy individuals without radiological evidence of lung disease served as controls. After lung and airway segmentation, the ratio between the weight of interstitial opacities [densities between −500 and +50 Hounsfield units (HU)] and the total lung weight (densities between −1,000 and +50 HU) was used as an ILD indicator (ILD[%] $= 100 \times [LW_{(-500\text{ to }+50HU)}/LW_{(-1,000\text{ to }+50HU)}]$). The cutoff of normality between controls and SSc was determined with a receiver operator characteristic curve. The severity of pulmonary involvement in SSc patients was also assessed by calculating *Z* scores of ILD relative to the average interstitial opacities in controls. Accordingly, SSc-ILD was classified as SSc Limited-ILD (Z score < 3) and SSc Extensive-ILD (Z score ≥ 3 or FVC $< 70\%$).

Results: Seventy-eight (83%) SSc patients were classified as presenting SSc-ILD (optimal ILD threshold of 23.4%, 0.83 sensitivity, 0.92 specificity, and 0.94 area under the receiver operator characteristic curve, 95% CI from 0.89 to 0.96, 0.93 positive predictive value, and 0.81 negative predictive value, $p < 0.001$) and exhibited radiological attenuations compatible with interstitial pneumonia dispersed in the lung parenchyma.

Thirty-six (38%) patients were classified as SSc Extensive-ILD (ILD threshold $\geq$ 29.6% equivalent to a Z score $\geq$ 3) and 42 (45%) as SSc Limited-ILD. Eighteen (50%) patients with SSc Extensive-ILD presented FVC < 70%, being only five patients classified exclusively based on FVC. SSc Extensive-ILD also presented lower DL_{CO} (57.9 $\pm$ 17.9% vs. 73.7 $\pm$ 19.8%; $p < 0.001$) and total lung volume (2,916 $\pm$ 674 vs. 4,286 $\pm$ 1,136, $p < 0.001$) compared with SSc Limited-ILD.

Conclusion: The proposed method seems to provide an alternative to identify and quantify the extension of ILD in patients with SSc, mitigating the subjectivity of semiquantitative analyzes based on visual scores.

Keywords: systemic sclerosis, interstitial lung disease, chest computed tomography, quantitative chest CT-analysis, densitometry

KEY RESULTS

- Quantitative analysis of chest CT scans by densitometry was able to quantify the extent of interstitial lung disease associated with systemic sclerosis (SSc).
- Extensive pulmonary involvement in SSc subjects was associated with pulmonary function impairment.
- Interstitial lung disease almost completely involves lung parenchyma in patients classified as with SSc extensive—interstitial lung disease.

INTRODUCTION

Systemic sclerosis (SSc) is a rare multisystemic disease with heterogeneous clinical presentation characterized by extensive fibrosis and autoimmune and vascular dysfunction that may progress to multiple organ dysfunction including skin, lung, heart, and kidney involvement (1).

SSc clinical evolution is commonly insidious, progressive, and irreversible with considerable morbidity and mortality (2). The most common imaging and histopathologic pattern observed on computed tomography (CT) and surgical lung biopsy is nonspecific interstitial pneumonia (NSIP) (3, 4). On histopathology, this pattern is characterized by a relatively homogeneous thickening of the alveolar walls caused by inflammation (cellular-NSIP) and/or fibrosis (fibrotic-NSIP). In cellular-NSIP, alveolar septa are thickened by infiltration of lymphocytes and plasma cells, whereas in fibrotic-NSIP, the thickening is more related to collagen deposition (5). Chest CT findings usually reflect the histological pattern and are mainly characterized by ground-glass opacities, especially in cellular-NSIP. Interstitial reticular thickening with traction bronchiectasis and some focal consolidation are more frequently observed in fibrotic-NSIP (2).

As ILD associated with SSc (SSc-ILD) occurs in more than half of SSc patients (6) and as the extent of pulmonary involvement is quite variable, the severity of symptoms ranges from subclinical symptoms up to respiratory failure and death (7). Assuming that SSc-ILD considerably impacts morbidity and mortality, the early identification of patients with pulmonary involvement might help to mitigate both disease progression and severity of respiratory symptoms (2, 6).

CT is the gold standard for SSc-ILD detection (8). However, the visual quantification of ILD extension by CT generally results in low agreement even among experienced radiologists (9, 10). On the other hand, the quantitative assessment of chest CT, using dedicated software and methods, might overcome the observational limitation by quantifying the lung volume and tissue fraction in a voxel-by-voxel basis, allowing a more accurate calculation of the degree of pulmonary involvement (11, 12).

The main objective of this study was to assess whether the ratio between the weight of the interstitial opacities [densities between −500 and +50 Hounsfield units (HU)] and the total lung weight (LW) (densities between −1,000 and +50 HU) expressed in percentage values can be used as an ILD indicator. It is also intended to investigate the association between ILD severity and lung function impairment based on the assessment of forced vital capacity (FVC) and carbon monoxide diffusion capacity (DL_{CO}).

MATERIALS AND METHODS

Patients

This study reviewed CT and pulmonary function tests from 94 patients with SSc followed up at the Policlínica Piquet Carneiro da Universidade do Estado do Rio de Janeiro, Rio de Janeiro, Brazil, and at Centro Hospitalar Universitário do Porto, Porto, Portugal.

Patients had been diagnosed in accordance with ACR/EULAR criteria (13). Patients with clinical instability, history of respiratory infection 3 weeks before CT, who were previously or are currently smoking, with evidence of overlapping of scleroderma with other connective tissue diseases, and with a report of previous tracheal or pleuropulmonary disease not related to scleroderma were not included.

Cutaneous involvement was classified as limited (lc-SSc; thickening of the skin distal to the elbows and knees and proximal to the clavicles, including the face) or diffuse (dc-SSc; thickening of the proximal skin as well as of the skin distal to the elbows and knees and including the trunk and face) (14).

Anti-topoisomerase I (Scl-70) and anti-centromere (ACA) antibodies were determined by indirect immunofluorescence using Hep-2 cells as substrates, and autoantibody specificities were further assessed by ELISA (Shield, Dundee, UK).

Seventy-three none smoking healthy individuals with no chronic tracheal or pleuropulmonary diseases, chest CT scans without radiological abnormalities, and matched anthropometrically with SSc patients served as controls.

The protocol was approved at the Research Ethics Committee from the Universidade do Estado do Rio de Janeiro (CAAE-50752615.9.0000.5259) and Centro Hospitalar Universitário do Porto (reference number 2019.353, 288-DEFI/307-CE), and it complied with the current national and international standards.

Pulmonary Function Tests

FVC, DL_{CO}, and DL_{CO} adjusted to alveolar volume (DL_{CO}/VA) were reviewed and expressed as percentages of the predicted values (15–18). Additionally, FVC(%)/DL_{CO}(%) ratio was calculated in subjects with severe reduced DL_{CO} (<55% predicted) to assess isolated pulmonary hypertension (19). The maximal accepted interval between pulmonary function and CT acquisition was 3 months in SSc patients.

Chest Computed Tomography Acquisition

CT scans were performed on a 64-channel multi-slice (Brilliance 40 scanner, Philips Medical Systems, Cleveland, OH, USA, and General Electrics Lightspeed VCT, Chicago Illinois, USA). The acquisitions were gathered in the axial plane with patients in the supine position with 120 kV and 120–300 mA (these parameters varied according to the biotype of the patient), slice thickness of 2 mm with 50% superposition. After the acquisition, all images were reconstructed with a matrix of 512 × 512/728 × 728 voxels using standard reconstruction algorithms.

Imaging Processing

Lung segmentation and airway segmentation were performed (20), and images were then exported to an in-house developed software (QUALI) written in MATLAB® (MathWorks®, Natick, MA, USA).

Before densitometry calculation, the average densities expressed in HU of air inside the trachea (HU_{Air}) and blood in the descending aorta (HU_{Tissue}) were measured (QUALI software). The intensity values of all voxels in lung parenchyma were then linearly rescaled, considering that HU_{Air} and HU_{Tissue} should be equal to −1,000 and +50 HU, respectively (21, 22).

Total lung volume (TLV) was calculated as previously described (23). LW, in grams, was calculated as:

$$\text{LW (g)} = [(\text{HU} - \text{HU}_{\text{Air}})/(\text{HU}_{\text{Aorta}} - \text{HU}_{\text{Air}})] \times \text{voxel volume} \times 1.04\ \text{g/ml} \quad (1)$$

where 1.04 mg/ml means lung tissue density, and HU is voxel density in an HU (21).

Additionally, LW related to hyperinflated (−1,000 to −901 HU), normally aerated (−900 to −501 HU), and to interstitial opacities (−500 to +50 HU) areas were also calculated and normalized to the whole LW (23).

Regional Densitometry Assessment

LW was calculated in three sub-volumes equally divided considering the number of slices, from the basal to the apical (basal, middle, and apical lung thirds), and was used for regional densitometry assessment. LW at regions of interest generated by an erosion process performed from the outermost layer of the 10-mm-thick pulmonary parenchyma, progressing to the hilar

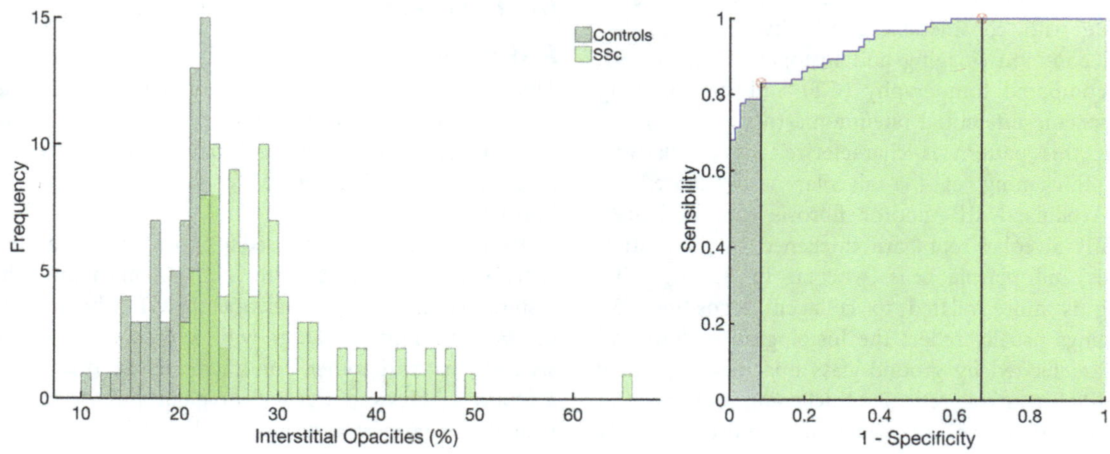

FIGURE 1 | Left panel: histograms of the frequency of occurrence of interstitial opacities in the control group (light green) and in patients with systemic sclerosis (SSc, in dark green). Right panel: receiver operator characteristic curve with the area under the curve (AUC) hatched in light green. Vertical lines mark the normality cutoff (equivalent to 23.4% of total lung weight represented by interstitial opacites) and the *Z* score = 3 (equivalent to 29.6% of the total lung weight and used to classify SSc patients as with extensive interstitial lung disease, SSc-Extensive ILD). Between the normality cutoff up to *Z* score < 3, SSc patients were classified as with limited interstitial lung disease. Use of interstitial opacities as an indicator of ILD presented 0.83 sensitivity, 0.92 specificity, with an receiver operator characteristic curve with the area under the curve of 0.94; 95% from CI 0.89–0.96 ($p < 0.001$) and 0.93 positive predictive value and 0.81 negative predictive value.

regions in 10-mm steps, until the entire pulmonary parenchyma was also calculated.

Identification of Systemic Sclerosis Patients With Interstitial Lung Disease

After lung and airway segmentation, the ratio between the weight of voxels with densities between −500 and +50 HU and the total LW ($100 \times [LW_{(-500\ to\ +50HU)}/LW_{(-1{,}000\ to\ +50HU)}]$) was defined as an indicator of ILD. The cutoff of normality between controls and SSc was determined with a receiver operator characteristic (ROC) curve (**Figure 1**). The severity of pulmonary involvement in SSc patients was also assessed by calculating *Z* scores of ILD relative to the average interstitial opacities in controls. Accordingly, SSc-ILD patients were classified as SSc Limited-ILD (Z score < 3) and SSc Extensive-ILD (Z score ≥ 3). To increase sensitivity, all SSc patients with FVC < 70% were reclassified as SSc Extensive-ILD (24).

Statistical Analysis

The normality of the data (Kolmogorov–Smirnov test with Lilliefors' correction) and the homogeneity of variances (Levene median test) were tested. As both conditions were always satisfied, all data are presented as mean and standard deviation.

From the ROC curve, the threshold limit, sensitivity, specificity, the area under the ROC curve, and bootstrapped 95% confidence intervals (CIs) (bias-corrected and accelerated), as well as positive and negative predictive values were assessed.

SSc-ILD and SSc without (SSc No-ILD) ILD were compared with a Student's *t*-test for independent samples. An ANOVA test followed by Bonferroni *post hoc* test assessed statistical differences among SSc Extensive-ILD, SSc Limited-ILD, and SSc No-ILD. Spearman correlation coefficient (r) was calculated to evaluate the associations between FVC, DL_{CO}, and DL_{CO}/VA with ILD-Extent in SSc patients. The criterion for determining significance was 5%. Statistical analysis was performed using Matlab® software (MathWorks®, Natick, MA, USA).

TABLE 1 | Demographic characteristics, clinical features, pulmonary function tests, and densitometry of the control group and scleroderma patients.

	SSc (94)	Control group (73)	*p*-value
Demographic data			
Females	87 (92.5%)	64 (87.7%)	
Age (years)	54.5 ± 13.5	57.9 ± 20.0	0.19
BMI (kg/m²)	25.4 ± 5.5	26.2 ± 4.3	0.27
SSc cutaneous involvement			
lc-SSc	64 (68.1%)	–	–
dc-SSc	30 (31.9%)	–	–
Type of antibody			
Anti-topoisomerase I antibody	13 (13.8%)	–	–
Anti-centromere antibody	50 (53.2%)	–	–
Anti-RNA polymerase III	3 (3.2%)	–	–
Autoantibody not identified	28 (29.8%)	–	–
Lung function			
FVC (% predicted)	98.0 ± 26.9	–	–
DL_{CO}/VA (% predicted)	81.3 ± 18.6	–	–
DL_{CO} (% predicted)	69.9 ± 20.8	–	–
Densitometry			
TLV (ml)	**3,804.8 ± 1,160.9**	**4,170.7 ± 755.3**	**0.021**
Total $LT_{Fraction}$ (g)	**738.8 ± 156.1**	**611.4 ± 144.9**	**<0.001**
Hyperinflated (%)	**7.9 ± 4.7**	**18.0 ± 8.6**	**<0.001**
Normally aerated (%)	62.6 ± 7.1	62.0 ± 10.2	0.651
Interstitial opacities (%)	**29.5 ± 8.1**	**20.0 ± 3.2**	**<0.011**

Values are presented as mean ± standard deviation or number (percentage value). Bold characters indicate statistically significant differences. BMI, body mass index; lc-SSc, limited skin form; dc-SSc, diffuse skin form; FVC (%), forced vital capacity expressed as predicted values; DL_{CO}/VA, carbon monoxide diffusion capacity adjusted for alveolar volume expressed as predicted values; DL_{CO} (%), carbon monoxide diffusion capacity expressed as predicted values; TLV, total lung volume; Total $LT_{Fraction}$, lung tissue fraction related to densities from −1,000 to +50 Hounsfield units (HU); Hyperinflated, tissue fraction related to densities from −1,000 to −901 HU; Normally Aerated, tissue fraction related to densities from −900 to −501 HU; Interstitial Opacities, lung weight related to densities from −500 to +50 HU.

RESULTS

In SSc patients, the mean age at CT review was 54.5 ± 13.5 years, and 87 (92.5%) were women ($p = 0.19$ vs. controls). The disease durations were 4.21 ± 2.50 years from the onset of the non-Raynaud phenomenon and 9.65 ± 5.13 years from the onset of the Raynaud phenomenon. Sixty-four patients (68.1%) had lc-SSc, and 30 (31.9%) presented dc-SSc. Anti-topoisomerase I (Scl-70) antibody, anti-centromere antibody (ACA), and anti-RNA polymerase III were positive in 13 (13.8%), 50 (53.2%), and 3 (3.2%) patients, respectively. Twenty-eight patients (29.8%) did not present autoantibodies (**Table 1**).

SSc presented a significant reduction in TLV, whereas total LW and LW related to hyperinflated and interstitial opacities were significantly higher in SSc compared with those in controls (**Table 1**).

Seventy-eight (83%) SSc patients were classified as presenting SSc-ILD based on the ROC curve with an optimal ILD threshold of 23.4%, 0.83 sensitivity, 0.92 specificity, and 0.94 area under the ROC curve; 95% from CI 0.89–0.96 ($p < 0.001$), 0.93 positive predictive value, and 0.81 negative predictive value (**Figure 1**).

Thirty-six (38%) patients were classified as SSc Extensive-ILD (ILD threshold of 29.6%, 0.32 sensitivity, and 1.00 specificity) and exhibited radiological attenuations compatible with interstitial pneumonia diffusely distributed in the lung parenchyma (**Figure 2**, uppermost row). Forty-two (45%) patients were classified as SSc Limited-ILD, and radiological attenuations were mainly distributed in basal and middle lung thirds (**Figure 2**, second row). In SSc patients, SSc-ILDs, color-coded in green, were therefore interpreted, in addition to the peribronchial vessels, as ground-glass opacities, reticular consolidations, and possible compressed tissues broadly spread over the lung parenchyma (**Figure 2**, rightmost column). Note that the pattern of involvement of lung parenchyma differed between Extensive- and Limited-ILDs.

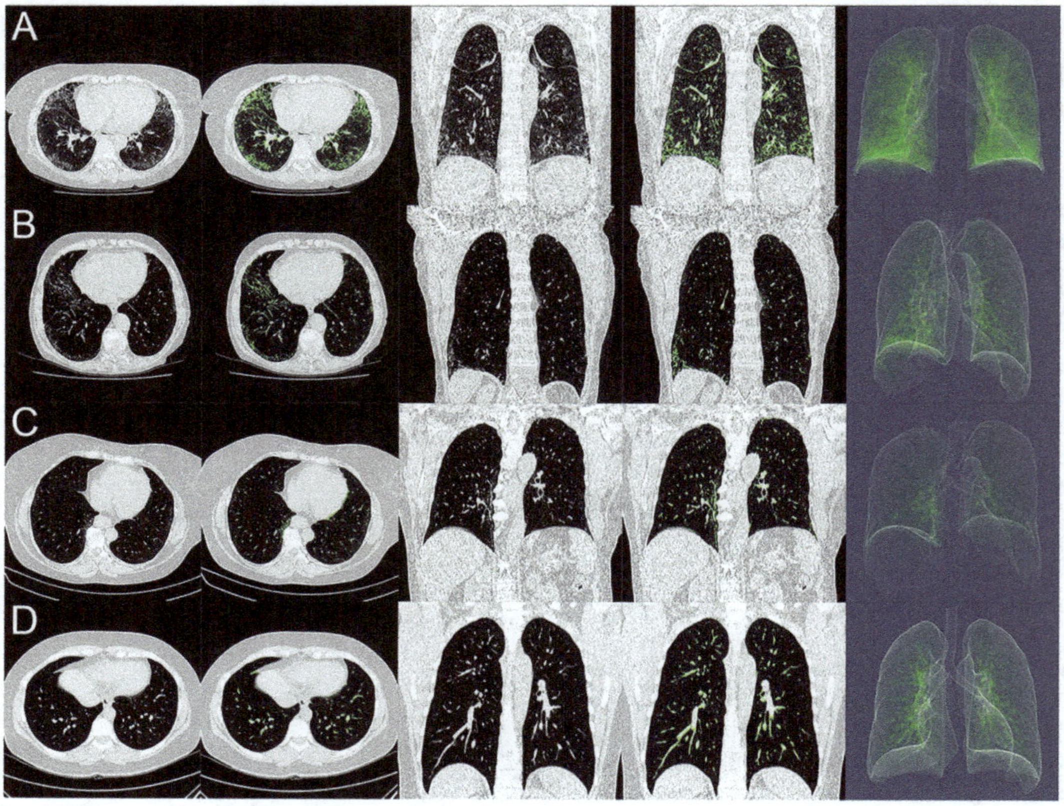

FIGURE 2 | (A–D) Show axial (columns 1 and 2) and coronal (columns 3 and 4) CT scans and three-dimensional rendering (column 5) of the lung of systemic sclerosis classified as with extensive interstitial lung disease (SSc Extensive-ILD, **A**), as with limited interstitial lung disease (SSc Limited-ILD, **B**), as with no interstitial lung disease (SSc No-ILD, **C**), and controls **(D)**. Note, in **(A)**, predominance of ground glass/reticular consolidation and compressed tissue likely related to cellular/fibrotic nonspecific interstitial pneumonia at basal lung third. Those in green are represented interstitial opacities with densities ranging from −500 and +50 HU that would represent the extent of pulmonary involvement.

In controls, interstitial opacities mainly represented peribronchial vessels and some ground glass (**Figure 2**, lowermost row), especially in dorsal–basal-dependent regions in older subjects (age $\geq$ 60 years) being quite comparable with SSc No-ILD patients (**Figure 2**, third row).

Eighteen (50%) patients with SSc Extensive-ILD presented FVC $< 70\%$, being five patients initially classified as SSc Limited-ILD, and in only three SSc (8%) Extensive-ILD, a severe restrictive pattern (FVC $< 50\%$) was observed. Moreover, SSc Extensive-ILD presented lower DL_{CO} (57.9 $\pm$ 17.9% vs. 73.7 $\pm$ 19.8%; $p < 0.001$) and TLV (2,916 $\pm$ 674 vs. 4,286 $\pm$ 1,136, $p < 0.001$), hyperinflated, and normally aerated tissue fraction, but not lower DL_{CO}/VA and total LW compared with those in SSc Limited-ILD (**Table 2**).

Moreover, the proportion of FVC/DL_{CO} ratio higher than 1.4 in subjects with severe DL_{CO} reduction ($DL_{CO} < 55\%$) was very similar to that in patients with Extensive- and Limited-ILDs (22 and 21%, respectively).

Noteworthy, in five (31%) SSc No-ILD patients, a moderate reduction in DL_{CO} ($55\% < DL_{CO} < 80\%$) was observed with DL_{CO} ranging from 62 to 76% despite presenting no evidence of a restrictive pattern in spirometry. Additionally, the frequencies of occurrence of positive anti-topoisomerase I (ATA-1) and anti-centromere antibodies (ACA) were quite similar among SSc patients with no apparent relationship with ILD extent (**Table 2**).

In **Figure 3**, volume and tissue fractions are plotted against densities in HU. A reduction in the peak of volume and tissue fractions at densities related to normally aerated areas and a right-shift toward densities related to ground-glass opacities and consolidation were observed. In the **Supplementary Material**, videos of representative cases of SSc Extensive-ILD, Limited-ILD, and No-ILD are presented in axial and coronal slices (**Supplementary Videos 1–6**). Thus, it is possible to compare how tissue fractions vs. density relationships of patients with SSc differ from the control group, as the lung is visualized in axial and coronal sections.

Figure 4 presents the correlations between ILD extent, FVC (left panel), DL_{CO} (middle panel), and DL_{CO}/VA (right panel). A significant inverse and moderate to poor correlation were observed between ILD Extent and FVC ($r = -0.57$, $p < 0.001$) and between ILD extent and DL_{CO} ($r = -0.49$, $p < 0.001$) but not with DL_{CO}/VA ($r = 0.009$, $p = 0.99$).

Figure 5, upper panels, depicts ILD extent in the whole lung and the basal, middle, and apical thirds. Additionally, the extent of the pulmonary involvement from the subpleural layers to hilar

TABLE 2 | Demographic variables, pulmonary function tests, and densitometry considering scleroderma patients with less or greater pulmonary involvement.

	SSc-ILD (78)	**SSc No-ILD (16)**	***p*-value**	
	SSc extensive- ILD (36)	**SSc limited-ILD (42)**		
Demographic data				
Females	34 (94%)	38 (90%)	15 (94%)	
Age (years)	51.7 ± 14.6	58.9 ± 12.3	49.5 ± 11.0	
BMI (kg/m^2)	25.8 ± 5.9	25.0 ± 5.7	25.4 ± 4.4	
SSc cutaneous involvement				
lc-SSc	22 (23%)	30 (32%)	12 (13%)	
dc-SSc	14 (15%)	12 (13%)	4 (4%)	
Type of antibody				
Anti-topoisomerase I antibody	4 (4%)	5 (5%)	4 (4%)	
Anti-centromere antibody	23 (24%)	25 (27%)	2 (2%)	
Anti-RNA polymerase III	–	2 (2%)	1 (1%)	
Autoantibody not identified	9 (9%)	10 (11%)	9 (9%)	
Pulmonary function tests				
FVC (% predicted)	**74.6 ± 22.0[a,b]**	**112.1 ± 18.5**	**113.5 ± 17.0**	**<0.001[a,b]**
50% < FVC < 70%	18 (50%)	0 (0%)	0 (0%)	
FVC < 50%	3 (8%)	0 (0%)	0 (0%)	
DL_{CO}/VA (% predicted)	84.1 ± 20.2	76.2 ± 18.5	88.3 ± 11.4	
DL_{CO} (% predicted)	**57.9 ± 17.9[a,b]**	**73.7 ± 19.8[c]**	**87.0 ± 13.3**	**<0.001[a,b]** **0.04[c]**
DL_{CO} < 55%	17 (47%)	10 (24%)	0 (0%)	
55% < DL_{CO} < 80%	14 (39%)	12 (29%)	5 (31%)	
FVC(%)/DL_{CO}(%)	1.35 ± 0.38	1.62 ± 0.49	1.33 ± 0.25	**0.02[a]**
FVC(%)/DL_{CO}(%) > 1.4 and DL_{CO}(%) < 55%	8 (22%) **1.86 ± 0.28[a]**	9 (21%) **2.35 ± 0.48**	0 (0%)	**0.022**
CT densitometry				
TLV (mL)	**2,915.7 ± 673.9[a,b]**	**4,286.3 ± 1,136.5**	**4,541.0 ± 800.4**	**<0.001[a,b]**
Total lung weight (g)	723.3 ± 142.1	736.1 ± 158.7	780.7 ± 180.9	
Hyperinflated (%)	**4.6 ± 3.1[a,b]**	**9.8 ± 4.3**	**10.2 ± 4.5**	**<0.001[a,b]**
Normally aerated (%)	**58.7 ± 8.4[a,b]**	**63.9 ± 4.5**	**67.8 ± 4.9**	**0.002[a]** **<0.001[b]**
ILD Extent (%)	**36.7 ± 8.7[a,b]**	**26.3 ± 2.1[c]**	**22.0 ± 0.8**	**<0.001[a,b]** **0.03[c]**

Values are presented as mean ± standard deviation. Bold characters indicate statistically significant differences.
[a]Statistically significant difference between SSc Extensive-ILD and SSc Limited-ILD.
[b]Statistically significant difference between SSc Extensive-ILD and SSc No-ILD.
[c]Statistically significant difference between SSc Limited-ILD and SSc No-ILD.
SSc No-ILD, scleroderma with no interstitial lung disease (ILD ≤ 25%); SSc-ILD, scleroderma with interstitial lung disease; SSc Limited-ILD, scleroderma with interstitial lung disease between 25 and 35%; SSc Extensive-ILD, scleroderma with interstitial lung disease higher than 35%; BMI, body mass index; FVC (%), forced vital capacity expressed as predicted values; DL_{CO}/VA, carbon monoxide diffusion capacity adjusted for alveolar volume expressed as predicted values; DL_{CO} (%), carbon monoxide diffusion capacity expressed as predicted values; TLV, total lung volume; Total lung weight, lung tissue fraction related to densities from −1,000 to +50 Hounsfield units (HU); Hyperinflated, tissue fraction related to densities from −1,000 to −901 HU; Normally Aerated, tissue fraction related to densities from −900 to −501 HU; ILD Extent, extent of interstitial lung disease defined as lung weight related to interstitial opacities normalized by total lung weight.

regions could be observed in SSc No-ILD and SSc Limited- and Extensive-ILDs (**Figure 5**, lower panels).

DISCUSSION

The main findings of the present study were (1) an optimal threshold of 23.4% of LW assigned as interstitial opacities was determined by ROC curve and used to classify 78 SSc patients as presenting ILD; (2) 36 (38%) SSc patients were classified as SSc Extensive-ILD and 42 (45%) as SSc Limited-ILD based on the *Z* score for interstitial opacities in patients with SSc relative to controls; (3) ILD extent negatively and moderately to poorly correlated with FVC and DL_{CO}, but not with DL_{CO}/VA; and (4) in patients with SSc Extensive-ILD, pulmonary involvement dispersed in all lung parenchyma from apical to basal thirds and from the periphery to hilar regions.

In healthy subjects, CT interstitial opacities are mainly related to vascular peribronchial network and, especially in older

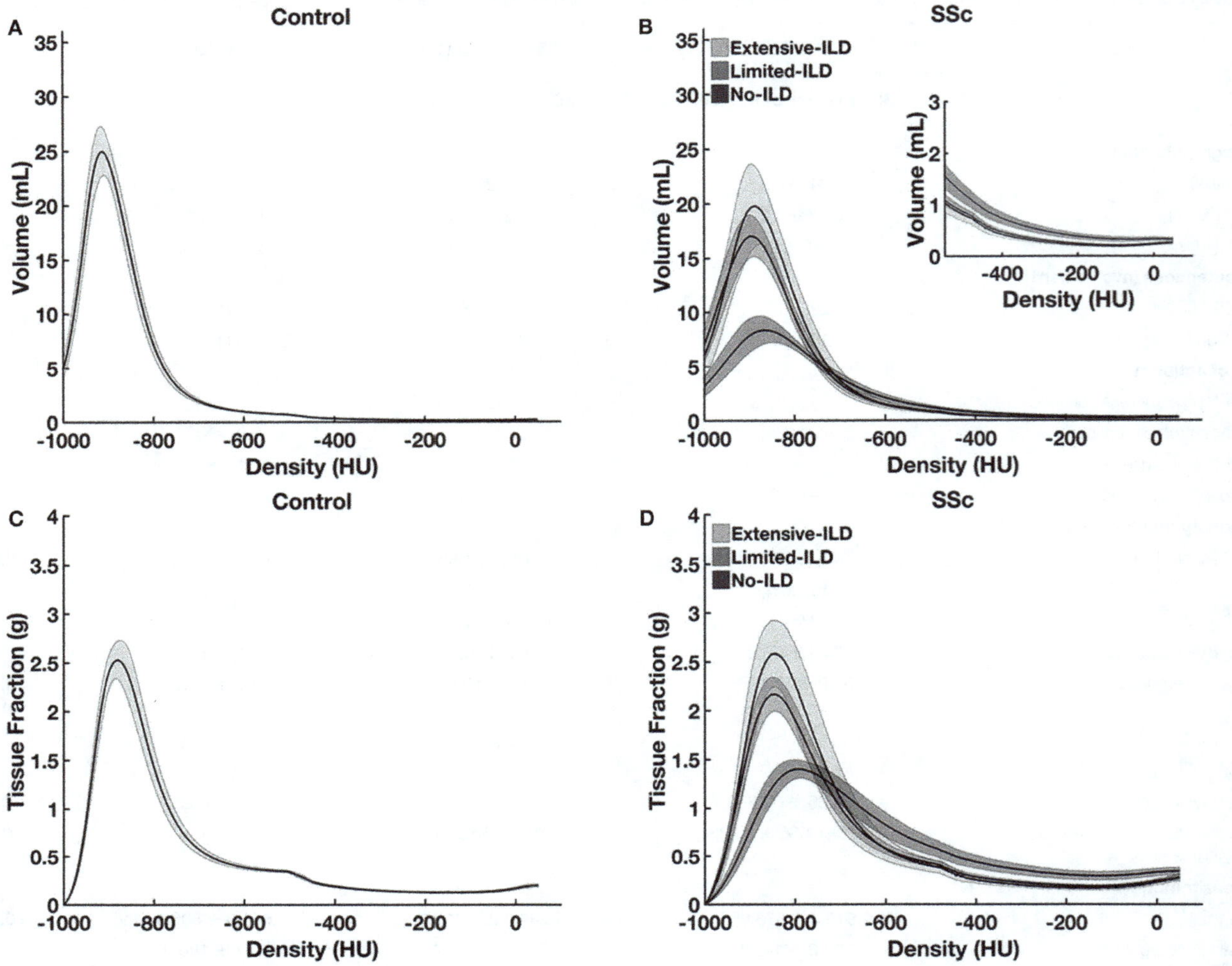

FIGURE 3 | Lung tissue volume **(A,C)** and lung tissue fraction **(B,D)** plotted against density in controls **(A,B)** and SSc-patients **(C,D)**. Note the peak volume and tissue fraction reduction and the right-shift of the histogram to higher densities from SSc No-ILD to SSc Extensive-ILD. Such aspect reflects lung volume reduction as well as tissue increase at higher densities, as ILD spreads through lung parenchyma. Graphs are presented with average, and the hatched areas correspond to the 95% coefficient interval.

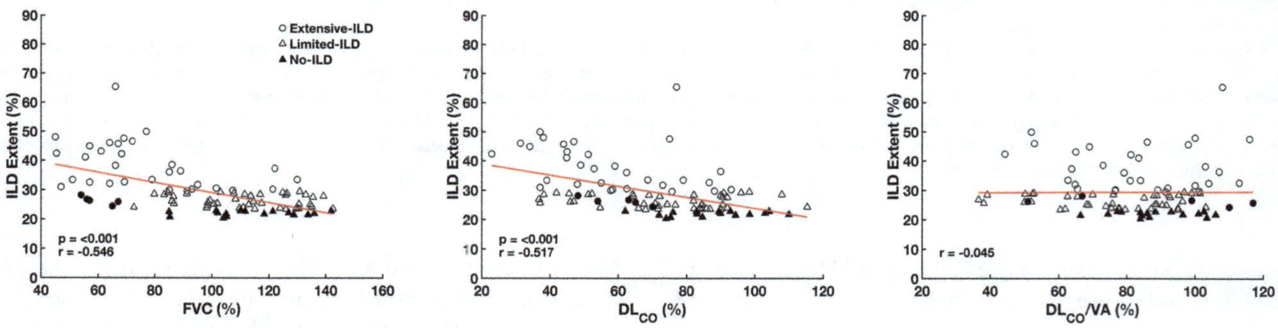

FIGURE 4 | Correlation between interstitial lung disease extent (ILD Extent), forced vital capacity (FVC), carbon monoxide diffusion capacity (DL_{CO}), and carbon monoxide diffusion capacity adjusted to alveolar volume (DL_{CO}/VA) expressed as predicted values considering all SSc patients. Circle symbols represent SSc Extensive-ILD, SSc Limited-ILD triangles, and SSc No-ILD patient filled triangles. Filled circles represent patients initially classified as SSc Limited-ILD but with an FVC < 70% being reclassified as SSc Extensive-ILD.

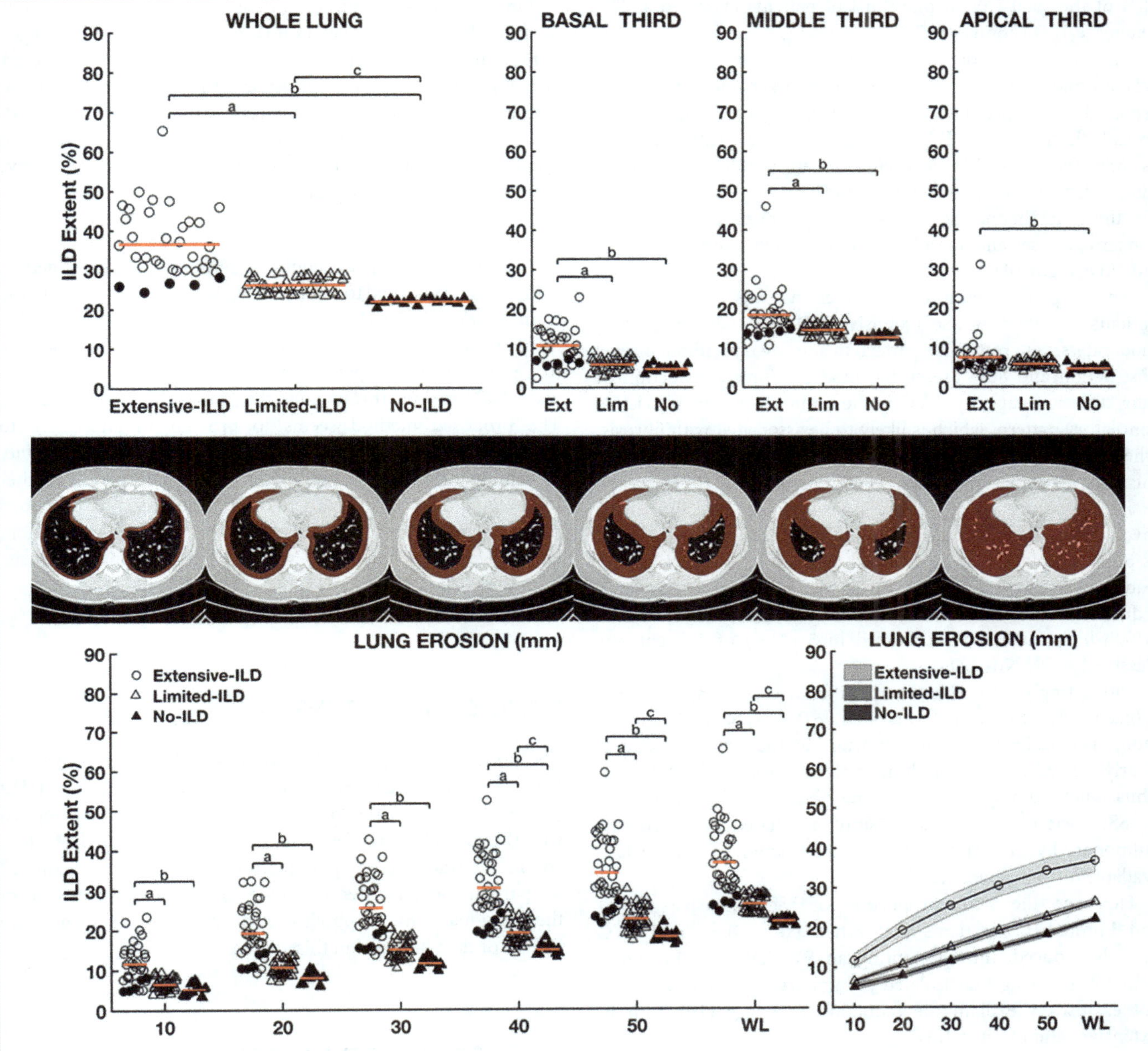

FIGURE 5 | Upper panels: Interstitial lung disease extent (ILD Extent) expressed as a percentage of total lung weight among groups considering the whole lung, basal, middle, and apical thirds. Lower panels: comparison between groups at different erosion depths from the outermost layer of the parenchyma hilar regions, outlined in the middle panels. Left panel shows ILD Extent in 10-mm steps, and right panel shows the continuous graphs with mean and 95% coefficient interval. Letters a, b, and c represent statistically significant differences between SSc Limited-ILD vs. No-ILD, SSc Diffuse-ILD vs. No-ILD, and SSc Diffuse-ILD vs. SSc Limited-ILD, respectively. Circle symbols represent SSc Extensive-ILD, SSc Limited-ILD and SSc No-ILD triangles, and patient filled triangles. Filled circles represent patients initially classified as SSc Limited-ILD but with an FVC < 70% being reclassified as SSc Extensive-ILD. Noteworthy, ILD Extent in SSc Extensive-ILD group was always significantly higher than in SSc Limited- and SSc No-ILD even in the subpleural surface (**Figure 4**, lower panels).

subjects and at dorsal-dependent regions, to areas with low ventilation/perfusion ratio (25–28). Thus, we speculate that tissue weight related to such opacities could be used as a potential indicator of ILD in SSc patients. Hence, the laborious exclusion of peribronchial vessels would not be necessary, and values above a certain normality threshold could be interpreted as ILD in patients with SSc.

The ROC curve from the weight of interstitial opacities in controls and SSc patients determined the optimal limit of normality of 23.4% of tissue weight related to interstitial opacities (**Figure 1**). The visual inspection of CT matched with computed interstitial opacities indicated that, in addition to peribronchial vessels, ground-glass opacities and reticular/focal consolidations were also identified (**Figure 2**) and could represent more than

40% of the total LW in one-third of patients classified as SSc Extensive-ILD (**Figures 1, 5**).

The prevalence of ILD based on our proposed criteria was around 83% and is just slightly larger than previously reported data (prevalence of SSc-ILD up to 80%) (29). A spread distribution of ILD was observed in patients classified as SSc Extensive-ILD involving basal, middle, and apical lung thirds as well as lung periphery and central regions. On the other hand, SSc Limited-ILD pulmonary involvement concerned basal and middle thirds more extensively than SSc No-ILD (**Figure 4**).

An impaired pulmonary function was observed in patients classified as SSc Extensive-ILD with 58% presenting moderate/severe restrictive pattern in spirometry without airway obstruction and 86% presenting moderate/severe reduction in lung diffusion capacity. FVC is the main marker of restrictive ventilatory pattern, which is likely to be associated with fibrosis, whereas DL_{CO} is an indicator of alveolitis, ventilation–perfusion mismatch, vascular involvement, and fibrosis (27).

DL_{CO} seems to be more sensitive in detecting lung involvement than FVC, although it is less specific regarding ILD, as pulmonary vascular disease and coexisting fibrosis may also lead to decreased DL_{CO} (27, 28). Thus, a moderate and isolated reduction in DL_{CO} may also indicate just subclinical alveolitis (19), which might have occurred in 5 (31%) of our patients classified as SSc No-ILD.

Interestingly, no significant differences among SSc-ILD subjects were observed in terms of DL_{CO}/VA (**Table 2**). DL_{CO}/VA more specifically represents diffusion, as the transfer factor is clearly related to available lung surface estimated by VA (27). Thus, one could speculate that the observed DL_{CO} reduction in SSc Extensive-ILD was mainly associated with isolated pulmonary hypertension and not to a reduction of lung surface available for gas exchange.

However, the same proportion of SSc Extensive- (22%) and Limited-ILD patients (21%) had both DL_{CO} and FVC severely reduced, thus presenting an FVC/DL_{CO} ratio higher than 1.4, stressing that isolated pulmonary hypertension could not exclusively explain the reduction in DL_{CO} (19) both in Extensive- and Limited-ILDs.

The main limitation of this study is the small number of SSc patients. This aspect could have an impact on the power of our study. However, patients included herein were well characterized clinically, radiographically, and functionally. Another important limitation is the need for a threshold of normality for ILD determination in SSc patients as well as a severity classification, with Z score mainly related to the average weight of interstitial opacities in controls. Although an impaired pulmonary function was observed in SSc Extensive-ILD, it is not yet possible to assess whether those classified as SSc Limited-ILD would benefit from any specific antifibrotic therapy (30).

Finally, the application of densitometry is not the only method for quantitative evaluation in chest CT images. Other methods based on deep-learning or even texture analysis (31, 32) have been successfully applied to similar subjects. However, densitometric assessment methods are computationally very simple and do not require prior preparation of libraries or image banks with their respective radiological pattern classification.

In conclusion, SSc-ILD could be automatically quantified by computing LW related to interstitial opacities in densities ranging from −500 to +50 HU. Patients with SSc, who had an ILD extent greater than about 30% of total LW, exhibited moderate to severe restrictive pattern and reduced diffusion capacity with ILD spread throughout the entire lung parenchyma. The proposed method seems to provide an alternative to estimate ILD in patients with SSc, mitigating the subjectivity of semiquantitative analyzes based on visual scores. Further follow-up studies of SSc patients using the presently described method could clarify the extent of pulmonary involvement and suggest the therapeutic window for pulmonary fibrosis-inhibiting drugs.

ETHICS STATEMENT

The protocol was approved at the Research Ethics Committee from the UERJ (CAAE-50752615.9.0000.5259) and from CHUP (reference number 2019.353, 288-DEFI/307-CE), and it complied with the current national and international standards. The ethics committee waived the requirement of written informed consent for participation. Written informed consent was obtained from the individual(s) for the publication of any potentially identifiable images or data included in this article.

AUTHOR CONTRIBUTIONS

AC: image processing and analysis of results, statistical evaluation, theoretical development of software, the computation method of voxel-to-voxel analysis, and writing of the text and submission of the article. AG: image processing and segmentation and statistical evaluation. FS and MF: capture and organization of clinical data and draft review. RR: capture and organization of clinical data, discussion of results, and draft review. BS, AL, and IA: capture and organization of clinical data. WZ: draft review. All authors contributed to the article and approved the submitted version.

REFERENCES

1. Doyle TJ, Dellaripa PF. Lung manifestations in the rheumatic diseases. *Chest.* (2017) 152:1283–95. doi: 10.1016/j.chest.2017.05.015
2. Saketkoo LA, Magnus JH, Doyle MK. The primary care physician in the early diagnosis of systemic sclerosis: the cornerstone of recognition and hope. *Am J Med Sci.* (2014) 347:54–63. doi: 10.1097/MAJ.0b013e3182a55d24
3. Desai SR, Veeraraghavan S, Hansell DM, Nikolakopolou A, Goh NSL, Nicholson AG, et al. CT features of lung disease in patients with systemic sclerosis: comparison with idiopathic pulmonary fibrosis and nonspecific interstitial pneumonia. *Radiology.* (2004) 232:560–7. doi: 10.1148/radiol.2322031223
4. Wells AU, Margaritopoulos GA, Antoniou KM, Denton C. Interstitial lung disease in systemic sclerosis. *Semin Respir Crit Care Med.* (2014) 35:213–21. doi: 10.1055/s-0034-1371541
5. Bouros D, Wells AU, Nicholson AG, Colby TV, Polychronopoulos V, Pantelidis P, et al. Histopathologic subsets of fibrosing alveolitis in patients with systemic sclerosis and their relationship to outcome. *Am J Respir Crit Care Med.* (2002) 165:1581–6. doi: 10.1164/rccm.2106012
6. Cappelli S, Bellando Randone S, Camiciottoli G, De Paulis A, Guiducci S, Matucci-Cerinic M. Interstitial lung disease in systemic sclerosis: where do we stand? *Eur Respir Rev.* (2015) 24:411–9. doi: 10.1183/16000617.000 02915
7. Hoffmann-Vold A-M, Aaløkken TM, Lund MB, Garen T, Midtvedt Ø, Brunborg C, et al. Predictive value of serial high-resolution computed tomography analyses and concurrent lung function tests in systemic sclerosis. *Arthritis Rheumatol.* (2015) 67:2205–12. doi: 10.1002/art.39166
8. Hansell DM, Goldin JG, King TE, Lynch DA, Richeldi L, Wells AU. CT staging and monitoring of fibrotic interstitial lung diseases in clinical practice and treatment trials: a position paper from the Fleischner Society. *Lancet Respir Med.* (2015) 3:483–96. doi: 10.1016/S2213-2600(15)00096-X
9. Walsh SLF, Calandriello L, Sverzellati N, Wells AU, Hansell DM, Observer Consort UIP. Interobserver agreement for the ATS/ERS/JRS/ALAT criteria for a UIP pattern on CT. *Thorax.* (2016) 71:45–51. doi: 10.1136/thoraxjnl-2015-207252
10. Watadani T, Sakai F, Johkoh T, Noma S, Akira M, Fujimoto K, et al. Interobserver variability in the CT assessment of honeycombing in the lungs. *Radiology.* (2013) 266:936–44. doi: 10.1148/radiol.12112516
11. Ariani A, Silva M, Bravi E, Saracco M, Parisi S, De Gennaro F, et al. Operator-independent quantitative chest computed tomography versus standard assessment of interstitial lung disease related to systemic sclerosis: a multi-centric study. *Modern Rheumatol.* (2015) 25:724–30. doi: 10.3109/14397595.2015.1016200
12. Tashkin DP, Volkmann ER, Tseng C-H, Kim HJ, Goldin J, Clements P, et al. Relationship between quantitative radiographic assessments of interstitial lung disease and physiological and clinical features of systemic sclerosis. *Ann Rheum Dis.* (2016) 75:374–81. doi: 10.1136/annrheumdis-2014-206076
13. van den Hoogen F, Khanna D, Fransen J, Johnson SR, Baron M, Tyndall A, et al. 2013 classification criteria for systemic sclerosis: an American College of Rheumatology/European League against Rheumatism collaborative initiative. *Ann Rheum Dis.* (2013) 72:2737–47. doi: 10.1136/annrheumdis-2013-204424
14. LeRoy EC, Black C, Fleischmajer R, Jablonska S, Krieg T, Medsger TA, et al. Scleroderma. (systemic sclerosis): classification, subsets and pathogenesis. *J Rheumatol.* (1988) 15:202–5.
15. Miller MR. General considerations for lung function testing. *Eur Respir J.* (2005) 26:153–61. doi: 10.1183/09031936.05.00034505
16. Neder JA, Andreoni S, Castelo-Filho A, Nery LE. Reference values for lung function tests. I Static volumes. *Braz J Med Biol Res.* (1999) 32:703–17. doi: 10.1590/S0100-879X1999000600006
17. Neder JA, Andreoni S, Peres C, Nery LE. Reference values for lung function tests. III Carbon monoxide diffusing capacity (transfer factor). *Braz J Med Biol Res.* (1999) 32:729–37. doi: 10.1590/S0100-879X19990006 00008
18. de Pereira CA, Sato T, Rodrigues SC. New reference values for forced spirometry in white adults in Brazil. *J Bras Pneumol.* (2007) 33:397–406. doi: 10.1590/S1806-37132007000400008
19. Steen VD, Graham G, Conte C, Owens G, Medsger TA. Isolated diffusing capacity reduction in systemic sclerosis. *Arthritis Rheum.* (1992) 35:765–70. doi: 10.1002/art.1780350709
20. Fedorov A, Beichel R, Kalpathy-Cramer J, Finet J, Fillion-Robin J-C, Pujol S, et al. 3D Slicer as an image computing platform for the Quantitative Imaging Network. *Magn Reson Imaging.* (2012) 30:1323–41. doi: 10.1016/j.mri.2012.05.001
21. Staring M, Bakker ME, Stolk J, Shamonin DP, Reiber JHC, Stoel BC. Towards local progression estimation of pulmonary emphysema using CT. *Med Phys.* (2014) 41:021905. doi: 10.1118/1.4851535
22. Stoel BC, Vrooman H, Stolk J, Reiber J. Sources of error in lung densitometry with CT. *Invest Radiol.* (1999) 303–9. doi: 10.1097/00004424-199904000-00008
23. Camilo GB, Carvalho ARS, Machado DC, Mogami R, Melo PL, Lopes AJ. CT pulmonary densitovolumetry in patients with acromegaly: a comparison between active disease and controlled disease. *Br J Radiol.* (2015) 88:20150315. doi: 10.1259/bjr.20150315
24. Goh NSL, Desai SR, Veeraraghavan S, Hansell DM, Copley SJ, Maher TM, et al. Interstitial lung disease in systemic sclerosis: a simple staging system. *Am J Respir Crit Care Med.* (2008) 177:1248–54. doi: 10.1164/rccm.200 706-877OC
25. Millar AB, Denison DM. Vertical gradients of lung density in supine subjects with fibrosing alveolitis or pulmonary emphysema. *Thorax.* (1990) 45:602–5. doi: 10.1136/thx.45.8.602
26. Sa RC, Cronin MV, Cortney Henderson A, Holverda S, Theilmann RJ, Arai TJ, et al. Vertical distribution of specific ventilation in normal supine humans measured by oxygen-enhanced proton MRI. *J Appl Physiol.* (2010) 109:1950–9. doi: 10.1152/japplphysiol.00220.2010
27. Behr J, Furst DE. Pulmonary function tests. *Rheumatology.* (2008) 47:v65–7. doi: 10.1093/rheumatology/ken313
28. Guttadauria M, Ellman H, Emmanuel G, Kaplan D, Diamond H. Pulmonary function in scleroderma. *Arthritis Rheum.* (1977) 20:1071–9. doi: 10.1002/art.1780200506
29. Taormina VJ, Miller WT, Gefter WB, Epstein DM. Progressive systemic sclerosis subgroups: variable pulmonary features. *AJR Am J Roentgenol.* (1981) 137:277–85. doi: 10.2214/ajr.137.2.277
30. Distler O, Highland KB, Gahlemann M, Azuma A, Fischer A, Mayes MD, et al. Nintedanib for systemic sclerosis-associated interstitial lung disease. *N Engl J Med.* (2019) 380:2518–28. doi: 10.1056/NEJMoa1 903076
31. Occhipinti M, Bosello S, Sisti LG, Cicchetti G, de Waure C, Pirronti T, et al. Quantitative and semi-quantitative computed tomography analysis of interstitial lung disease associated with systemic sclerosis: a longitudinal evaluation of pulmonary parenchyma and vessels. *PLoS ONE.* (2019) 14:e0213444. doi: 10.1371/journal.pone.0213444
32. Yabuuchi H, Matsuo Y, Tsukamoto H, Horiuchi T, Sunami S, Kamitani T, et al. Evaluation of the extent of ground-glass opacity on high-resolution

Permissions

All chapters in this book were first published by Frontiers; hereby published with permission under the Creative Commons Attribution License or equivalent. Every chapter published in this book has been scrutinized by our experts. Their significance has been extensively debated. The topics covered herein carry significant findings which will fuel the growth of the discipline. They may even be implemented as practical applications or may be referred to as a beginning point for another development.

The contributors of this book come from diverse backgrounds, making this book a truly international effort. This book will bring forth new frontiers with its revolutionizing research information and detailed analysis of the nascent developments around the world.

We would like to thank all the contributing authors for lending their expertise to make the book truly unique. They have played a crucial role in the development of this book. Without their invaluable contributions this book wouldn't have been possible. They have made vital efforts to compile up to date information on the varied aspects of this subject to make this book a valuable addition to the collection of many professionals and students.

This book was conceptualized with the vision of imparting up-to-date information and advanced data in this field. To ensure the same, a matchless editorial board was set up. Every individual on the board went through rigorous rounds of assessment to prove their worth. After which they invested a large part of their time researching and compiling the most relevant data for our readers.

The editorial board has been involved in producing this book since its inception. They have spent rigorous hours researching and exploring the diverse topics which have resulted in the successful publishing of this book. They have passed on their knowledge of decades through this book. To expedite this challenging task, the publisher supported the team at every step. A small team of assistant editors was also appointed to further simplify the editing procedure and attain best results for the readers.

Apart from the editorial board, the designing team has also invested a significant amount of their time in understanding the subject and creating the most relevant covers. They scrutinized every image to scout for the most suitable representation of the subject and create an appropriate cover for the book.

The publishing team has been an ardent support to the editorial, designing and production team. Their endless efforts to recruit the best for this project, has resulted in the accomplishment of this book. They are a veteran in the field of academics and their pool of knowledge is as vast as their experience in printing. Their expertise and guidance has proved useful at every step. Their uncompromising quality standards have made this book an exceptional effort. Their encouragement from time to time has been an inspiration for everyone.

The publisher and the editorial board hope that this book will prove to be a valuable piece of knowledge for researchers, students, practitioners and scholars across the globe.

List of Contributors

Garifallia Sakellariou
Division of Rheumatology, IRCCS Policlinico San Matteo Foundation, University of Pavia, Pavia, Italy

lessandra Bortoluzzi and Georgios Filippou
UOC e Sezione di Reumatologia - Dipartimento di Scienze Mediche, Università degli Studi di Ferrara, Ferrara, Italy

Carlo Alberto Scirè
UOC e Sezione di Reumatologia - Dipartimento di Scienze Mediche, Università degli Studi di Ferrara, Ferrara, Italy
Società Italiana di Reumatologia, Unità Epidemiologica, Milan, Italy

Antonella Adinolfi and Oscar Massimiliano Epis
Rheumatology Unit, Grande Ospedale Metropolitano Niguarda, Milan, Italy

Alberto Batticciotto
Rheumatology Unit, Department of Internal Medicine, ASST-Settelaghi, "Ospedale di Circolo - Fondazione Macchi", Varese, Italy

Andrea Delle Sedie
Rheumatology Unit, University of Pisa, Pisa, Italy

Orazio De Lucia
Unit of Clinical Rheumatology, Department of Rheumatology and Clinical Sciences, ASST Centro Traumatologico Ortopedico G. Pini - CTO, Milan, Italy

Luca Idolazzi
Rheumatology Unit, Ospedale Civile Maggiore, University of Verona, Verona, Italy

Andrea Picchianti Diamanti
Department of Clinical and Molecular Medicine, S. Andrea University Hospital, "Sapienza" University, Rome, Italy

Alen Zabotti
Department of Medical and Biological Science, Rheumatology Clinic, Azienda Sanitaria Universitaria Integrata, Udine, Italy

Annamaria Iagnocco
Academic Rheumatology Centre, Università degli Studi di Torino, Turin, Italy

Xuan Luo, Yu Peng, Panpan Zhang, Jieqiong Li, Zheng Liu, Hui Lu, Xuan Zhang, Xiaofeng Zeng, Fengchun Zhang, Yunyun Fei and Wen Zhang
Department of Rheumatology, Peking Union Medical College Hospital, Chinese Academy of Medical Sciences, Peking Union Medical College, Beijing, China
National Clinical Research Center for Dermatologic and Immunologic Diseases (NCRC-DID), Key Laboratory of Ministry of Health, Beijing, China

Gianluca Smerilli, Edoardo Cipolletta, Marco Di Carlo and Emilio Filippucci
Rheumatology Unit, Department of Clinical and Molecular Sciences, Polytechnic University of Marche, "Carlo Urbani" Hospital, Jesi, Ancona, Italy

Andrea Di Matteo
Rheumatology Unit, Department of Clinical and Molecular Sciences, Polytechnic University of Marche, "Carlo Urbani" Hospital, Jesi, Ancona, Italy
Leeds Institute of Rheumatic and Musculoskeletal Medicine, University of Leeds, Leeds, United Kingdom

Jiaqi Wu, Xianghong Chen, Yue Zhao, Xiaohong He, Yongliang Chu, Xiaodong Wu, Aihua Ou, Zehuai Wen and Qingchun Huang
The Second Affiliated Hospital of Guangzhou University of Chinese Medicine (Guangdong Provincial Hospital of Chinese Medicine), Guangzhou, China

Yuan Lv and Kaixin Gao
Second Clinical Medical College, Guangzhou University of Chinese Medicine, Guangzhou, China

Zehao Liu
Ruikang Hospital Affiliated to Guangxi University of Chinese Medicine, Guangxi, China

Xiumin Chen and Runyue Huang
The Second Affiliated Hospital of Guangzhou University of Chinese Medicine (Guangdong Provincial Hospital of Chinese Medicine), Guangzhou, China
Second Clinical Medical College, Guangzhou University of Chinese Medicine, Guangzhou, China
Guangdong Provincial Key Laboratory of Clinical Research on Traditional Chinese Medicine Syndrome, and State Key Laboratory of Dampness Syndrome of Chinese Medicine, The Second Affiliated Hospital of Guangzhou University of Chinese Medicine, Guangzhou, China

Jianyong Zhang
Shenzhen Hospital of Traditional Chinese Medicine, Shenzhen, China

Jianhong Peng
Dongguan Hospital of Traditional Chinese Medicine, Dongguan, China

Zhisheng Huang
Guangzhou Hospital of Integrated Traditional Chinese and Western Medicine, Huadu, China,

Per-Johan Jakobsson
Rheumatology Unit, Department of Medicine Solna, Karolinska Institutet, Karolinska University Hospital, Stockholm, Sweden

Mette B. Axelsen
Copenhagen Center for Arthritis Research and Center for Rheumatology and Spine Diseases, Centre of Head and Orthopaedics, Rigshospitalet, Glostrup, Denmark

Sin Ngai Ng
Copenhagen Center for Arthritis Research, Center for Rheumatology and Spine Diseases, Rigshospitalet, Glostrup, Denmark
Department of Medicine, Queen Elizabeth Hospital, Kowloon, Hong Kong

Merete L. Hetland
Copenhagen Center for Arthritis Research, Center for Rheumatology and Spine Diseases, Rigshospitalet, Glostrup, Denmark
Department of Clinical Medicine, Faculty of Health Sciences, University of Copenhagen, Copenhagen, Denmark

Iris Eshed
Department of Diagnostic Imaging, Sheba Medical Center, Tel Giborim Affiliated With Tel Aviv University, Tel Aviv, Israel

Jakob M. Møller
Department of Clinical Medicine, Faculty of Health Sciences, University of Copenhagen, Copenhagen, Denmark
Department of Radiology, Herlev-Gentofte Hospital, Copenhagen, Denmark

Francesca Ingegnoli, Lavinia Agra Coletto and Roberto Caporali
Division of Clinical Rheumatology, Gaetano Pini Hospital, Milan, Italy
Department of Clinical Sciences and Community Health, Research Center for Adult and Pediatric Rheumatic Diseases, Università degli Studi di Milano, Milan, Italy

Massimiliano Buoli and Cecilia Maria Esposito
Department of Neurosciences and Mental Health, Fondazione Istituto di Ricovero e Cura a Carattere Scientifico (IRCCS) Ca'Granda Ospedale Maggiore Policlinico, Milan, Italy
Department of Pathophysiology and Transplantation, Università degli Studi di Milano, Milan, Italy

Flavia Antonucci
Department of Medical Biotechnology and Translational Medicine (BIOMETRA), Università degli Studi di Milano, Milan, Italy
Department of Clinical Medicine, Faculty of Health and Medical Sciences, University of Copenhagen, Copenhagen, Denmark

Ashish J. Mathew
Copenhagen Center for Arthritis Research (COPECARE), Center for Rheumatology and Spine Diseases, Glostrup, Denmark
Department of Clinical Medicine, Faculty of Health and Medical Sciences, University of Copenhagen, Copenhagen, Denmark
Clinical Immunology and Rheumatology, Christian Medical College, Vellore, India
Centre for Prognosis Studies in the Rheumatic Diseases, Krembil Research Institute, University Health Network, University of Toronto, Toronto, ON, Canada

Alice Bartoletti, Elisa Bellis and Carlomaurizio Montecucco
Rheumatology Department, IRCCS Policlinico S. Matteo Foundation, University of Pavia, Pavia, Italy

Sara Monti and Paolo Delvino
Rheumatology Department, IRCCS Policlinico S. Matteo Foundation, University of Pavia, Pavia, Italy
PhD in Experimental Medicine, University of Pavia, Pavia, Italy

Martin Brom, Ignacio J. Gandino, Johana B. Zacariaz Hereter, Marina Scolnik, Florencia B. Mollerach, Leandro G. Ferreyra Garrott, Josefina Marin, Santiago O. Ruta, Javier E. Rosa and Enrique R. Soriano
Rheumatology Department, Hospital Italiano de Buenos Aires, Buenos Aires, Argentina

Cláudia Quaresma, Barbara Lopes and Carla Quintão
Instrumentation, Biomedical Engineering and Radiation Physics Laboratory (LIBPhys-UNL), Physics Department, NOVA School of Science and Technology, NOVA University of Lisbon, Caparica, Portugal
Physics Department, NOVA School of Science and Technology, NOVA University of Lisbon, Caparica, Portugal

Ricardo D. García-Mónaco
Radiology Department, Hospital Italiano de Buenos Aires, Buenos Aires, Argentina

Jorge Jacinto, Tiago Robalo and Mariana Matos
Rehabilitation Medicine Center of Alcoitão, Alcabideche, Portugal

Inge Juul Sørensen and Uffe Møller Døhn
Copenhagen Center for Arthritis Research and Center for Rheumatology and Spine Diseases, Centre of Head and Orthopaedics, Rigshospitalet, Glostrup, Denmark

Sengul Seven, Susanne Juhl Pedersen, Mikkel Østergaard, Sara Kamp Felbo and Lene Terslev
Copenhagen Center for Arthritis Research and Center for Rheumatology and Spine Diseases, Centre of Head and Orthopaedics, Rigshospitalet, Glostrup, Denmark
Department of Clinical Medicine, University of Copenhagen, Copenhagen, Denmark

Dan Ma and Liyun Zhang
Department of Rheumatology, Shanxi Bethune Hospital, Shanxi Academy of Medical Sciences, Shanxi Bethune Hospital Affiliated to Shanxi Medical University, Taiyuan, China

Nana Liang
First Hospital/First Clinical Medical College of Shanxi Medical University, Taiyuan, China

Rasmus Klose-Jensen and Ellen-Margrethe Hauge
Department of Rheumatology, Aarhus University Hospital, Aarhus, Denmark
Department of Clinical Medicine, Faculty of Health, Aarhus University, Aarhus, Denmark

Justin J. Tse and Sarah L. Manske
Cumming School of Medicine, McCaig Institute for Bone and Joint Health, University of Calgary, Calgary, AB, Canada
Department of Radiology, Cumming School of Medicine, University of Calgary, Calgary, AB, Canada

Kresten Krarup Keller
Diagnostic Centre, Silkeborg Regional Hospital, Silkeborg, Denmark
Department of Medicine, Cumming School of Medicine, University of Calgary, Calgary, AB, Canada

Andrew J. Burghardt
Department of Radiology and Biomedical Imaging, University of California, San Francisco, San Francisco, CA, United States

Stephanie Finzel
Department of Rheumatology and Clinical Immunology, Medical Centre - University of Freiburg, Freiburg, Germany
Faculty of Medicine, University of Freiburg, Freiburg, Germany

Lai-Shan Tam
Department of Medicine and Therapeutics, The Chinese University of Hong Kong, Hong Kong, China

Kathryn S. Stok
Department of Biomedical Engineering, The University of Melbourne, Parkville, VIC, Australia

Walter Grassi, Maria Chiara Fiorentino, Irene Guidotti and Emanuele Frontoni
Department of Information Engineering, Polytechnic University of Marche, Ancona, Italy

Sara Moccia
Department of Information Engineering, Polytechnic University of Marche, Ancona, Italy
Department of Advanced Robotics, Italian Institute of Technology, Genoa, Italy

Richard J. Wakefield and Ai Lyn Tan
Leeds Institute of Rheumatic and Musculoskeletal Medicine, Chapel Allerton Hospital, University of Leeds, Leeds, United Kingdom
NIHR Leeds Biomedical Research Centre, Leeds Teaching Hospitals NHS Trust, Leeds, United Kingdom

Matthew Farrow
Leeds Institute of Rheumatic and Musculoskeletal Medicine, Chapel Allerton Hospital, University of Leeds, Leeds, United Kingdom
NIHR Leeds Biomedical Research Centre, Leeds Teaching Hospitals NHS Trust, Leeds, United Kingdom
School of Pharmacy and Medical Sciences, University of Bradford, Bradford, United Kingdom

John Biglands
NIHR Leeds Biomedical Research Centre, Leeds Teaching Hospitals NHS Trust, Leeds, United Kingdom
Medical Physics and Engineering, Leeds Teaching Hospitals NHS Trust, Leeds, United Kingdom

Abdulrahman M. Alfuraih
Radiology and Medical Imaging Department, Prince Sattam Bin Abdulaziz University, Al-Kharj, Saudi Arabia

Maria João Jacinto
Patient Innovation, Lisbon, Portugal
Católica-Lisbon School of Business and Economics, Universidade Católica Portuguesa, Lisbon, Portugal

Pedro Oliveira
Patient Innovation, Lisbon, Portugal
Copenhagen Business School, Copenhagen, Denmark
Nova School of Business and Economics, Universidade Nova de Lisboa, Lisbon, Portugal

Helena Canhão
Patient Innovation, Lisbon, Portugal
CHRC, Comprehensive Health Research Center, NOVA Medical School, UNL, Lisbon, Portugal
EpiDoC Unit, Chronic Diseases Research Centre, Nova Medical School, Universidade Nova de Lisboa, Lisbon Portugal
National School of Public Health, Universidade Nova de Lisboa, Lisbon, Portugal

Sayam R. Dubash, Gabriele De Marco, Richard J. Wakefield, Dennis McGonagle and Helena Marzo-Ortega
NIHR Leeds Biomedical Research Centre, Leeds Teaching Hospitals Trust, Leeds, United Kingdom
Leeds Institute of Rheumatic and Musculoskeletal Medicine, University of Leeds, Leeds, United Kingdom

Chao-Yi Wu
Division of Allergy, Asthma, and Rheumatology, Department of Pediatrics, Chang Gung Memorial Hospital and Chang Gung University College of Medicine, Taoyuan, Taiwan

Chun-Chun Gau
Division of Allergy, Asthma, and Rheumatology, Department of Pediatrics, Chang Gung Memorial Hospital and Chang Gung University College of Medicine, Taoyuan, Taiwan
Division of Pediatric General Medicine, Department of Pediatrics, Chang Gung Memorial Hospital and Chang Gung University College of Medicine, Taoyuan, Taiwan
Department of Pediatrics, Chang Gung Memorial Hospital at Keelung, Keelung, Taiwan

Min-Hua Tseng
Division of Nephrology, Department of Pediatrics, Chang Gung Memorial Hospital and Chang Gung University College of Medicine, Taoyuan, Taiwan

Huang-Yu Yang
Department of Nephrology, Chang Gung Memorial Hospital, College of Medicine, Chang Gung University, Taoyuan, Taiwan

Jing-Long Huang
Division of Allergy, Asthma, and Rheumatology, Department of Pediatrics, Chang Gung Memorial Hospital and Chang Gung University College of Medicine, Taoyuan, Taiwan
Department of Pediatrics, New Taipei Municipal TuCheng Hospital, Chang Gung Memorial Hospital and Chang Gung University, New Taipei City, Taiwan

Michaela Köhm
Division of Rheumatology, Goethe-University Frankfurt, Frankfurt, Germany
Clinical Research, Fraunhofer Institute for Molecular Biology and Applied Ecology IME, Branch for Translational Medicine and Pharmacology TMP, Frankfurt, Germany
Fraunhofer Cluster of Excellence Immune-Mediated Diseases CIMD, Frankfurt, Germany

Lukas Zerweck and Phuong-Ha Ngyuen
Fraunhofer Cluster of Excellence Immune-Mediated Diseases CIMD, Frankfurt, Germany
Fraunhofer Institute for Applied Information Technology FIT, St. Augustin, Germany

Harald Burkhardt and Frank Behrens
Division of Rheumatology, Goethe-University Frankfurt, Frankfurt, Germany
Clinical Research, Fraunhofer Institute for Molecular Biology and Applied Ecology IME, Branch for Translational Medicine and Pharmacology TMP, Frankfurt, Germany
Fraunhofer Cluster of Excellence Immune-Mediated Diseases CIMD, Frankfurt, Germany
Centre of Innovative Diagnostics and Therapeutics Rheumatology/Immunology CIRI, Frankfurt, Germany

Hsin-Hua Chen
Department of Medical Research, Taichung Veterans General Hospital, Taichung, Taiwan
Division of Allergy, Immunology and Rheumatology, Department of Internal Medicine, Taichung Veterans General Hospital, Taichung, Taiwan
Institute of Biomedical Science and Rong Hsing Research Centre for Translational Medicine, Chung Hsing University, Taichung, Taiwan
Department of Industrial Engineering and Enterprise Information, Tunghai University, Taichung, Taiwan
Institute of Public Health and Community Medicine Research Center, National Yang-Ming University, Taipei, Taiwan

Ching-Heng Lin
Department of Medical Research, Taichung Veterans General Hospital, Taichung, Taiwan
Department of Industrial Engineering and Enterprise Information, Tunghai University, Taichung, Taiwan
Department of Healthcare Management, National Taipei University of Nursing and Health Sciences, Taipei, Taiwan
Department of Public Health, College of Medicine, Fu Jen Catholic University, New Taipei City, Taiwan

Wen-Cheng Chao
Department of Critical Care Medicine, Taichung Veterans General Hospital, Taichung, Taiwan
Department of Computer Science, Tunghai University, Taichung, Taiwan
Department of Automatic Control Engineering, Feng Chia University, Taichung, Taiwan

Peter Salat
Department of Radiology, Cumming School of Medicine, University of Calgary, Calgary, AB, Canada
Cumming School of Medicine, McCaig Institute for Bone and Joint Health, University of Calgary, Calgary, AB, Canada

Scott C. Brunet
Department of Radiology, Cumming School of Medicine, University of Calgary, Calgary, AB, Canada
Cumming School of Medicine, McCaig Institute for Bone and Joint Health, University of Calgary, Calgary, AB, Canada
Biomedical Engineering Graduate Program, Schulich School of Engineering, University of Calgary, Calgary, AB, Canada

Glen S. Hazlewood and Cheryl Barnabe
Cumming School of Medicine, McCaig Institute for Bone and Joint Health, University of Calgary, Calgary, AB, Canada
Division of Rheumatology, Department of Medicine, Cumming School of Medicine, University of Calgary, Calgary, AB, Canada

Daniel B. Abrar, Christoph Schleich, Anja Müller-Lutz, Miriam Frenken and K. Ludger Radke
Department of Diagnostic and Interventional Radiology, Medical Faculty, University Dusseldorf, Düsseldorf, Germany

Stefan Vordenbäumen, Matthias Schneider, Benedikt Ostendorf and Philipp Sewerin
Department and Hiller Research Unit for Rheumatology, UKD, Heinrich Heine University Düsseldorf, Düsseldorf, Germany

Rusmir Husic, Angelika Lackner and Winfried Graninger
Department of Rheumatology and Immunology, Medical University Graz, Graz, Austria

Patrizia Katharina Kump and Christoph Högenauer
Department of Gastroenterology and Hepatology, Medical University Graz, Graz, Austria

Christian Dejaco
Department of Rheumatology, Medical University of Graz, Graz, Austria
Department of Rheumatology, Hospital of Brunico (Südtiroler Sanitätsbetrieb-Azienda Sanitaria dell'Alto Adige), Brunico, Italy

Alysson Roncally S. Carvalho
Department of Radiology, Medical School, Centro Hospitalar Universitário do Porto (CHUP), Instituto de Ciências Biomédicas Abel Salazar (ICBAS), Porto University, Porto, Portugal
Laboratory of Pulmonary Engineering, Biomedical Engineering Program, Alberto Luiz Coimbra Institute of Post-Graduation and Research in Engineering, Universidade Federal do Rio de Janeiro, Rio de Janeiro, Brazil
Laboratory of Respiration Physiology, Carlos Chagas Filho Institute of Biophysics, Universidade Federal do Rio de Janeiro, Rio de Janeiro, Brazil

Alan R. Guimarães
Laboratory of Pulmonary Engineering, Biomedical Engineering Program, Alberto Luiz Coimbra Institute of Post-Graduation and Research in Engineering, Universidade Federal do Rio de Janeiro, Rio de Janeiro, Brazil

Walter Araujo Zin
Laboratory of Respiration Physiology, Carlos Chagas Filho Institute of Biophysics, Universidade Federal do Rio de Janeiro, Rio de Janeiro, Brazil

Flávio R. Sztajnbok
Division of Pediatric Rheumatology, State University of Rio de Janeiro, Rio de Janeiro, Brazil

Rosana Souza Rodrigues
Department of Radiology, Universidade Federal do Rio de Janeiro, Rio de Janeiro, Brazil
IDOR - D'Or Institute for Research and Education, Rio de Janeiro, Brazil

Bruno Rangel Antunes Silva and Agnaldo José Lopes
Graduate Program in Medical Sciences, School of Medical Sciences, State University of Rio de Janeiro, Rio de Janeiro, Brazil

Isabel Almeida
Clinical Immunology Unit, Deptartment of Medicine, Centro Hospitalar Universitário do Porto (CHUP), Instituto de Ciências Biomédicas Abel Salazar (ICBAS), Porto University, Porto, Portugal

Manuela Maria França
Radiology Department, Centro Hospitalar Universitário do Porto (CHUP), Instituto de Ciências Biomédicas Abel Salazar (ICBAS), Porto University, Porto, Portugal

Index

S

T

U